Practical Medical and Surgical Management of Chronic Rhinosinusitis

Pete S. Batra • Joseph K. Han
Editors

Practical Medical and Surgical Management of Chronic Rhinosinusitis

Springer

Editors
Pete S. Batra
Department of Otorhinolaryngology
Head and Neck Surgery
Rush Center for Skull Base
and Pituitary Surgery
Rush University Medical Center
Chicago, IL
USA

Joseph K. Han
Department of Otolaryngology
Head and Neck Surgery
Eastern Virginia Medical School
Norfolk, VA
USA

ISBN 978-3-319-16723-7 ISBN 978-3-319-16724-4 (eBook)
DOI 10.1007/978-3-319-16724-4

Library of Congress Control Number: 2015943505

Springer Cham Heidelberg New York Dordrecht London

Printed on acid-free paper

Springer International Publishing AG Switzerland is part of Springer Science+Business Media (www.springer.com)

Preface

Any physician in clinical practice over the past 25 years has witnessed rapid expansion of the field of rhinology. Indeed, our ability to offer more sophisticated medical and surgical solutions for chronic sinusitis has immensely improved the care of our patients. However, important knowledge gaps persist that can lead to differences in expert opinion and variations in delivery of care. Further, better translation of the available information into practical knowledge is required to optimize patient care and streamline clinical care pathways. With this in mind, it is with great enthusiasm that we introduce the first edition of *Practical Medical and Surgical Management of Chronic Rhinosinusitis*. The focus of this textbook is to offer practicing otolaryngologists and trainees state-of-the-art information on management of this challenging group of patients. Recognized rhinologic experts from around the globe have convened to provide clinically practical tips to enhance medical and surgical management of chronic sinusitis.

The textbook is arranged in three parts to facilitate an easy to follow readable format. The first part will focus on core principles in chronic sinusitis, its subtypes and related disease processes. The second part will outline key categories of medical therapies, including established and innovative treatments, utilized in this patient population. The third part will delineate surgical nuances of endoscopic sinus surgery targeting specific sinuses and special clinical scenarios. The hope is to provide readily usable practical information to further care of patients with sinonasal disease. We are grateful to the contributors for their excellent contributions to help construct an important textbook in the field of rhinology. We are also thankful to the Springer staff for their tireless work on this textbook. Whether you are a practicing clinician, trainee, nurse, or a student, we hope that this useful information will augment care of your sinus patients.

Chicago, USA — Pete S. Batra
Norfolk, USA — Joseph K. Han

Acknowledgements

I dedicate this textbook to my loving wife Michele for her enduring support and patience and our wonderful children Gia and Sam who give meaning to our lives. I will be eternally thankful to my parents for their encouragement and support in pursuit of my dreams. I am grateful to my mentors Donald Lanza and Martin Citardi who have been instrumental in my journey in academic rhinology.

Pete S. Batra

I would like to thank God who made all things possible. I dedicate this textbook to my wife Caroline who is my inspiration and source of passion. I want to thank my parents, Paul and Sarah, for their continuous support and prayer. To my brilliant and unconditionally loving children, Joshua and Alicia, I love you very much and thank you for the countless hours of joy and happiness you give me. To my many mentors and friends, I would not be where I am without your wisdom and guidance. Specifically I would like to mention Peter Hwang, Charlie Gross, Tim Smith, and Andrew Kim.

Joseph K. Han

Contents

Part II Medical Therapy of Chronic Rhinosinusitis

Part III Surgical Therapy of Chronic Rhinosinusitis

Contributors

Jeremiah A. Alt, MD, PhD Division of Otolaryngology – Rhinology, Sinus and Skull Base Surgery Program, Otolaryngology, University of Utah, Salt Lake City, UT, USA

Kristen L. Baugnon, MD Department of Radiology and Imaging Sciences, Emory University, Atlanta, GA, USA

Pete S. Batra, MD, FACS, FARS Department of Otorhinolaryngology – Head and Neck Surgery, Rush Center for Skull Base and Pituitary Surgery, Rush University Medical Center, Chicago, IL, USA

Andrew C. Birkeland, MD Department of Otolaryngology – Head and Neck Surgery, University of Michigan Health System, Ann Arbor, MI, USA

Larry Borish, MD Department of Medicine (Allergy and Immunology) and, Microbiology University of Virginia Health System, Charlottesville, VA, USA

Joseph Brunworth, MD Department of Otolaryngology, St. Louis University Hospital, St. Louis, MO, USA

Kathleen Buchheit, MD Department of Allergy and Immunology, Brigham and Women's Hospital, Boston, MA, USA

Sean B. Bury, MD Division of Otolaryngology – Head and Neck Surgery, George Washington University Hospital, Washington, DC, USA

Marie Bussières, MD, FRCSC Division of Otolaryngology – Head and Neck Surgery, Université de Sherbrooke, Sherbrooke, QC, Canada

Katherine N. Cahill, MD Department of Medicine/Division of Rheumatology, Immunology, and Allergy, Brigham and Women's Hospital/Harvard Medical School, Boston, MA, USA

Eric T. Carniol, MD, MBA Department of Otolaryngology – Head and Neck Surgery, Rutgers New Jersey Medical School, Newark, NJ, USA

Justin T. Casey, MD Department of Otolaryngology – Head and Neck Surgery, University of Colorado School of Medicine, Aurora, CO, USA

Rakesh K. Chandra, MD Department of Otolaryngology – Head and Neck Surgery, Vanderbilt University School of Medicine, Nashville, TN, USA

Martin J. Citardi, MD Department of Otorhinolaryngology – Head and Neck Surgery, University of Texas Medical School at Houston, Houston, TX, USA

John Craig, MD Department of Otolaryngology, Henry Ford Hospital, Detroit, MI, USA

Dana L. Crosby, MD Division of Otolaryngology – Head and Neck Surgery, Southern Illinois University School of Medicine, Springfield, IL, USA

Opeyemi O. Daramola, MD Department of Otolaryngology – Head and Neck Surgery, Northwestern University Feinberg School of Medicine, Chicago, IL, USA

Nathan A. Deckard, MD Division of Otolaryngology – Head and Neck Surgery, Department of Surgery, Cooper University Hospital, Camden, NJ, USA

John M. DelGaudio, MD, FACS, FARS Department of Otolaryngology – Head and Neck Surgery, Emory University, Atlanta, GA, USA

Jean Anderson Eloy, MD, FACS Department of Otolaryngology – Head and Neck Surgery, Rutgers New Jersey Medical School, Newark, NJ, USA

Department of Neurological Surgery, Rutgers New Jersey Medical School, Newark, NJ, USA

Center for Skull Base and Pituitary Surgery, Neurological Institute of New Jersey, Rutgers New Jersey Medical School, Newark, NJ, USA

Carrie E. Flanagan, MD Department of Otolaryngology – Head and Neck Surgery, Emory University, Atlanta, GA, USA

Wytske Fokkens, MD, PhD Department of Otorhinolaryngology, Academic Medical Centre, Amsterdam, NH, The Netherlands

Rachel Georgopoulos, MD Department of Otolaryngology – Head and Neck Surgery, Temple University Hospital, Philadelphia, PA, USA

Anne E. Getz, MD Department of Otolaryngology – Head and Neck Surgery, University of Colorado School of Medicine, Aurora, CO, USA

Andrew N. Goldberg, MD, MSCE, FACS Division of Rhinology and Sinus Surgery, Department of Otolaryngology – Head and Neck Surgery and Neurological Surgery, University of California, San Francisco, San Francisco, CA, USA

Parul Goyal, MD, MBA Syracuse Otolaryngology, Syracuse, NY, USA

Jessica W. Grayson, MD Department of Surgery/Division of Otolaryngology – Head and Neck Surgery, University of Alabama at Birmingham, Birmingham, AL, USA

Ashleigh A. Halderman, MD Section of Rhinology, Sinus and Skull Base Surgery, Head and Neck Institute, Cleveland Clinic Foundation, Cleveland, OH, USA

Joseph K. Han, MD, FARS, FAAOA, FACS Division of Allergy, Division of Rhinology Endoscopic Sinus and Skull Base Surgery, Department of Otolaryngology – Head and Neck Surgery, Eastern Virginia Medical School, Norfolk, VA, USA

Richard Harvey, MD Department of Otolaryngology Head and Neck Surgery, St Vincent's Hospital, Sydney, NSW, Australia

Department of Otolaryngology Head and Neck Surgery, Rhinology and Skull Base, Applied Medical Research Centre, University of New South, Sydney, NSW, Australia

Australian School of Advanced Medicine, Macquarie University, Sydney, NSW, Australia

Chase M. Heaton, MD Department of Otolaryngology – Head and Neck Surgery, University of California, San Francisco, San Francisco, CA, USA

Eric H. Holbrook, MD Department of Otolaryngology, Harvard Medical School, Boston, MA, USA

Division Chief of Rhinology, Massachusetts Eye and Ear Infirmary, Boston, MA, USA

Benjamin P. Hull, MD, MHA Department of Otolaryngology – Head and Neck Surgery, Eastern Virginia Medical School, Norfolk, VA, USA

Peter H. Hwang, MD Division of Rhinology and Endoscopic Skull Base Surgery, Department of Otolaryngology – Head and Neck Surgery, Stanford University School of Medicine, Stanford, CA, USA

Niall Jefferson, MBBCh, BAO, FRACS (OHNS) Department of Otolaryngology – Head and Neck Surgery, St. Vincent's Hospital, Sydney, NSW, Australia

Michael C. Kao, MD Department of Otolaryngology – Head and Neck Surgery, University of Washington, Seattle, WA, USA

David W. Kennedy, FACS, FRCSI, MD Department of Otorhinolaryngology – Head and Neck Surgery, Perelman School of Medicine, University of Pennsylvania, Philadelphia, PA, USA

Todd T. Kingdom, MD Department of Otolaryngology – Head and Neck Surgery, University of Colorado School of Medicine, Aurora, CO, USA

C. Carrie Liu, MD Division of Otolaryngology – Head and Neck Surgery, Department of Surgery, Foothills Medical Centre, University of Calgary, Calgary, AB, Canada

Phillip S. LoSavio, MD, MS Section Head – Sleep Surgery, Department of Otorhinolaryngology – Head and Neck Surgery, Rush University Medical Center, Chicago, IL, USA

Amber Luong, MD, PhD Department of Otorhinolaryngology – Head and Neck Surgery, University of Texas Medical School at Houston, Houston, TX, USA

R. Peter Manes, MD, FACS Section of Otolaryngology, Department of Surgery, Yale University School of Medicine, New Haven, CT, USA

Stanley W. McClurg, MD Department of Otolaryngology/Head and Neck Surgery, University of North Carolina – Chapel Hill, Chapel Hill, NC, USA

Caitlin McLean, MD Department of Otolaryngology – Head and Neck Surgery, Temple University School of Medicine, Philadelphia, PA, USA

Josh Meier, MD Nevada ENT and Hearing Associates, Reno, NV, USA

Richard R. Orlandi, MD Division of Otolaryngology – Rhinology, Sinus and Skull Base Surgery Program, Otolaryngology, University of Utah, Salt Lake City, UT, USA

Thomas R. O'Toole, MD Department of Otorhinolaryngology – Head and Neck Surgery, Rush University Medical Center, Chicago, IL, USA

Sanjay R. Parikh, MD, FACS Department of Otolaryngology – Head and Neck Surgery, Seattle Children's Hospital, University of Washington, Seattle, WA, USA

Drew P. Plonk, MD Department of Otolaryngology, Wake Forest University School of Medicine, Medical Center Boulevard, Winston-Salem, NC, USA

David M. Poetker, MD, MA Department of Otolaryngology, Zablocki VA Medical Center, Medical College of Wisconsin, Milwaukee, WI, USA

Vishal Pundir, MS, MRCS Department of Otorhinolaryngology, Academic Medical Centre, Amsterdam, The Netherlands

Hassan H. Ramadan, MD, MSc, FACS Department of Otolaryngology – Head and Neck Surgery, RCBHSCS, West Virginia University, Morgantown, WV, USA

Luke Rudmik, MD, MSc Division of Otolaryngology – Head and Neck Surgery, Department of Surgery, Foothills Medical Centre, University of Calgary, Calgary, AB, Canada

Brent A. Senior, MD, FACS, FARS Division of Rhinology, Allergy and Endoscopic Skull Base Surgery, Department of Otolaryngology/Head and Neck Surgery, University of North Carolina – Chapel Hill, Chapel Hill, NC, USA

Raj Sindwani, MD Section of Rhinology, Sinus and Skull Base Surgery, Head and Neck Institute, Cleveland Clinic Foundation, Cleveland, OH, USA

Ameet Singh, MD Division of Otolaryngology – Head and Neck Surgery, George Washington University Hospital, Washington, DC, USA

Timothy L. Smith, MD, MPH Division of Rhinology and Sinus Surgery, Department of Otolaryngology – Head and Neck Surgery, Oregon Sinus Center, Oregon Health and Science University, Portland, OR, USA

Janalee Stokken, MD Section of Rhinology, Sinus and Skull Base Surgery, Head and Neck Institute, Cleveland Clinic Foundation, Cleveland, OH, USA

Peter F. Svider, MD Department of Otolaryngology – Head and Neck Surgery, Wayne State University School of Medicine, Detroit, MI, USA

Neville W.Y. Teo, MBBS, MRCS Department of Otolaryngology, Singapore General Hospital, Singapore, Singapore

Brian D. Thorp, MD Department of Otolaryngology/Head and Neck Surgery, University of North Carolina – Chapel Hill, Chapel Hill, NC, USA

Elina Toskala, MD, PhD Department of Otolaryngology – Head and Neck Surgery, Temple University, School of Medicine, Philadelphia, PA, USA

Alejandro Vazquez, MD Department of Otolaryngology – Head and Neck Surgery, Rutgers New Jersey Medical School, Newark, NJ, USA

Kevin C. Welch, MD, FACS Department of Otolaryngology – Head and Neck Surgery, Feinberg School of Medicine, Northwestern University, Chicago, IL, USA

Joshua Wiedermann, MD Division of Otolaryngology – Head and Neck Surgery, George Washington University Hospital, Washington, DC, USA

Bradford A. Woodworth, MD, FACS Department of Surgery/Division of Otolaryngology – Head and Neck Surgery, Gregory Fleming James Cystic Fibrosis Research Center, University of Alabama at Birmingham, Birmingham, AL, USA

Carolyn Word, MD Department of Allergy and Immunology, University of Virginia Health System, Charlottesville, VA, USA

Peter John Wormald, FRACS, FCS(SA), FRCS(Ed), MD Department of Otolaryngology – Head and Neck Surgery, The Queen Elizabeth Hospital, Woodville South, SA, Australia

Erin D. Wright, MDCM, MEd Division of Otolaryngology – Head and Neck Surgery, University of Alberta, Edmonton, AB, Canada

Mark A. Zacharek, MD, FACS Department of Otolaryngology – Head and Neck Surgery, University of Michigan Health System, Ann Arbor, MI, USA

Part I

Overview of Chronic Rhinosinusitis

Epidemiology and Pathophysiology of Chronic Rhinosinusitis

1

Eric T. Carniol, Peter F. Svider, Alejandro Vázquez, and Jean Anderson Eloy

Key Take-Home Points

- CRS is defined as inflammation of the sinonasal tract lasting at least twelve consecutive weeks.
- CRS afflicts approximately 31 million patients (12.5 % of the population) annually in the USA, resulting in a substantial economic and noneconomic burden.
- Economic figures have been cited noting approximately 20 million outpatient visits annually attributed to CRS sequelae and greater than $5 billion in associated healthcare expenditures.
- CRS patients with asthma, nasal polyposis, aspirin sensitivity, or inhalant allergy tend to have greater disease burden.
- CRS represents a common end point of a heterogeneous group of pathophysiologic processes, influenced by various environmental, anatomic, congenital, immune, and infectious factors.

E.T. Carniol, MD, MBA • A. Vázquez, MD
Department of Otolaryngology – Head and Neck Surgery, Rutgers New Jersey Medical School, 90 Bergen St., Suite 8100, Newark, NJ 07103, USA
e-mail: ericcarniol@gmail.com; avazquez84@gmail.com

P.F. Svider, MD
Department of Otolaryngology – Head and Neck Surgery, Wayne State University School of Medicine, 4201 St. Antoine, 5E UHC, Detroit, MI 48201, USA
e-mail: psvider@gmail.com

J.A. Eloy, MD, FACS (✉)
Department of Otolaryngology – Head and Neck Surgery, Rutgers New Jersey Medical School, 90 Bergen St., Suite 8100, Newark, NJ 07103, USA

Department of Neurological Surgery, Rutgers New Jersey Medical School, Newark, NJ, USA

Center for Skull Base and Pituitary Surgery, Neurological Institute of New Jersey, Rutgers New Jersey Medical School, Newark, NJ, USA
e-mail: jean.anderson.eloy@gmail.com

P.S. Batra, J.K. Han (eds.), *Practical Medical and Surgical Management of Chronic Rhinosinusitis*, DOI 10.1007/978-3-319-16724-4_1

Definitions

In 1997, Lanza and Kennedy published a definition and classification scheme for adult rhinosinusitis. Endorsed by the American Academy of Otolaryngology-Head and Neck Surgery (AAO-HNS), the American Academy of Otolaryngic Allergy (AAOA), and the American Rhinologic Society (ARS), the terminology, classification system, and diagnostic criteria proposed gained wide acceptance. Affirming recommendations made by the AAO-HNS Task Force on rhinosinusitis the previous year, the term *sinusitis* was abandoned in favor of the more descriptive *rhinosinusitis*, which was defined as "an inflammatory response involving…the mucous membranes (possibly including the neuroepithelium) of the nasal cavity and paranasal sinuses, fluids within these cavities, and/or underlying bone." Moreover, the authors established a temporal classification of rhinosinusitis that is still used today, recognizing acute, subacute, and chronic forms of the disease on the basis of symptom duration. Finally, guidelines for the diagnosis of rhinosinusitis were issued, based on the presence of certain major and minor criteria (Table 1.1) [3–5].

According to the 2007 AAO-HNS clinical practice guidelines, CRS is defined as inflammation of the sinonasal tract lasting at least twelve consecutive weeks. The cardinal *symptoms* of CRS include nasal obstruction (present in 81–95 % of cases), facial pain, pressure, fullness or congestion (70–85 %), mucopurulent drainage (51–83 %), and hyposmia (61–69 %) [3–5]. A diagnosis of CRS requires the presence of *at least two* of these symptoms, in addition to sinonasal inflammation documented by *one or more* of the following means [6]:

- Purulent or discolored rhinorrhea on endoscopy
- Edema in the middle meatus or ethmoid region on endoscopy
- Polyps in the nasal cavity or middle meatus on endoscopy
- Radiographic imaging showing inflammation of the paranasal sinuses

Table 1.1 Factors associated with the diagnosis of chronic rhinosinusitis [3–5]

Major factors		Minor factors	
Facial pain/pressure*	53–83 %	Headache	51–83 %
Facial congestion/fullness	70–85 %	Fever	8.8–33 %
Nasal obstruction/blockage	81–95 %	Halitosis	37–53 %
Nasal discharge/ purulence/discolored postnasal drainage	70–85 %	Fatigue	67–84 %
Hyposmia/anosmia	61–69 %	Dental pain	23–50 %
Purulence in nasal cavity on exam	10.5 %	Cough	39–65 %
		Ear pain/pressure/fullness	68 %

The European Position Paper on Rhinosinusitis and Nasal Polyps (EPOS 2012) [7] defines CRS in adults as the presence of sinonasal inflammation for at least twelve weeks. A diagnosis of CRS requires the presence of *two or more* of the following symptoms:

- Nasal obstruction (syn., blockage or congestion) *OR* nasal discharge (syn., anterior/posterior nasal drip) [*at least one of these is required*]
- Facial pain/pressure
- Reduction or loss of smell

The EPOS further defines CRS as either *CRS with nasal polyps* (*CRSwNP*) or *CRS without nasal polyps* (*CRSsNP*), depending on whether polyps are visualized in the middle meatus during nasal endoscopy.

By way of comparison, it is worthwhile to briefly mention three related entities: acute bacterial rhinosinusitis (ABRS), recurrent acute rhinosinusitis (RARS), and acute exacerbation on chronic rhinosinusitis. ABRS is a disease process that lasts up to four weeks and is characterized by purulent rhinorrhea with either nasal obstruction or facial pain/pressure/fullness. RARS is characterized by four or more discrete episodes of ABRS separated by symptom-free intervals [6, 8, 9]. Finally, patients with CRS may also have flare-ups or exacerbations of symptoms, termed *acute-on-chronic rhinosinusitis*. During these exacerbations, patients experience either new symptoms or worsening of existing symptoms, which, when treated, should improve and return to baseline CRS symptoms [10].

Epidemiology

According to the 1996 National Health Institute Survey, CRS afflicts approximately 31 million patients (12.5 % of the population) annually [11]. In 1997, there were an estimated 18 to 22 million office visits to physicians for CRS and over half a million visits to the emergency department [12]. In 2001, over 50 % of the visits were to either family practitioners or pediatricians, and less than 10 % were to otolaryngologists. It is important to note that, unlike acute rhinosinusitis, CRS cannot be diagnosed by symptoms alone; objective findings are important to differentiate CRS from related entities that can cause similar symptoms. Despite uncertainty regarding the true prevalence of CRS, economic figures have been cited noting approximately 20 million outpatient visits annually attributed to CRS sequelae and greater than $5 billion in associated healthcare expenditures [1, 13].

As there is a strong familial incidence for CRS, there is believed to be a strong genetic predisposition. In one analysis from France of patients with CRSwNP, 53 % of patients had a family history of nasal polyposis, while 44 % had a family history of asthma [14].

A wide variety of comorbidities have been found among CRS patients. In a focused retrospective review of patients with refractory CRS, Batra et al. noted significant prevalence of asthma, nasal polyposis, aspirin sensitivity, and inhalant allergy, with greater disease burden among CRS patients with these comorbidities [1]. Several analyses have also suggested that laryngopharyngeal reflux (LPR) may be associated with CRS. For example, one evaluation of 77 patients confirmed to have gastroesophageal reflux disease found significantly higher SNOT-20 scores compared to controls (22.1 vs. 9.4), a difference that was noted to be statistically significant [15]. Furthermore, a separate analysis by Wise et al. found increased reporting of CRS symptoms, particularly postnasal drip, among those with LPR [16]. Despite this potential association with LPR, no direct pathophysiologic mechanisms have been described in the literature.

Geographic patterns in the distribution of CRS have also been reported. Most notably, Southeastern USA has a far higher prevalence of allergic fungal subtypes, ranging as high as one in five cases requiring operative intervention [17, 18].

Pathophysiology

In their 1997 article on the definition of adult rhinosinusitis, Lanza and Kennedy suggest that rhinosinusitis could be conceptualized as a syndrome rather than a disease, given that it is an entity whose characteristics are not well established. Although this comment alludes to the heterogeneity of its clinical features, it further attests to the complexity of the pathophysiologic processes underlying CRS.

In recent years, there has been a trend toward considering CRS as two related but distinct disease processes: CRS with nasal polyps (CRSwNP) and CRS without nasal polyps (CRSsNP). The former is thought to represent primarily a Th2-mediated inflammatory process, with strong association to asthma and aspirin sensitivity. CRSsNP, on the other hand, is thought to be primarily related to Th1-mediated inflammation [19].

In many cases, CRS represents a common end point of a heterogeneous group of pathophysiologic processes, influenced by various environmental, anatomic, congenital, immune, and infectious factors. Independent of the precipitants, chronic inflammation is the common endpoint and hallmark of this disease. In the sections that follow, a variety of extrinsic and intrinsic factors that have been implicated in the pathogenesis of CRS are reviewed.

Anatomic and Physiologic Abnormalities

Any anatomic derangements that interfere with mucociliary clearance may potentially cause chronic mucus stasis that facilitates inflammation and leads to a CRS-type state. Severe septal deflections or large spurs may cause lateralization of the middle turbinate or otherwise grossly impair drainage from the middle meatus. Variant pneumatization of certain structures, such as the concha bullosa, agger nasi cell, or Haller cell, may obstruct outflow from the ostiomeatal complex. In cases where a clear anatomic cause can be identified, either clinically or radiographically, correction of this offending abnormality may potentially alleviate CRS depending on duration of preceding symptoms and underlying genetic susceptibility. However, the majority of CRS cases will not be attributable to a singular anatomic abnormality. In most cases, the pathophysiologic mechanisms underlying CRS are far more complex, and an anatomic abnormality, if present, may represent only one confounding factor.

At the cellular level, the sinonasal mucosa produces a mucociliary "escalator" that forms part of the innate immune system in the upper respiratory tract. This mechanism is based on (1) the production of mucus and (2) effective ciliary beating in an organized fashion. The mucus produced contains immunoglobulins, enzymes, and other factors for trapping and/or eliminating microbes, allergens, pollutants, and other particles. This clearance can be affected by a multitude of host, environmental, and infectious factors.

In response to pollutants, the mucosa of the sinuses and nasal cavity upregulates mucus production [20, 21]. With infection and chronic inflammation, the mucociliary transport system may become impaired. The mucous takes on a more viscous state, which is more difficult to clear from the paranasal sinuses [22]. This thicker mucous also does not cover the sinonasal mucosa as effectively, leading to decreased barrier function [23]. This impairment propagates the infectious and inflammatory state by preventing the egress of the bacteria and inflammatory cytokines [24]. With age, mucociliary transport malfunctions as the cilia become increasingly dysfunctional due to microtubular construction errors and slower ciliary beat frequency, possibly leading to more frequent sinus infections in elderly patients [25]. Primary ciliary dyskinesia is discussed further later in this chapter.

It should be noted that benign or malignant neoplastic lesions may lead to obstruction of paranasal sinus outflow tract and thus result in CRS. This possibility should be kept in mind, particularly when evaluating unilateral or single-subsite disease.

Environmental Irritants

Tobacco Smoke

Similar to other airway irritants, tobacco smoke causes inflammation and increased mucus production. Patients that are chronic smokers have been found to have markedly increased mucociliary transport times. Increased clearance time leads to mucostasis, which allows for increased inflammation in the nasal cavity and paranasal sinuses [26]. Heavy smokers (i.e., those who smoke more than 5 packs per week) are believed to have even greater mucociliary clearance times than less avid smokers [27]. In addition to the changes in mucus viscosity and volume, ciliary beat frequency significantly decreases in these patients [28]. These findings have led to the identification of tobacco smoke and second-hand smoke as independent risk factors for CRS [29].

Immune System Dysregulation

Sinonasal Polyposis

Several alterations in the immune response have been implicated in the development of sinonasal polyposis. While sinonasal polyposis is estimated to affect approximately 4 % of the general population, its prevalence is 2–4 times greater in patients with asthma [30–32]. Moreover, sinonasal polyposis has been noted to be associated with an increased incidence in patients with aspirin intolerance, conjunctivitis, urticaria, eczema, food and other allergies, and current smokers. These disorders share a common pathophysiologic mechanism, namely, a predominance of a type 2 helper T-cell-mediated (or Th2-mediated) response. Certain studies have demonstrated an upregulation in Th2-mediated immunity, downregulation of Th1-mediated immunity, and reduction (up to 50 %) in toll-like receptor (TLR) 9 gene expression [33]. The decrease of this TLR (which helps recognize bacterial DNA) has been directly correlated with severity of CRSwNP [34]. An upregulation of B-cell activating factor of the TNF family (BAFF) has been recognized in CRSwNP. It is this upregulation that is believed to upregulate B-cell production of IgA which may also contribute to the eosinophilia of nasal polyps [34]. Ongoing basic and translational research will continue to elucidate our understanding of nasal polyposis.

Asthma and Chronic Rhinosinusitis: Unified Airway Disease

Asthma is caused by lower airway inflammation, immune dysregulation, and airway wall remodeling. The pathophysiologic changes in asthma mirror those of CRS and allergic rhinitis. The high degree of coexistence and shared causative mechanisms has led to the postulation of the concept termed *the unified airway* (and, consequently, *unified airway disease*). In unified airway disease, the Th2-mediated immune response produces local hypereosinophilia and elevated levels of immunoglobulin E (IgE), as well as elevated Th2-type cytokines, including TGF-ß [35]. This eosinophil-dominated response leads to airway remodeling. TGF-ß1 activation and regulation has been found to play important physiologic role in CRS and differ in its subtypes [35, 36]. Although exact mechanisms are still under investigation, the difference in activity of plasminogen activator inhibitor 1 (PAI-1) and fibrinolytic pathways may help differentiate either CRSwNP or CRSsNP [37].

Aspirin-Sensitive (ASA) Triad

The clinical triad of nasal polyposis, asthma, and aspirin intolerance was first described by Samter and Beers in 1968 [38]. Aspirin hypersensitivity is believed to be related to the inhibition of cyclooxygenase enzyme and increases in lipoxygenase, leading to an elevation of leukotriene synthesis. The leukotrienes then induce increased nasal mucosal edema, mucus secretion, bronchoconstriction, and eosinophilic migration [39]. Symptomatically, these patients have more severe clinical presentation of CRS and asthma [40]. They are at high risk for treatment failure and recurrence of polyps following endoscopic sinus surgery (ESS) and often require multiple subsequent procedures. While only 4.6 % of patients undergoing ESS have ASA triad, Kim and Kountakis noted that these patients had undergone ten times as many surgeries as the non-ASA triad counterparts [40].

Role of Bacteria in Chronic Rhinosinusitis

The role of bacterial infection in CRS remains to be fully elucidated; however, a majority of experts believe that bacteria play an important role in CRS as evidenced by the fact that antimicrobial therapy forms an integral part of most CRS management strategies [10, 41]. Inconclusive evidence exists regarding whether bacteria are the inciting event in CRS or simply a modifier worsening the disease process. Nonetheless, *Staphylococcus aureus*, gram negative rods, and anaerobic bacteria have been noted to be significant pathogens in CRS, especially when considering their relative infrequency among uncomplicated acute rhinosinusitis cases [42].

Bacterial Biofilms

Bacterial biofilms have been theorized to play a role in both CRSwNP and CRSsNP. A biofilm is an organized aggregation of bacteria that adheres to mucosal surfaces and expresses a molecular profile unique from that expressed by the individual planktonic bacteria. Biofilm is associated with an extracellular matrix material that facilitates genetic alterations, increases resistance to antibiotics, and enhances capabilities to resist host immunity [13, 43]. One mechanism attributed to biofilms is quorum sensing [44, 45]. This encompasses the responsiveness of these bacterial aggregates to produce hormone-like molecules that are controlled by water channels found in the biofilm and function in an autocrine fashion [44]. Patients with biofilm formation exhibit a clinical course characterized by chronic infections with periods of marked worsening of symptoms [46].

Multiple studies have noted mucosal biofilms in the majority of samples among the CRS patient population [43, 47–49]. Further supporting the role of biofilms in the development of CRS is the fact that numerous analyses have noted a relative absence of biofilms in healthy controls not affected by sinus disease [43, 50–52].

Singhal et al. evaluated the role of biofilms in patients undergoing ESS for CRS [50]. Consistent with prior reports, 71 % of their 51 CRS patients had bacterial biofilms. Following surgery, this cohort of patients had significantly worse sinus symptoms and nasal endoscopy findings than individuals without biofilms, supporting the concept that biofilms may be an important contributor to treatment-resistant CRS [34, 53].

The relationship between *S. aureus* and biofilms has been studied in the context of CRS, as certain strains of *S. aureus* have a propensity for biofilm formation through increased expression of immunosuppressive proteins (relative to non-biofilm-forming *S. aureus* strains) [54, 55]. However, it should be noted that even in the biofilm state, *S. aureus* can differentiate into free-living bacteria that are thought to be responsible for acute exacerbations [44].

Pathogen-Mediated Immunomodulation and the Superantigen Hypothesis

Recent studies also illustrate that *S. aureus* may survive intracellularly within nasal epithelial cells, mucus-producing cells, and antigen-presenting cells [56, 57]. One theory of CRS pathogenesis posits that intracellular *S. aureus* releases toxins that activate lymphocytes and thus drives inflammation [58].

It has been postulated that *S. aureus* exotoxins may function as superantigens. A superantigen is a substance that can activate T cells nonspecifically, resulting in polyclonal (rather than monoclonal) activation of T cells, as well as eosinophilic activation, leading to a vigorous immune response. Activation of immune cells in this manner within the sinonasal tract stimulates the release of IL-4, IL-5, and IL-13, which skew the response toward a Th2 phenotype seen in CRSwNP. This is consistent with the fact that *S. aureus* may be found in greater numbers in CRSwNP than CRSsNP. Krysko et al. noted that phagocytosis of *S. aureus* by antigen-presenting cells, specifically macrophages, may be impaired in CRSwNP, promoting chronic inflammation [59]. Definitive evidence for the superantigen hypothesis is still lacking as approximately 50 % of patients will express superantigen-specific IgE and approximately one third will demonstrate superantigen-specific T-cell changes [34].

The Role of Osteitis

The role of inflammation of the bone (i.e., osteitis) in the development of CRS has been extensively studied. Proponents of osteitis as a pathogenic factor in CRS cite computed tomography (CT) findings of bony thickening with neo-osteogenesis in refractory disease as potential evidence [60]. Histologic sections demonstrate thickened bone with neo-osteogenesis, further perpetuating mucosal fibrosis. It is important to differentiate osteitis from osteomyelitis, as the latter signifies infection of bone marrow, while the former specifically refers to inflammation of the bone. As sinuses are devoid of marrow, osteitis is the correct nomenclature [61]. Kennedy et al. analyzed ethmoid bone samples which were found to histologically resemble lesions seen in patients suffering from osteomyelitis; further, debridement of this inflamed bone led to resolution of overlying mucosal inflammation [62]. Animal models support this hypothesis and suggest that inflammation in the bone disseminates through the Haversian canal system [60, 63]. Turning to more clinical evaluations of the role of the bone in CRS, greater disease burden has been demonstrated on the CT scans of those with neo-osteogenesis compared to controls [60, 64, 65], as well as worse endoscopically documented disease severity and increased rates of dysosmia [60, 66].

Systemic Diseases with Chronic Rhinosinusitis as Common End Point

Several systemic diseases can lead to chronic inflammation of the sinonasal tract and, consequently, to a clinical picture that is indistinguishable from more conventional CRS. In many cases, CRS can be the initial presenting feature of a serious systemic disorder. Oftentimes, workup for an underlying disorder will not be considered until after the patient has undergone (and failed) standard treatment for CRS. Historical or physical features that might distinguish this group of patients from conventional CRS may be subtle, or even absent. For this reason, a high index of suspicion is necessary when an underlying systemic disorder is suspected in the setting of CRS refractory to conventional treatment modalities, especially in patients who may have seen multiple practitioners or undergone multiple previous surgical procedures and/or courses of medical therapy.

Congenital Disorders

Primary Ciliary Dyskinesia

Primary ciliary dyskinesia (PCD), also referred to as *immotile cilia syndrome*, is a primarily autosomal recessive genetic condition which affects the structure or function of cilia, thereby resulting in impaired mucociliary clearance. Patients with PCD are usually afflicted by chronic, recurrent lower respiratory tract infections. Early descriptions of PCD identified a clinical picture of sinusitis, bronchiectasis, and situs inversus that eventually came to be known as the Kartagener triad [67]. In a report of 78 subjects diagnosed with PCD, Noone et al. identified a 100 % frequency of chronic rhinitis/sinusitis. These patients were also noted to have very low levels of nasal nitric oxide production relative to normal subjects [68]. The mechanism for this alteration in nitric oxide is unknown, but proposed theories include altered ciliary activity, altered expression of nitric oxide synthase, or another aspect of chronic sinonasal inflammation itself [69].

Cystic Fibrosis

Cystic fibrosis (CF) is an autosomal recessive genetic disorder which disrupts the transport of chloride ions across cell membranes (via the CF transmembrane conductance regulator, or CFTR), leading to an abnormally low level of water in mucous secretions. Mucous secretions become abnormally viscous, and, as a consequence, mucociliary transport is severely altered [70]. Patients with classic CF have an incidence of CRS that approaches 100 %. In these patients, the incidence of sinonasal polyposis can be as high as 48 % [71]. CF is often associated with decreased pneumatization or frank hypoplasia of the paranasal sinuses, as well as mucocele formation. Active CRS may also impact the frequency of serious lower respiratory tract infections. Traditionally, patients have been treated with a combination of systemic antibiotics, corticosteroids, and ESS. However, the precise roles of these treatment modalities remain the subject of controversy. Several novel therapeutic agents aimed at rescuing CFTR function at the molecular level are currently in clinical trials.

Rheumatologic and Autoimmune Disorders

Granulomatosis with Polyangiitis (or Wegener Granulomatosis)

Granulomatosis with polyangiitis (GPA) is an autoimmune disorder characterized by a necrotizing vasculitis of small- to medium-sized vessels. Sinonasal complaints are quite common. In a retrospective analysis of 120 patients with GPA referred for otolaryngologic evaluation, Cannady et al. found that 89 % of patients exhibited sinonasal involvement, including nasal crusting (69 %), CRS (61 %), nasal obstruction (58 %), bloody rhinorrhea (52 %), and septal perforation (33 %) [72]. The inflammatory reaction characteristic of this disease typically arises from the nasal septum and inferior turbinates and then spreads bilaterally to the rest of the nasal cavity and sinuses. If left untreated, this disease can lead to erosion of the sinonasal architecture, leading to a common cavity [73, 74]. The mainstay of therapy for GPA is to induce and then maintain remission using immunosuppressive agents. Many of the regimens include methotrexate, cyclophosphamide, azathioprine, corticosteroids, TNF-alpha blockers (including infliximab), and rituximab [75].

Sarcoidosis

Sarcoidosis is an idiopathic disorder that can affect multiple organ systems. It exhibits a broad range of severity, ranging from an essentially asymptomatic radiographic abnormality to a life-threatening condition. Unlike GPA, the granulomatosis seen in sarcoidosis is non-necrotizing. The precise incidence of CRS in sarcoidosis is unclear. However, it is thought to be low, on the order of <1 % [76]. A retrospective analysis of 36 patients with sarcoid rhinosinusitis identified nasal obstruction as the most frequent symptom (86 %), followed by nasal crusting (47 %), anosmia (44 %), epistaxis (28 %), and nasal polyposis (25 %) [77].

Eosinophilic Granulomatosis with Polyangiitis (or Churg-Strauss Syndrome)

Eosinophilic granulomatosis with polyangiitis (EGPA) is a rare disorder characterized by a necrotizing, eosinophilic vasculitis of small- to medium-sized vessels. "Paranasal sinusitis" is among the six diagnostic criteria established by the American College of Rheumatology in 1990; approximately 61 % of patients exhibit this complaint at the time of diagnosis [78]. The sinonasal inflammation seen in EGPA responds to systemic corticosteroids.

Relapsing Polychondritis

Relapsing polychondritis is a recurrent inflammation of cartilaginous tissue. The most common manifestations of this disease are ocular edema, auricular inflammation (possibly leading to cauliflower deformity), nasal inflammation (possibly leading to saddle nose deformity), or intranasal inflammation. The diagnostic criteria for this disease are three of the following six findings: auricular chondritis, seronegative nonerosive inflammatory polyarthritis, nasal chondritis, ocular inflammation, respiratory chondritis, and audiovestibular damage. Although relapsing polychondritis can lead to rhinitis, it is typically localized to the anterior nasal cavity and not a true rhinosinusitis [37].

Systemic Lupus Erythematosus

Systemic lupus erythematosus (SLE) is an autoimmune connective tissue of unknown etiology, which can affect superficial tissues exclusively or cause multiorgan dysfunction. This disorder which is often recognized for its malar rash can lead to granulomatous inflammation with edema and nasal crusting and can progress to septal perforation. Rhinitis may occur initially at presentation or later in the clinical course, while the patient undergoes immunosuppressive therapy [79].

Infectious Diseases

Fungal

Various forms of rhinosinusitis can be attributed either to direct invasion by fungal pathogens or immune system reactivity to fungal antigens. Fungal rhinosinusitis can be classified as *invasive fungal rhinosinusitis* (either *acute* [AIFRS] or *chronic*

[CIFRS]), *noninvasive fungal rhinosinusitis* (*saprophytic overgrowth* or *fungal ball*), or *allergic fungal rhinosinusitis* (AFRS). A detailed discussion of these entities is found in Chapter 7. AIFRS is typically seen in immunocompromised patients, usually with hematologic malignancies, poorly controlled diabetes mellitus, chronic corticosteroid therapy, or acquired immunodeficiency syndrome [80]. Although geographic variations exist, pathogens usually belong to the genus *Aspergillus*. However, a wide variety of fungal species can exhibit invasive behavior in the setting of immunocompromise. CIFRS, also known as indolent invasive fungal rhinosinusitis, exhibits a slower course than AIFRS. It is a rare disorder in the USA with *Aspergillus flavus* implicated in many cases.

AFRS is considered to be the sinonasal analogue of allergic bronchopulmonary aspergillosis, an eosinophilic disorder that affects the lower airways. It is characterized by typical histopathologic findings, including the presence of eosinophils, Charcot-Leyden crystals (a by-product of eosinophil breakdown), necrotic inflammatory cells, and hyphal elements. Although the precise mechanism of AFRS remains to be elucidated, recent studies have implicated a strong Th2 response, triggered by respiratory epithelial cell-derived factors such as interleukin (IL)-25, IL-33, and thymic stromal lymphopoietin [81].

Syphilis

Although the overall incidence of syphilis has fallen in the USA, the importance of recognizing the manifestations of syphilis should be emphasized. While the first stage of syphilis is characterized by a painless chancre and regional lymphadenopathy that may go unrecognized, later stages affect the mucosa of the nose, mouth, lips, palate, tongue, tonsils, and throat. The treponemal infection can affect the sinonasal microvasculature, causing necrosis and even collapse, and predisposing the sinuses and nasal cavities to infection [79].

Human Immunodeficiency Virus (HIV)

Human immunodeficiency virus (HIV) infection progresses to the acquired immunodeficiency syndrome (AIDS) once CD4+ T-cell counts are sufficiently depleted (i.e., below 200 cells/mm^3). AIDS causes increased vulnerability to various infections [82]. Patients with AIDS have been found to have increased serum levels of IgE production, prolonged mucociliary transport times, and a higher incidence of CRS [82–84].

Rhinoscleroma

Rhinoscleroma is a rare, chronic sinonasal infection caused by *Klebsiella rhinoscleromatis*. It is characterized by the formation of nasal granulomas. In the first stage of rhinoscleroma (the atrophic or catarrhal stage), rhinorrhea, nasal obstruction, purulent discharge, and nasal crusting are common. This can progress to the hypertrophic (or granulomatous) stage with formation of nasal nodules and destruction of nasal cartilage. The third stage (the sclerotic stage) is characterized by fibrosis and intranasal scarring [85]. This stage can affect the respiratory tract from the nose and mouth to the bronchi, causing destruction and often stenosis. It is more common in Central and South America, Central Europe, and the Middle East, Asia, and Africa; in the USA, incidence is higher in travelers and immigrants from these regions.

Atypical Mycobacteria

In patients with refractory CRS, diagnostic studies for mycobacteria may be useful [86]. Risk factors for atypical mycobacterial infection include foreign bodies in the sinonasal tract, non-HIV immunodeficiency, history of chemoradiation therapy for sinonasal malignancy, sinus irrigation from contaminated water supplies, and possibly previous endoscopic sinus surgery [87–89]. In a series by Solyar et al. of 37 patients with recalcitrant CRS with a positive acid-fast bacilli test, the most frequently isolated species of mycobacteria included *M. abscessum, M. avium-intercellulare* complex, and *M. chelonae* (57.1, 14.3, and 14.3 % respectively) [88].

Toxin-Related Disorders

Cocaine

Intranasal drug abuse can also contribute to CRS. Messinger et al. demonstrated an incidence of 4.8 % of nasal complications among a cohort of intranasal cocaine users [90]. Cocaine causes mucosal complications due to a combination of chemical irritation, vasoreactivity, and trauma from the instrumentation [91]. The vasoreactivity includes vasoconstriction, which leads to ischemic necrosis, followed by rebound vasodilation. The end result is necrotic mucosa and local tissue atrophy, as well as osteocartilaginous erosion. The granulomatous necrotic tissue provides a healthy medium for bacterial colonization and growth. It has also been noted that midline cocaine-induced destructive lesions can be c-ANCA positive [92].

Conclusion

CRS exacts a considerable toll upon society, significantly impacting both quality of life in individuals and raising costs associated with healthcare delivery. CRS represents a common end point for a heterogeneous group of pathophysiologic processes. Although significant strides have been made over the past decades in our understanding of disease mechanisms in CRS, a great number of questions have yet to be answered. Ongoing basic science and translational research is crucial to continue to shed light on these key unanswered questions.

Financial Disclosures None
Conflicts of Interest None

References

1. Batra PS, Tong L, Citardi MJ. Analysis of comorbidities and objective parameters in refractory chronic rhinosinusitis. Laryngoscope. 2013;123 Suppl 7:S1–11.
2. Senior BA, Glaze C, Benninger MS. Use of the Rhinosinusitis Disability Index (RSDI) in rhinologic disease. Am J Rhinol. 2001;15:15–20.
3. Bhattacharyya N. The economic burden and symptom manifestations of chronic rhinosinusitis. Am J Rhinol. 2003;17:27–32.
4. Lanza DC, Kennedy DW. Adult rhinosinusitis defined. Otolaryngol Head Neck Surg. 1997;117:S1–7.
5. Orlandi RR, Terrell JE. Analysis of the adult chronic rhinosinusitis working definition. Am J Rhinol. 2002;16:7–10.
6. Rosenfeld RM, Andes D, Bhattacharyya N, et al. Clinical practice guideline: adult sinusitis. Otolaryngol Head Neck Surg. 2007;137:S1–31.
7. Fokkens WJ, Lund VJ, Mullol J, et al. EPOS 2012: European position paper on rhinosinusitis and nasal polyps 2012. A summary for otorhinolaryngologists. Rhinology. 2012;50:1–12.
8. Rosenfeld RM. Clinical practice guideline on adult sinusitis. Otolaryngol Head Neck Surg. 2007;137:365–77.
9. Meltzer EO, Hamilos DL. Rhinosinusitis diagnosis and management for the clinician: a synopsis of recent consensus guidelines. Mayo Clin Proc. 2011;86:427–43.
10. Benninger MS, Ferguson BJ, Hadley JA, et al. Adult chronic rhinosinusitis: definitions, diagnosis, epidemiology, and pathophysiology. Otolaryngol Head Neck Surg. 2003; 129:S1–32.
11. Adams PF, Hendershot GE, Marano MA. Current estimates from the National Health Interview Survey, 1996. Vital and health statistics Series 10, Data from the National Health Survey; 1999. p. 1–203.
12. Schappert SM. Ambulatory care visits to physician offices, hospital outpatient departments, and emergency departments: United States, 1997. Vital and health statistics Series 13, Data from the National Health Survey; 1999. p. i–iv, 1–39.
13. Cohen M, Kofonow J, Nayak JV, et al. Biofilms in chronic rhinosinusitis: a review. Am J Rhinol Allergy. 2009;23:255–60.
14. Rugina M, Serrano E, Klossek JM, et al. Epidemiological and clinical aspects of nasal polyposis in France; the ORLI group experience. Rhinology. 2002;40:75–9.
15. Katle EJ, Hart H, Kjaergaard T, Kvaloy JT, Steinsvag SK. Nose- and sinus-related quality of life and GERD. Eur Arch Otorhinolaryngol. 2012;269:121–5.
16. Wise SK, Wise JC, DelGaudio JM. Association of nasopharyngeal and laryngopharyngeal reflux with postnasal drip symptomatology in patients with and without rhinosinusitis. Am J Rhinol. 2006;20:283–9.
17. Hamilos DL. Chronic rhinosinusitis: epidemiology and medical management. J Allergy Clin Immunol. 2011;128:693–707; quiz 708–699.
18. Ferguson BJ, Barnes L, Bernstein JM, et al. Geographic variation in allergic fungal rhinosinusitis. Otolaryngol Clin North Am. 2000;33:441–9.
19. Banerji A, Piccirillo JF, Thawley SE, et al. Chronic rhinosinusitis patients with polyps or polypoid mucosa have a greater burden of illness. Am J Rhinol. 2007;21:19–26.
20. Antunes MB, Cohen NA. Mucociliary clearance – a critical upper airway host defense mechanism and methods of assessment. Curr Opin Allergy Clin Immunol. 2007;7:5–10.
21. Chen B, Shaari J, Claire SE, et al. Altered sinonasal ciliary dynamics in chronic rhinosinusitis. Am J Rhinol. 2006;20:325–9.
22. Girod S, Zahm JM, Plotkowski C, Beck G, Puchelle E. Role of the physiochemical properties of mucus in the protection of the respiratory epithelium. Eur Respir J. 1992;5:477–87.
23. Atsuta S, Majima Y. Nasal mucociliary clearance of chronic sinusitis in relation to rheological properties of nasal mucus. Ann Otol Rhinol Laryngol. 1998;107:47–51.

24. Jorissen M, Willems T, De Boeck K. Diagnostic evaluation of mucociliary transport: from symptoms to coordinated ciliary activity after ciliogenesis in culture. Am J Rhinol. 2000;14:345–52.
25. Ho JC, Chan KN, Hu WH. The effect of aging on nasal mucociliary clearance, beat frequency, and ultrastructure of respiratory cilia. Am J Respir Crit Care Med. 2001;163:983–8.
26. Briggs RD, Wright ST, Cordes S, Calhoun KH. Smoking in chronic rhinosinusitis: a predictor of poor long-term outcome after endoscopic sinus surgery. Laryngoscope. 2004;114:126–8.
27. Mahakit P, Pumhirun P. A preliminary study of nasal mucociliary clearance in smokers, sinusitis and allergic rhinitis patients. Asian Pac J Allergy Immunol. 1995;13:119–21.
28. Agius AM, Smallman LA, Pahor AL. Age, smoking and nasal ciliary beat frequency. Clin Otolaryngol Allied Sci. 1998;23:227–30.
29. Reh DD, Higgins TS, Smith TL. Impact of tobacco smoke on chronic rhinosinusitis: a review of the literature. Int Forum Allergy Rhinol. 2012;2:362–9.
30. Klossek JM, Neukirch F, Pribil C, et al. Prevalence of nasal polyposis in France: a cross-sectional, case–control study. Allergy. 2005;60:233–7.
31. Hedman J, Kaprio J, Poussa T, Nieminen MM. Prevalence of asthma, aspirin intolerance, nasal polyposis and chronic obstructive pulmonary disease in a population-based study. Int J Epidemiol. 1999;28:717–22.
32. Larsen K. The clinical relationship of nasal polyps to asthma. Allergy Asthma Proc. 1996;17:243–9.
33. Ramanathan Jr M, Lee WK, Dubin MG, Lin S, Spannhake EW, Lane AP. Sinonasal epithelial cell expression of toll-like receptor 9 is decreased in chronic rhinosinusitis with polyps. Am J Rhinol. 2007;21:110–6.
34. Hsu J, Peters AT. Pathophysiology of chronic rhinosinusitis with nasal polyp. Am J Rhinol Allergy. 2011;25:285–90.
35. Frieri M. Asthma linked with rhinosinusitis: an extensive review. Allergy Rhinol (Providence). 2014;5:41–9.
36. Kou W, Hu GH, Yao HB, et al. Regulation of transforming growth factor-beta1 activation and expression in the tissue remodeling involved in chronic rhinosinusitis. ORL J Otorhinolaryngol Relat Spec. 2012;74:172–8.
37. Önerci TM. Nasal Physiology and Pathophysiology of Nasal Disorders. Heidelberg: Springer; 2013.
38. Samter M, Beers Jr RF. Intolerance to aspirin. Clinical studies and consideration of its pathogenesis. Ann Intern Med. 1968;68:975–83.
39. Antczak A, Montuschi P, Kharitonov S, Gorski P, Barnes PJ. Increased exhaled cysteinyl-leukotrienes and 8-isoprostane in aspirin-induced asthma. Am J Respir Crit Care Med. 2002;166:301–6.
40. Kim JE, Kountakis SE. The prevalence of Samter's triad in patients undergoing functional endoscopic sinus surgery. Ear Nose Throat J. 2007;86:396–9.
41. Bhattacharyya N, Kepnes LJ. The microbiology of recurrent rhinosinusitis after endoscopic sinus surgery. Arch Otolaryngol Head Neck Surg. 1999;125:1117–20.
42. Hwang PH. Staph aureus has long been recognized as being more prevalent in cultures from patients with chronic rhinosinusitis(CRS) compared to those with acute rhinosinusitis. Int Forum Allergy Rhinol. 2013;3:81–2.
43. Foreman A, Jervis-Bardy J, Wormald PJ. Do biofilms contribute to the initiation and recalcitrance of chronic rhinosinusitis? Laryngoscope. 2011;121:1085–91.
44. Madeo J, Frieri M. Bacterial biofilms and chronic rhinosinusitis. Allergy Asthma Proc. 2013;34:335–41.
45. Al-Mutairi D, Kilty SJ. Bacterial biofilms and the pathophysiology of chronic rhinosinusitis. Curr Opin Allergy Clin Immunol. 2011;11:18–23.
46. Donlan RM, Costerton JW. Biofilms: survival mechanisms of clinically relevant microorganisms. Clin Microbiol Rev. 2002;15:167–93.
47. Korkmaz H, Ocal B, Tatar EC, et al. Biofilms in chronic rhinosinusitis with polyps: is eradication possible? Eur Arch Otorhinolaryngol. 2014;271:2695–702.

48. Tatar EC, Tatar I, Ocal B, et al. Prevalence of biofilms and their response to medical treatment in chronic rhinosinusitis without polyps. Otolaryngol Head Neck Surg. 2012;146:669–75.
49. Bezerra TF, Padua FG, Gebrim EM, Saldiva PH, Voegels RL. Biofilms in chronic rhinosinusitis with nasal polyps. Otolaryngol Head Neck Surg. 2011;144:612–6.
50. Singhal D, Psaltis AJ, Foreman A, Wormald PJ. The impact of biofilms on outcomes after endoscopic sinus surgery. Am J Rhinol Allergy. 2010;24:169–74.
51. Foreman A, Psaltis AJ, Tan LW, Wormald PJ. Characterization of bacterial and fungal biofilms in chronic rhinosinusitis. Am J Rhinol Allergy. 2009;23:556–61.
52. Sanclement JA, Webster P, Thomas J, Ramadan HH. Bacterial biofilms in surgical specimens of patients with chronic rhinosinusitis. Laryngoscope. 2005;115:578–82.
53. Li H, Wang D, Sun X, Hu L, Yu H, Wang J. Relationship between bacterial biofilm and clinical features of patients with chronic rhinosinusitis. Eur Arch Otorhinolaryngol. 2012;269:155–63.
54. Quinn GA, Tarwater PM, Cole AM. Subversion of interleukin-1-mediated host defence by a nasal carrier strain of Staphylococcus aureus. Immunology. 2009;128:e222–9.
55. Cole AM, Tahk S, Oren A, et al. Determinants of Staphylococcus aureus nasal carriage. Clin Diagn Lab Immunol. 2001;8:1064–9.
56. Plouin-Gaudon I, Clement S, Huggler E, et al. Intracellular residency is frequently associated with recurrent Staphylococcus aureus rhinosinusitis. Rhinology. 2006;44:249–54.
57. Clement S, Vaudaux P, Francois P, et al. Evidence of an intracellular reservoir in the nasal mucosa of patients with recurrent Staphylococcus aureus rhinosinusitis. J Infect Dis. 2005;192:1023–8.
58. Tomassen P, Van Zele T, Zhang N, et al. Pathophysiology of chronic rhinosinusitis. Proc Am Thorac Soc. 2011;8:115–20.
59. Krysko O, Holtappels G, Zhang N, et al. Alternatively activated macrophages and impaired phagocytosis of S. aureus in chronic rhinosinusitis. Allergy. 2011;66:396–403.
60. Bhandarkar ND, Sautter NB, Kennedy DW, Smith TL. Osteitis in chronic rhinosinusitis: a review of the literature. Int Forum Allergy Rhinol. 2013;3:355–63.
61. Sethi N. The significance of osteitis in rhinosinusitis. Eur Arch Otorhinolaryngol 2014;272(4):821–6.
62. Kennedy DW, Senior BA, Gannon FH, Montone KT, Hwang P, Lanza DC. Histology and histomorphometry of ethmoid bone in chronic rhinosinusitis. Laryngoscope. 1998;108:502–7.
63. Perloff JR, Gannon FH, Bolger WE, Montone KT, Orlandi R, Kennedy DW. Bone involvement in sinusitis: an apparent pathway for the spread of disease. Laryngoscope. 2000;110:2095–9.
64. Georgalas C, Videler W, Freling N, Fokkens W. Global Osteitis Scoring Scale and chronic rhinosinusitis: a marker of revision surgery. Clin Otolaryngol. 2010;35:455–61.
65. Lee JT, Kennedy DW, Palmer JN, Feldman M, Chiu AG. The incidence of concurrent osteitis in patients with chronic rhinosinusitis: a clinicopathological study. Am J Rhinol. 2006;20:278–82.
66. Bhandarkar ND, Mace JC, Smith TL. The impact of osteitis on disease severity measures and quality of life outcomes in chronic rhinosinusitis. Int Forum Allergy Rhinol. 2011;1:372–8.
67. Popatia R, Haver K, Casey A. Primary ciliary dyskinesia: an update on new diagnostic modalities and review of the literature. Pediatr Allergy Immunol Pulmonol. 2014;27:51–9.
68. Noone PG, Leigh MW, Sannuti A, et al. Primary ciliary dyskinesia: diagnostic and phenotypic features. Am J Respir Crit Care Med. 2004;169:459–67.
69. Deja M, Busch T, Bachmann S, et al. Reduced nitric oxide in sinus epithelium of patients with radiologic maxillary sinusitis and sepsis. Am J Respir Crit Care Med. 2003;168:281–6.
70. Egan M. Cystic fibrosis (Chapter 395). In: Kliegman EA, editor. Nelson Textbook of Pediatrics. 19th ed. Philadelphia: Elsevier Saunders; 2011.
71. Chaaban MR, Kejner A, Rowe SM, Woodworth BA. Cystic fibrosis chronic rhinosinusitis: a comprehensive review. Am J Rhinol Allergy. 2013;27:387–95.
72. Cannady SB, Batra PS, Koening C, et al. Sinonasal Wegener granulomatosis: a single-institution experience with 120 cases. Laryngoscope. 2009;119:757–61.

73. Woywodt A, Haubitz M, Haller H, Matteson EL. Wegener's granulomatosis. Lancet. 2006;367:1362–6.
74. Lloyd G, Lund VJ, Beale T, Howard D. Rhinologic changes in Wegener's granulomatosis. J Laryngol Otol. 2002;116:565–9.
75. Bosch X, Guilabert A, Espinosa G, Mirapeix E. Treatment of antineutrophil cytoplasmic antibody – associated vasculitis: a systematic review. JAMA. 2007;298:655–69.
76. Kirsten AM, Watz H, Kirsten D. Sarcoidosis with involvement of the paranasal sinuses – a retrospective analysis of 12 biopsy-proven cases. BMC Pulm Med. 2013;13:59.
77. Reed J, de Shazo RD, Houle TT, Stringer S, Wright L, Moak 3rd JS. Clinical features of sarcoid rhinosinusitis. Am J Med. 2010;123:856–62.
78. Guillevin L, Cohen P, Gayraud M, Lhote F, Jarrousse B, Casassus P. Churg-Strauss syndrome. Clinical study and long-term follow-up of 96 patients. Medicine. 1999;78:26–37.
79. Thaler ER, Kennedy DW. Rhinosinusitis: A Guide for Diagnosis and Management: Springer. 2008.
80. Parikh SL, Venkatraman G, DelGaudio JM. Invasive fungal sinusitis: a 15-year review from a single institution. Am J Rhinol. 2004;18:75–81.
81. Plonk DP, Luong A. Current understanding of allergic fungal rhinosinusitis and treatment implications. Curr Opin Otolaryngol Head Neck Surg. 2014;22:221–6.
82. Prasad HK, Bhojwani KM, Shenoy V, Prasad SC. HIV manifestations in otolaryngology. Am J Otolaryngol. 2006;27:179–85.
83. Milgrim LM, Rubin JS, Small CB. Mucociliary clearance abnormalities in the HIV-infected patient: a precursor to acute sinusitis. Laryngoscope. 1995;105:1202–8.
84. Godofsky EW, Zinreich J, Armstrong M, Leslie JM, Weikel CS. Sinusitis in HIV-infected patients: a clinical and radiographic review. Am J Med. 1992;93:163–70.
85. Kim NR, Han J, Kwon TY. Nasal rhinoscleroma in a nonendemic area: a case report. J Korean Med Sci. 2003;18:455–8.
86. Hamilos DL. Host-microbial interactions in patients with chronic rhinosinusitis. J Allergy Clin Immunol. 2014;133:640–53.e4.
87. Suh JD, Ramakrishnan VR, Tajudeen B, Reger C, Kennedy DW, Chiu AG. Identification and treatment of nontuberculous Mycobacterium sinusitis. Am J Rhinol Allergy. 2011;25:421–4.
88. Solyar A, Lee AS, Przybyszewski B, Lanza DC. Atypical mycobacterium detection in refractory chronic rhinosinusitis. Otolaryngol Head Neck Surg. 2012;146:1012–6.
89. Tichenor WS, Thurlow J, McNulty S, Brown-Elliott BA, Wallace Jr RJ, Falkinham 3rd JO. Nontuberculous Mycobacteria in household plumbing as possible cause of chronic rhinosinusitis. Emerg Infect Dis. 2012;18:1612–7.
90. Messinger E. Narcotic septal perforations due to drug addiction. JAMA. 1962;179:964–5.
91. Gupta A, Hawrych A, Wilson WR. Cocaine-induced sinonasal destruction. Otolaryngol Head Neck Surg. 2001;124:480.
92. Fuchs HA, Tanner SB. Granulomatous disorders of the nose and paranasal sinuses. Curr Opin Otolaryngol Head Neck Surg. 2009;17:23–7.

Microbiology of Chronic Rhinosinusitis

2

R. Peter Manes

Key Take-Home Points

- Thorough understanding of the microbiology of chronic rhinosinusitis is a requisite in the management of CRS patients.
- The most common cultured organisms in chronic rhinosinusitis are *Staphylococcus aureus*, coagulase-negative *Staphylococcus*, and gram-negative rods.
- *S. aureus* is the most common organism seen in chronic rhinosinusitis. Its presence at the time of endoscopic sinus surgery has been demonstrated to be a strong predictor of postoperative *S. aureus* infection and impaired mucosal healing.
- *Pseudomonas aeruginosa* is the most commonly cultured gram-negative rod and can be associated with biofilm formation.
- *Stenotrophomonas maltophilia* is a multidrug-resistant gram-negative bacteria seen in patients with previous FESS and prior antimicrobial treatment.

Introduction

Chronic rhinosinusitis (CRS) represents one of the most common healthcare problems in the United States, afflicting approximately 31 million Americans [1]. CRS is a clinical syndrome associated with persistent inflammation of the mucosa of the nose and paranasal sinuses for 12 weeks or longer [2, 3]. It is known to cause significant physical impairment, adversely impacting patient quality of life and psychosocial well-being. Despite its prevalence, CRS remains a challenging and, at

R.P. Manes, MD, FACS
Section of Otolaryngology, Department of Surgery, Yale University School of Medicine, 333 Cedar Street, PO Box 208041, New Haven, CT 06520, USA
e-mail: rpeter.manes@yale.edu

P.S. Batra, J.K. Han (eds.), *Practical Medical and Surgical Management of Chronic Rhinosinusitis*, DOI 10.1007/978-3-319-16724-4_2

times, controversial disease entity. The etiologic mechanisms of CRS continue to be a source of much debate, and as such, different schools of thought exist on the optimal management strategy. The purpose of this chapter is to describe the different proposed pathophysiologic mechanisms of CRS, with a focus on the microbiology associated with CRS.

Accurate diagnosis of CRS rests on the ability to identify signs and symptoms associated with the disease process, such as nasal obstruction, purulent discharge, and/or facial pain, as well as objective evidence of mucosal inflammation, either by nasal endoscopy and/or computerized tomography [4]. However, it is also important to recognize that this is a heterogeneous disease spectrum, subject to further subclassifications. Patients with CRS may be divided into CRS with nasal polyps (CRSwNP) and CRS without nasal polyps (CRSsNP). This distinction leads to both clinical and pathologic differences. CRSwNP is predominantly mediated by eosinophils, as well as increased levels of histamine, interleukin (IL)-5, and IL-13 [5]. In contrast, CRSsNP seems, at first glance, to be predominantly mediated by neutrophilic inflammation [6]. However, some CRSsNP cases may also exhibit extensive eosinophilic infiltration. Therefore, the distinction between CRS with and without polyps is not as clear as originally thought. In addition, CRS must be clearly differentiated from systemic processes that lead to sinonasal mucosal inflammation. Clinical entities, such as cystic fibrosis, sarcoidosis, Wegener's granulomatosis, and primary immunodeficiency (PID), may present with sinus involvement as a component of the multisystem process. Some cases of PID can be relatively mild and manifest primarily as sinusitis without pneumonia or other more serious systemic infections. The prevalence of PID in patients with recalcitrant CRS varies widely in the literature, from 0 to 19 %. Furthermore, secondary CRS may arise as a result of local, discrete processes such as tumor, mycetoma, and foreign-body reaction. A recent study even suggests a potential causal relationship between tobacco smoke exposure and the development of CRS [7]. The primary focus of this review is to discuss CRS as a primary disease process in the absence of systemic or local predisposing factors.

Etiology of CRS

Bacteria likely represent the main underlying cause of acute rhinosinusitis (ARS), with the most commonly identified bacteria being *Streptococcus pneumoniae*, *Moraxella catarrhalis*, and *Haemophilus influenzae* [8]. In contrast, the central pathophysiology of CRS remains elusive to date. A variety of possible etiologic mechanisms have been proposed, including microbes (viruses, bacteria, fungi), allergy, osteitis, biofilm formation, staphylococcal superantigen, and derangements in innate and adaptive immunity. Though the exact role of bacteria in the disease process remains to be fully elucidated, it is likely that bacterial infection plays an important role in CRS, either as a causative or an exacerbating factor [9].

Bacteria

The microbiology of CRS varies greatly from ARS. Nadel et al. evaluated 507 endoscopically guided cultures in 265 patients [10]. The predominant organisms identified include *Staphylococcus aureus (31.3%)*, coagulase-negative *Staphylococcus* (SCN) (44.2 %), and gram-negative rods (34.3 %). A multitude of gram-negative organisms were cultured, with the most common being *Pseudomonas aeruginosa*, *Stenotrophomonas maltophilia*, *Escherichia coli*, and *Serratia marcescens*. Kingdom and Swain analyzed 182 total cultures with 257 isolates in 101 patients at the time of sinus surgery. The microbiologic yield was similar; the most common isolates were SCN (45 %), gram-negative rods (25 %), and *Staphylococcus aureus* (24 %) [11]. Comparative analysis between primary and revision sinus surgery cases demonstrated no differences in the bacterial yield or types. Bhattacharyya and Gopal have demonstrated that while approximately half of the bacteria cultured in CRS are found in isolation, the rest exhibit polymicrobial growth, with two or more bacterial species present [12]. See Table 2.1 for key bacteria and fungi identified in CRS.

Staphylococcus aureus

S. aureus is a ubiquitous microorganism, occupying the nasal vestibule of nearly one-third of the human population at any given time. *S. aureus* has emerged as an important pathogen in community- and hospital-acquired infections, resulting in sepsis, bacteremia, endocarditis, and soft tissue infections. *S. aureus* is commonly assayed in cultures performed for CRS [10, 11, 13, 14]. Nadel et al. and Kingdom and Swain reported its presence in 23.1 and 25 % of sinus cultures, respectively [10, 11]. Though the exact role in pathogenesis is a matter of debate, the presence of *S. aureus* infection at the time of sinus surgery has been demonstrated to be a strong predictor of postoperative *S. aureus* infection and impaired mucosal healing.

A variety of novel mechanisms of pathogenicity have also been implicated, including biofilm formation and intracellular residency [15]. Foreman et al. characterized bacterial biofilm by fluorescence in situ hybridization in 50 CRS patients. Biofilms were detected in 36 of 50 patients, with *S. aureus* being the most common biofilm-forming organism [16]. The capacity to form biofilms may confer the ability to create a recalcitrant infectious state unresponsive to conventional antimicrobial therapies.

Table 2.1 Key microbes cultured in chronic rhinosinusitis [8]

Aerobic	Anaerobic	Fungus
Staphylococcus aureus	*Fusobacterium* spp.	*Aspergillus fumigatus*
Coagulase-negative *Staphylococcus*	*Pigmented Prevotella* and *Porphyromonas* spp.	*Aspergillus niger*
Pseudomonas aeruginosa	*Peptostreptococcus* spp.	*Aspergillus flavus*
Stenotrophomonas maltophilia		
Haemophilus influenzae		
Streptococcus pneumoniae		

An increase in the recovery of methicillin-resistant *Staphylococcus aureus* (MRSA) has recently been noted in acute and chronic rhinosinusitis and anterior nares of normal individuals [17]. Brook et al. compared MRSA rates in chronic maxillary sinusitis between two time periods. *S. aureus* was found in 15 (15 %) of the patients between 2001 and 2003, four (27 %) of which were MRSA. *S. aureus* was cultured in 23 (20 %) of the patients between 2004 and 2006, with 14 (61 %) being MRSA. Indeed, MRSA represents a treatment challenge in the setting of CRS, given paucity of optimal treatment options. Oral antibiotics that may be effective include doxycycline, trimethoprim/sulfamethoxazole, and clindamycin. Topical mupirocin irrigations may also serve as an important adjunct in the postoperative CRS patient [18].

Staphylococcal Superantigens

The superantigen hypothesis proposes that *S. aureus* secretes high molecular weight proteins known as enterotoxins. These enterotoxins have significant stimulatory activity that can foster the characteristic tissue response seen in patients with nasal polyps. Approximately 50 % of CRSwNP patients show lymphocyte responses consistent with superantigen exposure [19]. In addition, staphylococcal toxin-specific IgE antibodies have been detected in 18 of 23 patients with nasal polyps [20]. It is unclear, however, whether *S. aureus* superantigens represent an etiologic agent or a disease modifier. The link between superantigens and CRSsNP has not yet been established.

Coagulase-Negative *Staphylococcus*

The exact role of SCN in CRS remains to be determined, as its reported incidence varies widely [11]. It has been posited to be a contaminant, supported by previous work that found CNS in the middle meatus of 56 % of healthy patients and in only 20 % of patients with CRS [21]. Moreover, the microbe is ubiquitous on human skin; thus, contamination may occur readily without proper sterile precautions during culture technique. However, different strains of CNS may have differing abilities to cause disease. Recent studies evaluating CNS in indwelling devices have shown that bacterial pathogenicity is dependent on genes associated with biofilm formation, which are only found in certain strains [22]. The mere presence of SCN may not indicate infection, as a specific strain may be necessary for such an infection to develop. Nonetheless, endoscopically acquired cultures have consistently identified SCN in multiple studies in CRS. Bolger found SCN in 17 %, Hsu et al. in 42 %, and Nadel et al. in 35 % of cultures [10, 13, 14]. One possible method to ascertain significance of SCN culture is based on the quantitative growth on culture, along with presence of leukocytosis on the gram stain result. Scant or light growth, especially with a paucity of gram-positive rods or white blood cells (WBCs) on gram stain, likely represents contamination. In contrast, moderate to heavy growth, with large number of WBCs on gram stain, should alert the clinician of the possibility of a true infection.

Pseudomonas aeruginosa

Gram-negative rods are often identified in CRS cultures, more commonly in patients who have undergone endoscopic sinus surgery [10, 13, 14]. However, their role in patients with CRS without previous surgery should also not be underestimated. Kingdom and Swain found GNRs in 31 % of cultures in a group of patients at the time of primary sinus surgery [11]. Nadel et al. found GNRs in 9.5 % of cultures taken from patients without previous sinus surgery [10]. *P. aeruginosa* has long been recognized as an important pathogen in the upper and lower airway in cystic fibrosis patients. It also represents a common and problematic organism in CRS. Rates of assay in CRS cultures have been reported between 9 and 16 % [10, 11]. Nadel et al. noted that *P. aeruginosa* was most commonly cultured in patients with previous FESS and irrigation usage [10]. *P. aeruginosa* also has the capability of biofilm formation which may in part contribute to its refractory nature in CRS patients. Further, the presence of *P. aeruginosa* biofilm has been associated with poor evolution after FESS [23]. Fluoroquinolones are the only orally administered antibiotic group with efficacy against *P. aeruginosa*. Quinolone resistance has become more problematic, with limited alternate proven oral antimicrobial therapies for *Pseudomonas* rhinosinusitis.

Stenotrophomonas maltophilia

Stenotrophomonas maltophilia is a multidrug-resistant gram-negative bacillus most often encountered as a nosocomial pathogen in immunocompromised and intensive care unit patients. Infection with *S. maltophilia* most frequently involves the respiratory tract, bloodstream, wounds, and genitourinary tract. *S. maltophilia* has also been cultured from the paranasal sinuses, often in the setting of prior antimicrobial treatment and sinus surgery. The exact implication of *S. maltophilia* cultures in the paranasal sinuses is unclear. Whether this represents a true infection by an atypical microorganism or colonization that surfaces after eradication of other microbes by antimicrobial therapy merits additional research. Despite its multidrug-resistant nature, trimethoprim/sulfamethoxazole and fluoroquinolone monotherapy has been employed with improvement of symptoms and endoscopic findings in CRS patients [24].

Viruses

Patients with CRS frequently report that their symptoms initially started after an acute viral event [25]. Furthermore, viruses can cause multiple changes on a cellular level, facilitating an infectious and inflammatory milieu of CRS, such as increase in bacterial adhesion and production of inflammatory mediators by nasal epithelial cells [26, 27]. Multiple studies have evaluated the presence of respiratory viruses in samples taken from patients with CRS. Ramadan and colleagues found RSV present in 20 % of samples collected from patients with CRS [28]. However, this study did not report a control group or the timing of the specimen collection, as the presence of RSV is much greater in the winter months in the general population. Jang et al. reported a similar study with a control group and collected specimens during the summer months [29]. Rhinovirus was identified in 21 % of samples from CRS patients and 0 % in the control group. However, these samples were taken from the inferior turbinates and not the paranasal sinus mucosa. In contrast to the above studies, Wood et al. collected sinus mucosa samples from 13 CRS patients and 2 controls [25]. No respiratory viruses, including RSV and rhinovirus, were identified in any of the samples. While viruses may be implicated in the initial or ongoing stimulus of inflammation, their exact role in CRS is not clearly defined.

Fungus

It is clear that fungus is responsible for some forms of sinusitis, in both invasive and noninvasive forms. Though a wide variety of fungi have been identified in the sinuses of CRS patients, the central etiologic role of fungus in CRS has not been clearly demonstrated. In 1999, positive fungal cultures from nasal mucus were used as the basis to posit that eosinophilic infiltration and fungal presence provided the main inciting event for CRS [30]. However, further studies found a similar percentage of positive cultures in normal control patients [31]. In addition, a double-blind, placebo-controlled randomized multicenter trial has failed to identify any benefit of topical antifungal therapy in objective and subjective outcome measures in patients with CRS [32]. A subset of CRS, allergic fungal rhinosinusitis (AFRS), is characterized by type I hypersensitivity to fungi, nasal polyposis, eosinophilic mucin, hyperdensities on CT imaging, and positive fungal stain or culture with the absence of diabetes, immunodeficiency, or an invasive fungal process [33]. Furthermore, patients with AFRS have been shown to have elevated levels of total serum IgE and IgG anti-*Alternaria* antibodies when compared to patients with CRS [34]. While fungus does play a role in specific subtypes of CRS, its role as a central pathophysiologic mechanism of CRS is not corroborated in the literature.

Osteitis

Osteitis is another possible etiologic factor for CRS. Patients with CRS often show areas of irregular bony thickening on CT imaging. It has been proposed that this irregular thickening and increased bone density may be a sign of inflammation in the bone, resulting in persistent inflammation of the overlying mucosa [35]. Osteitis is marked by varying degrees of osteoclast-osteoblast activity, leading to disruption of organized lamellar bone and formation of immature woven bone [36]. Entry of inflammatory infiltrate into the Haversian canal system may act as a potential pathway for spread of inflammation and, as such, mucosal disease. The prevalence of osteitis is estimated between 36 and 53 % in CRS patients, based on CT findings or pathologic evaluation [37]. This concept of osteitis, an inflammation of the bone, should be differentiated from osteomyelitis, as direct bacterial invasion of the bone in CRS has not yet been demonstrated in studies.

Innate and Adaptive Immune Dysfunction

The innate immune system provides the first line of defense against pathogens through both physical barriers, such as ciliated mucosa, and the expression of several antimicrobial molecules, including S100 and surfactant protein A. The data on these antimicrobial molecules has been somewhat inconsistent. Some studies have not shown consistent changes in these antimicrobial molecules in patients with CRS [38, 39]. Other, more recent studies have shown more consistent changes, specifically in the S100 proteins [40]. These have direct antimicrobial effects as well as aid in recruitment of neutrophils and lymphocytes. These proteins are decreased in patients with CRS compared to controls. The dysfunction of the innate immune system remains a strong area of ongoing research to determine its true role in the pathophysiology of CRS.

Dysfunction in the adaptive immune system may also play a role in the development of CRS. The epithelium serves an important role in the adaptive immune system, mediating communication through cell surface molecules that regulate activation of T cells, as well as producing cytokines and chemokines that activate B cells and T cells and enable their migration. Dysregulation of the interaction between epithelial cells and the adaptive immune system may also play an important role in the development of CRS. Moreover, free light chains, which are thought to be involved in mast cell-dependent immune responses, have been found to be increased in nasal secretions and mucosal tissue of patients with CRS [41]. This increase is most prominent in CRSwNP. The increased free light chains suggest a possible role in mediating the local immune dysregulation in CRS.

Allergy

Allergy may represent a confounding factor in the development of CRS. Allergy often manifests as swelling of nasal mucous membranes, leading to sinus ostia narrowing and obstruction. Such obstruction can lead to retained mucus, decreased ventilation, and infection. Furthermore, positive allergy skin prick tests are highly associated with CRS. Benninger reported 54 % of patients with CRS had positive skin prick tests [42]. This is in keeping with multiple other studies, showing rates of positive skin prick tests in 50–84 % of patients with CRS undergoing sinus surgery [43, 44]. However, others studies point toward no increase in CRS in patients with positive allergic responses. Despite the lack of a clear etiologic role for allergy in CRS, it likely represents a contributing factor that should be addressed in the overall treatment strategy.

Anatomic Factors

Anatomic factors have been theorized to play a role in the development of CRS. These include a pneumatized middle turbinate (concha bullosa), septal deviation, and variations in configuration of the uncinate process. Despite the proposed mechanisms of anatomic variability leading to CRS, multiple studies have shown no difference in prevalence of anatomic variations between patients with and without CRS [45, 46]. In contrast, a systematic review on the role of septal deviation in CRS concluded that increasing angles of septal deflection were associated with a small, but significant, increasing prevalence of CRS [47]. Based on current information, the exact role of anatomic variations in CRS is unclear. It would seem that altered sinus ventilation may result from anatomic variants, but this alone is likely insufficient for the development and propagation of CRS.

Conclusion

This snapshot of etiologic information highlights the inherent difficulties in managing the infectious aspects of CRS. Though coagulase-negative *Staphylococcus*, *S. aureus*, and *P. aeruginosa* predominate in microbiologic studies, multitude of gram-negative rods and other atypical organisms may also be cultured in refractory CRS, especially in the setting of previous sinus surgery. Furthermore, other factors including immune derangements, osteitis, fungus, viruses, allergy, and anatomic factors may also play a role in the etiology of CRS. Ongoing research in pathophysiologic mechanisms and treatment schemes is absolute imperatives to continue to enhance patient care.

References

1. National Center for Health Statistics. National ambulatory medical care survey 1990–1995. Hyattsville: US Public Health Service; 1997. Series 13 [CD-ROM].
2. Fokkens W, Lund V, Mullol J, et al. European position paper on rhinosinusitis and nasal polyps 2012. Rhinol Suppl. 2012;50:1–299.
3. Meltzer EO, Hamilos DL. Rhinosinusitis diagnosis and management for the clinician: a synopsis of recent consensus guidelines. Mayo Clin Proc. 2011;86:427–43.
4. Benninger MS, Ferguson BJ, Hadley JA, et al. Adult chronic rhinosinusitis: definitions, diagnosis, epidemiology and pathophysiology. Otolaryngol Head Neck Surg. 2003;129:S1–32.
5. Drake-Lee AB, McLaughlan P. Clinical symptoms, free histamine and IgE in patients with nasal polyposis. Int Arch Allergy Appl Immunol. 1982;69:268–71.
6. Pawankar R, Nanoka M. Inflammatory mechanisms and remodeling in chronic rhinosinusitis and nasal polyps. Curr Allergy Asthma Rep. 2007;7:202–8.
7. Reh DD, Higgins TS, Smith TL. Impact of tobacco smoke on chronic rhinosinusitis: a review of the literature. Int Forum Allergy Rhinol. 2012;2(5):362–9.
8. Brook I. Microbiology of sinusitis. Proc Am Thorac Soc. 2011;8:90–100.
9. Biel MA, Brown CA, Levinson RM, et al. Evaluation of the microbiology of chronic maxillary sinusitis. Ann Otol Rhinol Laryngol. 1998;107:942–5.
10. Nadel DM, Lanza DC, Kennedy DW. Endoscopically guided cultures in chronic sinusitis. Am J Rhinol. 1998;12:233–41.
11. Kingdom TT, Swain RE. The microbiology and antimicrobial resistance patterns in chronic rhinosinusitis. Am J Otolaryngol. 2004;25:323–8.
12. Bhattacharyya N, Gopal HV. Microbiology of the ethmoid sinus following endoscopic sinus surgery. Ear Nose Throat J. 2002;81:558–61.
13. Bolger WE. Gram negative sinusitis: an emerging clinical entity? Am J Rhinol. 1994;8:279–84.
14. Hsu J, Lanza DC, Kennedy DW. Antimicrobial resistance in bacterial chronic sinusitis. Am J Rhinol. 1998;12:243–7.
15. Lowy FD. Staphylococcal aureus infections. N Engl J Med. 1998;339:520–32.
16. Foreman A, Psaltis AJ, Tan LW, Wormald PJ. Characterization of bacterial and fungal biofilms in chronic rhinosinusitis. Am J Rhinol Allergy. 2009;23:556–61.
17. Brook I, Foote PA, Hausfeld JN. Increase in the frequency of recovery of methicillin-resistant *Staphylococcus aureus* in acute and chronic maxillary sinusitis. J Med Microbiol. 2008;57:1015–7.
18. Solares CA, Batra PS, Hall GS, Citardi MJ. Treatment of chronic rhinosinusitis exacerbations due to methicillin-resistant Staphylococcus aureus with mupirocin irrigation. Am J Otolaryngol. 2006;27:161–5.

19. Bachert C, Zhang N, van Zele T, et al. Staphylococcus aureus enterotoxins as immune stimulants in chronic rhinosinusitis. Clin Allergy Immunol. 2007;20:163–75.
20. Tripathi A, Conley DB, Grammer LC, et al. Immunoglobulin E to staphylococcal and streptococcal toxins in patients with chronic sinusitis/nasal polyposis. Laryngoscope. 2004;114:1822–6.
21. Araujo E, Palombini BC, Cantarelli V, et al. Microbiology of middle meatus in chronic rhinosinusitis. Am J Rhinol. 2003;17:9–15.
22. Larson DA, Han JK. Microbiology of sinusitis: does allergy or endoscopic sinus surgery affect the microbiologic flora? Curr Opin Otolaryngol Head Neck Surg. 2001;19:199–203.
23. Bendouah Z, Barbeau J, Hamad WA, Desrosiers M. Biofilm formation by Staphylococcus aureus and Pseudomonas aeruginosa is associated with an unfavorable evolution after surgery for chronic sinusitis and nasal polyposis. Otolaryngol Head Neck Surg. 2006;134:991–6.
24. Grindler D, Thomas C, Hall GS, Batra PS. The role of *Stenotrophomonas maltophilia* in refractory chronic rhinosinusitis. Am J Rhinol Allergy. 2010;24:200–4.
25. Wood AJ, Antoszewska H, Fraser J, Douglas RG. Is chronic rhinosinusitis caused by persistent respiratory virus infection? Int Forum Allergy Rhinol. 2011;1(2):95–100.
26. Wang JH, Kwon HJ, Jang YJ. Rhinovirus enhances various bacterial adhesions to nasal epithelial cells simultaneously. Laryngoscope. 2009;119:1406–11.
27. Wang J, Watanabe S, Matsukura S, et al. Double-stranded RNA poly (I:C) enhances matrix metalloproteinase mRNA expression in human nasal polyps epithelial cells. Acta Otolaryngol Suppl. 2009;562:105–9.
28. Ramadan HH, Farr RW, Wetmore SJ. Adenovirus and respiratory syncytial virus in chronic sinusitis using polymerase chain reaction. Laryngoscope. 1997;107:923–5.
29. Jang YJ, Kwon HJ, Park HW, et al. Detection of rhinovirus in turbinate epithelial cells of chronic sinusitis. Am J Rhinol. 2006;20:634–6.
30. Ponikau JU, Sherris DA, Kern EB, et al. The diagnosis and incidence of allergic fungal sinusitis. Mayo Clin Proc. 1999;74:877–84.
31. Braun H, Buzina W, Freudenschuss K, et al. Eosinophilic fungal rhinosinusitis: a common disorder in Europe? Laryngoscope. 2003;113:264–9.
32. Ebbens FA, Scadding GK, Badia L, et al. Amphotericin B nasal lavages: not a solution for patients with chronic rhinosinusitis. J Allergy Clin Immunol. 2006;118:1149–56.
33. Bent III JP, Kuhn FA. Diagnosis of allergic fungal sinusitis. Otolaryngol Head Neck Surg. 1994;111:580–8.
34. Hutcheson PS, Schubert MS, Slavin RG. Distinctions between allergic fungal rhinosinusitis and chronic rhinosinusitis. Am J Rhinol Allergy. 2010;24:405–8.
35. Kennedy DW, Senior BA, Gannon FH, et al. Histology and histomorphometry of ethmoid bone in chronic rhinosinusitis. Laryngoscope. 1998;108:502–7.
36. Giacchi RJ, Lebowitz RA, Yee HT, et al. Histopathologic evaluation of ethmoid bone in chronic sinusitis. Am J Rhinol. 2001;15:193–7.
37. Lee JT, Kennedy DW, Palmer JN, et al. The incidence of concurrent osteitis in patients with chronic rhinosinusitis: a clinicopathological study. Am J Rhinol. 2006;20:278–82.
38. Lee HM, Kang HJ, Woo JS, et al. Upregulation of surfactant protein A in chronic rhinosinusitis. Laryngoscope. 2006;116:328–30.
39. Psaltis AJ, Bruhn MA, Ooi EH, et al. Nasal mucosa expression of lactoferrin in patients with chronic rhinosinusitis. Laryngoscope. 2007;117:2030–5.
40. Tieu DD, Kern RC, Schleimer RP. Alterations in epithelial barrier function and host defense responses in chronic rhinosinusitis. J Allergy Clin Immunol. 2009;124:37–42.
41. Groot Kormelink T, Calus L, de Ruyck N, et al. Local free light chain expression is increased in chronic rhinosinusitis with nasal polyps. Allergy. 2012;67:1165–72.
42. Benninger M. Rhinitis, sinusitis and their relationship to allergies. Am J Rhinol. 1992;6:37–43.
43. Emanuel IA, Shah SB. Chronis rhinosinusitis: allergy and sinus computed tomography relationships. Otolaryngol Head Neck Surg. 2000;123:687–91.

44. Grove R, Farrior J. Chronic hyperplastic sinusitis in allergic patients: a bacteriologic study of 200 operative cases. J Allergy Clin Immunol. 1990;11:271–6.
45. Jones NS. CT of the paranasal sinuses: a review of the correlation with clinical, surgical and histopathological findings. Clin Otolaryngol. 2002;27:11–7.
46. Jones NS, Strobl A, Holland I. A study of the CT findings in 100 patients with rhinosinusitis and 100 controls. Clin Otolaryngol. 1997;22:47–51.
47. Orlandi RR. A systematic analysis of septal deviation associated with rhinosinusitis. Laryngoscope. 2010;120:1687–95.

Endoscopic Diagnosis of Chronic Rhinosinusitis

3

Joshua Wiedermann, Sean B. Bury, and Ameet Singh

Key Take-Home Points

- Nasal endoscopy is a essential tool in the diagnosis of chronic sinusitis.
- Endoscopic findings of polyps and/or mucopurulent secretions combined with the patient's clinical history permit diagnosis of chronic sinusitis.
- Proper endoscopic technique is essential to obtaining an accurate diagnosis of chronic sinusitis.

History of Nasal Endoscopy

The use of the endoscope for examination of the nasal cavity was introduced in the early twentieth century, when a modified cystoscope was used to examine the nasal cavity [1]. In 1925, Maxwell Maltz described the "sinuscope," used to examine the internal nasal anatomy in detail [2]. He concluded that his sinuscope allowed excellent visualization of the maxillary sinus enabling the practitioner to determine the "operative case from the non-operative case" [2]. It was not until the innovation of the rod-lens optical system by Harold Hopkins in 1959 that the potential of endoscopic sinus procedures began to be realized. Although his invention was novel, it was only with the help of Karl Storz's experience and knowledge of optics that allowed the Hopkins' rod to become revolutionary in sinus endoscopy [3]. Walter Messerklinger, a physician conducting research on patterns of mucociliary clearance in sinusitis, was one of the first to use the Storz-Hopkins endoscope [3, 4]. Internal nasal structures could be directly visualized, contributing to the current

J. Wiedermann, MD (✉) • S.B. Bury, MD • A. Singh, MD
Division of Otolaryngology – Head and Neck Surgery, George Washington University Hospital, 2021 K Street, Suite 206, Washington, DC 20006, USA
e-mail: josh.wiedermann@gmail.com; seanbury@mac.com; dr.ameetsingh.ent@gmail.com

P.S. Batra, J.K. Han (eds.), *Practical Medical and Surgical Management of Chronic Rhinosinusitis*, DOI 10.1007/978-3-319-16724-4_3

anatomy and terminology (e.g., osteomeatal unit) of the paranasal sinuses. Messerklinger's success with the endoscope set the stage for its importance in the diagnosis of rhinosinusitis [5].

Messerklinger's growing appreciation of internal nasal anatomy from direct visualization led him to perform many internal nasal surgeries, later termed functional endoscopic sinus surgery (FESS). His work was adopted and modified elsewhere in Europe and Japan, but it was not until 1985 that it was first introduced in English literature by David Kennedy et al. [4]. Kennedy suggested that preoperative evaluation with accurate endoscopic diagnosis of sinus disease, correlated with the gold standard of computed tomography (CT), could produce successful FESS outcomes. However, this hypothesis was not formally explored until the late 1990s, and endoscopy did not enter into guidelines for diagnosis of chronic rhinosinusitis (CRS) until 2007 [6].

Role of Nasal Endoscopy in Chronic Rhinosinusitis

Nasal endoscopy is a useful adjunctive tool in the diagnosis and management of CRS. It provides a visual correlation of the patient's sinonasal symptoms and the inflammation represented on CT scans. Ultimately, the incorporation of this technology has become widely accepted and has altered the algorithmic approach to diagnosis of this disease. Future studies may seek to delineate exact parameters for endoscopic diagnosis of this disease.

Chronic Rhinosinusitis

In Chap. 1, the authors gave a superlative explanation of the diagnosis of CRS. Nevertheless, a review of the criteria will enable a thorough understanding of the role of nasoendoscopy. In brief, chronic rhinosinusitis is a diagnosis based on patient-described symptoms and diagnostic studies. The American Academy of Otolaryngology has defined the criteria for the diagnosis of chronic rhinosinusitis [6] (see Table 3.1). Crucial to the diagnosis is the temporal aspect of symptoms and documented diagnostic study findings.

Individually, patient's symptoms can be nasal obstruction, congestion, purulent nasal discharge, and hyposmia which are found in an outstanding number of cases. Thus, the sensitivity for diagnosing CRS based on symptoms is very high, but the high prevalence of these symptoms results in a low specificity [6]. Consequently, documented physical exam findings or inflammation on imaging is required in addition to persistence of symptoms.

CT Scan

CT imaging is currently the gold standard for documenting paranasal sinus inflammation. CT scans accurately demonstrate the anatomy of the sinuses and clearly show mucosal thickening associated with the inflammatory state (see Fig. 3.1a, b).

Table 3.1 Chronic rhinosinusitis criteria [6]

Symptomatic criteria	Twelve (12) weeks or longer of two or more of the following:
	Mucopurulent drainage
	Nasal congestion
	Facial pain, pressure, and fullness
	Decreased sense of smell
	And objective documentation by one or more of the following:
Endoscopic criteria	Purulent (not clear) mucous or edema in the middle meatus or ethmoid region
	Polyps in nasal cavity or the middle meatus
Radiologic criteria	Radiographic imaging showing inflammation of the paranasal sinuses

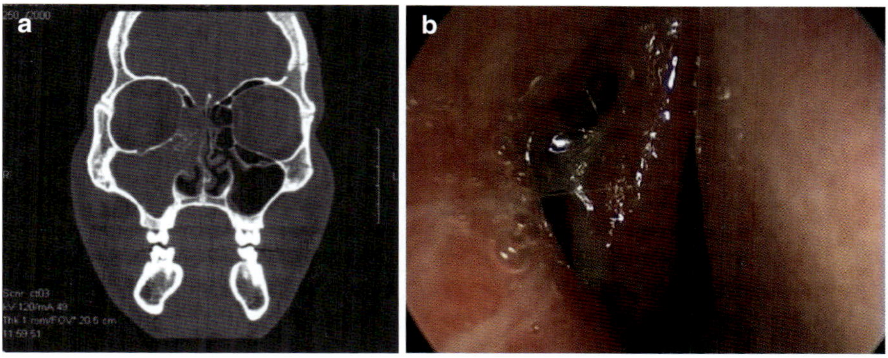

Fig. 3.1 (**a**) CT scan demonstrating maxillary and ethmoid opacification. (**b**) Endoscopy finding of bulging right maxillary sinus. This is the endoscopic visualization of the CT finding from (**a**) and demonstrates the role of endoscopy. In some cases endoscopy may reveal the same pathology but without associated radiation and cost

This inflammatory state may be graded using one of several systems, the progenitor of which and most commonly applied is the Lund-Mackay. In the Lund-Mackay system, individual sinuses and osteomeatal complexes are evaluated for inflammation. If inflammation occupies 0 % of a sinus on CT, a score of 0 is assigned; a maximum score of 2 is assigned when inflammation occupies 100 % of the sinus on CT. All other degrees of inflammation are scored as 1. Subsites include bilateral maxillary, ethmoid, sphenoid, frontal, and osteomeatal complexes. Scores are summed for a graded total of 0–24. This scoring allows for efficient and reliable total CT comparison [7, 8].

Although the scoring system is reliable, there are concerns over CT scans yielding false positives, and there is controversy surrounding the corroboration of imaging with the patient's perception of symptoms. Henceforth, CT imaging has not been recommended as the sole diagnostic tool.

Supporting this negative assertion, Flinn evaluated CT scans of 100 patients and observed sinus opacification in 27 % of patients scanned for unrelated findings [9]. This figure and its implications on specificity for the diagnosis of CRS effectively argue against CT scan being the sole diagnostic tool.

Flinn's conclusions were refuted by Calhoun et.al. in a subsequent study of 182 CT scan images [10]. He surmised that although CT scans of patients without symptoms of sinus disease do show some incidental sinus abnormalities, the incidence of such abnormalities is significantly greater in patients with a history of "sinus-type symptoms." The apparently contradictory implications of Flinn's and Calhoun's conclusions demand a more complete diagnostic algorithm for a CRS diagnosis than a CT scan may be able to deliver alone.

Furthermore, with regard to corroboration of symptoms and CT scan findings, Bhattarcharyya et al. completed an exhaustive study with 586 patients. He concluded there was no observed link between severity of symptoms and degree of inflammation on CT imaging because patients who presented with facial pain or pressure were as likely to have abnormal results on CT scan as patients who presented without these symptoms [11].

In contrast to Bhatacharyya's conclusions, Kenny et al. asserted that there was a correlation between CT scan and severity of other sinus symptoms. Prospective analysis of 304 patients demonstrated a link of the severity of CT scan and the severity of reported fatigue, sleep disturbance, nasal discharge or postnasal drip, nasal blockage, and decreased sense of smell [12].

Analysis of the aforementioned studies will show that while the data does not conflict, the conclusions do. This derived ambiguity ultimately supports the necessity for another tool besides CT imaging for the diagnosis of many cases of suspected CRS.

Nasal Endoscopy

Nasal endoscopy allows direct visualization of the entire nasal cavity and nasopharynx. This complete visualization may allow for the diagnosis of CRS in patients with sinonasal symptoms and nasal polyps (see Fig. 3.2) or purulent mucus in the middle meatus (see Fig. 3.3) or ethmoid region. As these findings may be subjective or not present at all, endoscopy is typically used to support a diagnosis of CRS, rather than define it. Alternately, it can be stated that the specificity of endoscopy demonstrates its utility, but the sensitivity of endoscopy limits its utility.

There have been multiple studies investigating the role of endoscopy in the diagnosis of CRS compared to CT imaging. The specificity of these investigative tools has found to be similar. Casiano found that clinical staging of CRS based on endoscopy findings was as predictive of CT staging of CRS (see Fig. 3.1b). The author determined the overall specificity of endoscopy for the diagnosis of CRS to be 84 % [13]. Stankiewicz et al. corroborated these findings, noting that nasal endoscopy had a specificity of 86 % [14].

Bhattacharyya evaluated patient symptoms and endoscopic findings compared to CT findings. In patients meeting the symptom criteria for CRS, the sensitivity of symptoms alone was 88–96 %, but specificity was abysmal with a range of 9–12 %. However, when a positive endoscopic finding was added, specificity rose to a more acceptable 84 %. Even more interesting, for those patients not meeting the symptom

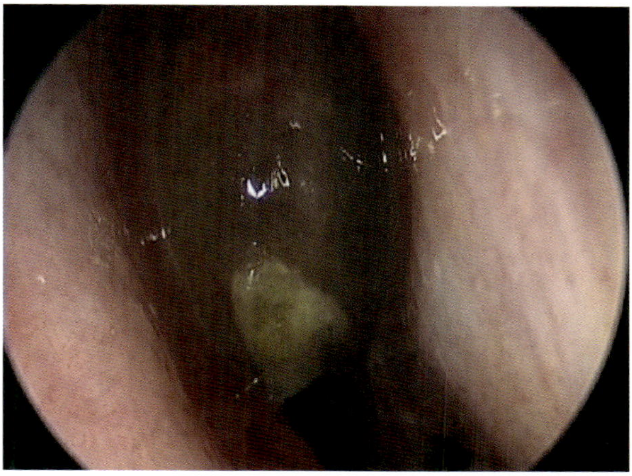

Fig. 3.2 Obstructive nasal polyp

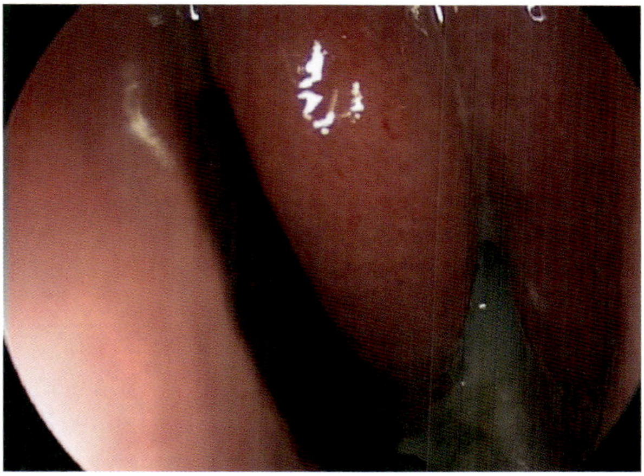

Fig. 3.3 Purulence in the left middle meatus

guideline criteria, a positive finding on endoscopy had a specificity of 90 %, although this was not statistically significant [15]. These results placed emphasis on the role of nasal endoscopy in the accurate diagnosis of CRS.

Several otolaryngology researchers critiqued the conclusive support given to the specificity of endoscopy, arguing that positive findings on nasal endoscopy were flawed given the subjective interpretation required. Annamalai's study in 2004 revealed that inter-rater agreement of mucosal edema was only "moderate" when compared to "very good" agreement for presence of discharge or polyps [16]. Annamalai suggested that polyps and purulence are clear physical findings, but mucosal changes require some subjective interpretation and therefore were less reliable as a diagnostic criterion.

Support for Annamalai's findings was provided by two separate studies conducted by Raithatha and McCoul independently. Both found calculated inter-rater reliability was strong for gross abnormalities such as atypical lesions or polyps (see Fig. 3.4) but much weaker for more nuanced findings such as mucosal changes or middle turbinate obstruction [17, 18].

The aforementioned conclusions are consistent with reports detailing the limited sensitivity (Table 3.2) [19] of nasoendoscopy. Ultimately, for those patients meeting symptom criteria but having negative endoscopic findings, a CT scan should be considered if clinical suspicion for CRS is high. Despite its limits, the role of endoscopy has been recognized [6]. Patients that meet symptom criteria of CRS and have polyps or purulent mucosa may be confidently diagnosed with endoscopy without the use of CT imaging.

Procedure

Effective clinical use of nasal endoscopes requires familiarity with the technology, knowledge of its limitations, expanded applications, and technical training in procedural methods. Technologic familiarity should encompass critical evaluation of strengths and weaknesses of rigid and fixed endoscopes, angulation of endoscopic lenses, and diameter of endoscopic rods. An astute clinician will be able to select

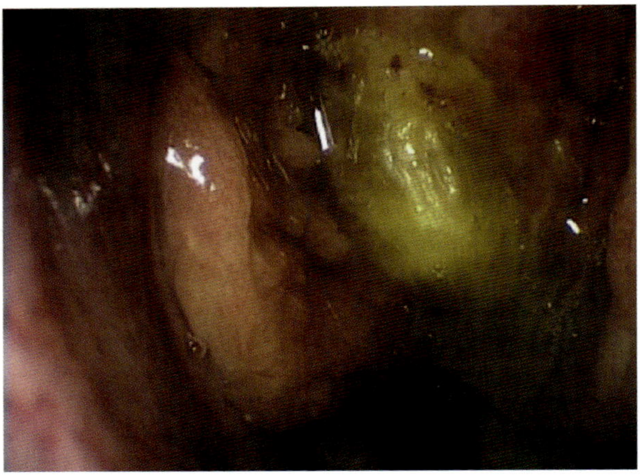

Fig. 3.4 Gross lesions such as polyps with eosinophilic mucin have high inter-rater agreement

Table 3.2 Sensitivity and specificity of nasal endoscopy

	Bhattacharyya	Stankiewicz	Agius
Sensitivity	0.46	0.46	.91 or .51
Specificity	0.84	0.86	0.71
Positive predictive value	0.66	0.74	0.62
Negative predictive value	0.7	0.64	0.71

appropriate instrumentation for most cases with knowledge and experience with these categories.

Furthermore, an endoscopist will understand that instrument use may exceed diagnostic purposes. For example, endoscopy permits the physician to gauge response to treatment and prescribe culture-directed antibiotics. Additionally, the use of endoscopy in teaching should not be understated, as it has a clear role in patient and resident education.

Like any procedure, technical training is essential, and contraindications though rare are present. Awareness and prophylactic mitigation of potential complications such as epistaxis or vasovagal response may ensure a successful exam. The generated exam findings are most useful when used in documented endoscopic staging systems.

Equipment

As with most procedures, endoscopy has a broad set of equipment with equally broad applications. There are utilitarian devices (i.e., 0° rigid 4.0 mm endoscope) with features that may be useful in most settings, and there are specialized instruments (i.e., 70° endoscopes, flexible endoscopes) that are more useful for obtaining optimal results in patients with altered anatomy. Rigidity, diameter, and lens angulation are the defining criteria of endoscope technology. Thus knowledge of categorical advantages and disadvantages are necessary for endoscope selection.

Rigid and Flexible Endoscopes

Rigid endoscopes are available in multiple diameters (2.7–4 mm) and divergent angles (0–70°). By virtue of their protected optic fibers and increased diameter, these endoscopes provide superior clarity and magnification allowing easy visualization of signs of chronic rhinosinusitis. Rigid endoscopy may be performed with one hand thereby allowing the clinician to perform procedures such as debridement, biopsies, and polypectomies. Furthermore, it has been posited that clinical examination with the rigid endoscope familiarizes trainees with its use for endoscopic sinus surgery. Some have suggested that rigid endoscopes may prove uncomfortable for patients [20], while others have shown that patients feel more discomfort with flexible scopes [21].

Alternatively, flexible endoscopes may be used to evaluate the nasal cavity. Their thin, flexible body and tip can be angulated up or down to help maneuver the scope. Although these maneuvers help visualize areas that cannot be seen with a rigid endoscope, such as the floor of the maxillary sinuses or superior aspects of the frontal sinuses, they may not be useful in all situations. This was confirmed in a prospective randomized study by Midwinter et al. who found that rigid endoscopes allow for increased visualization of most sinonasal structures, the exception being the nasopharynx [21]. Thus most patients benefit from rigid endoscopic examination, but those with obstructing anatomy or concurrent laryngeal/pharyngeal complaints may benefit from nasal examination with a flexible fiber-optic endoscope.

An unavoidable major disadvantage of flexible endoscopes is the decreased quality of images necessitated by the bending of optic fibers and necessary limits of diameter demanded by mobility. Also, patients may find the sensation of a moving tip uncomfortable [21]. Furthermore, using the flexible scope eliminates the ability to perform two-handed techniques such as nasal cavity debridement following sinus surgery. The increased cost of flexible endoscopes can also be a deterrent to their use [21].

Diameter

Large-diameter endoscopes (4.0 mm) provide a wide panoramic view with excellent clarity and magnification and the resulting ability to ascertain subtle rhinologic pathology. These qualities ensure that the 4.0 mm scope is the benchmark endoscopic examination tool for adults. Disadvantages of large-diameter endoscopes include the possibility of patient discomfort, a higher risk of mucosal trauma, and inability to view pathology in patients with anatomic abnormalities.

The 2.0 and 2.7 mm endoscopes possess the advantageous ability to perform endoscopy in patients with significant mucosal hypertrophy or those with anatomic limitations such as severely deviated septums, large concha bullosa, and massive polyposis. Smaller endoscopes are also utilized for nasal endoscopy in pediatric patients. Unfortunately, the smaller diameter presents a limited view with decreased photo-documentation quality. These scopes are also fragile, and slight angulation of the rod produces significant shadowing on the video screen. This fragility can contribute to the fracturing of internal glass rods, requiring costly repair.

Angulation

In our experience, the 0° scope is the workhorse of endoscopic diagnosis of CRS. While angled scopes may be useful in surgery and examination of certain pathologies (e.g., maxillary mucus recirculation), the 0° scope provides visualization of most significant structures involved in CRS including the nasal floor, middle meatus, and Eustachian tubes. Technique and experience may play a role in ensuring complete examination.

Mastery of 30°, 45°, and 70° angled endoscopes requires practice and complete understanding of sinonasal anatomy due to the divergent visual angles. Some [20] believe the 30° angle provides the most practical visualization for nasal examination, as most of the important pathology will lie superior or lateral to the plane of endoscopy. The 30° and 45° scope can provide excellent views of the sphenoid ostium and cribriform plate. Also, with rotation of the 30° or 45° scope to the right or left, the septum and lateral nasal walls can be visualized. The 70° scope is not standard for endoscopy and may be disorienting to the novice. It can provide views of the roof of the frontoethmoidal region, frontal sinus, floor of the maxillary sinus [22], and hypopharynx. Ultimately, selection of the angulation will depend on a balance of the examiner's skill and familiarity and the patient's anatomy and pathology.

Other Uses

As previously discussed, nasal endoscopy may evaluate for CRS-related symptoms. Additionally, after initial evaluation endoscopy may be used to track response to medical therapy. In monitoring of chronic sinus disease, physical exam findings such as edema, hyperplastic mucosa, hypertrophy of the turbinates, and polyps are functions where endoscopy proves truly beneficial.

Another potential use of endoscopy is to assist in middle meatal mucus samples. These samples are used in culture-directed antibiotics which are increasingly beneficial given the rising trend of resistance to empiric antibiotics. Studies have found an 85.7–90.5 correlation rate [23, 24] between endoscopic cultures and direct antral cultures, confirming endoscopy as a viable and simpler method of sampling. Furthermore, it has been shown there is a greater risk of adverse events with sinus puncture and aspiration than endoscopy [25].

An additional but often overlooked use of the endoscope is the preservation of exam images. When endoscopy is performed with a high-quality light source and a photo-documentation system is employed, the retained images may improve patient education and academic teaching.

Contraindications

Endoscopy is an uncomfortable but well-tolerated procedure, and very few contraindications exist. As with all procedures, a detailed history and physical is mandatory with particular attention paid to history of anxiety or vasovagal response. It can be very disconcerting to induce a vasovagal response, and physicians should be able to differentiate this reaction from more serious events (cardiac or cerebrovascular incidents). Smelling salts and a safe resting area should be available for treatment under these circumstances. Furthermore, an evaluation of bleeding disorders and anticoagulant use is recommended to minimize any risk of procedural bleeding. Careful attention to technique should allow examination in most patients though.

Method

Proper method and technique in nasal endoscopy permits the examination to successfully contribute to patient care. Thus, the importance of training and experience cannot be overstated. Procedural method can be subdivided into premedication and endoscopy technique. Once the procedure is completed, a standardized report of findings should be generated as this allows for consistent patient care. The literature on technical aspects of endoscopy is generally instructional and anecdotal, but studies have evaluated the effects of premedication and the reliability of systematic grading of findings.

Premedication

The discomfort associated with nasal endoscopy has been addressed with a variety of topical anesthetics and vasoconstrictors including phenylephrine, pontocaine, lidocaine, oxymetazoline, xylometazoline, and cocaine. It is postulated that the sensation of discomfort comes from mucosal drag and friction created when the endoscope is passed along mucosal surfaces. In general, patients are better able to tolerate mucosal contact with the inferior turbinate than contact with the nasal septum. Topical lidocaine may not prevent this sensation, whereas oxymetazoline theoretically reduces the likelihood of mucosal drag to occur. These two medications are often combined into an atomizer which allows for a gentle misting of the nasal cavity.

A Cochrane Review conducted by Sunkareni and Jones investigated the use of nasal anesthetic in flexible nasopharyngeal endoscopy and reinforced its optional nature [26]. One evaluated study suggested the use of a vasoconstrictor (xylometazoline) alone reduced the level of "general unpleasantness" of the procedure but that the use of a local anesthetic increased scores for unpleasant taste [27]. Five of the eight reported studies did not see any benefit from premedication of the nares before endoscopy, and one study suggested avoidance may be beneficial due to the medications' unpleasant taste and risk of allergic reaction [26–31].

Technique

The examination should proceed with a standard anterior rhinoscopy just before nasal decongestant is administered, if used. The anterior rhinoscopy allows appreciation for mucosa and anterior anatomy in its natural state. Topical agents are typically fast acting with an onset of action in minutes. Before exposing the endoscope to the heated, humid air of the nasal cavity, a "de-fog" agent should be applied (ethyl alcohol, hot water, etc.).

With the patient in the sitting position, the physician sits facing the patient. A right-handed physician may feel most comfortable just to the right of the patient. Either the 0° or the 30° endoscope [20] should be placed in the non-dominant hand, and the dominant hand should be used to guide advancement of the scope. The dominant hand can also be used to maintain position of the patient's head with gentle pressure and guidance exerted on the patient's nasal dorsum. Keeping the endoscope in the non- dominant hand also allows the dominant hand to remain available for instrumentation if needed. There are many ways to complete the endoscopic evaluation of the nasal cavity.

In general, the examination should be performed with delicacy, and the endoscope should *never* be forced into a particular area. The nasal cavity mucosa is sensitive, and rough movements will be met with patient discomfort and a poor examination will result [32]. The examination can be completed utilizing the "three-pass technique" [20, 33] as follows:

1. Advance the endoscope along the inferior meatus/floor of the nasal cavity taking care not to brush up against the nasal septum. The nasal septum is one of the most sensitive areas of the nasal cavity. If there is limited room along the floor of the nasal cavity due to a septal spur or deviation, the scope may be passed between the middle and inferior turbinates. Once the choana is visualized, a number of structures can be assessed: the posterior inferior turbinate, the fossa of Rosenmüller, the Eustachian tube, and the nasopharynx. Purulence in this area suggests sinusitis but does not localize its origin.
2. The next step involves angling the endoscope superiorly to visualize the sphenoethmoid recess. Visualization of this area as well as the sphenoid ostium may be improved with a 30° endoscope. Although the sphenoid ostium may not be visualized depending on the location of the turbinates, purulence can be visualized along the anterior wall of the sphenoid suggesting sphenoid sinus disease. Additionally, polyps in the superior meatus suggest ethmoid and sphenoid sinusitis. Purulence can also be visualized at the root of the middle turbinate further suggesting posterior ethmoid disease.

3. While retracting the endoscope, gently roll under the middle turbinate to visualize the middle meatus. While in this position, visualize under the ethmoid bulla to see if there is purulence draining from the maxillary sinus. If an ostium is visualized, it is usually the accessory ostium as the uncinate process often hides the true maxillary ostium. Rolling the endoscope to the left and right will help visualize around the uncinate and under the middle turbinate for evidence of polyps or purulence.
4. Finally, the endoscope can be tilted up, once again, to visualize the frontal recess. Pathology visualized here points to frontal sinus disease.

Complications

With appropriate technique and due diligence, complications are rare. In our experience, vasovagal events and epistaxis are the most common complications. Reports have detailed the possibility of CSF leak associated with skull base injury during examination of the middle meatus and the singular incident of a fatal hemorrhage during endoscopic-assisted biopsy of the internal carotid. Thus while endoscopy is generally one of the safer procedures, it must be performed with respect for the anatomy and the patient.

Findings

With the rise of evidence-based medicine, there has been a trend toward quantification of findings. To this purpose endoscopic scoring systems [34–37] have been proposed, notably the Lund-Kennedy (LK) system [35]. This system was originally intended for postoperative sinus surgery cases but has since been adapted for diagnostic purposes. Exam findings are graded according to degree of scarring, crusting, edema, polyps, and discharge. Unfortunately there is a discrepancy when comparing LK scores to quality of life and described symptoms in patient questionnaires; some studies demonstrated a positive correlation [34, 38, 39], and other studies found a lack of correlation [34, 40]. This may be due to the original postsurgical focus (i.e., scarring and crusting) of the LK system. Thus modified systems have been proposed [34, 37], but the LK system is still frequently used.

Conclusion

Nasal endoscopy is the culmination of decades of research and innovation in optical science. Data has shown endoscopy is a useful adjunctive tool in diagnosis and management of CRS. Specifically, it has been recognized to clarify patient-reported symptoms and in certain cases permit diagnosis without the added expense and associated radiation exposure of CT scans. Successful examination is dependent on correct choice of equipment and technical expertise. As our knowledge continues to grow, we may seek to further quantify endoscopic findings and expand endoscopic applications.

References

1. Hirschmann A. Uber Endoskopie der Nase und deren Nebenhohlen. Arch Laryngol Rhinol. 1903;14:195–202.
2. Maltz M. New instrument: the sinuscope. Laryngoscope. 1925;35:805–11.
3. Linder TE, Simmen D, Stool SE. Revolutionary inventions in the 20th century: the history of endoscopy. Arch Otolaryngol Head Neck Surg. 1997;123(11):1161–3.
4. Kennedy DW, Zinreich SJ, Rosenbaum AE, Johns ME. Functional endoscopic sinus surgery. Theory and diagnostic evaluation. Arch Otolaryngol. 1985;111(9):576–82.
5. Messerklinger W. Endoscopy of the nose. Baltimore: Urban & Schwarzenberg; 1978.
6. Rosenfeld RM, Andes D, Bhattacharyya N, Cheung D, Eisenberg S, Ganiats TG, et al. Clinical practice guideline: adult sinusitis. Otolaryngol Head Neck Surg. 2007;137(3 Suppl):S1–31.
7. Okushi T, Nakayama T, Morimoto S, Arai C, Omura K, Asaka D, et al. A modified Lund-Mackay system for radiological evaluation of chronic rhinosinusitis. Auris Nasus Larynx. 2013;40(6):548–53. Epub 2013 Jun 14.
8. Lund VJ, Mackay IS. Staging in rhinosinusitis. Rhinology. 1993;31(4):183–4.
9. Flinn J, Chapman ME, Wightman AJ, Maran AG. A prospective analysis of incidental paranasal abnormalities on CT head scans. Clin Otolaryngol. 1994;19:287–9.
10. Calhoun K, Waggenspack G. CT Evaluation of the paranasal sinuses in symptomatic and asymptomatic populations. Otolaryngol Head Neck Surg. 1991;104:480–3.
11. Bhattacharyya T, Piccirillo J, Wippold 2nd FJ. Relationship between patient-based descriptions of sinusitis and paranasal sinus computed tomographic findings. Arch Otolaryngol Head Neck Surg. 1997;123(11):1189–92.
12. Kenny TJ, Duncavage J, Bracikowski J, Yildirim A, Murray JJ, Tanner SB. Prospective analysis of sinus symptoms and correlation with paranasal computed tomography scan. Otolaryngol Head Neck Surg. 2001;125:40–3.
13. Casiano R. Correlation of clinical examination with computer tomography in paranasal sinus disease. Am J Rhinol. 1997;11:193–6.
14. Stankiewicz JA, Chow JM. Nasal endoscopy and the definition and diagnosis of chronic rhinosinusitis. Otolaryngol Head Neck Surg. 2002;126:623–7.
15. Bhattacharyya N, Fried MP. The accuracy of computed tomography in the diagnosis of chronic rhinosinusitis. Laryngoscope. 2003;113:125–9.
16. Annamalai S, Davis J, Kubba H. How subjective is nasal endoscopy? A study of interrater agreement using the Lund and Mackay scoring system. Am J Rhinol. 2004;18(5):301–3.
17. McCoul ED, Smith TL, Mace JC, Anand VK, Senior BA, Hwang PH, et al. Interrater agreement of nasal endoscopy in patients with a prior history of endoscopic sinus surgery. Int Forum Allergy Rhinol. 2012;2(6):453–9.
18. Raithatha R, Anand VK, Mace JC, Smith TL, Schaberg MR, Nyquist GG, et al. Interrater agreement of nasal endoscopy for chronic rhinosinusitis. Int Forum Allergy Rhinol. 2012;2(2):144–50.
19. Shargorodsky J, Bhattacharyya N. What is the role of nasal endoscopy in the diagnosis of chronic rhinosinusitis? Laryngoscope. 2013;123(1):4–6.
20. Batra PS. The role of endoscopy in the allergist's office. Curr Allergy Asthma Rep. 2006;6(3):228–31. Review.
21. Midwinter KI, Ahmed A, Willatt D. A randomised trial of flexible versus rigid nasendoscopy in outpatient sinonasal examination. Clin Otolaryngol Allied Sci. 2001;26:281–3.
22. Kuhn FA. Role of endoscopy in the management of chronic rhino-sinusitis. Ann Otol Rhinol Laryngol. 2004;193(Suppl):15–8.
23. Gold SM, Tami TA. Role of middle meatus aspiration culture in the diagnosis of chronic sinusitis. Laryngoscope. 1997;107(12 Pt 1):1586–9.
24. Vogan JC, Bolger WE, Keyes AS. Endoscopically guided sinonasal cultures: a direct comparison with maxillary sinus aspirate cultures. Otolaryngol Head Neck Surg. 2000;122(3):370–3.

25. Talbot GH, Kennedy DW, Scheld WM, Granito K, Endoscopy Study Group. Rigid nasal endoscopy versus sinus puncture and aspiration for microbiologic documentation of acute bacterial maxillary sinusitis. Clin Infect Dis. 2001;33(10):1668–75. Epub 2001 Oct 5.
26. Sunkaraneni VS, Jones SE. Topical anaesthetic or vasoconstrictor preparations for flexible fibre-optic nasal pharyngoscopy and laryngoscopy. Cochrane Database Syst Rev. 2011;(3):CD005606.
27. Sadek SAA, De R, Scott A, White AP, Wilson PS, Carlin WV. The efficacy of topical anaesthesia in flexible nasendoscopy: a double-blind randomised controlled trial. Clin Otolaryngol. 2001;26:25–8.
28. Cain AJ, Murray DP, McClymont LG. The use of topical nasal anaesthesia before flexible nasendoscopy: a double-blind, randomized controlled trial comparing cophenylcaine with placebo. Clin Otolaryngol. 2002;27:485–8.
29. Georgalas C, Sandhu G, Frosh A, Xenellis J. Cophenylcaine spray vs placebo in flexible nasendoscopy: a prospective double-blind randomised controlled trial. Int J Clin Pract. 2005;59(2):130–3.
30. Leder SB, Ross DA, Briskin KB, Sasaki CT. A prospective, double-blind, randomized study on the use of a topical anesthetic, vasoconstrictor and placebo during transnasal flexible fiberoptic endoscopy. J Speech Lang Hear Res. 1997;40:1352–7.
31. Singh V, Brockbank MJ, Todd GB. Flexible transnasal endoscopy: is local anaesthetic necessary? J Laryngol Otol. 1997;111:616–8.
32. Pownell PH, Minoli JJ, Rohrich RJ. Diagnostic nasal endoscopy. Plast Reconstr Surg. 1997;99(5):1451–8. Review.
33. Bolger WE, Kennedy DW. Nasal endoscopy in the outpatient clinic. Otolaryngol Clin North Am. 1992;25(4):791–802. Review.
34. Psaltis AJ, Li G, Vaezeafshar R, Cho KS, Hwang PH. Modification of the Lund-Kennedy endoscopic scoring system improves its reliability and correlation with patient-reported outcome measures. Laryngoscope. 2014;124(10):2216–23.
35. Lund VJ, Kennedy DW. Quantification for staging sinusitis. The Staging and Therapy Group. Ann Otol Rhinol Laryngol Suppl. 1995;167:17–21.
36. Wright ED, Agrawal S. Impact of perioperative systemic steroids on surgical outcomes in patients with chronic rhinosinusitis with polyposis: evaluation with the novel Perioperative Sinus Endoscopy (POSE) scoring system. Laryngoscope. 2007;117:1–28.
37. Durr ML, Pletcher SD, Goldberg AN, Murr AH. A novel sinonasal endoscopy scoring system: the discharge, inflammation, and polyps/edema (DIP) score. Int Forum Allergy Rhinol. 2013;3:66–72.
38. Giger R, Dulguerov P, Quinodoz D, et al. Chronic panrhinosinusitis without nasal polyps: long-term outcome after functional endoscopic sinus surgery. Otolaryngol Head Neck Surg. 2004;131:534–41.
39. Toros SZ, Bolukbasi S, Naiboglu B, et al. Comparative outcomes of endoscopic sinus surgery in patients with chronic sinusitis and nasal polyps. Eur Arch Otorhinolaryngol. 2007;264:1003–8.
40. Mace JC, Michael YL, Carlson NE, et al. Correlations between endoscopy score and quality of life changes after sinus surgery. Arch Otolaryngol Head Neck Surg. 2010;136:340–6.

Radiographic Diagnosis of Chronic Rhinosinusitis

4

Carrie E. Flanagan, Kristen L. Baugnon, and John M. DelGaudio

Key Take Home Points

- The view obtained from CT in the coronal plane most closely resembles intranasal anatomy when viewed endoscopically and has become essential in preoperative planning because it provides critically relevant surgical information and can be used for intraoperative navigation.
- CT findings should always be interpreted in conjunction with clinical and endoscopic findings as mucosal thickening is an extremely common incidental finding, which is not necessarily related to infection.
- Indications for MRI include cases of aggressive sinus infection with ocular and/or intracranial complication, developmental lesions (i.e., meningoencephalocele), or for the evaluation of a sinonasal mass.
- Involvement of the skull base and orbits with exophthalmos or optic nerve compression is not uncommon in allergic fungal sinusitis, with 56 % having radiographic evidence of skull base or lamina papyracea erosion.

C.E. Flanagan, MD • J.M. DelGaudio, MD, FACS, FARS (✉)
Department of Otolaryngology – Head and Neck Surgery, Emory University, 550 Peachtree Street NE, Suite 1135, Atlanta, GA 30308, USA
e-mail: ceflan3@comcast.net; jdelgau@emory.edu

K.L. Baugnon, MD
Department of Radiology and Imaging Sciences, Emory University, 1364 Clifton Road, Atlanta, GA 30322, USA
e-mail: kmlloyd@emory.edu

P.S. Batra, J.K. Han (eds.), *Practical Medical and Surgical Management of Chronic Rhinosinusitis*, DOI 10.1007/978-3-319-16724-4_4

Introduction

The American Academy of Otolaryngology – Head Neck Surgery has defined chronic rhinosinusitis (CRS) as rhinosinusitis that persists for greater than 12 weeks. Diagnosis is primarily symptom-based, and patients should be suspected of having CRS if they manifest two or more of the following signs or symptoms for a duration of greater than 12 weeks: (1) mucopurulent nasal drainage; (2) nasal obstruction or congestion; (3) facial pain, pressure, or fullness; or (4) a decreased sense of smell (dysosmia). In those patients with suspected CRS, diagnostic confirmation must be made by physical exam, which often requires nasal endoscopy, or radiologic findings to document sinonasal inflammation [1–4]. Consensus opinion has also defined CRS as radiologic evidence of persistent sinus disease after maximal medical therapy. CRS is commonly diagnosed and has a complex and multifactorial etiology. Contributing factors include environmental exposures, genetic or immunologic abnormalities or deficiencies, or several anatomic variants that may predispose patients to developing CRS.

CRS is divided into various subtypes including CRS without polyps, CRS with polyps, and fungal sinusitis. Fungal sinusitis can be further divided into fungus ball (mycetoma), allergic fungal sinusitis, and invasive fungal sinusitis. These divisions have been created based on both clinical and pathologic findings, which despite unclear underlying etiologies, seem to be inherently different entities. Radiologic imaging has become increasingly utilized for diagnostic purposes, and differences in the radiographic appearance of the various types of CRS do exist. However, radiographic evaluation cannot be used as the sole modality to arrive at a particular diagnosis.

Historically, plain X-rays were used to aid in the diagnosis of CRS. A standard radiographic sinus series consisted of four views: lateral (frontal, maxillary, and sphenoid sinuses), Caldwell (frontal sinus), Waters (maxillary sinus), and submentovertex/base (sphenoid and anterior and posterior wall of frontal sinuses). Overlapping structures on plain films limit evaluation of the ostiomeatal complex (OMC) and the individual paranasal sinuses. They also fail to provide sufficient detail regarding the osseous framework of the sinonasal cavity or the extent of nasal and sinus pathology [5]. Plain films are of limited value in the setting of CRS due to the lack of sufficient diagnostic sensitivity [2].

Computed Tomography (CT)

CT has become the imaging modality of choice for diagnosing CRS for several reasons [4, 6]. Improvements in CT technology have greatly improved with respect to speed, safety, and image resolution. CT provides the best overall bony anatomic detail of the paranasal sinuses and adjacent structures [5–7]. It has increased sensitivity for detecting mucosal thickening and the ability to delineate other pathological features compared to plain films [4]. CT scan exhibits excellent test-retest reliability over time and has good to excellent diagnostic accuracy in the diagnosis of CRS with good positive and negative predictive values [2, 8]. Concurrent to technological advances, sinus surgery has evolved from external approaches to endoscopic techniques, which require more detailed and precise anatomic delineation for surgical planning. The view obtained from CT in the coronal plane most closely resembles intranasal anatomy when viewed endoscopically and has become essential in preoperative planning because it provides critically relevant surgical information and can be used for intraoperative navigation [9, 10].

Sinus mucosal inflammation results in submucosal edema, which is visible on CT imaging as mucosal thickening. Mucosal thickening on CT imaging is almost always considered an abnormal radiographic finding if it is present within the sinuses. The mucosal lining is considered normal if its thickness is less than 4 mm in the maxillary, less than 2 mm in the ethmoid sinuses, and not visible in the frontal or sphenoid sinuses [5, 11]. Chronic inflammatory sinus disease is often associated with mucosal thickening, retention cysts, and polyps, and this will appear as a variable amount of mucosal thickening, or partial or complete opacification of a sinus [3, 5]. Chronic sinusitis may also be associated with thickened, sclerotic, or hyperostotic bone of the chronically inflamed sinuses. Chronic secretions vary in fluid and protein content, which results in areas of variable density on CT [12] (Fig. 4.1a–c).

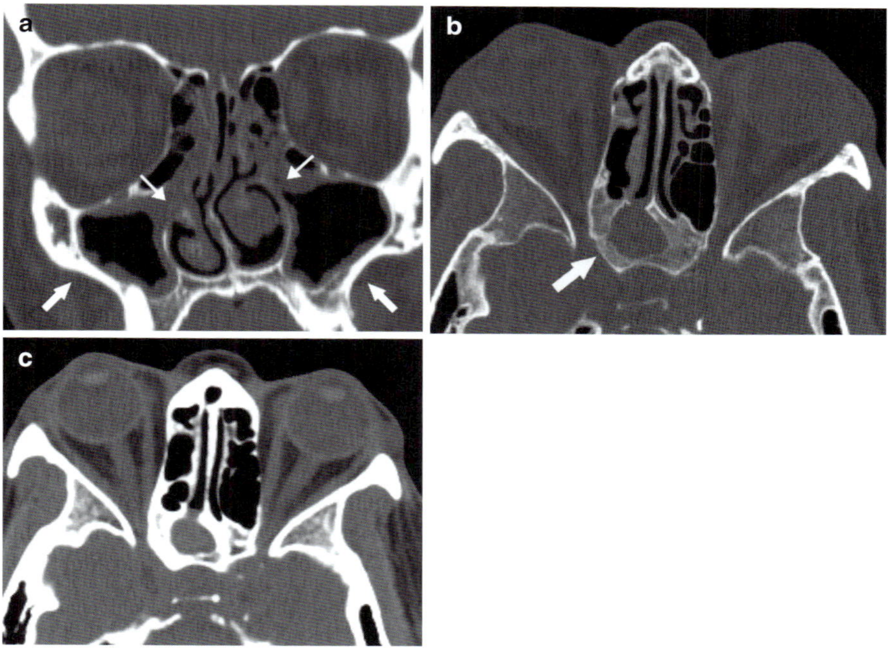

Fig. 4.1 Varied appearance of chronic sinusitis. (**a**) Coronal image showing bilateral maxillary sinus mucosal thickening, extending into the outflow tracts (*thin arrows*). Note the sclerosis and thickening of the surrounding maxillary sinus walls (*thick arrow*). Axial images in bone window (**b**) and soft tissue window (**c**), demonstrating chronic right sphenoid sinusitis, recurrent postoperatively, with opacification with high-density secretions extending through the sphenoid ostium and sclerosis and hyperostosis of the surrounding bone (*thick arrow*)

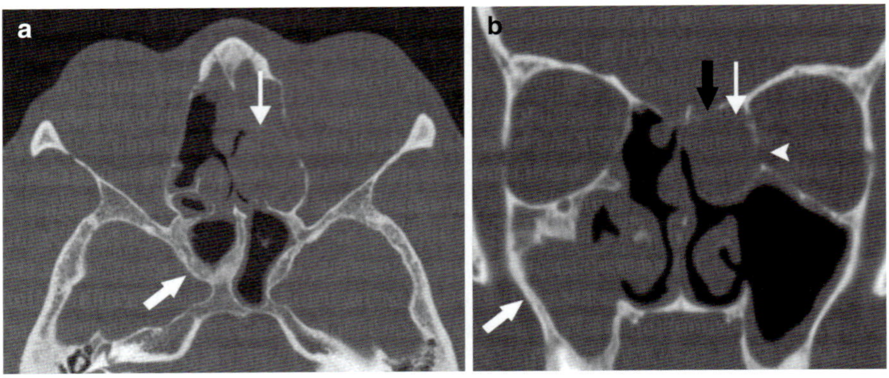

Fig. 4.2 Bony changes associated with chronic sinusitis. Axial (**a**) and coronal (**b**) images of a patient with recurrent chronic sinusitis after endoscopic sinus surgery, with thickening and sclerosis surrounding chronic sinusitis within the sphenoid and the right greater than the left maxillary sinuses (*thick arrows*), as well as bony remodeling and expansion surrounding an opacified left ethmoid air cell, compatible with mucocele (*thin arrow*). Note the thinning and dehiscence of the left lateral lamella (*black arrow*) and the left lamina papyracea (*arrowhead*) from the expansion of the mucocele

Acute infections can cause demineralization of the wall of the sinus when severe, and when the process becomes chronic, reactive sclerosis of the sinus walls occurs [3]. Sclerotic changes often indicate the presence of osteitis, but may also indicate a reactive process [3, 13, 14]. Bony erosion of the sinus margins and lamellae can also occur with aggressive infections, such as invasive fungal sinusitis, or malignancy. Bony remodeling is usually indicative of slow, progressive inflammatory pathology such as mucocele formation or allergic fungal sinusitis, but can also be seen in less aggressive malignancies [13] (Fig. 4.2a, b).

CT findings should always be interpreted in conjunction with clinical and endoscopic findings as mucosal thickening is an extremely common incidental finding, which is not necessarily related to infection [4, 5]. Over 80 % of patients with minor URIs have abnormal findings on CT scan [4, 6, 12]. Additionally, patient symptoms and quality of life do not necessarily correlate with extent of disease on imaging [1]. CT findings are important for excluding more serious pathology, such as neoplasm or malignancy that may mimic CRS [1]. Primary indications for imaging include recurrent or refractory disease and unilateral symptoms [14]. Although inflammatory processes can result in unilateral sinus opacification on imaging, when unilateral disease is present, the likelihood of neoplasm should be considered [15]. When a diagnosis of CRS is certain, imaging is usually reserved for refractory sinusitis, complicated sinusitis, CRS with atypical symptoms, for defining sinus anatomy when surgery is planned, or for intraoperative navigation [6, 7]. Most recommend obtaining CT after a course of adequate medical therapy; some also recommend use of a nasal decongestant prior to imaging [3, 13].

Technique

There are many modalities available for obtaining CT images, and these vary in radiation dose, cost, and image quality. Historically, conventional and single slice scanning was previously performed with the patient in the prone position with neck extension, with images obtained in the coronal plane from the anterior wall of the frontal sinus through the posterior wall of the sphenoid sinus, so-called "direct coronal" image acquisition. Axially acquired coronal reconstructed images on single slice scanners were previously inferior to direct coronal helical images because of "Stair-step" artifacts [6, 9]. However, current generation multi-slice, multichannel CT scanners can acquire submillimeter axial slices with contiguous coverage of the entire volume, allowing excellent quality reconstructed images from the same data set in any desired plane [9, 16]. Scanning in the axial plane with multiplanar reformations in coronal and sagittal planes is now considered the standard of care, which is preferable, as the supine position is more comfortable for the patient, and reconstructed coronal images are free of dental amalgam artifacts [9]. In recent years, the use of cone-beam CT has been expanded to in-office use for sinonasal evaluation. Advantages include patient convenience, decreased cost, and significant reduction in radiation exposure. However, disadvantages include diminished soft tissue visibility, increased propensity for X-ray scatter/artifact, and a concern for over usage when scanning is so readily available [6, 17].

The appearance of CT images is affected by window width and level that are arranged according to Hounsfield units. A Hounsfield unit (HU) is defined as a unit of X-ray attenuation based on water where air has a value of −1,000, water has a value of 0, and compact bone/metallic density has a value of +1,000. To obtain the highest bony definition of the paranasal sinuses, the windows of the scan are set between 1,500 and 2,000 HU with a center, or level, of +100 to +300 HU, so-called bone windows. Separate images reconstructed with soft tissue window settings are helpful in assessing sinonasal masses, fungal sinus disease, or complications of sinusitis [5, 11].

The three main planes of imaging include coronal, axial, and sagittal. Each plane of imaging can be helpful in defining paranasal sinus anatomy. The coronal view optimally demonstrates the OMC, the ethmoid roof, and the relationship of ocular structures, and it best correlates with the endoscopic surgical approach. Axial views are particularly useful in determining the drainage pathway of the frontal sinus and the course of the sphenoid septum. The parasagittal view is indispensible to a surgeon's ability to assess the complex frontal recess anatomy and is helpful when assessing the pneumatization pattern of the sphenoid. Therefore, for every sinus CT in patients with chronic rhinosinusitis, the study should contain thin section axial bone window images through the sinuses, with thin reconstructed coronal and sagittal reconstructions, as well as axial soft tissue window images reconstructed with increased slice thickness, for improved soft tissue resolution (Fig. 4.3a–d).

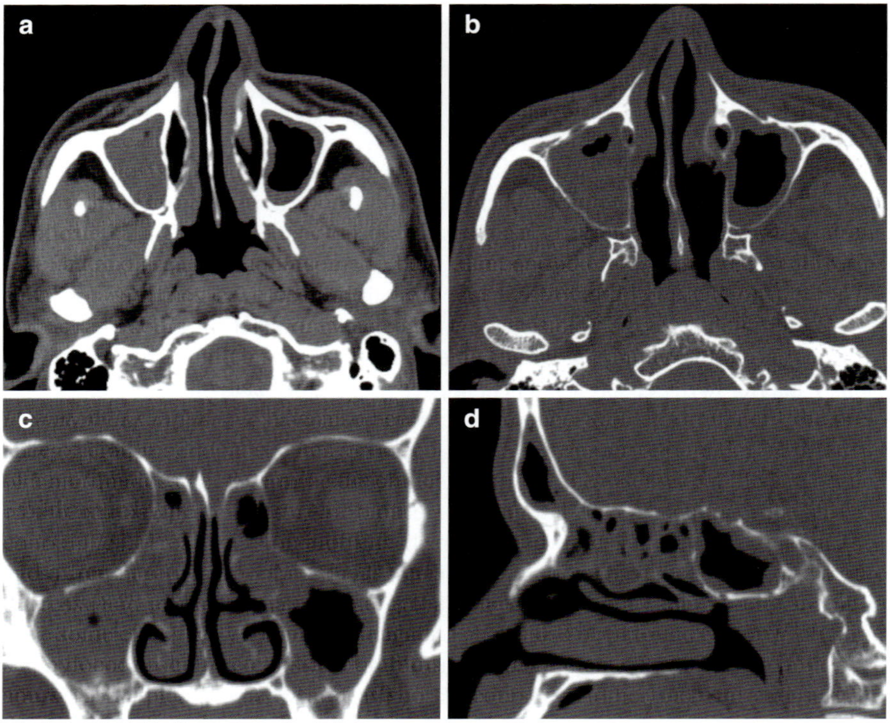

Fig. 4.3 Images generated and sent to PACS for every sinus CT performed should include: (**a**) axial soft tissue window images in thicker slices for improved soft tissue resolution, i.e., 2.5 mm thickness, (**b**) axial thin section bone window images reconstructed at thin submillimeter (i.e., 0.625 mm) thickness, and (**c**) coronal, and (**d**) sagittal thin section bone window images reconstructed at submillimeter to 1 mm thickness. Images should include the facial soft tissues and tip of the nose, without tape or tubing distorting facial soft tissues, so that images may be used for image guidance software

Staging

There are multiple radiographic staging systems (Lund–Mackay, Kennedy, Harvard, May) that have been used to assess radiographic disease severity. Notably, they are not designed to be used to diagnose CRS. The Lund–Mackay staging system (Table 4.1) is the most commonly used system. Its use has been recommended by the American Academy of Otolaryngology Task Force on Rhinosinusitis for staging and has been found to be useful in determining radiographic cutoffs for a truly "diseased" paranasal sinus CT scan. This system quantifies disease severity on a scale from 0 to 2 for six regions, which are scored bilaterally, for a potential total score of 24 [4]. Despite a widespread consensus that staging for chronic rhinosinusitis would be helpful, the utility of radiographic staging has been difficult to demonstrate [8]. Symptom scores for CRS typically fail to correlate with CT scan findings and thus with CT scan stage

Table 4.1 Lund–Mackay CT scoring system

Regions	Score
Maxillary sinus	0 – No evidence of opacification
Anterior ethmoid sinuses	1 – Partial opacification
Posterior ethmoid sinuses	2 – Complete opacification
Frontal sinus	**OMC is scored 0 if occluded or 2 if not occluded
Sphenoid sinus	
Ostiomeatal complex	

**Vary from rest of staging system

[8]. Investigators have suggested that radiographic cutoffs for an abnormal CT scan should be based on a score of 4 or greater in the presence of appropriately related sinonasal symptoms [2]. These cutoffs have shown a sensitivity of greater than 85 % and a positive predictive value greater than 80 % in the diagnosis of CRS [2].

Radiation

One of the main concerns associated with CT scanning is radiation exposure and its anticipated effects on other organ systems. Cumulative exposure to radiation correlates with an increase in the incidence of malignancies. With respect to sinus CT scans, the primary concerns are thyroid cancer and cataract formation [5, 7, 18]. The exact dose of radiation to which a patient is exposed is dependent on patient size and is also largely a function of the parameters that are often set by the manufacturer of the scanner or the scanning institution. These settings are often higher than necessary to achieve a comparable image and vary greatly across manufacturers and institutions [9, 16, 19, 20]. Although the risk of malignancy or other adverse effect is perceived to be small, the availability of CT imaging technology usage has greatly increased, and over usage is a concern. It has been suggested that up to 2 % of cancers in the US could be attributable to radiation exposure associated with CT imaging [20]. The age of exposure is highly relevant, with younger patients having an increased risk for cancer incidence and mortality [18, 21].

A standard head CT has an estimated effective radiation dose of 2 mSv (chest X-ray – 0.1 mSv), which is equivalent to approximately the natural background radiation an individual would be exposed to in 8 months [22]. The mean dose to the lens when obtaining images in the axial plane has been shown to be 24.5 mGy compared to 35.1 mGy in the coronal plane [9]. There is a threshold dose of 0.5–2 Gy for detectable lens opacities, with cataracts occurring after dosages of 2–10 Gy [9, 18]. Studies have shown that even after multiple CT examinations, the radiation dose to the lens is still well below the known thresholds of clinical damage [5]. The mean dose for the thyroid gland has been shown to be 1.4 mGy in the axial plane compared to 2.9 mGy in the coronal plane [9]. Various studies have documented maintenance of image quality with a reduction in radiation dose [9]. Multi-slice axial imaging reduces radiation exposure when compared to direct coronal imaging, and cone-beam technology is believed to substantially decrease effective dose [9].

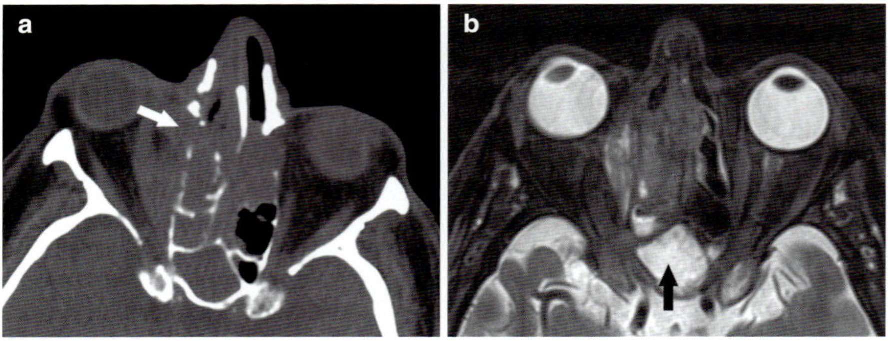

Fig. 4.4 (**a**) Axial CT images showing a polypoid soft tissue mass centered in the right sinonasal cavity, crossing midline to the left, with extrasinus extension into the right orbit and destructive non-expansile bony changes (*arrow*). This is concerning for an aggressive process (malignancy or aggressive infection in the appropriate clinical scenario). MRI should be obtained. (**b**) Axial T2w MR images showing an infiltrative mass centered in the right ethmoid air cells, extending into the right orbit, relatively T2 hypointense compared to the benign post-obstructive sinonasal secretions in the sphenoid sinus (*black arrow*). This was a case of sinonasal melanoma

Magnetic Resonance Imaging (MRI)

MRI has been used as a complementary exam to CT for the evaluation of the paranasal sinuses. Its advantages include superior soft tissue characterization and no radiation exposure. It is not routinely used for the assessment of CRS due to cost, longer imaging time, and lack of bone detail [5–7, 11]. MRI has also been found to be potentially overly sensitive to mucosal thickening. At least 20–40 % of patients undergoing MRI of the head are found to have edematous tissue of the paranasal sinuses as an incidental finding [3]. However, MRI has been shown to correlate very well with CT when paired CT and MR images of the paranasal sinuses were assessed with the Lund–Mackay system. Further studies are needed to establish the role for MRI in the diagnosis of CRS [2, 6].

Indications for MRI include cases of aggressive sinus infection with ocular and/or intracranial complication, developmental lesions (i.e., meningoencephalocele), or for the evaluation of a sinonasal mass [5, 6]. Any sinonasal mass that does not appear typical for benign sinonasal polyposis should undergo further investigation with MRI, as it can discriminate neoplasm and other nonneoplastic masses from retained mucous or inflammatory disease and can occasionally separate mucosal thickening from retained secretions (Fig. 4.4a, b). It is particularly valuable in assessing for dural or orbital invasion or extension [3, 23]. It has also been shown to be useful for the evaluation of patients who have undergone prior osteoplastic flap with obliteration with ongoing symptoms.

A standard MRI protocol includes obtaining thin section T1-weighted (T1w) images before and after gadolinium administration, with fat saturation on the postcontrast images, and T2-weighted (T2w) images in the axial and coronal planes. MRI signals of sinonasal secretions have been related to multiple properties such as viscosity, fat, metal content, and protein concentration. In general, watery secretions appear hypointense on T1w images and hyperintense on T2w images. As the protein concentration increases and free water decreases, the signal intensity on T2w images decreases, presumably due to cross-linking between glycoprotein molecules [11, 12, 24]. Thus, sinonasal secretions in acute sinusitis, which consist of 95 % water and 5 % proteins, usually demonstrate low intensity on T1w and high intensity on T2w images [12]. In contrast, in chronic sinusitis, secretions often have a higher protein concentration and less free water, and this may result in different patterns of MRI signal intensity [5]. Generally speaking, four signal intensity patterns in CRS are possible:

- Hypointense T1; hyperintense T2 – total protein concentration < 10 %
- Hyperintense T1; hyperintense T2 –total protein concentration 20–25 %
- Hyperintense T1; hypointense T2 – total protein concentration 25–30 %
- Hypointense T1; hypointense T2 – total protein concentration > 30 % and inspissated secretions in almost solid form [25].

Notably, inspissated secretions or fungal colonization may produce signal voids on T1w and T2w images, which may result in a signal void and appear identical to normally aerated sinuses [12, 23]. Peripheral, linear enhancement is suggestive of infection, whereas central enhancement is more likely consistent with neoplasm [5, 12]. Additionally, tumor, particularly hypercellular malignant tumors are typically relatively hypointense on T2w images compared to benign sinonasal mucosal disease, allowing the combination of T2 and postcontrast images to help differentiate sinonasal neoplasm from benign mucosal disease (Fig. 4.4a, b).

Ultrasound (US)

Ultrasound (US) has been used in the diagnosis of rhinosinusitis, usually acute sinusitis, primarily in Europe. Its advantages include a lack of radiation, low cost, and wide availability; however, it has poor sensitivity compared with CT. US is not recommended for the evaluation of sinusitis [7, 11].

Normal Anatomic Variants

Although not a direct cause of CRS, many anatomic variations of normal structures in and around the sinuses exist that may predispose to sinus obstruction and inflammation [11, 26]. Knowledge of variant sinus anatomy will also help to avoid complications during surgery [27]. Some of the more common variants will be discussed further below.

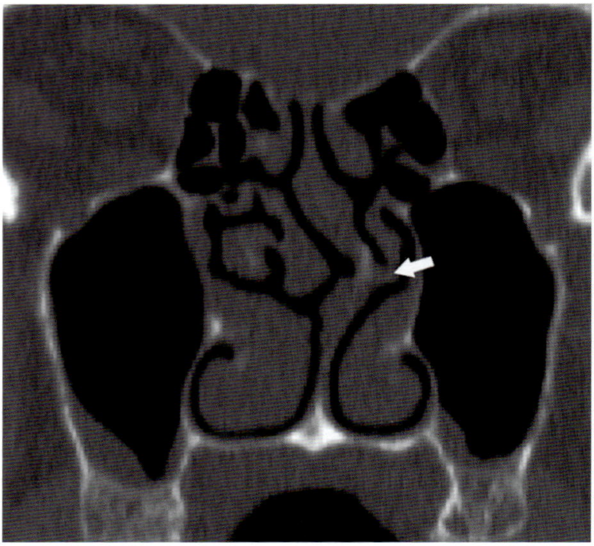

Fig. 4.5 Coronal CT image demonstrating severe leftward nasal septal deviation with spur contacting and deforming the left middle turbinate (*arrow*), possibly contributing to osteomeatal unit obstruction in this patient with chronic sinusitis

OMC/Maxillary Sinus

Septal deviation is one of the most common anatomic variations and is present in 20–79 % of the population, but is often not clinically relevant [26, 28]. However, severe deviation may narrow the middle meatus, impacting the OMC [28] (Fig. 4.5). It may also alter the airflow pattern, which may negatively impact ciliary clearance [11]. Pneumatization of the nasal septum may occur, which is also often not clinically significant, but may narrow the sphenoethmoidal recess [28].

A *paradoxical middle turbinate* has been shown to be present in approximately 3–26 % of the population [26]. It is believed that this anatomic variant can contribute to the development of sinusitis if particularly large [28, 29]. *Concha bullosa*, an aerated middle turbinate, is relatively common, is often bilateral, and has been shown to be present in up to 24–55 % of patients [26, 28] (Fig. 4.6). An *uncinate bulla*, a rare entity with a prevalence of less than 5 %, refers to an extension of air cells into the uncinate process [26, 27, 29]. The *ethmoid bulla*, the largest and most prominent anterior ethmoid air cell, can be enlarged or extensively pneumatized forming a "giant bulla" [5, 28, 29] (Fig. 4.7). These variants may result in narrowing of the ostiomeatal complex, potentially affecting drainage patterns of the maxillary and frontal sinuses, with a combination of anomalies possibly increasing the pathogenic effect more than any single variant would cause [27]. *Pneumatization of the inferior and superior turbinates* can also occur, but this is relatively rare with an incidence of <3 % and is usually clinically insignificant because of little impact on drainage patterns [26–28].

Haller cells, or infraorbital ethmoid cells, are located along the anterosuperomedial maxillary sinus, just inferior to the orbital floor, and are typically in close

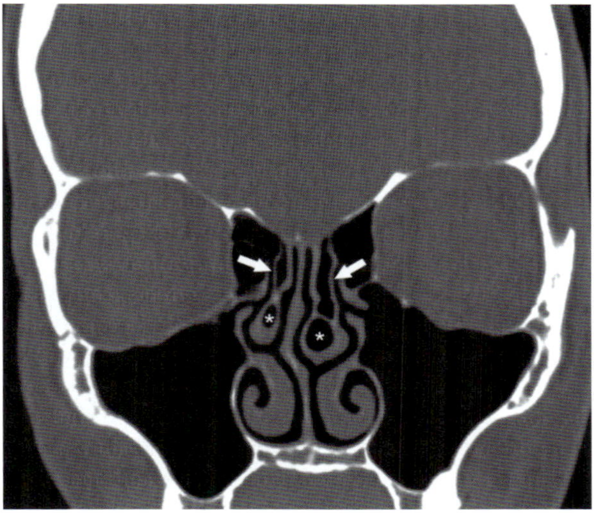

Fig. 4.6 Coronal CT image demonstrating bilateral middle turbinate concha bullosae (*), as well as incidental pneumatization of the vertical insertion of the middle turbinates bilaterally (*arrows*)

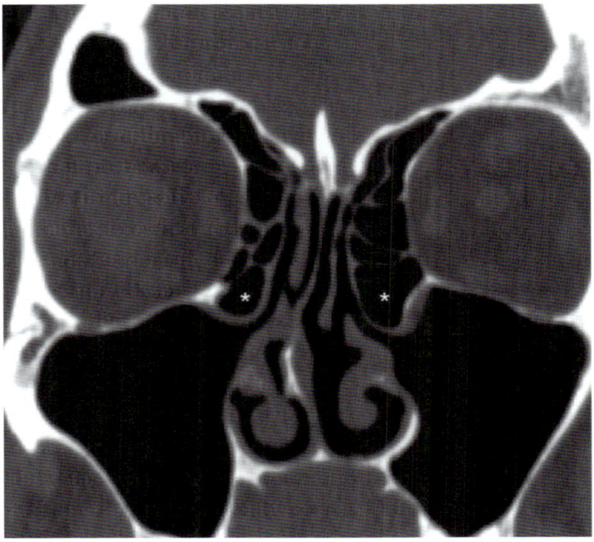

Fig. 4.7 Coronal CT images showing bilateral large ethmoid bullae (*) prolapsing into the maxillary sinus outflow tracts

proximity to the maxillary sinus ostium (Fig. 4.8). They are estimated to be present in approximately 10–45 % of patients. Bilateral Haller cells are rare. They may contribute to sinonasal inflammatory disease if they result in obstruction of the ethmoidal infundibulum or ostium of the maxillary sinus [5, 26–28].

Ten to thirty percent of people have an *accessory maxillary ostium* in the posterior fontanelle (Fig. 4.9a, b). This can cause nasal mucous recirculation and result in recurrent sinusitis. Surgically, if the two ostia are close together, it is important to consider joining the natural and accessory ostia to prevent recirculation [5, 13, 28].

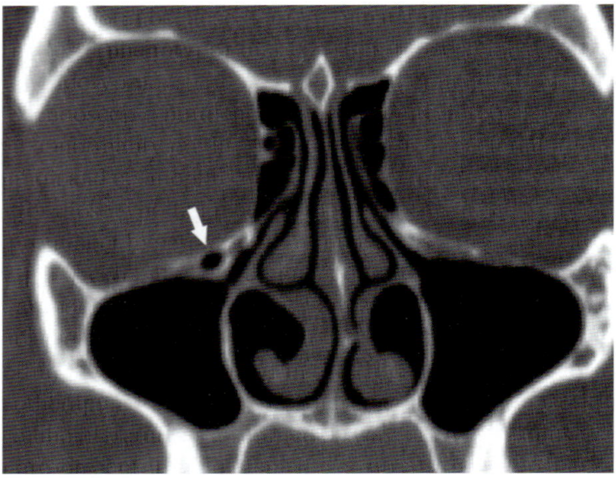

Fig. 4.8 Coronal CT image showing a right non-opacified Haller cell, or infraorbital ethmoid cell, narrowing the maxillary sinus ostium (*arrow*). Probable opacified tiny Haller cell present on the left as well

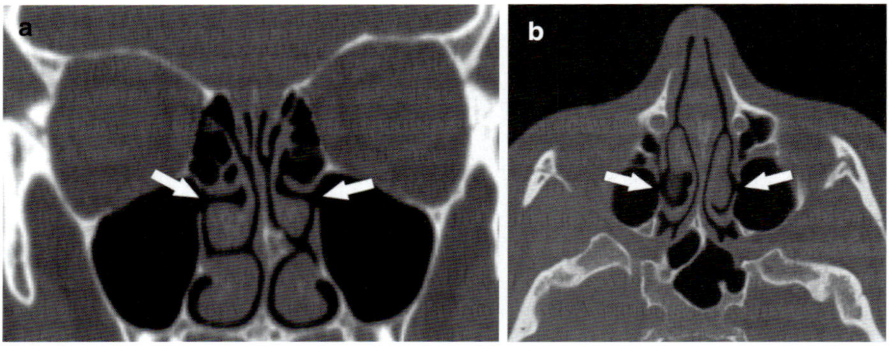

Fig. 4.9 Coronal (**a**) and axial (**b**) CT images of bilateral accessory maxillary sinus ostia (*arrows*), just posterior and inferior to the native maxillary sinus outflow tract

Congenital hypoplasia of the maxillary sinus can occur, which will cause lateralization of the uncinate process. The primary risk of surgery in a case of maxillary hypoplasia is inadvertent penetration of the orbit [5, 28].

Ethmoid

Anatomic variants in the ethmoid region are usually more important for preoperative planning. Careful evaluation of a sinus CT scan for the presence or absence of mucosal thickening in the ethmoid sinuses, as well as the pattern of ethmoid involvement, is important. The presence of *ethmoid roof or lamina papyracea dehiscences* should be noted to avoid inadvertent intracranial or orbital entry. The lamina

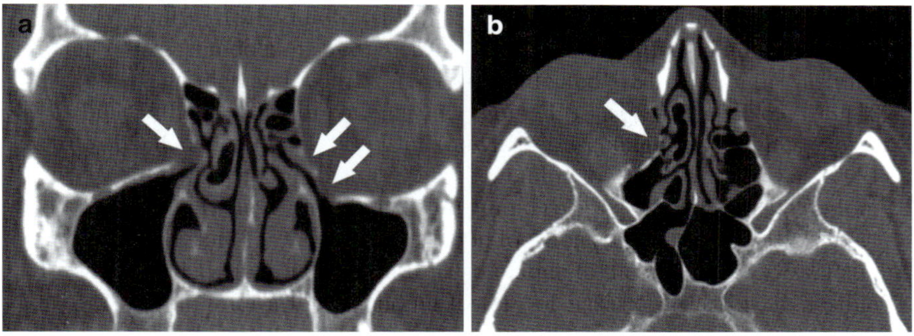

Fig. 4.10 Coronal (**a**) and axial (**b**) CT images demonstrating bilateral, right greater than left, inferior lamina papyracea, and orbital floor defects from prior trauma (*arrows*), with fat herniating through the defect on the right, prolapsing into the maxillary sinus outflow tract

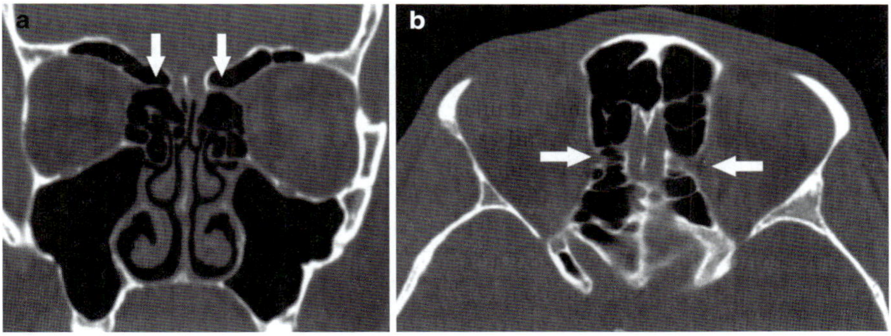

Fig. 4.11 Coronal (**a**) and axial (**b**) CT images demonstrating a common appearance of the anterior ethmoid artery canal which is located on a mesentery extending through the ethmoid air cells (*arrows*). Notice the tapering of the canal as it extends medially, located just medial to the superior oblique muscle, at the level on the coronal view just beyond the globe. Note the lamina papyracea defect on the left associated with the canal

Table 4.2 Keros classification

Category	Olfactory fossa depth (mm)
Keros 1	1–3
Keros 2	4–7
Keros 3	8–16

papyracea has been noted to have areas of focal dehiscence in 0.5–10 % of the population [13] (Fig. 4.10a, b). The most common area of dehiscence is at the anterior ethmoid foramen (Fig. 4.11a, b).

Additionally, variations in the *height of the ethmoid roof* in comparison to the cribriform plate are also important to consider preoperatively. The Keros classification (Table 4.2) [13, 29] classifies olfactory fossa height according to depth and is often used to assess and quantify the steepness of the ethmoid roof, with a higher likelihood of penetration of the lateral lamella of the lamina cribrosa with increasing height [26].

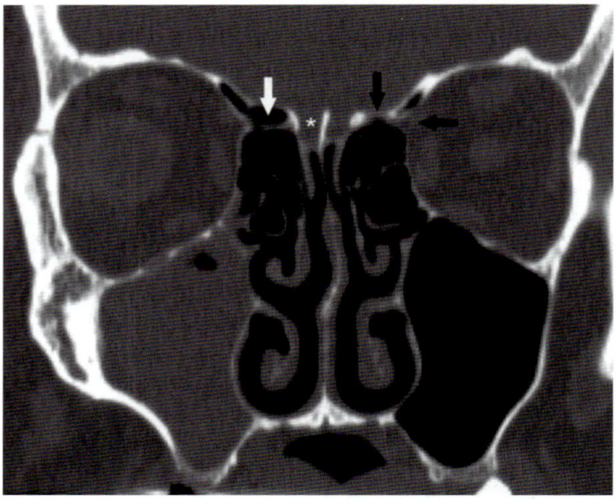

Fig. 4.12 Mildly asymmetric and low-lying right cribriform plate (*), with asymmetric anterior ethmoid artery canals, which extend through the ethmoid air cells on a mesentery on the right (*white arrow*), and along the skull base on the left (*black arrows*)

There may be asymmetry to the height of the ethmoid roof, or the roof may be particularly low, both of which should be noted preoperatively as inadvertent penetration of the skull base may occur if these are not anticipated. The location of the *anterior ethmoid arteries* should also be noted as to whether they are positioned in the bony skull base or hanging lower in a mesentery, where they may be at risk for injury during surgery when clearing remaining anterior ethmoid cells toward the frontal outflow tract. The anterior ethmoid artery is usually near the insertion of the ethmoid bulla into the skull base. It can be identified on CT as a "pinching" of the medial orbital wall on coronal views just posterior to the globe proper and where the medial rectus and superior oblique muscles are seen in the same cut (Figs. 4.11a, b and 4.12).

Sphenoid

The superior turbinate is often used as a surgical landmark to identify the sphenoid ostium. A *pneumatized superior turbinate* may cause obstruction of the sphenoid ostium, predisposing to sinusitis of the sphenoid. However, symptomatic pneumatization is extremely rare [27].

A *sphenoethmoidal cell, or Onodi cell*, is a posterior ethmoid air cell that pneumatizes lateral and superior to the sphenoid sinus [27] (Fig. 4.13a–c). It has an incidence of 8–14 % [26, 27]. Knowledge of the presence of an Onodi cell is of paramount importance during endoscopic sinus surgery due to its close association with the carotid artery and optic nerve [5]. A sphenoethmoidal cell, if not anticipated, may cause disorientation to the surgeon and increase the potential risk of injury to the optic nerve. The risk of blindness is high if the optic nerve is damaged within the sinus [27]. If unrecognized, entry into a sphenoethmoidal cell may be mistaken for entry into the sphenoid sinus, leaving the sphenoid sinus obstructed. *Isolated mucoceles of a sphenoethmoidal cell* have been reported, but are rare [27]. Optic neuropathy due to paranasal sinus disease of an Onodi cell has been reported [27].

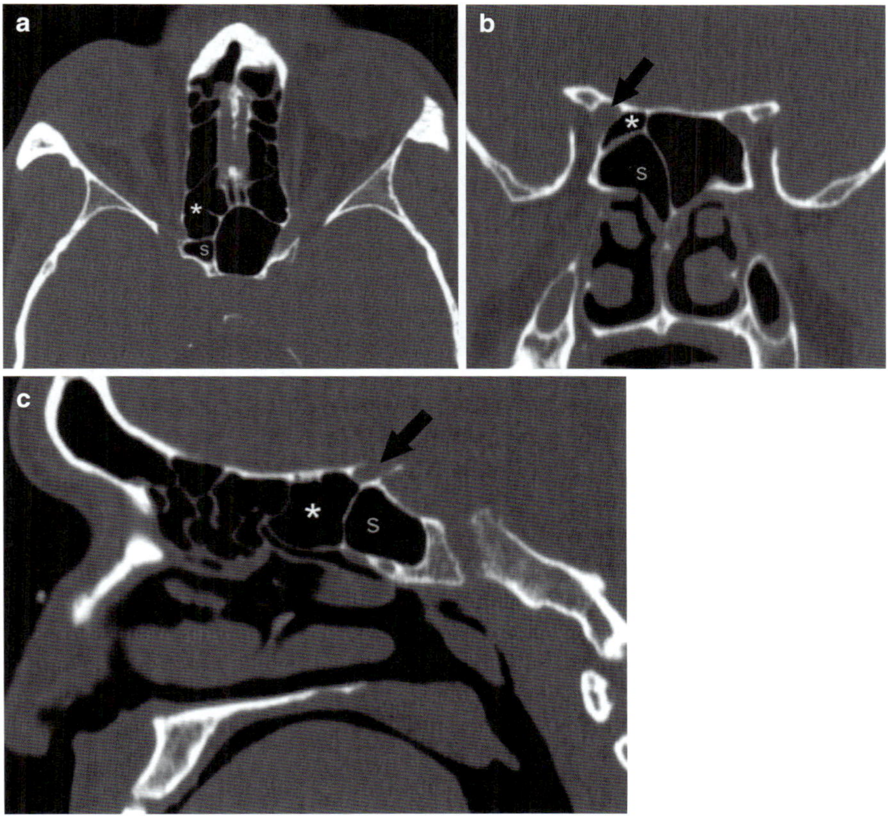

Fig. 4.13 Axial (**a**), coronal (**b**), and sagittal (**c**) CT images demonstrating a right Onodi cell, or sphenoethmoidal cell (*), pneumatized superiorly and laterally to the native sphenoid sinus (*s*). Note how the cell borders the optic nerve canal (*black arrow*)

The extent of *sphenoid pneumatization* and the presence of *carotid artery or optic nerve dehiscence* should be identified preoperatively. Pneumatization of the anterior clinoid process, which occurs in 6–13 % of cases, is more commonly associated with optic nerve dehiscence [28, 29]. Carotid dehiscence is estimated to be between 5 and 25 %, while optic nerve dehiscence occurs in approximately 4–24 % of cases [5, 30, 13]. The *intersphenoid septum* often deviates to one side and may attach to the bony wall over the carotid artery or optic nerve. Avulsion of the septum may result in injury to either of these structures [29] (Fig. 4.14a, b).

Frontal Sinus

The frontal sinus develops from the extension of anterior ethmoidal air cells into the frontal bone. *Frontal sinus aplasia or hypoplasia* has been shown to occur in approximately 4–10 % of patients [28].

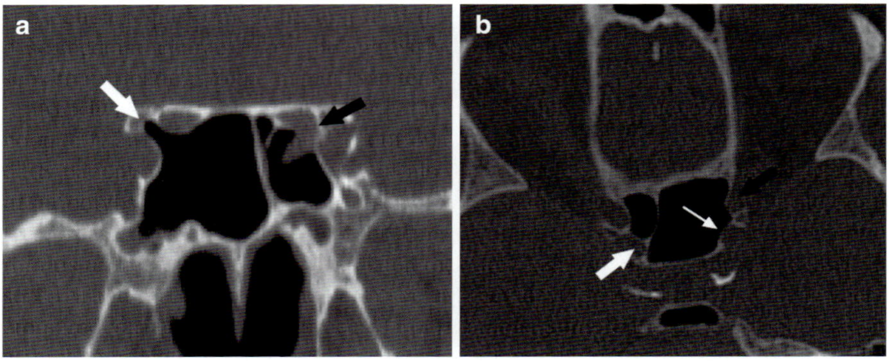

Fig. 4.14 (**a**) Coronal CT demonstrating dehiscence of the optic nerve canal on the left (*black arrow*), with adjacent mucosal disease in the sphenoid sinus. Note the pneumatization of the sphenoid sinus on the right extending into the clinoid process (*white arrow*). (**b**) Axial CT images through the sphenoid sinus demonstrating dehiscence of the left carotid canal (*white arrow*), and thinning of the adjacent left optic nerve canal (*black arrow*). Also note that the intersphenoidal sinus septum inserts on the right carotid canal (*thick arrow*)

Table 4.3 Frontal cell Kuhn classification

Kuhn classification	
Type I	Single cell superior to the agger nasi cell that does not extend into the frontal sinus
Type II	Two or more cells superior to the agger nasi cell that may or may not extend into the frontal sinus
Type III	Single frontal cell superior to the agger nasi cell that extends into the frontal sinus
Type IV	Cell completely contained in the frontal sinus

The frontal sinus drains into the frontal recess, also known as the frontal outflow tract, and is usually quite narrow with a mean anterior-posterior diameter of 13 mm [28]. The anatomy of the frontal recess is very complex and variable. However, the *agger nasi cell (ANC)* is present in almost all patients [13, 26, 27, 29]. The ANC is the most anterior ethmoid cell, located anterior, inferior, and lateral to the frontal recess [27]. The degree of pneumatization of the ANC affects the size of the frontal sinus ostium and the shape of the frontal outflow tract. Enlargement of the ANC can contribute to blockage of the frontal sinus outflow tract, contributing to chronic sinusitis [5, 28]. Additional structures or cells that may populate the outflow of the frontal sinus depending on their size, location, and pattern of pneumatization, include the superior attachment of the uncinate process, *frontal bullar cells, supraorbital* and *suprabullar ethmoid cells*, *intersinus septal cells*, and *frontal cells* (Tables 4.3 and 4.4) [13, 28] (Fig. 4.15). Frontal sinus cells are present in approximately 25–40 %, with type I cells being the most common, and intersinus septal cells in 12 % of patients. Preoperative awareness to the presence of any of these cells is of utmost importance so that they can be removed to provide the widest recess possible. Failure to adequately remove these cells may lead to persistent or recurrent frontal sinus disease [31].

Table 4.4 Frontal ethmoidal cell Wormald classification

Wormald classification	
Type I	Single cell superior to the agger nasi cell that does not extend into the frontal sinus
Type II	Two or more cells superior to the agger nasi cell that may or may not extend into the frontal sinus
Type III	Single frontal ethmoidal cell that pneumatizes cephalad into the frontal ostium but not extending > 50 % of the vertical height of the frontal sinus on the CT scan
Type IV	Single frontal ethmoidal cell that pneumatizes cephalad into the frontal ostium > 50 % of the vertical height of the frontal sinus on CT scan

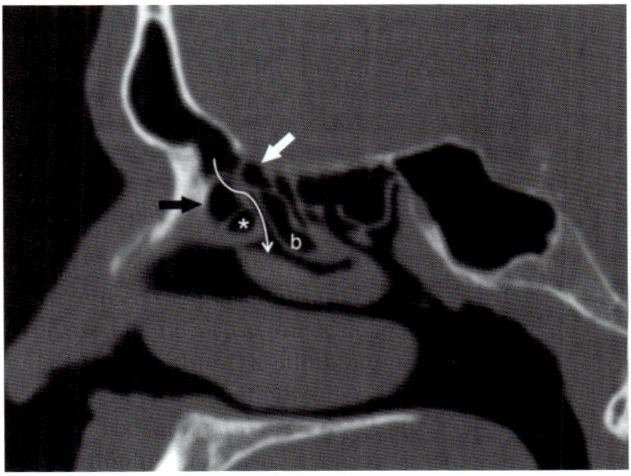

Fig. 4.15 Sagittal CT images are the best to define the anatomy of the frontal recess, as in this case, showing the frontal sinus outflow tract (*curved arrow*), bordered anteriorly and inferiorly by the agger nasi cell (*), and posteriorly and inferiorly by the ethmoid bulla (*b*). Frontal cells (*black arrow*) are located anteriorly, above the agger nasi cell, whereas bullar cells (i.e., suprabullar cell, in this case, *white arrow*) are located posteriorly above the ethmoid bulla

Types of Chronic Sinusitis

Mucous Retention Cyst

Mucous retention cysts occur in 10–30 % of the population and are the most common radiologic findings [12]. They are usually an asymptomatic, incidental finding [11]. The maxillary sinus floor is the most common location; the sphenoid floor is the second most common [3]. They result from inflammatory obstruction of a single seromucinous gland within the sinus mucosal lining with resultant accumulation of serous fluid in the submucosal space [3, 5]. The contents may be serous or mucoid [12]. They have a characteristic smoothly marginated, convex appearance arising from the wall of a sinus and do not cause bony remodeling. They are homogeneous and hypodense to isodense of water or soft tissue density on CT scan and do not

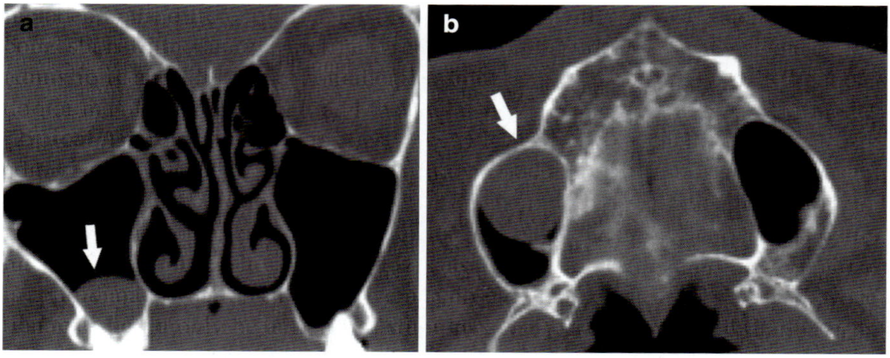

Fig. 4.16 Coronal (**a**) and axial (**b**) CT images demonstrating an incidental mucous retention cyst in a very common location within the alveolar recess of the right maxillary sinus (*arrows*). Note the smoothly marginated convex appearance, without bony remodeling. However, in a symptomatic patient with a finding in this location, one should ensure that there is no adjacent odontogenic disease

enhance with contrast [3, 12] (Fig. 4.16a, b). On MRI, they usually show low signal intensity on T1w images and high signal intensity on T2w images [3]. Treatment is usually not necessary unless they are large enough to obstruct the sinus ostium.

Polyps

Polyps result from local inflammation and edema of the sinus mucosa with mucous membrane hyperplasia caused by chronic inflammation. They can exist as a single polyp, such as an *antrochoanal polyp*, which develops from an expanding intramural cyst that arises within the maxillary sinus and extends through the maxillary sinus ostium, or occasionally through an accessory ostium, into the posterior nasal cavity [3, 5, 12] (Fig. 4.17a–c). They can also occur as multiple polyps located throughout the sinonasal cavity, such as in *severe polyposis*. They often result in symptoms because of their ability to cause local obstruction. Polyps most commonly occur in the anterior ostiomeatal unit [12].

On CT, polyps are soft tissue or fluid-density lesions and may be indistinguishable from a retention cyst. If a study with contrast is obtained, unlike retention cysts, polyps will demonstrate marked contrast enhancement [3, 6]. If multiple polyps exist, sinus secretions may become entrapped between polyps; depending on the concentration of entrapped secretions, CT attenuation rises, and chronic polyposis may show mixed CT attenuation with areas of increased density [3]. Chronic polyposis may be associated with extensive opacification of the sinuses, bone thinning, and remodeling with expansion of outflow tracts [5]. Bony remodeling is commonly observed at the ethmoid infundibula, which are widened, which may be a useful sign of polyposis [12] (Fig. 4.18a–c). Bone erosion is not common unless polyps are long-standing and aggressive [3]. It may be impossible to distinguish between

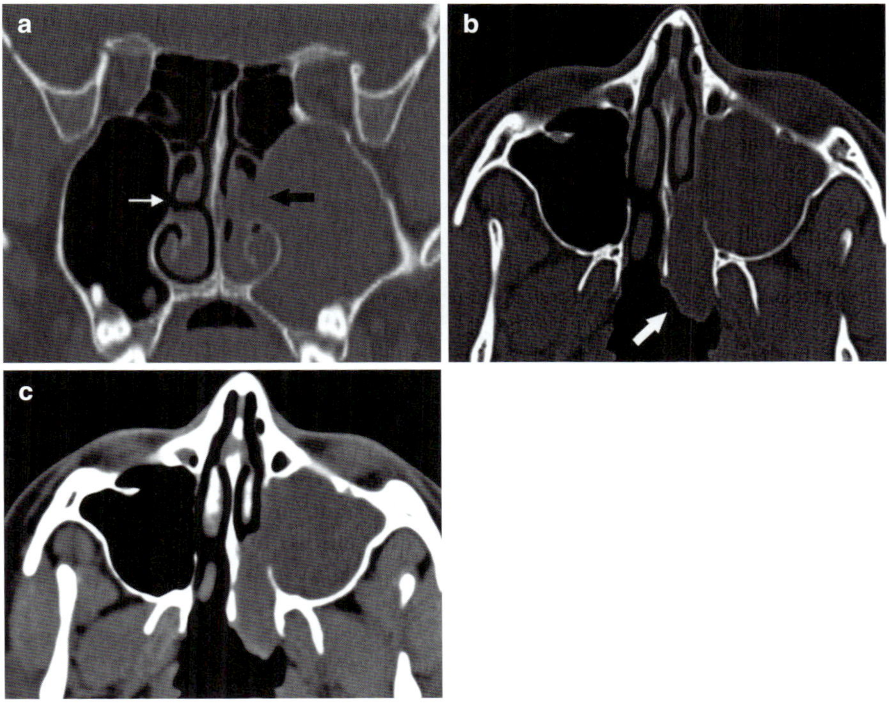

Fig. 4.17 Coronal (**a**) and axial (**b**) bone window CT images demonstrating a polypoid mass originating from the left maxillary sinus, extending into the mid and posterior left nasal cavity, through an accessory ostium (*black arrow*), and prolapsing through the choana into the nasopharynx (*thick arrow*). Note the benign appearing expansion of the ostium compared to the other side (*white arrow*). In isolation, this is compatible with an antrochoanal polyp. (**c**) Soft tissue windows demonstrate the mass to be low density on CT, which correlates with a watery appearance on MRI (bright on T2) and pink appearance of polyposis on endoscopy. Conversely a lesion which may also be considered in this location, inverted papilloma, is often more solid appearing on endoscopy and soft tissue windows and often associated with more bone erosion on CT

mucoceles and multiple polyps on CT imaging, and it is not uncommon for the two to coexist [3]. Polyps are usually bright on T2w MRI scans and exhibit avid contrast enhancement on post-gadolinium sequences [12].

Mucocele

A mucocele consists of a dilated, mucus-filled sinus that is lined with sinus mucosa and is believed to result from a chronically obstructed sinus ostium. It is most commonly caused by inflammatory obstruction, but can also be secondary to trauma, tumors, or postsurgical changes [3, 5]. They usually cause gradual pressure atrophy, erosion, and expansion of the surrounding bone as they enlarge, with bony

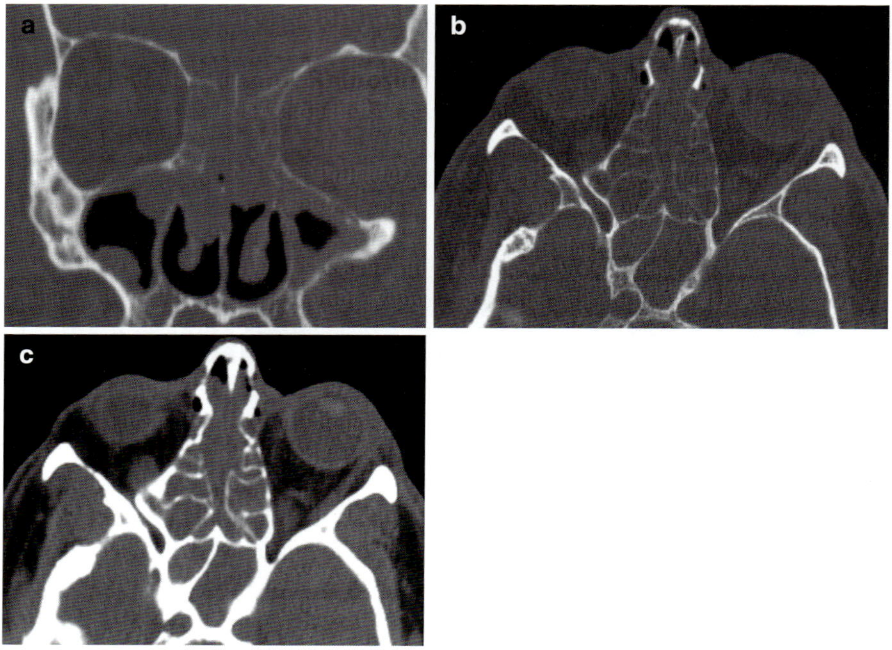

Fig. 4.18 Sinonasal polyposis and chronic sinusitis. (**a**) Coronal CT image demonstrating polypoid nondependent soft tissue filling and expanding the nasal cavity bilaterally, particularly within the olfactory recesses, as well as along the frontal recess and maxillary sinus outflow tracts. Polypoid mucosal thickening is also noted in bilateral maxillary sinuses. (**b**) Axial CT bone window images demonstrating diffuse post-obstructive secretions within the ethmoid and sphenoid sinuses, with surrounding sclerosis and thickening of the bones, compatible with chronic sinusitis. (**c**) Axial soft tissue windows demonstrating increased density within the sinuses, compatible with chronic inspissated secretions

remodeling and expansion being essential features [3, 5 12]. 66 % occur in the frontal sinus; 25 % occur in the ethmoid sinuses; 10 % in the maxillary sinus; their occurrence in the sphenoid is rare [3, 11].

On CT, a mucocele appears as a hypodense nonenhancing mass that fills and expands the sinus cavity and occasional peripheral calcification [3]. The MRI appearance is variable on T1w and T2w images and dependent on the protein concentration of the obstructed mucoid secretions. Secretions within a mucocele often desiccate over time and become increasingly dense [3, 5]. Typically a mucocele is hypointense, or less frequently hyperintense, on T1w images and hyperintense on T2w images [3] (Fig. 4.19a–c). MRI may be better at assessing the interface of a mucocele with intraorbital and intracranial structures. An infected mucocele, a mucopyocele, often contains more proteinaceous secretions resulting in increased intensity on T1w images and decreased intensity on T2w images [12]. Rim enhancement can occur, but would be more suggestive of a mucopyocele. Internal enhancement would be more suggestive of a solid mass [5].

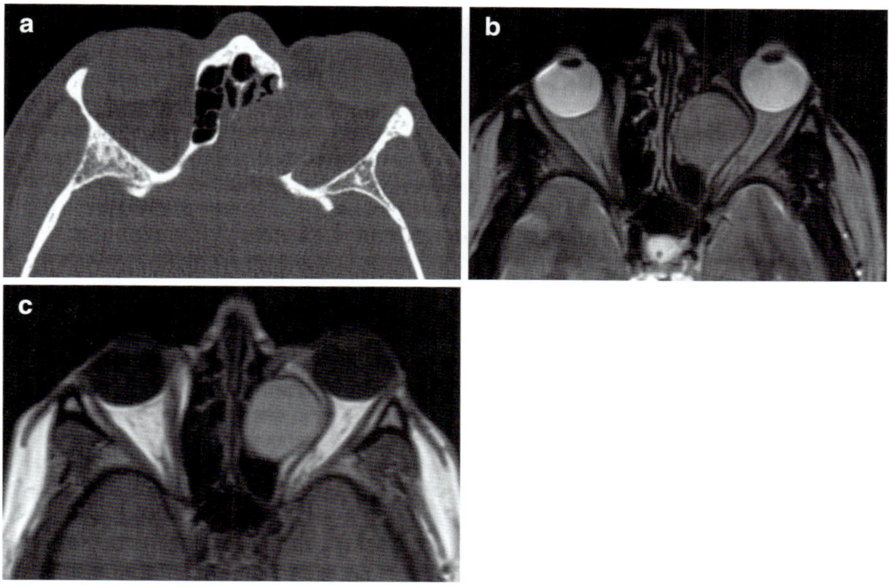

Fig. 4.19 (**a**) Axial CT images demonstrating an expanded opacified left ethmoid air cell, with bony remodeling and dehiscence, with soft tissue bulging into the left orbit and anterior cranial fossa. MRI was recommended to define the intraorbital and intracranial extent of disease and to exclude the possibility of an atypical low-grade neoplasm. MR images demonstrate the mass to be hyperintense on T2w images (**b**) and hyperintense on T1w pre-contrast images (**c**), compatible with proteinaceous cystic contents of a mucocele

Maxillary Silent Sinus Syndrome (SSS)

Chronic maxillary sinusitis with ostial obstruction may lead to persistent negative pressure, resulting in retraction of the sinus walls and orbital floor with a reduction of sinus volume. Initially asymptomatic, it is often characterized by the eventual development of enophthalmos and facial asymmetry [5]. It usually occurs in the third to fifth decades, but can occur at any time [11, 27]. This entity can be distinguished from maxillary sinus hypoplasia by pneumatization of the malar eminence and the maxillary alveolus, which is absent in a hypoplastic sinus. The earliest finding is lateralization of the uncinate process with approximation to the inferomedial wall of the orbit and possibly even adherence to the lamina papyracea [32].

Continued obstruction causes downward bowing of the orbital floor, causing increased orbital volume that can result in enophthalmos (Fig. 4.20a–c). Severe SSS can cause facial asymmetry due to collapse of the face of the maxilla causing loss of anterior maxillary projection. Failure to recognize this anomaly either pre- or intraoperatively may result in inadvertent penetration of the orbit due to the inferior displacement of the orbital floor and difficulty identifying the ostium of the maxillary sinus [27].

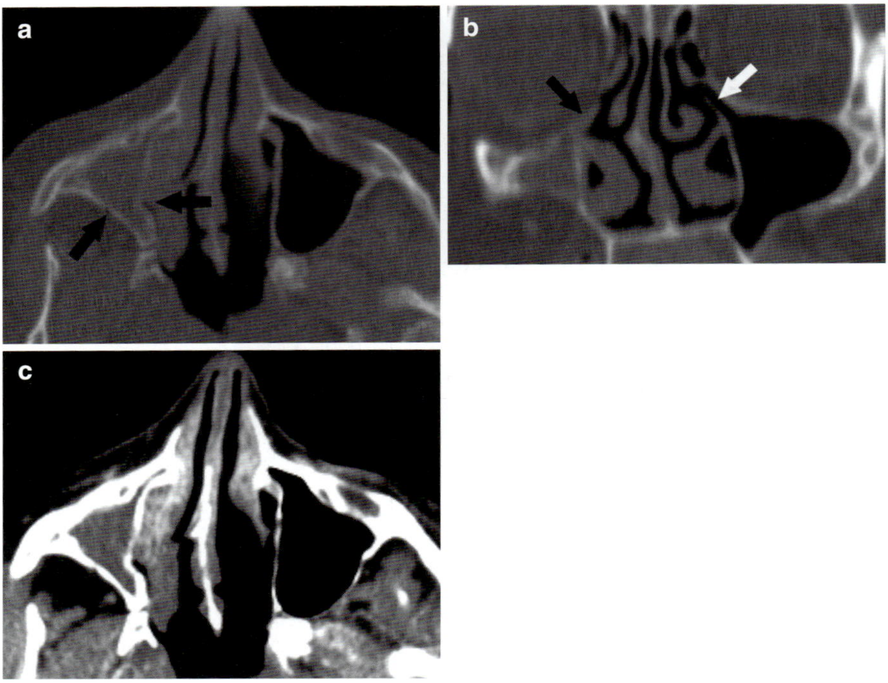

Fig. 4.20 Silent sinus syndrome. (**a**) Axial bone window CT images demonstrating chronic appearing complete opacification of a small right maxillary sinus, with atelectasis or inward bowing of the medial and posterior walls of the sinus (*arrows*). (**b**) Coronal CT images showing atelectasis and lateralization of the uncinate process on the right (*black arrow*), which approximates the floor of the orbit, putting the orbit at risk for injury. Compare to the more normal position of the uncinate process on the left, along a vertical line with the lamina papyracea (*thick arrow*). Note the downward bowing of the right orbital floor and resultant increase in orbital volume. (**c**) Axial soft tissue CT windows demonstrating chronic high density secretions and surrounding thickening and sclerosis of the bone, compatible with chronicity

Odontogenic Infections

Periodontal disease increases the risk of maxillary sinusitis, and isolated infections of the maxillary sinus may be caused by dental caries in about 10–40 % of cases [3, 12, 33]. The peak incidence occurs in the fourth or fifth decade [33]. Common sinonasal symptoms are present in patients with odontogenic sinusitis and cannot distinguish odontogenic from other causes of sinusitis. Only about 30 % of patients with an odontogenic source complain of dental pain or hypersensitivity. The most characteristic finding of an odontogenic sinusitis is the presence of unilateral symptoms [7, 33].

Dental evaluations with only panoramic radiographs frequently fail to diagnose dental disease in patients with odontogenic sinusitis [7]. CT is highly sensitive for dental disease, and careful evaluation for *periapical lucencies* will reveal a dental source. However, they are often missed due to failure to capture the dentition in the

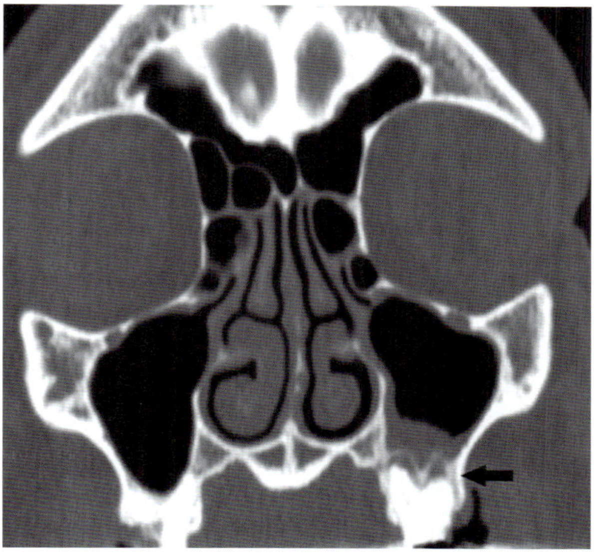

Fig. 4.21 Coronal sinus CT demonstrating periapical lucency around the root of a left maxillary molar (*black arrow*), with adjacent isolated unilateral mucosal thickening within the alveolar recess of the left maxillary sinus, findings suggestive of an odontogenic source of maxillary sinusitis

image field or failure to thoroughly evaluate the dentition on review of images. A high index of suspicion is needed to make this diagnosis [12, 33] (Fig. 4.21).

Fungal Sinusitis

Fungal sinusitis can be divided into noninvasive and invasive subtypes. Noninvasive forms include eosinophilic/allergic fungal sinusitis and fungal ball (mycetoma), while invasive types include acute and chronic invasive fungal sinusitis. Chronic noninvasive fungal sinusitis develops as a saprophytic growth in retained secretions in a sinus cavity [3]. A diagnosis of fungal sinusitis should be considered in patients with chronic inflammation that has not been responsive to antibiotics [5]. Imaging manifestations of fungal rhinosinusitis may be nonspecific or highly suggestive (punctate calcifications) of the presence of fungal infection and cannot be solely relied upon to make a diagnosis [5].

Fungal Ball

A fungus ball, or mycetoma, consists of the sequestration of fungal hyphal elements within a sinus without invasion or granulomatous reaction [12]. The

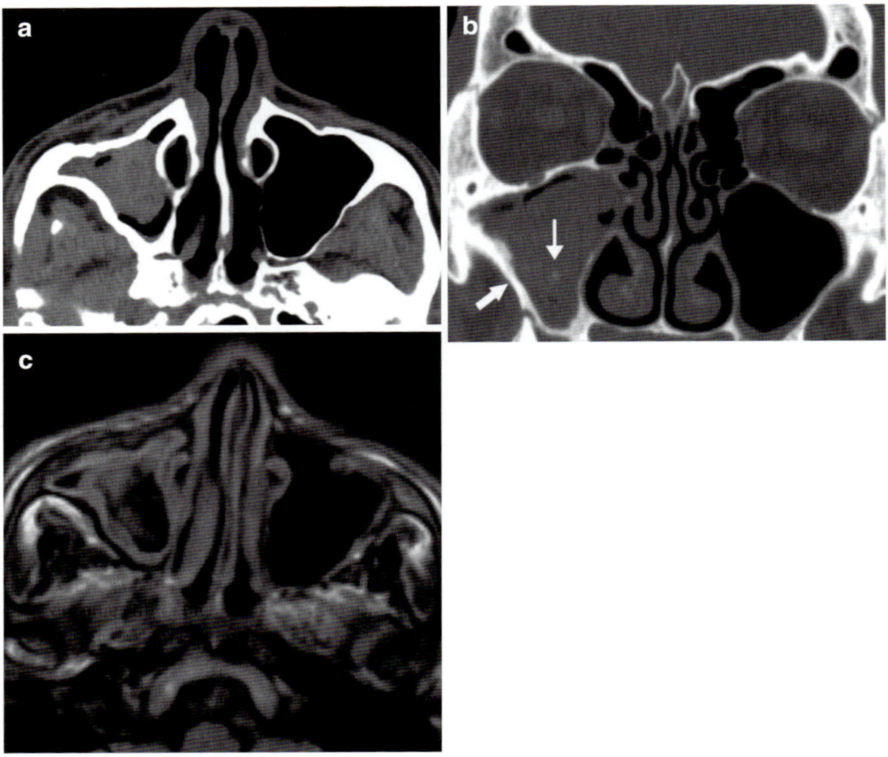

Fig. 4.22 Fungus ball or mycetoma. (**a**) Axial soft tissue window CT demonstrating a high-density soft tissue mass in the right maxillary sinus. (**b**) Coronal sinus CT demonstrates punctate calcifications within the mass (*white arrow*), as well as thickening and sclerosis of the surrounding maxillary sinus walls (*thick arrow*). (**c**) T2w FLAIR images through the right maxillary sinus demonstrating T2 hypointensity within the maxillary sinus mass, due to fungal elements and proteinaceous contents

most common sinus to be affected is the maxillary sinus (70–80 %), and the second most commonly affected sinus is the sphenoid. On CT scan, there is often complete or near complete opacification of a single sinus that may or may not be associated with punctate or large hyperdense masses free from the sinus walls [3, 34]. The increased density is believed to be caused by calcium phosphate and calcium sulfate deposits within necrotic areas of the mycelium [5]. Additionally, such a process may cause bony expansion or surrounding osteoneogenesis; bony erosion is rare [5, 34]. Fungal sinusitis on MRI is hypointense in all noncontrast sequences (T1 and T2) due to calcifications and paramagnetic metals [5, 12, 34]. Occasionally, increased iron and manganese, as well as the presence of calcium, will cause a signal void on T2w images [5] (Fig. 4.22a–c).

Table 4.5 Bent and Kuhn diagnostic criteria for AFS

Major	Minor
Type I hypersensitivity	Asthma
Nasal polyposis	Unilateral disease
Characteristic CT findings	Bone erosion
Eosinophilic mucin without invasion	Fungal cultures
Positive fungal stain	Charcot–Leyden crystals
	Serum eosinophilia

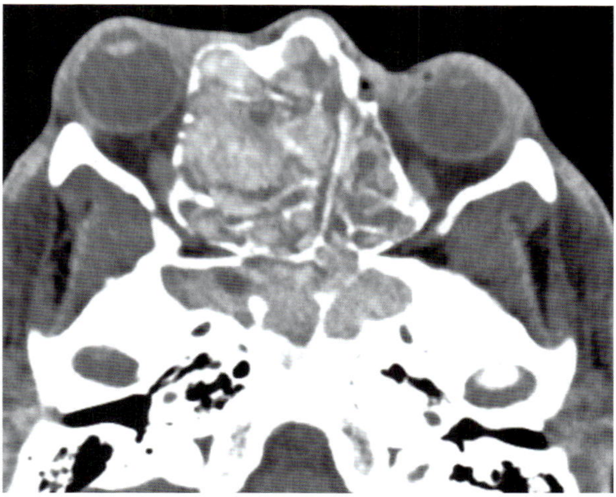

Fig. 4.23 Allergic fungal sinusitis (AFS). Axial noncontrast soft tissue window sinus CT demonstrating the characteristic imaging appearance of AFS with complete opacification of the sinonasal cavity with polypoid soft tissue and high density secretions, due to the proteinaceous eosinophilic mucin, associated with diffuse bony expansion, mucocele formation, and remodeling of the lamina papyracea and extension into the orbits

Allergic Fungal Sinusitis (AFS)

Allergic fungal sinusitis (AFS) is a form of polypoid CRS that is characterized by a type I hypersensitivity to aspergillus or dematiaceous fungi leading to inflammation resulting in the formation of sinonasal polyps and the accumulation of highly proteinaceous, inspissated eosinophilic mucin [3, 30]. As these materials accumulate within the sinus, bony demineralization of the sinus walls ensues secondary to the release of inflammatory mediators and pressure, resulting in expansion of the sinus and mucocele formation [3]. AFS may account for as high as 7–12 % of cases of CRS taken to surgery in the USA. It primarily affects younger patients. It more commonly occurs in patients with atopy or asthma.

The diagnosis of AFS requires a combination of clinical, radiographic, microbiologic, and histopathologic information, and the diagnosis of AFS cannot be made reliably until after surgical intervention. However, there is still no universally recognized set of diagnostic criteria for AFS, although the Bent and Kuhn criteria are often utilized (Table 4.5) [30]. The radiologic hallmarks of AFS on CT include multiple unilateral or bilateral opacified sinuses with central hyperdense secretions with associated bony erosion, remodeling, or expansion of the sinuses (Fig. 4.23). A heterogeneous signal is often due to the increased heavy metals and calcium salts. The maxillary or ethmoid sinuses are commonly involved.

Involvement of the skull base and orbits with exophthalmos or optic nerve compression is not uncommon with 56 % having radiographic evidence of skull base or lamina papyracea erosion (5 % in other forms of CRS). A radiologic staging system has been proposed that is similar to the Lund–Mackay staging system, but focuses on bony erosion and expansion, as these are considered characteristic of the disease [3, 5, 13, 24, 30, 34–36]. The appearance may occasionally mimic malignancy. Although not usually clinically necessary in the management of AFS unless complications are present, MRI has been shown to demonstrate a high specificity for AFS [24]. Due to the high protein concentration of allergic mucin (>28 %), MRI will often demonstrate a central low signal within the sinuses on T1w and T2w imaging corresponding to the mucin. However, the signal on T1 can be of variable intensity ranging from hypointense to hyperintense [30, 34]. Peripheral high intensity corresponds with inflamed mucosa [5, 24, 30].

Acute Invasive Fungal Sinusitis

Invasive fungal sinusitis is a rapidly progressive disease primarily seen in immunosuppressed, often neutropenic patients and poorly controlled diabetics that is associated with high morbidity and mortality. It requires prompt diagnosis and treatment, and a high index of suspicion should be maintained [6]. The infection nearly always involves the nasal cavity, most often at the middle turbinate and usually involves the maxillary and ethmoid sinuses. It may not be able to be distinguished from bacterial rhinosinusitis based on imaging alone. Early CT findings are nonspecific and include soft tissue thickening of the mucosa of the nasal floor, septum, and lateral nasal wall, as well as extrasinus extension of disease into the retroantral, premaxillary, or orbital soft tissues [37] (Fig. 4.24a, b). Late CT findings include bone erosion [5, 34] and significant orbital, intracranial, and cavernous sinus extension. MRI is of great value when assessing spread or invasion to these structures [5, 12]. Invasive spread of fungi by angioinvasion ultimately leads to necrosis of soft tissues, which can progress to nonenhancement on postcontrast MRI sequences. Enhancement within the involved soft tissues is variable (Fig. 4.25a–c). Angioinvasion can also result in intracranial vascular thrombosis and infarctions in late stage disease, which are visible on MRI. Sinus secretions may be very dark on all sequences, sometimes causing underestimation of disease extent. There is usually intermediate intensity on T1w images and low intensity on T2w images [34].

Chronic Invasive Fungal Sinusitis

Chronic invasive fungal sinusitis is a severe, indolent form of invasive fungal infection. It usually involves only a few sinuses and does not cause sinus expansion [30]. There is clinical and radiologic evidence of chronic sinusitis. On radiologic imaging, there is nonspecific soft tissue thickening often associated with erosion or remodeling of adjacent bone, with orbital invasion being common [5, 12]. The bone destruction can mimic a neoplastic lesion radiologically [34] (Fig. 4.26a–c).

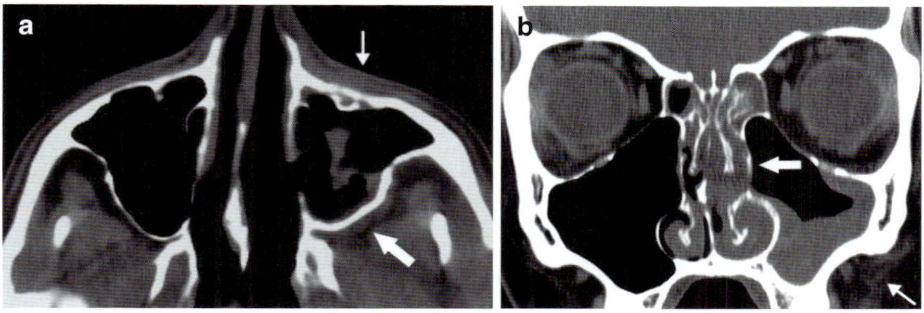

Fig. 4.24 CT findings in early invasive fungal sinusitis. (**a**) Neutropenic patient status post stem cell transplant, with nonspecific soft tissue, debris, and mucosal thickening in the left maxillary sinus, with abnormal asymmetric soft tissue thickening in the left premaxillary soft tissues (*thin white arrow*), and within the left retroantral soft tissues (*thick arrow*), proven to be invasive fungal sinusitis. (**b**) Another neutropenic patient with left eye swelling. Coronal CT images demonstrate abnormal asymmetric soft tissue in the left nasal cavity predominantly surrounding the middle turbinate (*thick arrow*), with nonspecific sinus disease, as well as adjacent extrasinus soft tissue swelling in the premaxillary soft tissues (*white arrow*)

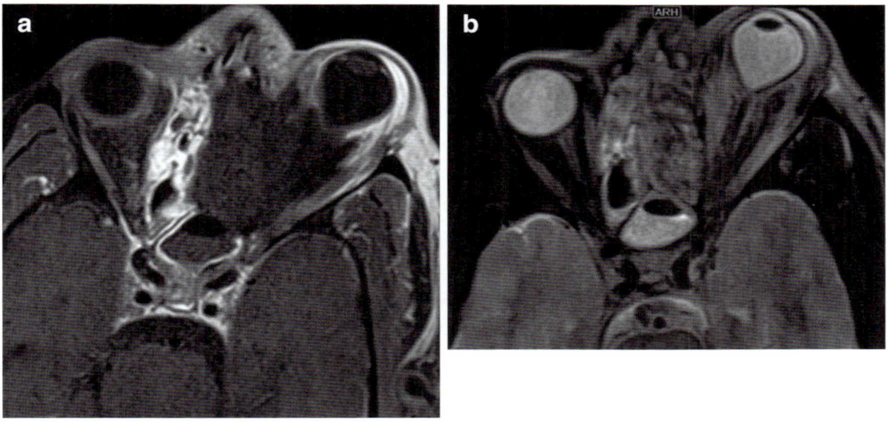

Fig. 4.25 Advanced invasive fungal sinusitis (mucormycosis) in a diabetic patient, demonstrating infiltration from the left ethmoid sinuses into the left orbit, as well as the superficial soft tissue overlying the nasal dorsum and left face. (**a**) Postcontrast fat-saturated MR images demonstrating large central area of necrotic nonenhancing and nonviable tissue. (**b**) Axial T2w images demonstrating relative T2 hypointense soft tissue in the area of greatest fungal involvement in the left ethmoid sinuses and orbit, mimicking malignancy. (**c**) Diffusion weighted image of the brain shows frank intracranial extension into the frontal lobes of the brain, causing resultant anterior cerebral artery distribution infarctions

Fig. 4.25 (continued)

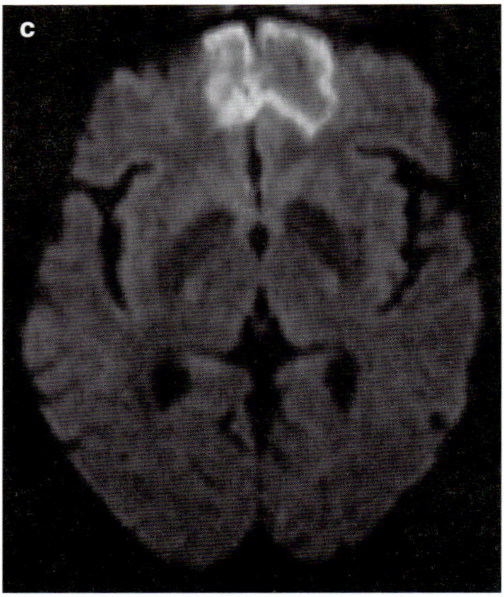

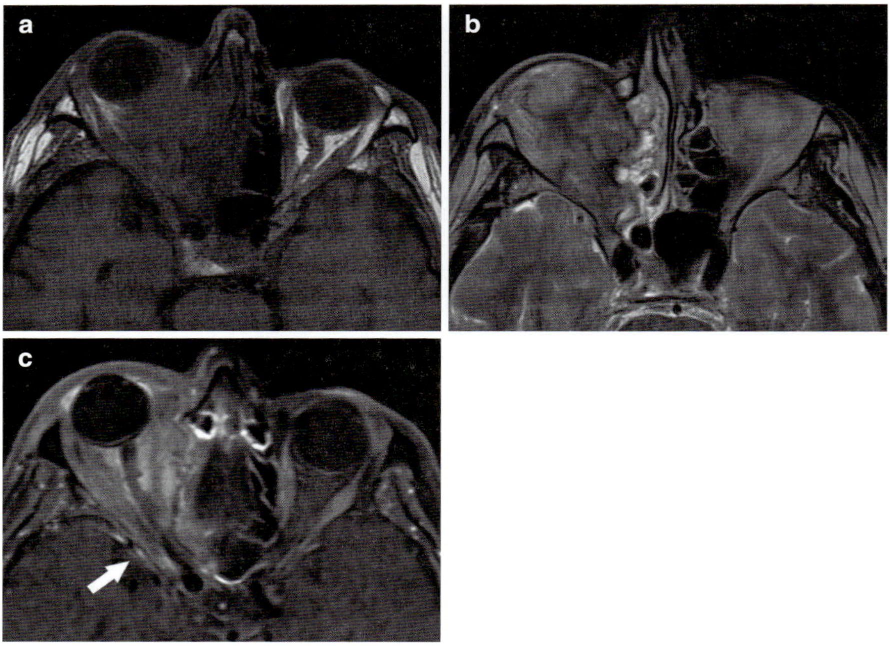

Fig. 4.26 Chronic invasive fungal sinusitis. (**a**) T1w pre-contrast images demonstrating aggressive appearing soft tissue mass within the right ethmoid sinuses, infiltrating into the orbit, causing proptosis, involving the optic nerve and posterior globe. (**b**) Axial T2w images showing relative T2 hypointensity of the lateral ethmoid and orbital component of the mass, with enhancement on the postcontrast fat-saturated sequences (**c**), which extends into the preseptal soft tissues and posteriorly along the orbital apex (*arrow*). The patient was immunocompetent with a relatively indolent disease course. This case mimicked malignancy. However tissue diagnosis confirmed chronic invasive fungal sinusitis

Conclusion

CRS is a commonly diagnosed condition that encompasses multiple variants of sinus inflammation or infection. CT is currently considered the gold standard imaging study because of its ability to delineate and clearly define the inherently complex sinus anatomy. MRI is used as an ancillary study that can compliment CT findings and is particularly useful when evaluating complications of sinusitis and extrasinus extension, or in the workup of an atypical or unilateral sinonasal mass. Although the diagnosis of CRS is primarily clinical, imaging can help to confirm the diagnosis, detect possible contributing anatomic variants, characterize the extent and pattern of sinus involvement, identify complications of sinusitis, potentially elucidate an etiology, and provide a roadmap during endoscopic sinus surgery.

References

1. Rosenfeld RM, Andes D, Bhattacharyya N, Cheung D, et al. Clinical practice guideline: adult sinusitis. Otolaryngol Head Neck Surg. 2007;137:S1–37.
2. Bhattacharyya N. The role of CT and MRI in the diagnosis of chronic rhinosinusitis. Curr Allergy Asthma Rep. 2010;10:171–4.
3. Mafee MF, Tran BH, Chapa AR. Imaging of rhinosinusitis and its complications: plain film, CT, and MRI. Clin Rev Allergy Immunol. 2006;30:165–85.
4. Bhattacharyya N, Fried MP. The accuracy of computed tomography in the diagnosis of chronic rhinosinusitis. Laryngoscope. 2013;113:125–9.
5. Dym RJ, Masri D, Shifteh K. Imaging of the paranasal sinuses. Oral Maxillofac Surg Clin North Am. 2012;24:175–89.
6. Cornelius RS, Martin J, Wippold FJ. ACR appropriateness criteria sinonasal disease. J Am Coll Radiol. 2013;10:241–6.
7. Setzen G, Ferguson BJ, Han JK, et al. Clinical consensus statement: appropriate use of computed tomography for paranasal sinus disease. Otolaryngol Head Neck Surg. 2012;147(5): 808–16.
8. Bhattacharyya N. Radiographic stage fails to predict symptom outcomes after endoscopic sinus surgery for chronic rhinosinusitis. Laryngoscope. 2006;116:18–22.
9. Zammit-Maempel I, Chadwick CL, Willis SP. Radiation dose to the lens of Eye and thyroid gland in paranasal sinus multislice CT. Br J Radiol. 2003;76:418–20.
10. Czechowski J, Janeczek J, Kelly G, et al. Radiation dose to the lens in sequential and spiral CT of the facial bones and sinuses. Eur Radiol. 2001;11:711–3.
11. Eggesbø HB. Radiological imaging of inflammatory lesions in the nasal cavity and paranasal sinuses. Eur Radiol. 2006;16:872–88.
12. Madani G, Beale TJ. Sinonasal inflammatory disease. Semin Ultrasound CT MR. 2009;30: 17–24.
13. Vaid S, Vaid N, Rawat S, et al. An imaging checklist for pre-FESS CT: framing a surgically relevant report. Clin Radiol. 2011;66:459–70.
14. Madani G, Beale TJ. Differential diagnosis in sinonasal disease. Semin Ultrasound CT MR. 2009;30:39–45.
15. Ahsan F, El-Hakim H, Ah-See KW. Unilateral opacification of paranasal sinus CT scans. Otolaryngol Head Neck Surg. 2005;133:178–80.
16. Abul-Kasim K, Strömbeck A, Sahlstrand-Johnson P. Low-dose computed tomography of the paranasal sinuses: radiation doses and reliability analysis. Am J Otolaryngol. 2011;32: 47–51.

17. Xu J, Reh DD, Mahesh M, et al. Technical assessment of a cone-beam CT scanner for otolaryngology imaging: image quality, dose, technique protocols. Med Phys. 2012;39(8):4932–42.
18. Goodman TR. Ionizing radiation effects and their risk to humans. American College of Radiology. 2010. http://www.imagewisely.org/Imaging-Modalities/Computed-Tomography/Imaging-Physicians/Articles/Ionizing-Radiation-Effects-and-Their-Risk-to-Humans.
19. Nauer CB, Eichenberger A, Dubach P, et al. CT radiation dose for computer-assisted endoscopic sinus surgery: dose survey and determination of dose-reduction limits. AJNR Am J Neuroradiol. 2009;30:617–22.
20. Schueler BA, Cody DD, Abbara S, et al. ACR appropriateness criteria – radiation dose assessment introduction. http://www.acr.org/~/media/ACR/Documents/AppCriteria/RadiationDoseAssessmentIntro.pdf. Updated Nov 2013. Accessed 17 Jan 2014.
21. http://www.fda.gov/Radiation-EmittingProducts/RadiationEmittingProductsandProcedures/MedicalImaging/MedicalX-Rays/ucm315011.htm. Updated 5 July 2013. Accessed 17 Jan 2014.
22. Radiation dose in X-Ray and CT exams. Radiologic Society of North America. http://radiologyinfo.org/en/safety/index.cfm?pg=sfty_xray. Updated 10 Oct 2013. Accessed 17 Jan 2014.
23. Chong VF, Fan YF. Comparison of CT and MRI features in sinusitis. Eur J Radiol. 1998;29:47–54.
24. Glass D, Amedee RG. Allergic fungal rhinosinusitis: a review. Ochsner J. 2011;11(3):271–5.
25. Som PM, Brandwein MS. Sinonasal cavities: inflammatory diseases. In: Som PM, Curton HD, editors. Head and neck imaging. 14th ed. St Louis: Mosby Year Book; 2003.
26. Arslan H, Aydinlioglu A, Bozkurt M, et al. Anatomic variations of the paranasal sinuses: CT examination for endoscopic sinus surgery. Auris Nasus Larynx. 1999;26:39–48.
27. Kantarci M, Karasen RM, Alper F, et al. Remarkable anatomic variations in paranasal sinus region and their clinical importance. Eur J Radiol. 2004;50:296–302.
28. Beale TJ, Madani G, Morley SJ. Imaging of the paranasal sinuses and nasal cavity: normal anatomy and clinically relevant anatomical variants. Semin Ultrasound CT MR. 2009;30:2–16.
29. Reddy UD, Dev B. Pictorial essay: anatomical variations of paranasal sinuses on multidetector computed tomography – How does it help FESS surgeons? Indian J Radiol Imaging. 2012;22(4):317–24.
30. Ryan MW. Allergic fungal rhinosinusitis. Otolaryngol Clin North Am. 2011;44:697–710.
31. DelGaudio JM, Hudgins PA, Venkatraman G, Beningfield A. Multiplanar computed tomographic analysis of frontal recess cells: effect on frontal isthmus dimensions and frontal sinusitis. Arch Otolaryngol Head Neck Surg. 2005;131:230–5.
32. Wise SK, Wojno TH, DelGaudio JM. Silent sinus syndrome: lack of orbital findings in early presentation. Am J Rhinol. 2007;21:489–94.
33. Patel NA, Ferguson BJ. Odontogenic sinusitis: an ancient but under-appreciated cause of maxillary sinusitis. Curr Opin Otolaryngol Head Neck Surg. 2012;20:24–8.
34. Ilica AT, Mossa-Basha M, Maluf F, et al. Clinical and radiologic features of fungal diseases of the paranasal sinuses. J Comput Assist Tomogr. 2012;36(5):570–6.
35. Wise SK, Venkatraman G, Wise JC, DelGaudio JM. Ethnic and gender differences in bone erosion in allergic fungal sinusitis. Am J Rhinol. 2004;18:397–404.
36. Wise SK, Rogers GA, Ghegan MD, Harvey RJ, DelGaudio JM, Schlosser RJ. Radiologic staging system for allergic fungal rhinosinusitis (AFRS). Otolaryngol Head Neck Surg. 2009;140:735–40.
37. DelGaudio JM, Swain RE, Kingdom TT, et al. Computed tomographic findings in patients with invasive fungal sinusitis. Arch Otolaryngol Head Neck Surg. 2003;129:236–40.

Classification of Chronic Rhinosinusitis and Its Subsets

5

Benjamin P. Hull and Joseph K. Han

Key Take-Home Points

- Not all forms of chronic rhinosinusitis are the same.
- Asthma and allergy can help differentiate the type of chronic rhinosinusitis.
- The diagnosis of aspirin triad should be considered in patients with chronic rhinosinusitis with nasal polyps and asthma but with little to no allergy.
- The phenotype and endotype can be used to differentiate the various forms of chronic rhinosinusitis.

Chronic rhinosinusitis (CRS) is a heterogeneous group of diseases that affects the nose and paranasal sinuses [1]. It was previously thought that the disease was caused by infection that leads to inflammation and clinical symptoms [2, 3]. Recently, attention has been focused on determining the etiology of CRS. Although the disease processes for various forms of CRS differ, "all definitions…seem to agree on one aspect of the disease"—that it involves sinonasal mucosal inflammation [4].

The effects of CRS are profound. In the United States, the annual estimated total cost due to CRS is approximately $6 billion [5, 6]. Direct costs of managing the disease in the United States include approximately 92 million annual health-care visits due to CRS [7] as well as about 200,000 sinus surgeries in 1994 [8]. Indirect

B.P. Hull, MD, MHA
Department of Otolaryngology – Head and Neck Surgery, Eastern Virginia Medical School, 600 Gresham Drive, Suite #1100, Norfolk, VA 23507, USA
e-mail: hullb@evms.edu

J.K. Han, MD, FARS, FAAOA, FACS (✉)
Division of Allergy, Division of Rhinology Endoscopic Sinus and Skull Base Surgery, Department of Otolaryngology – Head and Neck Surgery, Eastern Virginia Medical School, 600 Gresham Drive, Suite #1100, Norfolk, VA 23507, USA
e-mail: hanjk@evms.edu

P.S. Batra, J.K. Han (eds.), *Practical Medical and Surgical Management of Chronic Rhinosinusitis*, DOI 10.1007/978-3-319-16724-4_5

costs may be more expensive and are incurred due to lost work or school days and decreased workplace productivity and school learning [9]. The disease is also common. In the United States, approximately 16 % of the adult population is affected annually by CRS [6]. Similarly, CRS is prevalent in Western European societies with estimates ranging from 5 to 15 % of urban communities meeting the diagnostic criteria [10]. CRS also profoundly impacts a patient's quality of life. It has been shown that compared to patients with congestive heart failure, angina, chronic obstructive pulmonary disease (COPD), and back pain, patients with CRS who meet the criteria for endoscopic sinus surgery experience increased physical pain and negative effects on social functioning [11]. Furthermore, nasal polyps (a common manifestation of CRS) considerably impact a patient's quality of life, and their impact is compounded by the presence of allergy [12–14]. Patients with CRS and nasal polyposis have been shown to experience worse quality of life than patients with coronary artery disease [15], COPD [16], and asthma [17]. Alobid et al. compared the effect of CRS on quality of life with a healthy general population and found that CRS impacts all quality of life domains except for physical functioning [12, 13]. It should be noted, however, that the presence and severity of nasal symptoms do not always correlate with the results of quality of life questionnaires [18]. In short, CRS is a common disease with a significant impact on patients' quality of life and notable financial impact on society. Medical costs of CRS have been shown to be increasing over time [19], making this an important social issue, particularly in the current health-care climate.

Definition

As previously stated, the hallmark of CRS is sinonasal mucosal inflammation. In 1997, Lanza and Kennedy published a landmark paper defining the diagnostic criteria for CRS [20]. They used the time course of a constellation of symptoms to differentiate acute rhinosinusitis (ARS) from chronic rhinosinusitis. Patient-reported symptoms were divided into "major" and "minor" categories, with the former being more characteristic of CRS (see Table 5.1). The diagnosis of CRS required the presence of two major symptoms or one major symptom and two minor symptoms. Further research has attempted to clarify which symptoms are more, or less, characteristic of CRS. It has been shown that 58 % of adults with CRS and 80 % of children with CRS demonstrate rhinorrhea [21, 22]. Similarly, facial pain and pressure are less reliable for predicting the presence of objective findings of rhinosinusitis [23]. Finally, patients must demonstrate endoscopic and/or radiographic evidence of the disease [20, 24].

Acute Rhinosinusitis

Most episodes of sinonasal symptoms are caused by viral infections, which are a precipitator of ARS. A classic history for ARS is a week of nasal congestion

Table 5.1 Factors associated with the diagnosis of chronic rhinosinusitis

Major factors
Facial pain/pressure
Facial congestion/fullness
Nasal obstruction/blockage
Nasal discharge/purulence/discolored postnasal drainage
Hyposmia/anosmia
Purulence in nasal cavity on examination
Fever (acute rhinosinusitis only)
Minor factors
Headache
Fever (nonacute rhinosinusitis)
Halitosis
Fatigue
Dental pain
Cough
Ear pain/pressure/fullness

Reprinted by permission of SAGE Publications. Lanza and Kennedy [20]

and rhinorrhea that improves slightly and then returns with worsening symptoms several days later. This transition from viral rhinosinusitis to bacterial rhinosinusitis is variable and has been estimated to occur in only 0.5–2 % of cases [25]. Common bacterial pathogens associated with ARS have been identified as *Streptococcus pneumonia*, *Haemophilus influenzae*, *Moraxella catarrhalis*, and *Staphylococcus aureus* [26] (see Fig. 5.1). Most patients with ARS are successfully treated with broad-spectrum antibiotics and nasal care, although Rosenfeld et al. observed spontaneous resolution in 62–69 % of patients [24]. By definition, ARS manifests fewer than 4 weeks of clinical symptoms [9], after which the disease process is classified as *subacute rhinosinusitis*.

Chronic Rhinosinusitis

Symptoms that persist beyond 12 weeks despite maximum medical therapy are defined as CRS [20, 24]. Culture data from patients meeting the diagnostic criteria for CRS demonstrate a preponderance of *Staphylococcus aureus*, gram-negative species, as well as anaerobes [27]. All cases of rhinosinusitis (acute, subacute, and chronic) were initially believed to be infectious in nature, which has led to the prominent use of antibiotics and surgical drainage procedures as therapeutic modalities [2, 3]. However, it is likely that CRS is a chronic mucosal inflammatory process complicated by chronic infection.

The diagnosis of CRS requires careful consideration and integration of the details of the history, nasal endoscopy, and imaging data. The clinical history should elucidate the specific symptoms described by the patient and identify a pattern of symptoms, as well as precipitating or avoidable factors. Additionally, the previous

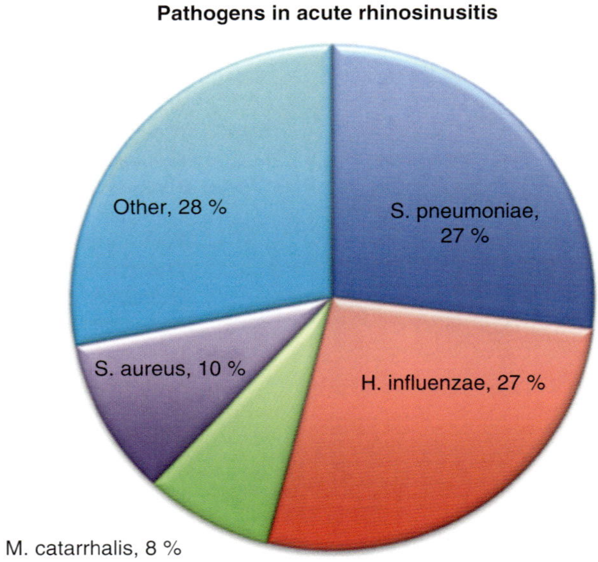

Fig. 5.1 Pathogens in acute rhinosinusitis (Reprinted from Payne and Benninger [26] by permission of Oxford University Press)

response to medical therapy, coexisting conditions, a detailed environmental history, and home and occupational exposures constitute important pieces of information [9]. The clinical history can also be very powerful. Benninger showed that the history may be more indicative of CRS than nasal endoscopy and recommended giving it more consideration if the diagnosis is unclear or if limited anterior rhinoscopy is all that is available to the treating physician [28].

Nasal endoscopy is an important part of the physical exam and is typically performed with a rigid nasal endoscope. For patients meeting clinical symptom criteria for CRS, nasal endoscopy has been shown to significantly improve diagnostic accuracy [29]. Typical endoscopic findings of CRS are pus or polyps [24]. One study reported that pus was only present in patients with CRS and never present in patients with negative radiographic computed tomography (CT) findings [30]. Rosbe and Jones found that 91 % of patients with positive endoscopic findings of CRS had CT scans consistent with CRS [23]. Dykewicz and Hamilos found nasal endoscopy was sufficient to establish the diagnosis of CRS but not sufficient to establish the extent of the disease unless the patient had undergone a previous sinus surgery [9]. In a study by Stankiewicz and Chow, positive endoscopic findings did not often correlate with positive CT findings, but the absence of endoscopic findings showed 78 % correlation with negative CT findings [31]. Despite some discrepancies, nasal endoscopy is an important part of the clinical exam and gives the practitioner the opportunity to culture or biopsy suspicious findings [32]. It can confirm CRS but by itself cannot rule out a diagnosis of CRS.

The imaging modality of choice for the diagnosis of CRS is a non-contrast CT scan. The most commonly used sinonasal grading metric for the evaluation of sinonasal

CT scans with a high degree of interobserver reliability is the Lund–Mackay score [33]. Radiographic evidence of CRS is important to the practitioner because it identifies the diseased sinuses and can help identify other contributing factors. For example, CT scans have been shown to be more accurate in diagnosing dental disease as the cause of maxillary sinusitis than a panorex, and more than 80 % of CT scans with a maxillary sinus fluid level greater than two thirds the height of the sinus with mucosal thickening have been shown to harbor dental pathology [34]. CT scans can also reveal other precipitating processes like benign sinonasal masses. They are not, however, recommended for the diagnosis of ARS unless a patient manifests with extra-sinus involvement [24]. Some discrepancies between the radiographic findings and patients' reported symptoms have been reported. Specifically, CT scan findings do not always correlate with the severity of nasal symptoms [35, 36], and Zheng et al. found that radiologic severity assessed by the Lund–Mackay score is weakly correlated by CRS severity as measured by patients' symptoms [37]. Despite these discrepancies, CT findings are still useful in that they are objective [38] and provide an important road map for surgical planning. Still, it is necessary when considering a diagnosis of CRS to consider the composite of patient's history, nasal endoscopic findings, and radiographic data to make an accurate diagnosis.

Differential Diagnosis

The differential diagnosis for CRS is broad. A patient's age is an important stratifier because some disease processes with similar symptoms are more common in children than adults (i.e., adenoid hypertrophy) [1, 9]. Children are also more likely to have nasal foreign bodies that may mimic CRS [1, 9]. Sinonasal tumors [1] like inverted papilloma, juvenile angiofibroma, antrochoanal polyps [9] and odontogenic sinus disease [34], and nasal carcinoma can present with similar symptoms as CRS. Anatomic abnormalities that predispose to recurrent sinus infections like nasal septal deviation may coexist with CRS and can mimic the symptoms of CRS [9].

Embryologic remnants like Thornwaldt cysts can also present similarly to CRS [1]. Furthermore, there is considerable overlap between sinus headaches and migraine or midfacial pain syndrome that can present with nasal congestion and rhinorrhea [39, 40]. Finally, systemic diseases like granulomatosis with polyangiitis (Wegener's), sarcoidosis, and Churg–Strauss disease can have prominent sinonasal manifestations. Thus, a comprehensive differential diagnosis with appropriate workup is paramount to accurately diagnose CRS.

Pathophysiology of Chronic Rhinosinusitis

The etiology of CRS is the subject of much current research. Because different forms of CRS have different pathophysiology, no single process or pathogen has been identified as the trigger for CRS [4]. Still, some of the immunologic factors involved in CRS are well understood. Histologic findings have furthered the immunologic understanding of disease processes. Other contributing factors like superantigens and nitric oxide have been suggested. More recent data demonstrates that pulmonary physiology in asthma has substantial similarities to sinonasal physiology in CRS [41]. All processes result in inflammatory changes that lead to decreased sinonasal mucociliary clearance and perpetuate the disease process. Instead of a coordinated beating action by millions of cilia that line the surface of the sinus epithelium and move particles toward the natural ostia, swelling and inflammation compromise this process and result in a decreased ciliary beat frequency. This in turn leads to stagnation of sinus secretions, lack of oxygen in the sinus, and further reduction of mucociliary clearance and nitric oxide production [27].

Because all forms of CRS manifest varying degrees of inflammation, an understanding of the immunologic processes driving them is critical to treating the disease. Allergy is a well-known risk factor for CRS. Consequently, patients with CRS and allergic rhinitis have been shown to have elevated levels of interleukin-5 (IL-5) [42]. Elevated levels of IL-5 have been discovered in the serum and secretions of patients with allergic rhinitis as well as that of non-allergic nasal polyps [43]. Aurora et al. showed that peripheral blood leukocytes isolated from patients with CRS responded to control lavage samples to produce IL-5. The same lavage samples when applied to leukocytes from healthy controls showed no production of IL-5 [44]. Interleukin-1 (IL-1), a cytokine responsible for increasing the presence of adhesion molecules that assist in neutrophil recruitment, has also been shown to be elevated in CRS [45–48]. CRS has also been associated with increased bone marrow eosinopoesis [42] leading to increased serum IgE, particularly in allergic forms of the disease [43]. Interleukin-8 (IL-8), another powerful cytokine whose expression has been elevated in CRS that is generated by neutrophils, has been found elevated in non-allergic forms of CRS [49]. It functions as a chemoattractant for other inflammatory mediators [45–48], and levels fivefold higher than healthy controls have been documented in nasal polyps and turbinates of patients with CRS [50]. The complex inflammatory milieu of CRS has received much attention and may hold the key to fully understanding the disease process.

Histologic findings of CRS have demonstrated that the epithelium and basement membrane of patients with CRS are thicker than that of healthy epithelium [51, 52], and one study reported that this finding was more pronounced in children [53]. Saitoh et al. reported that in patients with CRS and nasal polyps, the thickness of the basement membrane and epithelium correlated with the number of infiltrated eosinophils [52]. Other studies have also demonstrated increased tissue eosinophils in CRS [51, 54, 55]. These histologic sinonasal findings are similar to those found in pulmonary tissue of asthmatics [56–58], and they have been found to be unaffected histologically based solely on a patient's asthma status [52]. Additionally, tissue eosinophils have been found to be markedly increased in the sinonasal mucosa of asthmatics [59]. In asthmatics, eosinophilic infiltration was identified inside the subepithelial layer, and the amount of infiltration was related to the amount of epithelial damage and basement membrane thickness [59]. The amount of neutrophils was also increased in the subepithelial layer of the CRS sinonasal mucosa of these patients [59]. The histologic findings of the CRS mucosa suggest a link between upper and lower airway pathophysiology.

There are many similarities between asthma and CRS. The cytokine profile of CRS is similar to that of the lungs in asthma [57]. In fact, the inflammatory changes with epithelial shedding and thickening of the basement membrane identified in CRS are similar to the findings in asthmatic pulmonary tissue [51]. The discovery of neutrophils in CRS mirrors their discovery in asthma [4]. There are also clinical correlations between the lungs and sinuses indicating a link between the two. It has long been known that upper respiratory tract infections can precipitate asthma attacks [60]. Some have suggested that nasal obstruction, stasis of nasal secretions, and infections of the sinonasal mucosa may be a trigger for lower airway pathology in susceptible individuals [61].

Grünberg et al. demonstrated that after nebulization of a rhinovirus-16 suspension, asthma patients develop rhinitis symptoms with worsening of the asthma state [62]. Additionally, most patients with CRS who did not carry a diagnosis of asthma showed bronchial hyperreactivity when given a methacholine challenge [51]. Furthermore, the frequency of asthma in nasal polyp patients ranges from 17 to 31 % [63, 64], and the incidence of nasal polyps in asthmatics over age 40 years is 10–15 % [65]. Surgical treatment of CRS has been shown to have beneficial effects on asthma. Senior et al. demonstrated that after a mean of 6.5 years of follow-up, 90 % of asthmatics who underwent endoscopic sinus surgery (ESS) reported improvement in asthma, a lower number of asthma attacks, and less asthma medication usage [66]. Asthmatic children who underwent ESS reported fewer asthma-related hospitalizations and school days missed [67]. Finally, patients with CRS, nasal polyps, and asthma who underwent ESS had improvement in pulmonary function tests and required fewer systemic steroids for asthma control [65]. These studies have led to the conclusion that ESS in asthmatics is most often successful for sinonasal symptoms and may improve bronchial asthma symptoms as well as decrease medication use [68].

Nitric oxide (NO) has also been under investigation as a contributor to CRS [60]. NO is produced by the sinuses and functions as an innate immune mediator capable of killing bacteria, fungi, and viruses [27]. In cases of severe nasal obstruction, NO levels have been shown to be low, whereas inflammatory conditions are associated with a higher level of NO [69]. The clinical utility of NO has yet to be defined, but it has been proposed that it may be useful in assessing the response to treatment in CRS by gauging ostiomeatal complex (OMC) patency [70].

Biofilms have also been implicated as a cause of CRS [71], particularly refractory CRS. Biofilms are an organized community of bacteria adherent to a mucosal surface or foreign body and are situated in an extensive extracellular polymeric substance that is composed primarily of polysaccharides forming a glycocalyx [72]. This glycocalyx is a mixture of bacterial colonies of various phenotypes and serves as protection for its bacterial inhabitants while also modulating the microenvironment of the colonies through its numerous water channels via a process of interbacterial signaling called quorum sensing [72]. When in the form of a biofilm, infectious bacteria are difficult to detect and culture using conventional methods and are largely resistant to current antimicrobial therapy [73]. Antibiotics freely penetrate the bacterial biofilm, but the resistance is probably related to the slow growth conditions within the biofilm and sharing of multiple resistance genes within the members of the biofilm community [73]. Unfortunately, there is currently no simple, noninvasive clinical test for detecting biofilms; their identification relies on electron or confocal scanning laser microscopy or indirectly by identification of a DNA signature for presence of biofilm-forming genes [73]. In fact, in 2004, they were first discovered in sinonasal mucosa by using a scanning electron microscope to look at the mucosa from clinical nonresponders with CRS [71]. Since then, biofilms have been implicated in recurrent adenotonsillar infections, otitis media, and cholesteatoma [74, 75] and are thought by some to be present and likely contributors to all forms of CRS [76]. They have been identified in at least one third of CRS patients [73] and act as a source of bacteria which can be sources of antigens, superantigens, toxins, and other proinflammatory factors [76]. The most common bacteria identified in sinonasal biofilms is *Staphylococcus aureus*, but *Pseudomonas aeruginosa* and *Haemophilus influenzae* have also been identified [77–80]. Unfortunately, the presence of biofilms prognosticates a poor outcome after surgery [81, 82]. The presence of a biofilm does not determine the clinical course of the disease, but the persistence of the pathogenic organism via biofilm-forming capacity can impact the disease course [73]. Treatment for biofilms involves mechanical pressure irrigation [83] and different topical therapies [73]. Surfactant solutions have been tried with some success [84], and some data suggests that sinus rinses that contain baby shampoo have some effect [85]. Mupirocin irrigations have also been found to be effective for staphylococcal-cultured positive biofilms [86]. Treatment often requires prolonged courses of topical modalities after shorter courses of other medical and surgical therapies.

Other contributors to CRS have been proposed. Superantigens have been described in the literature, and enterotoxins from *Staphylococcus aureus*, a well-known pathogen in CRS, have been hypothesized to cause some forms of CRS [87]. Bachert et al. demonstrated that the presence of *Staphylococcus aureus* enterotoxin was associated with the upregulation of the production of polyclonal IgE antibodies [88]. Some suggest that hypoxia may be the etiology of CRS [89, 90]. Recently, it was hypothesized that fungi were responsible for CRS. It was thought that toxic mediators secreted by eosinophils that play an essential role in the elimination of sinonasal fungal infections also have an unwanted side effect of causing local tissue destruction and CRS-related symptoms [91, 92]. Later, a placebo-controlled study did not show any relevant effectiveness of antifungal treatment in the alleviation of CRS symptoms or on relevant mediators [93–96].

Risk Factors for Chronic Rhinosinusitis

Many factors contribute to the development of CRS. There is a tendency for CRS to run in families [97]. Cohen et al. reported that the severity of the disease process is proportional to the penetrance of an underlying genetic component [97]. Aspirin intolerance [98] and diseases that cause decreased mucociliary clearance [99] predispose to the development of CRS. Some forms of CRS are precipitated by anatomic deformities, specifically nasal septal deviation, concha bullosa, paradoxical middle turbinates, or Haller cells [9]. However, these anatomic variants are also seen in patients without CRS [100–103]. Smoking [104] and gastroesophageal reflux (GER) [1] have been associated with CRS. Smoke has been shown to inhibit the mucociliary clearance and epithelial regeneration of sinonasal mucosa [105], and GER has been associated with CRS, but direct causality has not been demonstrated [106].

Atopy has long been associated with CRS [104]. Although it is not causal in its relationship, there is a correlation between allergy and CRS. Newman et al. demonstrated that an increased serum total IgE level was associated with severe CRS [107]. Rachelefsky et al. reported that 53 % of people with allergic rhinitis had sinusitis [108], and other reports estimate that 25–58 % of people with sinusitis had allergic rhinitis [109, 110]. Allergic rhinitis without CRS has been shown to negatively impact a patient's quality of life compared to the general level of the US population [111]. Atopy with CRS is also a predictive factor for decreased quality of life and poorer surgical outcome for CRS patients [1]. CT scans in atopic CRS patients are also more likely to show increased inflammatory changes [107, 112, 113]. Steinke and Borish reported that more than 50 % of people with perennial allergic rhinitis have been shown to have abnormal CT scans [108, 114]. Berrettini et al. compared CT scans from adults with perennial allergic rhinitis with controls and found that 67.5 % of the atopic group had evidence of CRS compared with 33.4 % of controls [115]. CRS patients who required ESS were also more likely to be atopic. Tan et al. reported that 82 % of patients with CRS requiring ESS had positive skin tests which was similar to patients with allergic rhinitis (72 %) [116]. Emanuel and Shah showed that 84 % of patients who failed maximal medical therapy and required ESS tested positive for allergy [117]. Interestingly, more than 60 % of them had house dust mite allergy. It has also been reported that the most prevalent positive skin test in CRS and allergic rhinitis was to dust mites and that sensitivity to multiple allergens and perennial allergies put patients at a higher risk for chronic hyperplastic eosinophilic sinusitis [116]. Therefore, some have suggested that perennial allergy may be one of the underlying inflammatory factors for CRS [118]. Although some data suggests that atopic status is weakly associated with the severity of CRS [119–121], there is general consensus that management of allergy in CRS is important for proper disease control [1].

The mechanism by which allergy contributes to CRS is complex. Bacterial ARS can be due to allergic rhinitis, especially as mucosal inflammation causes occlusion of the sinus ostia with stagnation of secretions within the sinus cavities [109]. Moreover, the mucosal changes due to allergic rhinitis can alter mucociliary clearance, which can further predispose to CRS [1]. But this mechanism appears too simplistic to describe the relationship between CRS and allergy. Nasal allergen challenges in allergic patients have been shown to yield increased eosinophils and histamine in nasal and maxillary sinus specimens [122]. Furthermore, nasal allergen challenges in sensitive patients have demonstrated radiographic opacification in the maxillary sinus [123]. In 2004, Steinke and Borish described a potential mechanism between atopy and CRS that explains many of the observed relationships [124].

Environmental peptides are loaded onto dendritic cells associated with sinonasal cavities and migrate to nasal-associated lymphatic tissue. T-helper cells migrate from the nasal airway to the nasal lymphatic tissue and bone marrow. Some of the cells newly activated in the nasal airway may include locally produced eosinophil precursors. Once delivered to the bone marrow, these Th2-like cells stimulate the production of inflammatory cells, including basophils, eosinophils, and mast cell precursors. These inflammatory cells infiltrate susceptible tissues like sinuses and lungs. A process of selective recruitment takes place whereby tissues are induced to express appropriate adhesion molecules for inflammatory mediators. This process only occurs in the presence of preexisting disease. Subjects without preexisting sinusitis (or non-asthmatics) do not have adhesion molecules in their airways so their exacerbations of rhinitis do not spread to the sinuses (or lungs). Therefore, allergen-induced rhinitis or non-allergic rhinitis can cause increased systemic inflammation that may contribute to exacerbations of asthma frequently seen in individuals with these underlying conditions.

Leukotrienes have also been implicated in the pathology of allergy. Cysteinyl leukotrienes (cysLTs) have proinflammatory capabilities. Specifically, they induce chemotaxis, increase eosinophilic inflammation of the airways, increase smooth muscle hyperreactivity as well as vascular permeability, and increase mucous secretion, thereby reducing mucociliary clearance [125]. They have been found in elevated levels in the nasal polyps of patients with chronic hyperplastic eosinophilic sinusitis compared to tissue from patients with chronic inflammatory sinusitis and healthy sinus tissue [125].

Asthma is a well-known risk factor for CRS [41]. The incidence of asthma in CRS patients is 23 % compared with 5 % in the general population [126], and CRS has been estimated to coexist with asthma in 30–50 % of patients [127, 128]. Ponikau et al. demonstrated that up to 91 % of patients with CRS had asthma or bronchial hyperreactivity [51]. Many patients with asthma have also been shown to have radiographic findings suggestive of CRS. In adult asthmatics, 74–90 % had CT evidence of some degree of mucosal hyperplasia [107, 129, 130], and in patients with CRS and asthma, a higher Lund–Mackay score was associated with more severe asthma [38, 113, 131, 132]. Two forms of asthma have been described: a Th2 eosinophilic form and a Th2 non-eosinophilic form [59]. Similarly, asthma has been associated with an increase in eosinophils [59] that often correlates with the severity of asthma [133, 134] and a neutrophilic pulmonary infiltrate (rather than eosinophilic) [59]. Similar histologic observations have been made with CRS. Asthma with CRS is also associated with severe nasal polyposis [134].

A dual diagnosis of asthma and CRS has many clinical implications. While asthma alone was not shown to negatively impact a patient's quality of life, asthma with nasal polyps has been demonstrated to severely affect one's quality of life [12, 135]. In 2008, Staikuniene et al. reported that patients with CRS, asthma, and nasal polyps were more likely to be of older age, have a greater duration of nasal symptoms, undergone more previous sinus surgeries, present with worse CT scans, have a higher blood leukocyte and eosinophil count, have higher total IgE level, have increased bronchial obstruction, and have a higher incidence of allergic

Table 5.2 Immunodeficiency evaluation

Complete blood count with differential
Quantitative immunoglobulins: IgA, IgE, IgG, IgM
Immunoglobulin subclasses: secretory IgA, IgG1, IgG2, IgG3, IgG4
T-cell subpopulations: CD4, CD8
Pneumococcal antibody titers: before and 6 weeks after pneumococcal vaccination

Reprinted from Ferguson et al. [1], with permission from Elsevier

rhinitis [118]. Many studies also suggest that treatment of CRS in asthmatics improves asthma severity [38, 136–138]. In a study of 30 patients who had undergone FESS, 90 % reported asthma improvement, 74.1 % had fewer asthma attacks, 46 % described less inhaler usage, and 65 % reported decreased steroid requirement [66]. While the physiologic mechanism linking asthma to CRS is still debated, some potential mechanisms have been suggested [139]. Some have suggested that inflamed sinus secretions that are aspirated into the lower airways could precipitate an asthma attack. Others have proposed that enhanced vagal stimulation in the infected sinus could lead to bronchospasm. Finally, inflamed sinuses may produce cytokines that act as bronchoconstrictive mediators in the lower airways. As the mechanism is more completely defined, the treatment modalities for both CRS and asthma will hopefully improve. For now, it is clear that optimal treatment of CRS requires addressing a patient's asthma as well.

A common manifestation of immunodeficient patients is CRS. Some estimates report that 8–20 % of cases of persistent or recurrent ARS are due to immunodeficiency [1]. Similarly, deficient antibody production in response to vaccination or hypogammaglobulinemia was found in 12 % of adults with CRS with nasal polyps [140]. Therefore, chronic recalcitrant sinusitis should raise suspicion about the possibility of immunodeficiency [27]. Typically, these patients present with sinonasal symptoms that are responsive to antibiotic therapy but recur after their withdrawal [141]. This presentation is also common to other forms of CRS, so low index of suspicion is required. The most common primary immunodeficiency in adults is common variable immunodeficiency. It occurs in up to 10 % of patients with refractory CRS. General immunoglobulin deficiencies are seen in as many as 22 % of refractory CRS patients [142, 143]. Table 5.2 demonstrates appropriate lab tests to begin a workup for immunodeficiency. A multidisciplinary approach should be undertaken for these patients.

Classifications of Chronic Rhinosinusitis

The classification systems of CRS have mirrored our understanding of the disease processes that cause sinonasal inflammation. Much effort has been spent developing and refining different schema with a goal to improve patient outcomes. This is due in part to the difficulty associated with managing refractory CRS. Initial classification systems stratified CRS based on the presence or absence of nasal polyps [56, 144–147], and significant differences were discovered. CRS without nasal polyps demonstrated elevated levels of Th1 and Th2 mediators [145, 148, 149], with higher levels of neutrophils, IL-1, and IL-8 [45–48]. Furthermore, no difference was observed in epithelial IgE levels between CRS patients without nasal polyps and healthy controls [150]. On the other hand, CRS with nasal polyps demonstrates an immune profile with a Th2 skew with elevated levels of mast cells [151], IL-4 and IL-13 [152], and typically a preponderance of eosinophils [145, 148, 149, 153] with fewer observed neutrophils [153]. The prevalence of CRS with nasal polyps is estimated to be approximately 30 % in patients with CRS [38]. Approximately 80–90 % of all cases of nasal polyposis are characterized by eosinophilic infiltrates [154], particularly in Western cultures [155]. Curiously, Asian nasal polyps tend to be more neutrophilic [156] although they are macroscopically indistinguishable from their Caucasian counterparts [4]. Even in non-Asians, some nasal polyps do not contain elevated levels of eosinophils [157, 158]. Patients with CRS with nasal polyposis are also more likely to be associated with asthma [41, 159, 160]. Up to 7 % of asthmatics have nasal polyps [68], and CRS patients with nasal polyps are more likely to have aspirin sensitivity or asthma than the general population [1]. Although this classification provided some clinical value, it was still viewed by many as overly simplistic and incomplete.

Additional subclassification schemas have been introduced. Steinke and Borish [124] divided CRS into four subsets: CRS due to immunodeficiency, inflammatory CRS without prominent hyperplasia of immune cells, chronic hyperplastic eosinophilic sinusitis (CHES), and allergic fungal sinusitis (AFS). Two more categories were added later—aspirin-exacerbated respiratory disorder (AERD) and non-eosinophilic CRS [27]. CRS associated with immunodeficiency, AFS, and AERD are discussed later in this chapter. CHES is similar to most forms of CRS with nasal polyposis. CHES is often characterized by nasal polyposis [57, 161–165], activated eosinophils, fibroblasts, mast cells, and goblet cells [19, 161, 166]. The cytokine profile is also similar in that IL-3, IL-4, IL-5, IL-13, eotaxin, and GM-CSF levels are elevated [125].

Non-eosinophilic Sinusitis

Non-eosinophilic sinusitis (NES) is a more recently characterized category of CRS [167]. These patients do demonstrate levels of eosinophilia that are higher than controls, but lower than CHES [167]. The disease is due to chronic or recurrent occlusion of sinus ostia by viral rhinitis, allergic rhinitis, or anatomic predisposition [27, 145] and often predisposes to the formation of biofilms [158, 167]. Patients with NES present with recurrent and protracted sinonasal bacterial infections that cause barotrauma to the sinus cavity that in turn damages the respiratory epithelium resulting in ciliary dysfunction and mucous gland and goblet cell hyperplasia [27]. NES with nasal polyps shows similar histologic findings with a large mononuclear cell infiltrate, fibrosis, and mast cells [167, 168]. Mast cell concentration is increased in sinonasal connective tissue [167], and there is an interplay between fibroblasts and mast cells [169, 170] that results in more fibroblast recruitment and collagen deposition [27]. B-cell and plasma cell expression appears to be upregulated [158, 171]. The basement membrane of NES sinonasal mucosa is histologically thinner than that in eosinophilic nasal polyps [172], and it takes place in the absence of allergic disease [152]. Its pathophysiology is less due to Th1- or Th2-mediated processes; NES is thought to be more related to an innate immune response than atopy [152]. This is supported by the findings that lymphocytes expressing CCR5 (a Th1 marker) and CCR3 (a Th2 marker) were less frequently observed in NES than in eosinophilic sinus disease [172].

The cytokine profile of NES with nasal polyps is also markedly different than that of eosinophilic nasal polyps. In NES, there is no upregulation for genes associated with IL-4 and IL-13, two cytokines that are associated with eosinophilic allergic inflammation [152]. CXCL1, a cytokine with neutrophil chemoattractant activity, is upregulated in NES as are IL-6, IL-8, monocyte chemoattractant protein 1, and hypoxia-inducible factor-1α (HIF-1α) [152], an inducible transcription factor expressed in hypoxic conditions that is involved in the activation of glycolytic and inflammatory pathways [173]. NES has also been shown to be associated with decreased expression of cysLT2R protein [174], but some studies report that cysLT levels in NES sinonasal mucosa are similar to controls [125]. Tenascin-C is a cytokine that is expressed in transient acute tissue injury [175]. Its levels are elevated in NES with nasal polyps, and in the presence of chronic disease, it implies persistent acute injury; this may be responsible for the fibrotic characteristic of polyps associated with NES [175]. As the ostial obstruction is surgically corrected, the hypoxic conditions and resultant inflammation resolve, resulting in less barotrauma of the sinuses. Although much still remains to be learned about NES, it often appears to be a potentially surgically treatable disease.

In 2013, the senior author proposed a subclassification system that stratified patients based on two clinical variables, the presence of allergy and asthma [176]. This resulted from a prospective case–control study in which histopathologic findings and immunohistochemistry results of nasal polyps obtained from 84 patients were compared with nasal endoscopic findings and sinonasal CT scans. The result was the creation of seven subclasses of CRS (see Table 5.3): aspirin-exacerbated respiratory disease (AERD aka aspirin triad), asthmatic sinusitis with allergy (AScA), asthmatic sinusitis without allergy (ASsA), non-asthmatic sinusitis with allergy (NAScA), non-asthmatic sinusitis without allergy (NASsA), allergic fungal sinusitis (AFS), and cystic fibrosis (CF). Although this classification system may be

Table 5.3 Subclassifications of chronic rhinosinusitis [176]

Aspirin-exacerbated respiratory disease
Asthmatic sinusitis with allergy
Asthmatic sinusitis without allergy
Non-asthmatic sinusitis with allergy
Non-asthmatic sinusitis without allergy
Allergic fungal sinusitis
Cystic fibrosis

refined in subsequent studies, it is useful because it allows a patient to be characterized based on their clinical picture (phenotype) that can then be correlated to the immunohistochemical profile (endotype).

NASsA is characterized by endoscopic purulence without high CT scores. These patients often have a structural abnormality predisposing to persistent bacterial infections. Biofilms are not uncommon and eosinophils are sparse. Treatment involves oral antibiotics, steroids, and ESS for those who fail medical therapy. NASsA is similar to "inflammatory CRS without prominent hyperplasia of immune cells."

NAScA is mediated by helper T cells. It is driven by a combination of infectious and inflammatory processes and demonstrates a higher amount of eosinophils and mast cells than controls. The cause is thought to be due to an acute allergy exacerbation that led to mucosal swelling and often resulted in a cyclical sinusitis pattern. Treatment involved pharmacotherapy addressed at the allergy component of CRS.

AScA has been described in the literature as a "unified airway," in which sinusitis, allergic rhinitis, and asthma are present, but not aspirin sensitivity. These patients commonly have a pediatric history of allergy or asthma and often present with extensive nasal polyposis with little purulence on endoscopy. The pathophysiology of AScA is driven by a Th2 process, and eosinophils levels are very high in these nasal polyps. The connection between upper and lower airway has been proposed to involve the circulation of eosinophils that are activated in the sinus mucosa and then transported to the lungs via the circulatory system where they bind to adhesion molecules in pulmonary epithelial tissue and create a local inflammatory response. Treatment typically involves surgical debulking of the polyps with medical therapy in the form of topical budesonide and immunotherapy. AScA resembles "chronic hyperplastic eosinophilic sinusitis."

ASsA is thought to be a precursor to AERD. Patients typically do not have a history of pediatric atopy or asthma, and asthma in ASsA patients typically develops when they are adults. These patients should be counseled to avoid the use of NSAIDs and should undergo a workup for AERD. Management is similar to that of AERD.

Allergic Fungal Sinusitis

The first reported patient with AFS was thought to be suffering from allergic bronchopulmonary aspergillosis (ABPA) and had symptoms of nasal obstruction; hard, blood-tinged nasal casts; and nasal polyps. Sinonasal cultures demonstrated *Aspergillus fumigatus* [177]. In 1981, the sinus contents of these patients were compared to the bronchopulmonary mucus plugs characteristic of ABPA, resulting in the development of the term "allergic aspergillosis" to describe AFS [178]. In 1983, the allergic mucin of AFS was histologically compared to the pulmonary mucoid impactions and found to be identical [179]. Fungal hyphae were identified that were similar to those of *Aspergillus*; therefore, the term "allergic *Aspergillus* sinusitis" was coined. With the identification of other fungal species, the name was changed to "allergic fungal sinusitis," by which the disease process is currently known [180].

AFS typically affects adults with mean ages between 20 and 35 years [181], although it has been documented in children [99]. Those affected are immunocompetent [181], and men and women are equally affected [181]. In South Australia, it was estimated that 4–10 % of patients undergoing ESS have evidence of AFS [182]. The true prevalence of the disease is unknown because diagnosis requires examination of the surgical specimen and certain geographic locations are more affected by the disease [181]. In the United States, the humid river basins and coastal regions of the southeastern states are the most common locations to see AFS [150].

The signs and symptoms of AFS are also unique to the disease process. Patients with AFS present with a long-standing history of nasal obstruction, hyposmia or anosmia, and blowing out nasal casts [181]. Often the nasal obstruction is unilateral [27]. It is characterized by thick eosinophilic mucin, nasal polyps, and often painless proptosis and diplopia, with or without epiphora [181], especially in children [99]. In 1994, Bent and Kuhn defined the diagnostic criteria for AFS that are still used today [183] (see Table 5.4). Patients with AFS demonstrate a type 1 hypersensitivity, with positive sinonasal fungal stains/cultures, characteristic radiographic findings on CT, eosinophilic mucin without fungal tissue invasion, and nasal polyposis. The physiology of type 1 hypersensitivity depends on permanent sensitization of mast cells in the target organ where a high-affinity receptor of IgE is located. Specific allergens cause the receptors to cross-link, which results in the release of preformed and newly formed mediators that cause local inflammation and recruitment of leukocytes, including basophils and eosinophils, leading to the clinical symptoms and signs of the disease [181]. This is an exaggerated or inappropriate immune-mediated reaction to an antigen at a dose tolerated by normal subjects [184]. Diagnosis of type 1 hypersensitivity requires the detection of allergen-specific IgE in peripheral blood or a positive skin prick test to that allergen [185]. In AFS, up to 100 % of patients have fungal allergy [183, 186, 187], but not necessarily to the same species identified on culture [181].

The diagnosis of AFS requires the identification of fungi on culture or stains. Common fungi implicated with AFS include *Aspergillus*, *Alternaria*, *Bipolaris*, *Cladosporium*, *Curvularia*, *Drechslera*, and *Helminthosporium* [181]. Yet the mere presence of fungi does not imply an allergic response. The average person inhales millions of fungal spores daily. Furthermore, fungal allergy is not synonymous with AFS. In fact, a significant proportion of CRS patients have fungal allergy but do not have AFS [181]. Fungal allergy is estimated to affect 3–10 % of adults and children worldwide [188]. It may coexist with AFS and may exacerbate an underlying inflammatory disorder rather than be a major contributor to its pathogenesis [181].

Table 5.4 Bent and Kuhn criteria for allergic fungal sinusitis

Type 1 hypersensitivity
Positive fungal stain/culture
Characteristic radiographic findings
Presence of eosinophilic mucin without fungal invasion
Nasal polyposis

Reprinted by permission of SAGE Publications. Bent and Khun [183]

Eosinophilic mucin is a peculiar finding in AFS. Macroscopically, it is thick, viscous to almost solid, and colored. Often it is described as axle grease, peanut butter, or cottage cheese-like consistency [189]. It contains eosinophil breakdown products known as Charcot–Leyden crystals, other leukocytes, respiratory epithelial cells, and debris [190]. In 4–10 % of CRS patients with eosinophilic mucin in certain high-prevalence regions, fungal allergy is also present [182]. At this time, "it remains unclear whether CRS patients with eosinophilic mucin but no fungal elements or fungal allergy represent a different clinical and pathological entity from AFS patients" [181]. Eosinophilic mucin has an important role in the prognosis of CRS and signifies a distinct form of CRS associated with intense mucosal inflammatory response, a worse clinical course, and greater prevalence of lower respiratory tract disease [181].

The radiographic findings associated with sinonasal CT scans of AFS patients are unique. AFS has been shown to cause sinonasal expansion into adjacent structures and bony remodeling [191] but is also characterized by "double densities" on CT scans [192] (see Fig. 5.2). These CT scans demonstrate heterogeneous signal intensity within the sinuses caused by an increase in heavy metals including iron, manganese, and calcium that are associated with fungi [181].

Nasal polyps of AFS are thought to be due to fungi, enterotoxins, eosinophils, and IgE [88, 172, 193–195]. There are conflicting reports about the eosinophilia of the polyps themselves [88, 172].

The Bent and Kuhn criteria for AFS are still the gold standard in the diagnosis of AFS. More recently, variations in diagnostic criteria have been suggested. A recent international panel suggested that a CRS patient with histological confirmation of eosinophilic mucin and the presence of type 1 hypersensitivity meets the criteria for

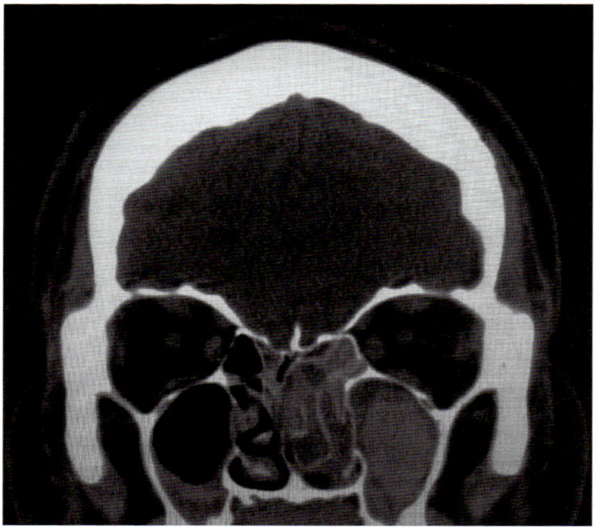

Fig. 5.2 Coronal non-contrast CT scan showing the "double densities" characteristic of AFS

the diagnosis of AFS [144]. Others question the need to demonstrate fungal allergy and suggest that the macroscopic presence of eosinophilic mucin is sufficient [182, 196, 197]. Additionally, a subclassification was proposed for patients with eosinophilic mucin and fungal allergy who did not meet the remaining diagnostic criteria [181]. At present, the gold standard for the diagnosis of AFS remains the Bent and Kuhn criteria.

The pathophysiology of AFS is still incompletely understood. However, there is evidence to suggest a predilection toward a Th2 cytokine profile with increased eosinophils and fungal and nonfungal IgE [150, 181]. Specifically, there is an increase in total serum IgE, peripheral blood eosinophils, serum eosinophil cationic protein, erythrocyte sedimentation rate, and often C-reactive protein [198, 199]. It has been suggested that AFS is driven by a local production of IgE [88]. In allergic rhinitis patients, there is an increased local sinonasal mucosal production of allergen-specific IgE [200, 201], and one study found increased antigen-specific fungal and nonfungal IgE in the sinus mucosa of AFS patients compared to controls [202]. Histologically, the subepithelium of AFS sinonasal mucosa demonstrates more IgE staining than the epithelium [150].

Initial treatment of AFS focused on the infectious process without much success. Current recommendations direct treatment toward the control of the atopic mechanisms [189]. Despite the name, there is no role for topical or systemic antifungal therapy in the treatment of AFS [203]. Initial treatment is aimed at surgical removal of polyps and eosinophilic mucin characteristic of this process. Systemic steroids are an important adjunct to this process. After the initial ESS, maintenance of the disease is performed by topically administered steroids in suspension [204] in the forms of irrigations and sprays. The benefit of fungal immunotherapy is still unclear [205]. However, the benefit of immunotherapy with nonfungal inhalant antigens has not been evaluated in this population [206, 207]. The long-term successful treatment for AFS has not been clearly defined although the use of topical steroid irrigation has been described [181], and many patients require additional surgeries since the patients maintain the inflammatory allergic disease despite surgery [27].

Aspirin-Exacerbated Respiratory Disease

Also known as aspirin triad, Samter's triad, or Widal's syndrome, AERD is a complex disease in which a very small single dose of aspirin or other COX-1 inhibitor can cause severe symptoms [1]. Aspirin-like compounds have been used since the time of Hippocrates (approximately 400 B.C.), when the bark of the white willow was used as an antipyretic agent. It was also used during Roman times and again in the 1700s as a treatment for fever [208]. The chemical structure was described and subsequently modified in the 1800s to produce the stable compound acetylsalicylic acid, which is now called aspirin. Bayer released this onto the market in 1899 as an analgesic and antipyretic agent. Soon thereafter, it was recognized that severe asthma attacks could occur after ingestion of aspirin. In 1922, Widal et al. [209] described the clinical symptoms of aspirin sensitivity, asthma, and nasal polyps and subsequently performed the first aspirin desensitization. Later, Samter and Beers described and characterized the aggressive mucosal disease associated with aspirin sensitivity, leading to the name "Samter's triad" [210].

AERD is an autosomal disorder [211, 212] with de novo development in adulthood [27] and a mean age of onset of 40–50 years [210]. Approximately 2–8 % of CRS patients with nasal polyps will also have AERD [120]. The classic triad of nasal polyps, asthma, and aspirin sensitivity characterizes AERD [210], although the disease develops gradually over time. Typically, patients will develop allergic rhinitis in their 30s, and 1–5 years later, they are diagnosed with asthma with aspirin sensitivity. Finally, within the next 5 years, they develop nasal polyps [213]. There are some variations to this process. For example, some patients may not develop asthma, while others may not manifest aspirin sensitivity during the initial progress of this disease. Therefore, a low index of clinical suspicion is required, especially in patients with recurrent polyps and intrinsic asthma with allergy that does not correlate to the severity of the atopic disease [69]. Additionally, there is a 30 % prevalence of aspirin sensitivity in people with asthma and nasal polyposis [214, 215], further necessitating a low index of suspicion.

AERD patients who ingest aspirin or NSAIDs classically develop a reproducible reaction within 20–120 min characterized by any of the following symptoms: facial flushing, perspiration, intense lethargy, rhinorrhea, nasal congestion, conjunctivitis, cough, bronchospasm, gastrointestinal symptoms, and even respiratory arrest and shock [27, 69, 213]. Once a patient develops aspirin sensitivity, they must avoid any NSAID, as aspirin sensitivity is often lifelong [216, 217]. Despite the "triad" of symptoms, patients with AERD seldom complain about sinus pressure or headaches [27]. Rather, anosmia is a more consistent complaint, and 65 % of aspirin-sensitive patients with CRS were reported as having olfactory impairment [27].

Asthma associated with AERD is a severe form that is often difficult to control and frequently associated with a progressive irreversible decrease in pulmonary function [218, 219]. Marquette et al. reported that 25 % of asthmatics requiring intubation for asthma had aspirin sensitivity. Ingestion of aspirin was not the cause of respiratory distress leading to intubation, suggesting that they may have an unstable disease despite appropriate avoidance measures [220]. Unfortunately, aspirin-induced asthma is not uncommon with estimates as high as one in ten asthmatics [60]. Aspirin-induced asthma is also present in up to 30 % of asthmatic patients with CRS and nasal polyps [27]. Non-AERD patients with aspirin-induced asthma also had a higher incidence of sinus disease, with one report suggesting an average of 5.5 episodes of sinusitis requiring antibiotics annually [217].

Nasal polyps in AERD are different from other types of polyps. They are more aggressive [27] and contain threefold higher concentration of eosinophils than other forms of polyps associated with CRS [167] and five times more eosinophils than asthmatic airways [221].

The pathophysiologic mechanism of AERD has been well defined (Fig. 5.3). Arachidonic acid is formed from the cell membrane. It can undergo conversion by cyclooxygenase-1 (COX-1) and cyclooxygenase-2 (COX-2) to prostaglandins and prostacyclins, or it can generate leukotrienes via the lipoxygenase pathway.

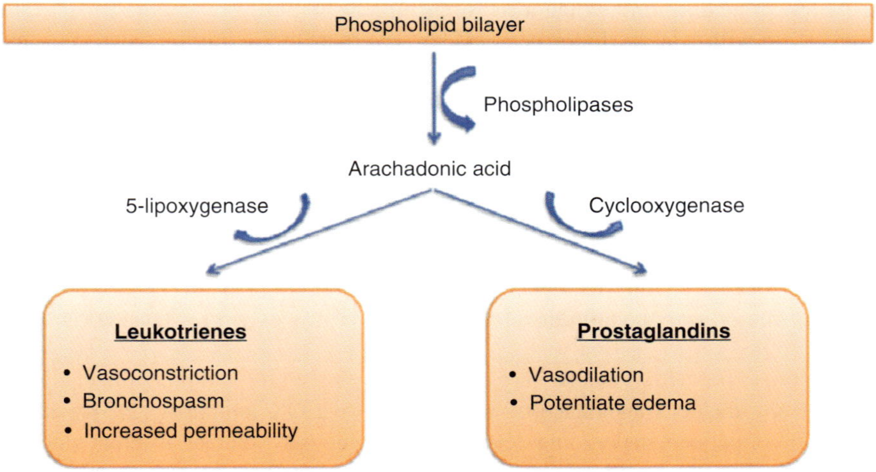

Fig. 5.3 Arachidonic acid pathway

Moorwood et al. described the physiology as follows [213]. COX-1 and COX-2 are constitutively expressed in the airway mucosa, and COX-2 is induced by proinflammatory signals. NSAIDs with COX-1 inhibitory activity all produce the aspirin reaction in sensitive individuals, but NSADs without COX-1 inhibition do not produce a reaction [222]. The reduction in COX-2 activity in aspirin-sensitive individuals, along with inhibition of COX-1 by aspirin, may together contribute to reduced prostaglandin-E2 (PGE2) production, resulting in clinical symptoms. There are some limitations with this model, but a decrease in PGE2 and COX-2 has been observed in AERD [163, 223] and PGE2 prevents activation of basophils, mast cells, and eosinophils. If a patient has a baseline deficiency of PGE2, they are susceptible to a massive inflammatory response [27]. Exogenously administered PGE2 has been shown to mitigate this response [224].

Patients with AERD have an overproduction of, and over-responsiveness to, cysLTs [125, 163]. CysLTs are lipid mediators that not only stimulate potent contractive activity of bronchial smooth muscle but also exert proinflammatory actions both in the upper and lower airways [174]. They act on target organs through specific receptors [174], and they are overexpressed in AERD [225, 226]. This correlates with the increased number of sinus mucosa infiltrated eosinophils observed in AERD [174]. Sinonasal tissue in AERD also demonstrates upregulation of 5-lipoxygenase and leukotriene C4 synthase [163, 221, 227]. Finally, the percentage of inflammatory leukocytes expressing cysLT1R is dramatically increased in the mucosa of patients with aspirin-sensitive asthma compared to aspirin-tolerant controls, which may explain the increased responsiveness of target organs in these patients [174, 225].

The diagnosis of AERD requires a high index of suspicion. Not only should it be suspected in patients with recurrent nasal polyps and asthma, it should also be included in the differential diagnosis for asthmatics with severe asthma and chronic congestion with watery rhinorrhea, sudden severe asthma with intensive care unit admissions, and adult-onset non-allergic asthma [213]. Interestingly, AERD patients do not manifest atopy [213], and their total IgE concentration tends to be modest [27]. An appropriate screening test for AERD is a nasal challenge. It is easily administered but requires a 4-h observation period [213]. If results are negative, an oral challenge is indicated [69]. Therefore, many practitioners immediately employ the oral provocation test, which is the current gold standard [1]. In patients with a history of aspirin sensitivity, it is 85 % sensitive [213]. The mean time for reaction is approximately 85 min, with an average dose of 67.5 mg [213]. The oral provocation test should only be administered in physician offices with resuscitation capabilities [69].

Treatment for AERD can be very challenging for patients and practitioners. First-line therapy includes avoidance of all nonselective COX inhibitors [213] with the exception of patients undergoing desensitization who may tolerate different amounts of NSAID. First-line medical treatment includes leukotriene receptor agonists [27]. Although they do not block the reaction in aspirin-sensitive individuals, they can convert the reaction from a predominant bronchospastic event to symptoms involving the upper airways [213]. Lipoxygenase inhibitors have also been beneficial for the treatment of AERD. In aspirin-sensitive patients, zileuton has been shown to improve asthma, reduce the corticosteroid requirement, reduce nasal polyps, and restore anosmia [228]. ESS is used to remove sinonasal polyps, but without proper medical management after surgery, nasal polyps universally recur [229]. For patients who require additional therapy, desensitization may be indicated. Current indications for desensitization include asthmatic patients who can only be controlled with progressively increasing amounts of corticosteroids, patients with recurrent polyposis requiring repeat ESS, and patients who need aspirin or NSAIDs to treat rheumatic or thrombotic conditions [213]. Aspirin desensitization has been shown to decrease the production of cysLTs and the expression of cysLT receptors [225, 230]. Stevenson et al. demonstrated that desensitization improved asthma control, led to fewer required corticosteroid bursts, improved (and in some cases restored) the sense of smell, decreased the need for repeat polypectomies, and markedly decreased the occurrence of bacterial superinfections [231]. Other studies have shown that desensitization lessens both upper and lower airway symptoms of AERD but did not lead to complete remission [232]. Unfortunately, up to 30 % of patients cannot tolerate the side effects of daily aspirin therapy [1]. The most common side effect with high-dose aspirin therapy is gastrointestinal bleeding [69]. In those cases, oral doses as low as 100 mg daily may also be effective and decrease the risk of complications [233].

Although patients with AERD should avoid NSAIDs, there is some data to suggest that selective COX-2 inhibitors appear to be safe. Still, some suggest that the first dose be given with monitoring for 2 h in a facility where resuscitative capabilities are available [69]. Acetaminophen is not always tolerated in AERD patients, but Szczeklik et al. demonstrated that single doses of up to 500 mg appear to be safe in up to 94 % of AERD patients [234].

Cystic Fibrosis

CF is a unique form of CRS. In the past, it was mainly a pediatric disease, but with better pulmonary treatments, patients with CF are living well into adulthood. It is an autosomal recessive disease caused by a mutation in the CF transmembrane receptor chloride channel (CFTR) [235]. Those with complete absence of the CFTR gene have more acute and severe rhinosinusitis, while those with mutations resulting in a partially functional channel have a milder form of CRS [236]. CF afflicts approximately 1 in 3,500 live births [237], and the carrier frequency in the general population is approximately 1 in 25. Reports have suggested that up to 8 % of patients with CRS are heterozygotes for CF [238].

All patients with CF will eventually develop CRS [235] as the impaired mucociliary transport predisposes the sinuses to colonization of bacteria [235]. The most common form of CRS in CF is similar to NES that results from blockage of the ostia [235]. A vicious cycle ensues in which functional obstruction (due to poor mucociliary transport) results in inflammation and remodeling [235]. Secondary inspissated mucous and biofilms often develop [235], and mononuclear cells and activated B cells with secondary germinal center formation have also been identified [149, 167]. Increased levels of IL-5 are seen in CF [4] as are nasal polyps, which are often the presenting complaint of CF patients [239]. The polyps associated with CF are unique in that they rarely demonstrate eosinophilia; rather, neutrophilia predominates [4, 235]. Some have speculated that nasal polyps associated with CF represent a subtype of non-eosinophilic nasal polyps given the histologic similarity [235].

One unique characteristic of CRS associated with CF is the higher concentration of DNA that was identified in CF mucin [235], along with the elevated concentration of IL-8 and neutrophils [145]. Steinke et al. [235] explained that extracellular DNA is derived from granulocytes, secreted as a component of neutrophils and eosinophils as part of their antibacterial response [240, 241]. Therefore, extracellular DNA represents cellular necrosis and the presence of inhibitors of phagocytosis of apoptotic bodies [242]. The resultant elevated content of DNA contributes to the viscosity of secretions and the inability to clear them. Attempts to reduce viscosity of the pulmonary secretions in CF patients respond best to DNAse [243–245]. Cimmino et al. demonstrated that administration of dornase alpha (a recombinant DNAse) between 4 weeks and 12 months after surgery was associated with improved nasal symptoms and rhinoscopic findings [244]. Furthermore, a double-blind placebo-controlled study found that dornase alpha improved the quality of life outcome measures in CF patients who had previously undergone ESS [246].

Treatment of CRS in CF involves a multidisciplinary approach as the physiology of the upper and lower airways is similar. Surgical treatment for CF typically requires aggressive measures to facilitate gravity-based drainage [247]. Unfortunately, despite the long-term benefits of aggressive surgical therapy, polyp regrowth is common necessitating revisions [248].

Other Forms of Chronic Rhinosinusitis

Granulomatous Chronic Rhinosinusitis

There are three granulomatous diseases that are not uncommonly associated with CRS: granulomatosis with polyangiitis (Wegener's), Churg–Strauss disease, and sarcoidosis. All cause local inflammatory processes in the sinonasal cavity and upper airways. An astute practitioner should consider them when evaluating a patient for sinonasal complaints.

Wegener's granulomatosis is a granulomatous disorder with a tendency to involve both the upper and lower respiratory tracts as well as the kidneys. The disease prevalence has been estimated at approximately 3 persons per 100,000, and approximately 97 % of patients are white with the average age of diagnosis between the ages of 50 and 60 years [249–251]. Sinonasal manifestations have been reported in up to 89 % of affected individuals [249] and typically include nasal obstruction, bloody rhinorrhea, epiphora, recalcitrant CRS, and nasal crusting [1]. More advanced manifestations include septal perforation, mucocele, orbital pseudotumor, and saddle nose deformities [1]. Definitive diagnosis requires histologic proof in the form of mucosal biopsy. Additionally, the serum cytoplasmic antineutrophil cytoplasmic autoantibody (c-ANCA) level is a sensitive blood test to confirm the diagnosis [252, 253]. Treatment of Wegener's involves a multidisciplinary approach that includes a nephrologist and rheumatologist [1], and sinonasal manifestations often require immunosuppressants; ESS is reserved for selected patients with refractory disease.

Churg–Strauss disease is an inflammatory multisystem disease of unknown etiology [1] characterized by an eosinophilic granulomatous vasculitis with a tendency to involve small- to medium-sized vessels [69]. The sinonasal manifestations of Churg–Strauss disease are similar to those of Wegener's, and up to 75 % of patients manifest them [1]. Patients with Churg–Strauss often have a more profound neuropathy [1] as well as severe asthma and nasal polyposis [69]. Diagnosis is facilitated by histopathology as well as the presence of serum perinuclear antineutrophil cytoplasmic autoantibody (p-ANCA), which is positive in at least half of the patients [69]. Treatment for Churg–Strauss disease is also multidisciplinary, often with a referral to a vasculitis clinic [69] with sinonasal treatments again typically consisting of immunosuppressants with judicious use of ESS.

Sarcoidosis is a unique multisystem inflammatory disorder of unknown etiology characterized by noncaseating granulomas [1]. Although almost any organ system can be involved, lungs are frequently involved. Estimates of sinonasal involvement range from 0.7 to 6 % of cases [254], and it classically manifests as mucosal hypertrophy, purple mucosa with granulomatous nodules, and lupus pernio [254]. Diagnosis requires histological confirmation provided by mucosal biopsy. Additionally, angiotensin-converting enzyme (ACE) levels are elevated, and chest x-ray findings often demonstrate hilar lymphadenopathy. Treatment of sarcoidosis requires oral steroids and often immunosuppressants. ESS is reserved for complicated cases as most cases respond to medical therapy [1].

Pediatric Chronic Rhinosinusitis

Pediatric CRS is a broad topic, and this chapter is meant to include only a brief synopsis since pediatric sinusitis will be covered in Chap. 9. Compared to adult CRS, pediatric CRS is characterized by fewer eosinophils and more neutrophils, lymphocytes, monocytes, and macrophages [255]. Some have suggested that because of the differences in cytokine profile, pediatric CRS may be a slightly different disease than its adult counterpart [53]. The prevalence of the disease is inversely related to the age of the patient [256]. Pediatric CRS has been shown to significantly affect the child's quality of life [257]. Furthermore, the radiographic standards for interpretation of pediatric sinonasal CT scans are different than that for adults. In adults, a normal Lund–Mackay score is zero, whereas in children, it is three. The diagnostic cutoff for an abnormal Lund–Mackay score in children is five [258, 259]. The same major and minor criteria apply to children as to adults [20, 24], but children often present differently than adults. For example, facial pain in a child may only manifest as irritability [99], and chronic cough is a common presenting symptom for pediatric CRS [260]. Additionally, any child that presents with nasal polyps should be referred for CF testing [69].

The pathophysiology of pediatric CRS has some significant differences from adult CRS. Both asthma and allergies are important risk factors for pediatric CRS. Whereas childhood asthmatics have been shown to be predisposed to CRS [99], allergic rhinitis has a less concrete relationship. Some studies reported that up to 70 % of children with CRS have allergic rhinitis [108, 261], but others suggest that the incidence of allergies in pediatric CRS is 30 %, which is similar to that in the general pediatric population [262, 263]. GER may have a stronger role in pediatric CRS than in the adult forms. It has been implicated as a cause of local inflammation [264, 265], and the prevalence of GER in children with medically refractory CRS is 63 % [266]. Additionally, patients with CRS due to impaired mucociliary clearance are more frequently children at the time of diagnosis than adults. Well-described conditions that demonstrate impaired mucociliary clearance include CF, primary ciliary dyskinesia, and Kartagener's syndrome. The CRS in these patients is typically very difficult to manage, and diagnosis is established by a biopsy of nasal or tracheal mucosa [99]. Perhaps the most obvious difference in physiology of pediatric and adult CRS deals with the adenoids in children. For a long time, large adenoids were thought to be causative of pediatric CRS [267]. Later studies showed that the size of the adenoids does not correlate with the diagnosis of CRS [99], and additional studies have suggested that the adenoids are unrelated to pediatric CRS [268–270]. This is less likely, given that they are often covered in biofilm and serve as a reservoir for bacteria [99]. Bernstein et al. demonstrated that cultures from the nasal wall and adenoids in children showed identical bacteria suggesting that adenoids do indeed serve as a reservoir for pediatric CRS [271]. Furthermore, pediatric sinonasal symptoms correlated with the amount of bacterial colonization [272, 273].

Medical treatment should be first-line unless there is an obvious anatomic cause of nasal obstruction [99]. Empiric treatment includes an oral antibiotic accompanied by an inhaled nasal steroid [274]. When possible, culture-directed therapy should be performed and should guide the choice of antibiotic. For example, cultures for methicillin-resistant *Staphylococcus aureus* might be treated with clindamycin and/or bactrim. Patients with known cystic fibrosis might be treated with a fluoroquinolone given the higher likelihood of *Pseudomonas* colonization [99]. Antibiotics are typically continued for 3–6 weeks before considering medical failure [99]. Inhaled nasal steroids do provide a modest benefit [275] and have been shown to have no effect on the growth or the pituitary axis of children [276, 277]. Oral steroids are typically reserved for cases in which inhaled nasal steroids failed to provide any benefit [278]. Wu et al. suggested that maximal medical therapy for pediatric CRS includes extended use of broad-spectrum antibiotics and inhaled nasal steroids with consideration for the use of oral antihistamines, oral mucolytics, and/or oral steroids. Children should also be encouraged to perform nasal saline irrigations as tolerated. Additionally, GER should be adequately controlled, and parents should be encouraged as much as possible to limit their children's exposure to inhaled irritants [99]. Surgical treatment for pediatric CRS often involves a stepwise approach. Notable exceptions include patients with immunodeficiency, impaired mucociliary clearance, or allergic fungal sinusitis [99]. Similarly, patients without large adenoids, asthmatics, or those with high Lund–Mackay scores may benefit from more aggressive initial interventions [99]. But in most cases of pediatric CRS, adenoidectomy is performed initially, not only to reduce the size of the tissue but also to remove the biofilm. Adenoidectomy alone has been shown to be effective in 50–70 % of pediatric CRS patients at relieving sinonasal symptoms [279–282]. If adenoidectomy fails to control a patient's symptoms, ESS should be considered. Before performing any ESS in children, a preoperative CT scan is recommended, and image guidance should be considered [99]. Initial sinus surgery should include a maxillary antrostomy and anterior ethmoidectomy [283], which has been shown to improve symptoms in 80–100 % of patients [284, 285]. Major complication rate for ESS in children has been shown to be approximately 0.6 % [285], and concerns that midfacial growth will be arrested have been disproven [286–288]. Postoperatively, maximum medical therapy is typically continued for several weeks [99], and whether to perform postoperative debridement in children remains controversial [289, 290].

Silent Sinus Syndrome

Silent sinus syndrome is a condition due to obstruction of the ostiomeatal complex. It typically involves the maxillary sinus and classically presents as unilateral enophthalmos. Patients are usually asymptomatic. Radiographic findings show an asymmetric sinus on a CT scan, often with inferior displacement of the orbital floor (Fig. 5.4). The affected sinus is smaller than its contralateral counterpart, and often obstruction can be visualized at the ostiomeatal complex. Treatment requires definitively relieving the obstruction. Over time, the enophthalmos resolves spontaneously without surgical correction.

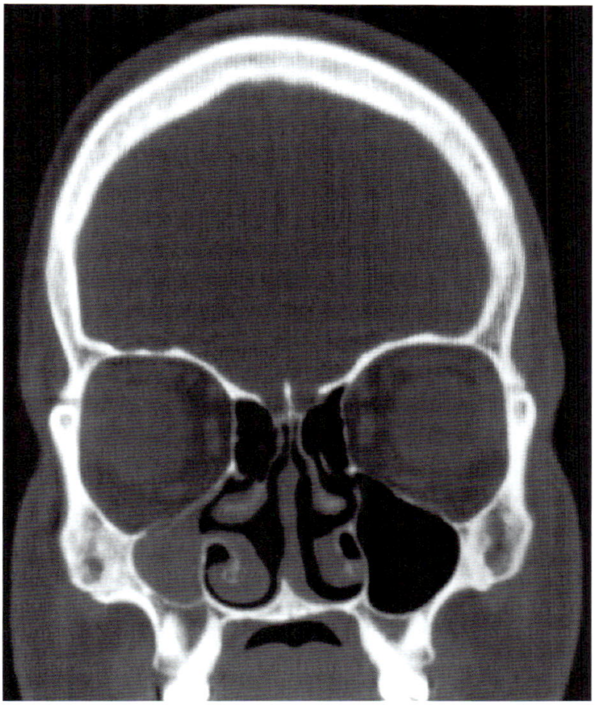

Fig. 5.4 Non-contrast coronal CT scan of silent sinus syndrome

References

1. Ferguson BJ, Otto BA, Pant H. When surgery, antibiotics, and steroids fail to resolve chronic rhinosinusitis. Immunol Allergy Clin North Am. 2009;29(4):719–32.
2. Orobello PW, Park RI, Belcher LJ, Eggleston P, Lederman HM, Banks JR, et al. Microbiology of chronic sinusitis in children. Arch Otolaryngol Head Neck Surg. 1991;117(9):980–3.
3. Wald ER. Microbiology of acute and chronic sinusitis in children and adults. Am J Med Sci. 1998;316(1):13–20.
4. van Drunen CM, Reinartz S, Wigman J, Fokkens WJ. Inflammation in chronic rhinosinusitis and nasal polyposis. Immunol Allergy Clin North Am. 2009;29(4):621–9.
5. Ray NF, Baraniuk JN, Thamer M, Rinehart CS, Gergen PJ, Kaliner M, et al. Healthcare expenditures for sinusitis in 1996: contributions of asthma, rhinitis, and other airway disorders. J Allergy Clin Immunol. 1999;103(3 Pt 1):408–14.
6. Anand VK. Epidemiology and economic impact of rhinosinusitis. Ann Otol Rhinol Laryngol Suppl. 2004;193:3–5.
7. Smith WM, Davidson TM, Murphy C. Regional variations in chronic rhinosinusitis, 2003–2006. Otolaryngol Head Neck Surg. 2009;141(3):347–52.
8. Hemmerdinger SA, Jacobs JB, Lebowitz RA. Accuracy and cost analysis of image-guided sinus surgery. Otolaryngol Clin North Am. 2005;38(3):453–60.
9. Dykewicz MS, Hamilos DL. Rhinitis and sinusitis. J Allergy Clin Immunol. 2010;125(2 Suppl 2):S103–15.

10. Melén I. Chronic sinusitis: clinical and pathophysiological aspects. Acta Otolaryngol Suppl. 1994;515:45–8.
11. Gliklich RE, Metson R. The health impact of chronic sinusitis in patients seeking otolaryngologic care. Otolaryngol Head Neck Surg. 1995;113(1):104–9.
12. Alobid I, Benítez P, Bernal-Sprekelsen M, Guilemany JM, Picado C, Mullol J. The impact of asthma and aspirin sensitivity on quality of life of patients with nasal polyposis. Qual Life Res. 2005;14(3):789–93.
13. Alobid I, Benítez P, Valero A, Berenguer J, Bernal-Sprekelsen M, Picado C, et al. The impact of atopy, sinus opacification, and nasal patency on quality of life in patients with severe nasal polyposis. Otolaryngol Head Neck Surg. 2006;134(4):609–12.
14. Radenne F, Lamblin C, Vandezande LM, Tillie-Leblond I, Darras J, Tonnel AB, et al. Quality of life in nasal polyposis. J Allergy Clin Immunol. 1999;104(1):79–84.
15. Failde I, Ramos I. Validity and reliability of the SF-36 Health Survey Questionnaire in patients with coronary artery disease. J Clin Epidemiol. 2000;53(4):359–65.
16. Alonso J, Prieto L, Ferrer M, Vilagut G, Broquetas JM, Roca J, et al. Testing the measurement properties of the Spanish version of the SF-36 Health Survey among male patients with chronic obstructive pulmonary disease. Quality of Life in COPD Study Group. J Clin Epidemiol. 1998;51(11):1087–94.
17. Espinosa De Los Monteros MJ, Alonso J, Ancochea J, González A. Quality of life in asthma: reliability and validity of the short form generic questionnaire (SF-36) applied to the population of asthmatics in a public health area. Arch Bronconeumol. 2002;38(1):4–9.
18. Wabnitz DA, Nair S, Wormald PJ. Correlation between preoperative symptom scores, quality-of-life questionnaires, and staging with computed tomography in patients with chronic rhinosinusitis. Am J Rhinol. 2005;19(1):91–6.
19. Kaliner MA, Osguthorpe JD, Fireman P, Anon J, Georgitis J, Davis ML, et al. Sinusitis: bench to bedside. Current findings, future directions. J Allergy Clin Immunol. 1997;99(6 Pt 3):S829–48.
20. Lanza DC, Kennedy DW. Adult rhinosinusitis defined. Otolaryngol Head Neck Surg. 1997;117(3 Pt 2):S1–7.
21. Friedman RL. Chronic sinusitis in children: a general overview. S Afr J Epidemiol Infect. 2011;26(1):13–7.
22. Bhattacharyya N. Clinical and symptom criteria for the accurate diagnosis of chronic rhinosinusitis. Laryngoscope. 2006;116(7 Pt 2 Suppl 110):1–22.
23. Rosbe KW, Jones KR. Usefulness of patient symptoms and nasal endoscopy in the diagnosis of chronic sinusitis. Am J Rhinol. 1998;12(3):167–71.
24. Rosenfeld RM, Andes D, Bhattacharyya N, Cheung D, Eisenberg S, Ganiats TG, et al. Clinical practice guideline: adult sinusitis. Otolaryngol Head Neck Surg. 2007;137(3 Suppl):S1–31.
25. Gwaltney JM. Acute community-acquired sinusitis. Clin Infect Dis. 1996;23(6):1209–23; quiz 24–5.
26. Payne SC, Benninger MS. Staphylococcus aureus is a major pathogen in acute bacterial rhinosinusitis: a meta-analysis. Clin Infect Dis. 2007;45(10):e121–7.
27. Payne SC, Borish L, Steinke JW. Genetics and phenotyping in chronic sinusitis. J Allergy Clin Immunol. 2011;128(4):710–20; quiz 21–2.
28. Benninger MS. Nasal endoscopy: its role in office diagnosis. Am J Rhinol. 1997;11(2):177–80.
29. Bhattacharyya N, Lee LN. Evaluating the diagnosis of chronic rhinosinusitis based on clinical guidelines and endoscopy. Otolaryngol Head Neck Surg. 2010;143(1):147–51.
30. Ferguson BJ, Narita M, Yu VL, Wagener MM, Gwaltney JM. Prospective observational study of chronic rhinosinusitis: environmental triggers and antibiotic implications. Clin Infect Dis. 2012;54(1):62–8.
31. Stankiewicz JA, Chow JM. Nasal endoscopy and the definition and diagnosis of chronic rhinosinusitis. Otolaryngol Head Neck Surg. 2002;126(6):623–7.
32. Shargorodsky J, Bhattacharyya N. What is the role of nasal endoscopy in the diagnosis of chronic rhinosinusitis? Laryngoscope. 2013;123(1):4–6.

33. Hopkins C, Browne JP, Slack R, Lund V, Brown P. The Lund-Mackay staging system for chronic rhinosinusitis: how is it used and what does it predict? Otolaryngol Head Neck Surg. 2007;137(4):555–61.
34. Bomeli SR, Branstetter BF, Ferguson BJ. Frequency of a dental source for acute maxillary sinusitis. Laryngoscope. 2009;119(3):580–4.
35. Stewart MG, Sicard MW, Piccirillo JF, Diaz-Marchan PJ. Severity staging in chronic sinusitis: are CT scan findings related to patient symptoms? Am J Rhinol. 1999;13(3):161–7.
36. Bhattacharyya T, Piccirillo J, Wippold FJ. Relationship between patient-based descriptions of sinusitis and paranasal sinus computed tomographic findings. Arch Otolaryngol Head Neck Surg. 1997;123(11):1189–92.
37. Zheng Y, Zhao Y, Lv D, Liu Y, Qiao X, An P, et al. Correlation between computed tomography staging and quality of life instruments in patients with chronic rhinosinusitis. Am J Rhinol Allergy. 2010;24(1):e41–5.
38. Lin DC, Chandra RK, Tan BK, Zirkle W, Conley DB, Grammer LC, et al. Association between severity of asthma and degree of chronic rhinosinusitis. Am J Rhinol Allergy. 2011;25(4):205–8.
39. Perry BF, Login IS, Kountakis SE. Nonrhinologic headache in a tertiary rhinology practice. Otolaryngol Head Neck Surg. 2004;130(4):449–52.
40. Cady RK, Schreiber CP. Sinus headache or migraine? Considerations in making a differential diagnosis. Neurology. 2002;58(9 Suppl 6):S10–4.
41. Pearlman AN, Chandra RK, Chang D, Conley DB, Tripathi-Peters A, Grammer LC, et al. Relationships between severity of chronic rhinosinusitis and nasal polyposis, asthma, and atopy. Am J Rhinol Allergy. 2009;23(2):145–8.
42. Denburg JA, Keith PK. Systemic aspects of chronic rhinosinusitis. Immunol Allergy Clin North Am. 2004;24(1):87–102.
43. Kramer MF, Ostertag P, Pfrogner E, Rasp G. Nasal interleukin-5, immunoglobulin E, eosinophilic cationic protein, and soluble intercellular adhesion molecule-1 in chronic sinusitis, allergic rhinitis, and nasal polyposis. Laryngoscope. 2000;110(6):1056–62.
44. Aurora R, Chatterjee D, Hentzleman J, Prasad G, Sindwani R, Sanford T. Contrasting the microbiomes from healthy volunteers and patients with chronic rhinosinusitis. JAMA Otolaryngol Head Neck Surg. 2013;139(12):1328–38.
45. Georgitis JW, Matthews BL, Stone B. Chronic sinusitis: characterization of cellular influx and inflammatory mediators in sinus lavage fluid. Int Arch Allergy Immunol. 1995;106(4):416–21.
46. Suzuki H, Takahashi Y, Wataya H, Ikeda K, Nakabayashi S, Shimomura A, et al. Mechanism of neutrophil recruitment induced by IL-8 in chronic sinusitis. J Allergy Clin Immunol. 1996;98(3):659–70.
47. Suzuki H, Shimomura A, Ikeda K, Oshima T, Takasaka T. Effects of long-term low-dose macrolide administration on neutrophil recruitment and IL-8 in the nasal discharge of chronic sinusitis patients. Tohoku J Exp Med. 1997;182(2):115–24.
48. Suzuki H, Ikeda K. Mode of action of long-term low-dose macrolide therapy for chronic sinusitis in the light of neutrophil recruitment. Curr Drug Targets Inflamm Allergy. 2002;1(1):117–26.
49. Rudack C, Sachse F, Alberty J. Chronic rhinosinusitis–need for further classification? Inflamm Res. 2004;53(3):111–7.
50. Ebbens FA, Rinia AB, Luiten S, et al. Increased neutrophil chemoattractant IL-8 is characteristic of all nasal polyp tissue specimens. In: Controversies in chronic rhinosinusitis. Thesis Ebbens FA. The Netherlands: University of Amsterdam; 2009, pp. 29–40.
51. Ponikau JU, Sherris DA, Kephart GM, Kern EB, Gaffey TA, Tarara JE, et al. Features of airway remodeling and eosinophilic inflammation in chronic rhinosinusitis: is the histopathology similar to asthma? J Allergy Clin Immunol. 2003;112(5):877–82.
52. Saitoh T, Kusunoki T, Yao T, Kawano K, Kojima Y, Miyahara K, et al. Relationship between epithelial damage or basement membrane thickness and eosinophilic infiltration in nasal polyps with chronic rhinosinusitis. Rhinology. 2009;47(3):275–9.

53. Chan KH, Abzug MJ, Coffinet L, Simoes EA, Cool C, Liu AH. Chronic rhinosinusitis in young children differs from adults: a histopathology study. J Pediatr. 2004;144(2):206–12.
54. Roche WR, Beasley R, Williams JH, Holgate ST. Subepithelial fibrosis in the bronchi of asthmatics. Lancet. 1989;1(8637):520–4.
55. Naylor B. The shedding of the mucosa of the bronchial tree in asthma. Thorax. 1962;17:69–72.
56. Fokkens W, Lund V, Mullol J, group EPPoRaNP. European position paper on rhinosinusitis and nasal polyps 2007. Rhinol Suppl. 2007;(20):1–136.
57. Hamilos DL, Leung DY, Wood R, Cunningham L, Bean DK, Yasruel Z, et al. Evidence for distinct cytokine expression in allergic versus nonallergic chronic sinusitis. J Allergy Clin Immunol. 1995;96(4):537–44.
58. Slavin RG. Asthma and sinusitis. J Allergy Clin Immunol. 1992;90(3 Pt 2):534–7.
59. Saitoh T, Kusunoki T, Yao T, Kawano K, Kojima Y, Miyahara K, et al. Role of interleukin-17A in the eosinophil accumulation and mucosal remodeling in chronic rhinosinusitis with nasal polyps associated with asthma. Int Arch Allergy Immunol. 2010;151(1):8–16.
60. Hellings PW, Hens G. Rhinosinusitis and the lower airways. Immunol Allergy Clin North Am. 2009;29(4):733–40.
61. Hens G, Vanaudenaerde BM, Bullens DM, Piessens M, Decramer M, Dupont LJ, et al. Sinonasal pathology in nonallergic asthma and COPD: 'united airway disease' beyond the scope of allergy. Allergy. 2008;63(3):261–7.
62. Grünberg K, Timmers MC, de Klerk EP, Dick EC, Sterk PJ. Experimental rhinovirus 16 infection causes variable airway obstruction in subjects with atopic asthma. Am J Respir Crit Care Med. 1999;160(4):1375–80.
63. Schenck NL. Nasal polypectomy in the aspirin-sensitive asthmatic. Trans Am Acad Ophthalmol Otolaryngol. 1974;78(3):ORL109–19.
64. Brown BL, Harner SG, Van Dellen RG. Nasal polypectomy in patients with asthma and sensitivity to aspirin. Arch Otolaryngol. 1979;105(7):413–6.
65. Batra PS, Kern RC, Tripathi A, Conley DB, Ditto AM, Haines GK, et al. Outcome analysis of endoscopic sinus surgery in patients with nasal polyps and asthma. Laryngoscope. 2003;113(10):1703–6.
66. Senior BA, Kennedy DW, Tanabodee J, Kroger H, Hassab M, Lanza DC. Long-term impact of functional endoscopic sinus surgery on asthma. Otolaryngol Head Neck Surg. 1999;121(1):66–8.
67. Manning SC, Wasserman RL, Silver R, Phillips DL. Results of endoscopic sinus surgery in pediatric patients with chronic sinusitis and asthma. Arch Otolaryngol Head Neck Surg. 1994;120(10):1142–5.
68. Hens G, Hellings PW. The nose: gatekeeper and trigger of bronchial disease. Rhinology. 2006;44(3):179–87.
69. Scadding GK, Durham SR, Mirakian R, Jones NS, Drake-Lee AB, Ryan D, et al. BSACI guidelines for the management of rhinosinusitis and nasal polyposis. Clin Exp Allergy. 2008;38(2):260–75.
70. Scadding G. Nitric oxide in the airways. Curr Opin Otolaryngol Head Neck Surg. 2007;15(4):258–63.
71. Cryer J, Schipor I, Perloff JR, Palmer JN. Evidence of bacterial biofilms in human chronic sinusitis. ORL J Otorhinolaryngol Relat Spec. 2004;66(3):155–8.
72. Costerton W, Veeh R, Shirtliff M, Pasmore M, Post C, Ehrlich G. The application of biofilm science to the study and control of chronic bacterial infections. J Clin Invest. 2003;112(10):1466–77.
73. Kilty SJ, Desrosiers MY. Are biofilms the answer in the pathophysiology and treatment of chronic rhinosinusitis? Immunol Allergy Clin North Am. 2009;29(4):645–56.
74. Manning SC. Basics of biofilm in clinical otolaryngology. Ear Nose Throat J. 2003;82(8 Suppl 2):18–20.
75. Chole RA, Faddis BT. Evidence for microbial biofilms in cholesteatomas. Arch Otolaryngol Head Neck Surg. 2002;128(10):1129–33.

76. Suh JD, Ramakrishnan V, Palmer JN. Biofilms. Otolaryngol Clin North Am. 2010;43(3):521–30, viii.
77. Sanclement JA, Webster P, Thomas J, Ramadan HH. Bacterial biofilms in surgical specimens of patients with chronic rhinosinusitis. Laryngoscope. 2005;115(4):578–82.
78. Ferguson BJ, Stolz DB. Demonstration of biofilm in human bacterial chronic rhinosinusitis. Am J Rhinol. 2005;19(5):452–7.
79. Bendouah Z, Barbeau J, Hamad WA, Desrosiers M. Use of an in vitro assay for determination of biofilm-forming capacity of bacteria in chronic rhinosinusitis. Am J Rhinol. 2006;20(5):434–8.
80. Sanderson AR, Leid JG, Hunsaker D. Bacterial biofilms on the sinus mucosa of human subjects with chronic rhinosinusitis. Laryngoscope. 2006;116(7):1121–6.
81. Zhang Z, Linkin DR, Finkelman BS, O'Malley BW, Thaler ER, Doghramji L, et al. Asthma and biofilm-forming bacteria are independently associated with revision sinus surgeries for chronic rhinosinusitis. J Allergy Clin Immunol. 2011;128(1):221–3.e1.
82. Psaltis AJ, Weitzel EK, Ha KR, Wormald PJ. The effect of bacterial biofilms on post-sinus surgical outcomes. Am J Rhinol. 2008;22(1):1–6.
83. Moussa FW, Gainor BJ, Anglen JO, Christensen G, Simpson WA. Disinfecting agents for removing adherent bacteria from orthopaedic hardware. Clin Orthop Relat Res. 1996;329:255–62.
84. Anglen JO, Gainor BJ, Simpson WA, Christensen G. The use of detergent irrigation for musculoskeletal wounds. Int Orthop. 2003;27(1):40–6.
85. Chiu AG, Palmer JN, Woodworth BA, Doghramji L, Cohen MB, Prince A, et al. Baby shampoo nasal irrigations for the symptomatic post-functional endoscopic sinus surgery patient. Am J Rhinol. 2008;22(1):34–7.
86. Le T, Psaltis A, Tan LW, Wormald PJ. The efficacy of topical antibiofilm agents in a sheep model of rhinosinusitis. Am J Rhinol. 2008;22(6):560–7.
87. Bernstein JM, Ballow M, Schlievert PM, Rich G, Allen C, Dryja D. A superantigen hypothesis for the pathogenesis of chronic hyperplastic sinusitis with massive nasal polyposis. Am J Rhinol. 2003;17(6):321–6.
88. Bachert C, Gevaert P, Holtappels G, Johansson SG, van Cauwenberge P. Total and specific IgE in nasal polyps is related to local eosinophilic inflammation. J Allergy Clin Immunol. 2001;107(4):607–14.
89. Early SB, Hise K, Han JK, Borish L, Steinke JW. Hypoxia stimulates inflammatory and fibrotic responses from nasal-polyp derived fibroblasts. Laryngoscope. 2007;117(3):511–5.
90. Matsune S, Kono M, Sun D, Ushikai M, Kurono Y. Hypoxia in paranasal sinuses of patients with chronic sinusitis with or without the complication of nasal allergy. Acta Otolaryngol. 2003;123(4):519–23.
91. Shin SH, Ponikau JU, Sherris DA, Congdon D, Frigas E, Homburger HA, et al. Chronic rhinosinusitis: an enhanced immune response to ubiquitous airborne fungi. J Allergy Clin Immunol. 2004;114(6):1369–75.
92. Wei JL, Kita H, Sherris DA, Kern EB, Weaver A, Ponikau JU. The chemotactic behavior of eosinophils in patients with chronic rhinosinusitis. Laryngoscope. 2003;113(2):303–6.
93. Ponikau JU, Sherris DA, Weaver A, Kita H. Treatment of chronic rhinosinusitis with intranasal amphotericin B: a randomized, placebo-controlled, double-blind pilot trial. J Allergy Clin Immunol. 2005;115(1):125–31.
94. Ebbens FA, Georgalas C, Luiten S, van Drunen CM, Badia L, Scadding GK, et al. The effect of topical amphotericin B on inflammatory markers in patients with chronic rhinosinusitis: a multicenter randomized controlled study. Laryngoscope. 2009;119(2):401–8.
95. Ebbens FA, Scadding GK, Badia L, Hellings PW, Jorissen M, Mullol J, et al. Amphotericin B nasal lavages: not a solution for patients with chronic rhinosinusitis. J Allergy Clin Immunol. 2006;118(5):1149–56.
96. Weschta M, Rimek D, Formanek M, Polzehl D, Podbielski A, Riechelmann H. Topical antifungal treatment of chronic rhinosinusitis with nasal polyps: a randomized, double-blind clinical trial. J Allergy Clin Immunol. 2004;113(6):1122–8.

97. Cohen NA, Widelitz JS, Chiu AG, Palmer JN, Kennedy DW. Familial aggregation of sinonasal polyps correlates with severity of disease. Otolaryngol Head Neck Surg. 2006;134(4):601–4.
98. Robinson JL, Griest S, James KE, Smith TL. Impact of aspirin intolerance on outcomes of sinus surgery. Laryngoscope. 2007;117(5):825–30.
99. Wu AW, Shapiro NL, Bhattacharyya N. Chronic rhinosinusitis in children: what are the treatment options? Immunol Allergy Clin North Am. 2009;29(4):705–17.
100. Lusk RP, McAlister B, el Fouley A. Anatomic variation in pediatric chronic sinusitis: a CT study. Otolaryngol Clin North Am. 1996;29(1):75–91.
101. Bolger WE, Butzin CA, Parsons DS. Paranasal sinus bony anatomic variations and mucosal abnormalities: CT analysis for endoscopic sinus surgery. Laryngoscope. 1991;101(1 Pt 1):56–64.
102. Jones NS, Strobl A, Holland I. A study of the CT findings in 100 patients with rhinosinusitis and 100 controls. Clin Otolaryngol Allied Sci. 1997;22(1):47–51.
103. Danese M, Duvoisin B, Agrifoglio A, Cherpillod J, Krayenbuhl M. Influence of naso-sinusal anatomic variants on recurrent, persistent or chronic sinusitis. X-ray computed tomographic evaluation in 112 patients. J Radiol. 1997;78(9):651–7.
104. Houser SM, Keen KJ. The role of allergy and smoking in chronic rhinosinusitis and polyposis. Laryngoscope. 2008;118(9):1521–7.
105. Tamashiro E, Xiong G, Anselmo-Lima WT, Kreindler JL, Palmer JN, Cohen NA. Cigarette smoke exposure impairs respiratory epithelial ciliogenesis. Am J Rhinol Allergy. 2009;23(2):117–22.
106. Passàli D, Caruso G, Passàli FM. ENT manifestations of gastroesophageal reflux. Curr Allergy Asthma Rep. 2008;8(3):240–4.
107. Newman LJ, Platts-Mills TA, Phillips CD, Hazen KC, Gross CW. Chronic sinusitis. Relationship of computed tomographic findings to allergy, asthma, and eosinophilia. JAMA. 1994;271(5):363–7.
108. Rachelefsky GS, Goldberg M, Katz RM, Boris G, Gyepes MT, Shapiro MJ, et al. Sinus disease in children with respiratory allergy. J Allergy Clin Immunol. 1978;61(5):310–4.
109. Savolainen S. Allergy in patients with acute maxillary sinusitis. Allergy. 1989;44(2):116–22.
110. Harlin SL, Ansel DG, Lane SR, Myers J, Kephart GM, Gleich GJ. A clinical and pathologic study of chronic sinusitis: the role of the eosinophil. J Allergy Clin Immunol. 1988;81(5 Pt 1):867–75.
111. Derebery MJ, Berliner KI. Allergy and health-related quality of life. Otolaryngol Head Neck Surg. 2000;123(4):393–9.
112. Krouse JH. Computed tomography stage, allergy testing, and quality of life in patients with sinusitis. Otolaryngol Head Neck Surg. 2000;123(4):389–92.
113. Ramadan HH, Fornelli R, Ortiz AO, Rodman S. Correlation of allergy and severity of sinus disease. Am J Rhinol. 1999;13(5):345–7.
114. Shapiro GG. Role of allergy in sinusitis. Pediatr Infect Dis. 1985;4(6 Suppl):S55–9.
115. Berrettini S, Carabelli A, Sellari-Franceschini S, Bruschini L, Abruzzese A, Quartieri F, et al. Perennial allergic rhinitis and chronic sinusitis: correlation with rhinologic risk factors. Allergy. 1999;54(3):242–8.
116. Tan BK, Zirkle W, Chandra RK, Lin D, Conley DB, Peters AT, et al. Atopic profile of patients failing medical therapy for chronic rhinosinusitis. Int Forum Allergy Rhinol. 2011;1(2):88–94.
117. Emanuel IA, Shah SB. Chronic rhinosinusitis: allergy and sinus computed tomography relationships. Otolaryngol Head Neck Surg. 2000;123(6):687–91.
118. Staikūniene J, Vaitkus S, Japertiene LM, Ryskiene S. Association of chronic rhinosinusitis with nasal polyps and asthma: clinical and radiological features, allergy and inflammation markers. Medicina (Kaunas). 2008;44(4):257–65.
119. Banerji A, Piccirillo JF, Thawley SE, Levitt RG, Schechtman KB, Kramper MA, et al. Chronic rhinosinusitis patients with polyps or polypoid mucosa have a greater burden of illness. Am J Rhinol. 2007;21(1):19–26.

120. Settipane GA. Epidemiology of nasal polyps. Allergy Asthma Proc. 1996;17(5):231–6.
121. Robinson S, Douglas R, Wormald PJ. The relationship between atopy and chronic rhinosinusitis. Am J Rhinol. 2006;20(6):625–8.
122. Baroody FM, Detineo M, Naclerio RM. Unilateral nasal allergic reactions increase bilateral sinus eosinophil infiltration. J Appl Physiol (1985). 2013;115(9):1262–7.
123. Pelikan Z, Pelikan-Filipek M. Role of nasal allergy in chronic maxillary sinusitis–diagnostic value of nasal challenge with allergen. J Allergy Clin Immunol. 1990;86(4 Pt 1):484–91.
124. Steinke JW, Borish L. The role of allergy in chronic rhinosinusitis. Immunol Allergy Clin North Am. 2004;24(1):45–57.
125. Steinke JW, Bradley D, Arango P, Crouse CD, Frierson H, Kountakis SE, et al. Cysteinyl leukotriene expression in chronic hyperplastic sinusitis-nasal polyposis: importance to eosinophilia and asthma. J Allergy Clin Immunol. 2003;111(2):342–9.
126. Seybt MW, McMains KC, Kountakis SE. The prevalence and effect of asthma on adults with chronic rhinosinusitis. Ear Nose Throat J. 2007;86(7):409–11.
127. Slavin RG. Sinusitis in adults and its relation to allergic rhinitis, asthma, and nasal polyps. J Allergy Clin Immunol. 1988;82(5 Pt 2):950–6.
128. Annesi-Maesano I. Epidemiological evidence of the occurrence of rhinitis and sinusitis in asthmatics. Allergy. 1999;54 Suppl 57:7–13.
129. Pfister R, Lütolf M, Schapowal A, Glatte B, Schmitz M, Menz G. Screening for sinus disease in patients with asthma: a computed tomography-controlled comparison of A-mode ultrasonography and standard radiography. J Allergy Clin Immunol. 1994;94(5):804–9.
130. Bresciani M, Paradis L, Des Roches A, Vernhet H, Vachier I, Godard P, et al. Rhinosinusitis in severe asthma. J Allergy Clin Immunol. 2001;107(1):73–80.
131. Dhong HJ, Kim HY, Chung YJ, Kim TW, Kim JH, Chung SK, et al. Computed tomographic assessment of chronic rhinosinusitis with asthma. Am J Rhinol. 2006;20(5):450–2.
132. Kountakis SE, Bradley DT. Effect of asthma on sinus computed tomography grade and symptom scores in patients undergoing revision functional endoscopic sinus surgery. Am J Rhinol. 2003;17(4):215–9.
133. Bousquet J, Chanez P, Lacoste JY, Barnéon G, Ghavanian N, Enander I, et al. Eosinophilic inflammation in asthma. N Engl J Med. 1990;323(15):1033–9.
134. Braunstahl GJ, Fokkens W. Nasal involvement in allergic asthma. Allergy. 2003;58(12):1235–43.
135. Alobid I, Benítez P, Bernal-Sprekelsen M, Roca J, Alonso J, Picado C, et al. Nasal polyposis and its impact on quality of life: comparison between the effects of medical and surgical treatments. Allergy. 2005;60(4):452–8.
136. Dhong HJ, Jung YS, Chung SK, Choi DC. Effect of endoscopic sinus surgery on asthmatic patients with chronic rhinosinusitis. Otolaryngol Head Neck Surg. 2001;124(1):99–104.
137. Dunlop G, Scadding GK, Lund VJ. The effect of endoscopic sinus surgery on asthma: management of patients with chronic rhinosinusitis, nasal polyposis, and asthma. Am J Rhinol. 1999;13(4):261–5.
138. Awad OG, Fasano MB, Lee JH, Graham SM. Asthma outcomes after endoscopic sinus surgery in aspirin-tolerant versus aspirin-induced asthmatic patients. Am J Rhinol. 2008;22(2):197–203.
139. Marney SR. Pathophysiology of reactive airway disease and sinusitis. Ann Otol Rhinol Laryngol. 1996;105(2):98–100.
140. Hamilos DL. Chronic rhinosinusitis patterns of illness. Clin Allergy Immunol. 2007;20:1–13.
141. Kainulainen L, Suonpää J, Nikoskelainen J, Svedström E, Vuorinen T, Meurman O, et al. Bacteria and viruses in maxillary sinuses of patients with primary hypogammaglobulinemia. Arch Otolaryngol Head Neck Surg. 2007;133(6):597–602.
142. Chee L, Graham SM, Carothers DG, Ballas ZK. Immune dysfunction in refractory sinusitis in a tertiary care setting. Laryngoscope. 2001;111(2):233–5.
143. Vanlerberghe L, Joniau S, Jorissen M. The prevalence of humoral immunodeficiency in refractory rhinosinusitis: a retrospective analysis. B-ENT. 2006;2(4):161–6.

144. Meltzer EO, Hamilos DL, Hadley JA, Lanza DC, Marple BF, Nicklas RA, et al. Rhinosinusitis: establishing definitions for clinical research and patient care. J Allergy Clin Immunol. 2004;114(6 Suppl):155–212.
145. Van Zele T, Claeys S, Gevaert P, Van Maele G, Holtappels G, Van Cauwenberge P, et al. Differentiation of chronic sinus diseases by measurement of inflammatory mediators. Allergy. 2006;61(11):1280–9.
146. Polzehl D, Moeller P, Riechelmann H, Perner S. Distinct features of chronic rhinosinusitis with and without nasal polyps. Allergy. 2006;61(11):1275–9.
147. Slavin RG, Spector SL, Bernstein IL, Kaliner MA, Kennedy DW, Virant FS, et al. The diagnosis and management of sinusitis: a practice parameter update. J Allergy Clin Immunol. 2005;116(6 Suppl):S13–47.
148. Kern RC, Conley DB, Walsh W, Chandra R, Kato A, Tripathi-Peters A, et al. Perspectives on the etiology of chronic rhinosinusitis: an immune barrier hypothesis. Am J Rhinol. 2008;22(6):549–59.
149. Cao PP, Li HB, Wang BF, Wang SB, You XJ, Cui YH, et al. Distinct immunopathologic characteristics of various types of chronic rhinosinusitis in adult Chinese. J Allergy Clin Immunol. 2009;124(3):478–84, 84.e1–2.
150. Ahn CN, Wise SK, Lathers DM, Mulligan RM, Harvey RJ, Schlosser RJ. Local production of antigen-specific IgE in different anatomic subsites of allergic fungal rhinosinusitis patients. Otolaryngol Head Neck Surg. 2009;141(1):97–103.
151. Carney AS, Tan LW, Adams D, Varelias A, Ooi EH, Wormald PJ. Th2 immunological inflammation in allergic fungal sinusitis, nonallergic eosinophilic fungal sinusitis, and chronic rhinosinusitis. Am J Rhinol. 2006;20(2):145–9.
152. Payne SC, Han JK, Huyett P, Negri J, Kropf EZ, Borish L, et al. Microarray analysis of distinct gene transcription profiles in non-eosinophilic chronic sinusitis with nasal polyps. Am J Rhinol. 2008;22(6):568–81.
153. Hamilos DL, Leung DY, Wood R, Meyers A, Stephens JK, Barkans J, et al. Chronic hyperplastic sinusitis: association of tissue eosinophilia with mRNA expression of granulocyte-macrophage colony-stimulating factor and interleukin-3. J Allergy Clin Immunol. 1993;92(1 Pt 1):39–48.
154. Drake-Lee AB, Price JM, Milford CM, Bickerton RC. Nasal mast cells: a preliminary report on their ultrastructure. J Laryngol Otol Suppl. 1987;13:1–17.
155. Hellquist HB. Nasal polyps update. Histopathology. Allergy Asthma Proc. 1996;17(5):237–42.
156. Zhang N, Van Zele T, Perez-Novo C, Van Bruaene N, Holtappels G, DeRuyck N, et al. Different types of T-effector cells orchestrate mucosal inflammation in chronic sinus disease. J Allergy Clin Immunol. 2008;122(5):961–8.
157. Steinke JW. The relationship between rhinosinusitis and asthma sinusitis. Curr Allergy Asthma Rep. 2006;6(6):495–501.
158. Berger G, Kattan A, Bernheim J, Ophir D. Polypoid mucosa with eosinophilia and glandular hyperplasia in chronic sinusitis: a histopathological and immunohistochemical study. Laryngoscope. 2002;112(4):738–45.
159. Dinis PB, Gomes A. Sinusitis and asthma: how do they interrelate in sinus surgery? Am J Rhinol. 1997;11(6):421–8.
160. Dejima K, Hama T, Miyazaki M, Yasuda S, Fukushima K, Oshima A, et al. A clinical study of endoscopic sinus surgery for sinusitis in patients with bronchial asthma. Int Arch Allergy Immunol. 2005;138(2):97–104.
161. Hamilos DL, Leung DY, Wood R, Bean DK, Song YL, Schotman E, et al. Eosinophil infiltration in nonallergic chronic hyperplastic sinusitis with nasal polyposis (CHS/NP) is associated with endothelial VCAM-1 upregulation and expression of TNF-alpha. Am J Respir Cell Mol Biol. 1996;15(4):443–50.
162. Finotto S, Ohno I, Marshall JS, Gauldie J, Denburg JA, Dolovich J, et al. TNF-alpha production by eosinophils in upper airways inflammation (nasal polyposis). J Immunol. 1994;153(5):2278–89.

163. Hamilos DL, Leung DY, Huston DP, Kamil A, Wood R, Hamid Q. GM-CSF, IL-5 and RANTES immunoreactivity and mRNA expression in chronic hyperplastic sinusitis with nasal polyposis (NP). Clin Exp Allergy. 1998;28(9):1145–52.
164. Bachert C, Wagenmann M, Hauser U, Rudack C. IL-5 synthesis is upregulated in human nasal polyp tissue. J Allergy Clin Immunol. 1997;99(6 Pt 1):837–42.
165. Minshall EM, Cameron L, Lavigne F, Leung DY, Hamilos D, Garcia-Zepada EA, et al. Eotaxin mRNA and protein expression in chronic sinusitis and allergen-induced nasal responses in seasonal allergic rhinitis. Am J Respir Cell Mol Biol. 1997;17(6):683–90.
166. Borrish L. Sinusitis and asthma: entering the realm of evidence-based medicine. J Allergy Clin Immunol. 2002;109(4):606–8.
167. Payne SC, Early SB, Huyett P, Han JK, Borish L, Steinke JW. Evidence for distinct histologic profile of nasal polyps with and without eosinophilia. Laryngoscope. 2011;121(10):2262–7.
168. Early SB, Han JW, Borish L, Steiner JW. Histologic examination reveals distinct disease subsets of chronic sinusitis. J Allergy Clin Immunol. 2007;119(1):S243.
169. Artuc M, Hermes B, Steckelings UM, Grützkau A, Henz BM. Mast cells and their mediators in cutaneous wound healing–active participants or innocent bystanders? Exp Dermatol. 1999;8(1):1–16.
170. Nishijima I, Sanai A, Yoshihara T. A relationship between mast cells and alpha-smooth muscle actin-positive cells in the nasal polyps of chronic rhinosinusitis. Acta Otolaryngol Suppl. 2009;562:110–4.
171. Kato A, Peters A, Suh L, Carter R, Harris KE, Chandra R, et al. Evidence of a role for B cell-activating factor of the TNF family in the pathogenesis of chronic rhinosinusitis with nasal polyps. J Allergy Clin Immunol. 2008;121(6):1385–92, 92.e1–2.
172. Kim JW, Hong SL, Kim YK, Lee CH, Min YG, Rhee CS. Histological and immunological features of non-eosinophilic nasal polyps. Otolaryngol Head Neck Surg. 2007;137(6):925–30.
173. Hu CJ, Wang LY, Chodosh LA, Keith B, Simon MC. Differential roles of hypoxia-inducible factor 1alpha (HIF-1alpha) and HIF-2alpha in hypoxic gene regulation. Mol Cell Biol. 2003;23(24):9361–74.
174. Ouyang Y, Kamijo A, Murata S, Okamoto A, Endo S, Katoh R, et al. Expression of cysLT1 and cysLT2 receptor in chronic hyperplastic eosinophilic sinusitis. Acta Histochem Cytochem. 2009;42(6):191–6.
175. Chiquet-Ehrismann R, Chiquet M. Tenascins: regulation and putative functions during pathological stress. J Pathol. 2003;200(4):488–99.
176. Han JK. Subclassification of chronic rhinosinusitis. Laryngoscope. 2013;123 Suppl 2:S15–27.
177. Safirstein BH. Allergic bronchopulmonary aspergillosis with obstruction of the upper respiratory tract. Chest. 1976;70(6):788–90.
178. Miller JW, Johnston A, Lamb D. Allergic aspergillosis of the maxillary sinuses. Thorax. 1981;36:710.
179. Katzenstein AL, Sale SR, Greenberger PA. Allergic aspergillus sinusitis: a newly recognized form of sinusitis. J Allergy Clin Immunol. 1983;72(1):89–93.
180. Robson JM, Hogan PG, Benn RA, Gatenby PA. Allergic fungal sinusitis presenting as a paranasal sinus tumour. Aust N Z J Med. 1989;19(4):351–3.
181. Pant H, Schembri MA, Wormald PJ, Macardle PJ. IgE-mediated fungal allergy in allergic fungal sinusitis. Laryngoscope. 2009;119(6):1046–52.
182. Collins MM, Nair SB, Wormald PJ. Prevalence of noninvasive fungal sinusitis in South Australia. Am J Rhinol. 2003;17(3):127–32.
183. Bent JP, Kuhn FA. Diagnosis of allergic fungal sinusitis. Otolaryngol Head Neck Surg. 1994;111(5):580–8.
184. Johansson SG, Hourihane JO, Bousquet J, Bruijnzeel-Koomen C, Dreborg S, Haahtela T, et al. A revised nomenclature for allergy. An EAACI position statement from the EAACI nomenclature task force. Allergy. 2001;56(9):813–24.
185. Coombs R, Gell P, Lachmann P. Classification of allergic reactions responsible for clinical hypersensitivity and disease. In: Gell P, Coombs R, Lachmann P, editors. Clinical aspects of immunology. Oxford: Blackwell Scientific; 1968. p. 575–96.

186. Manning SC, Mabry RL, Schaefer SD, Close LG. Evidence of IgE-mediated hypersensitivity in allergic fungal sinusitis. Laryngoscope. 1993;103(7):717–21.
187. Manning SC, Holman M. Further evidence for allergic pathophysiology in allergic fungal sinusitis. Laryngoscope. 1998;108(10):1485–96.
188. Horner WE, Helbling A, Salvaggio JE, Lehrer SB. Fungal allergens. Clin Microbiol Rev. 1995;8(2):161–79.
189. Marple BF. Allergic fungal rhinosinusitis: current theories and management strategies. Laryngoscope. 2001;111(6):1006–19.
190. Katzenstein AL, Sale SR, Greenberger PA. Pathologic findings in allergic aspergillus sinusitis. A newly recognized form of sinusitis. Am J Surg Pathol. 1983;7(5):439–43.
191. Nussenbaum B, Marple BF, Schwade ND. Characteristics of bony erosion in allergic fungal rhinosinusitis. Otolaryngol Head Neck Surg. 2001;124(2):150–4.
192. Mukherji SK, Figueroa RE, Ginsberg LE, Zeifer BA, Marple BF, Alley JG, et al. Allergic fungal sinusitis: CT findings. Radiology. 1998;207(2):417–22.
193. Weschta M, Rimek D, Formanek M, Polzehl D, Riechelmann H. Local production of Aspergillus fumigatus specific immunoglobulin E in nasal polyps. Laryngoscope. 2003;113(10):1798–802.
194. Pérez-Novo CA, Kowalski ML, Kuna P, Ptasinska A, Holtappels G, van Cauwenberge P, et al. Aspirin sensitivity and IgE antibodies to Staphylococcus aureus enterotoxins in nasal polyposis: studies on the relationship. Int Arch Allergy Immunol. 2004;133(3):255–60.
195. Sabirov A, Hamilton RG, Jacobs JB, Hillman DE, Lebowitz RA, Watts JD. Role of local immunoglobulin E specific for Alternaria alternata in the pathogenesis of nasal polyposis. Laryngoscope. 2008;118(1):4–9.
196. Ponikau JU, Sherris DA, Kern EB, Homburger HA, Frigas E, Gaffey TA, et al. The diagnosis and incidence of allergic fungal sinusitis. Mayo Clin Proc. 1999;74(9):877–84.
197. deShazo RD, Swain RE. Diagnostic criteria for allergic fungal sinusitis. J Allergy Clin Immunol. 1995;96(1):24–35.
198. Pant H, Kette FE, Smith WB, Macardle PJ, Wormald PJ. Eosinophilic mucus chronic rhinosinusitis: clinical subgroups or a homogeneous pathogenic entity? Laryngoscope. 2006;116(7):1241–7.
199. Ferguson BJ. Eosinophilic mucin rhinosinusitis: a distinct clinicopathological entity. Laryngoscope. 2000;110(5 Pt 1):799–813.
200. KleinJan A, Godthelp T, van Toornenenbergen AW, Fokkens WJ. Allergen binding to specific IgE in the nasal mucosa of allergic patients. J Allergy Clin Immunol. 1997;99(4):515–21.
201. KleinJan A, Vinke JG, Severijnen LW, Fokkens WJ. Local production and detection of (specific) IgE in nasal B-cells and plasma cells of allergic rhinitis patients. Eur Respir J. 2000;15(3):491–7.
202. Wise SK, Ahn CN, Lathers DM, Mulligan RM, Schlosser RJ. Antigen-specific IgE in sinus mucosa of allergic fungal rhinosinusitis patients. Am J Rhinol. 2008;22(5):451–6.
203. Ryan MW, Marple BF. Allergic fungal rhinosinusitis: diagnosis and management. Curr Opin Otolaryngol Head Neck Surg. 2007;15(1):18–22.
204. Schubert MS, Goetz DW. Evaluation and treatment of allergic fungal sinusitis. II. Treatment and follow-up. J Allergy Clin Immunol. 1998;102(3):395–402.
205. Marple BF, Mabry RL. Comprehensive management of allergic fungal sinusitis. Am J Rhinol. 1998;12(4):263–8.
206. Folker RJ, Marple BF, Mabry RL, Mabry CS. Treatment of allergic fungal sinusitis: a comparison trial of postoperative immunotherapy with specific fungal antigens. Laryngoscope. 1998;108(11 Pt 1):1623–7.
207. Mabry RL, Marple BF, Folker RJ, Mabry CS. Immunotherapy for allergic fungal sinusitis: three years' experience. Otolaryngol Head Neck Surg. 1998;119(6):648–51.
208. Kohl F. A pharmaceutical of the century will be 100. A historical vignette on the introduction of acetylsalicylic acid to the market in 1899. Schmerz. 1999;13(5):341–6.
209. Widal MF, Abrami P, Lermeyez J. Anaphylaxie et idiosyncrasies. Presse Med. 1922;30:189–92.

210. Samter M, Beers RF. Intolerance to aspirin. Clinical studies and consideration of its pathogenesis. Ann Intern Med. 1968;68(5):975–83.
211. Lockey RF, Rucknagel DL, Vanselow NA. Familial occurrence of asthma, nasal polyps and aspirin intolerance. Ann Intern Med. 1973;78(1):57–63.
212. Von Maur K, Adkinson NF, Van Metre TEJ, et al. Aspirin intolerance in a family. J Allergy Clin Immunol. 1974;54:380–95.
213. Morwood K, Gillis D, Smith W, Kette F. Aspirin-sensitive asthma. Intern Med J. 2005;35(4):240–6.
214. Settipane GA, Chafee FH. Nasal polyps in asthma and rhinitis. A review of 6,037 patients. J Allergy Clin Immunol. 1977;59(1):17–21.
215. Stevenson DD. Commentary: the American experience with aspirin desensitization for aspirin-sensitive rhinosinusitis and asthma. Allergy Proc. 1992;13(4):185–92.
216. Szczeklik A, Nizankowska E, Duplaga M. Natural history of aspirin-induced asthma. AIANE Investigators. European Network on Aspirin-Induced Asthma. Eur Respir J. 2000;16(3):432–6.
217. Berges-Gimeno MP, Simon RA, Stevenson DD. The natural history and clinical characteristics of aspirin-exacerbated respiratory disease. Ann Allergy Asthma Immunol. 2002;89(5):474–8.
218. ten Brinke A, Grootendorst DC, Schmidt JT, De Bruïne FT, van Buchem MA, Sterk PJ, et al. Chronic sinusitis in severe asthma is related to sputum eosinophilia. J Allergy Clin Immunol. 2002;109(4):621–6.
219. Mascia K, Haselkorn T, Deniz YM, Miller DP, Bleecker ER, Borish L, et al. Aspirin sensitivity and severity of asthma: evidence for irreversible airway obstruction in patients with severe or difficult-to-treat asthma. J Allergy Clin Immunol. 2005;116(5):970–5.
220. Marquette CH, Saulnier F, Leroy O, Wallaert B, Chopin C, Demarcq JM, et al. Long-term prognosis of near-fatal asthma. A 6-year follow-up study of 145 asthmatic patients who underwent mechanical ventilation for a near-fatal attack of asthma. Am Rev Respir Dis. 1992;146(1):76–81.
221. Cowburn AS, Sladek K, Soja J, Adamek L, Nizankowska E, Szczeklik A, et al. Overexpression of leukotriene C4 synthase in bronchial biopsies from patients with aspirin-intolerant asthma. J Clin Invest. 1998;101(4):834–46.
222. Szczeklik A. The cyclooxygenase theory of aspirin-induced asthma. Eur Respir J. 1990;3(5):588–93.
223. Schmid M, Göde U, Schäfer D, Wigand ME. Arachidonic acid metabolism in nasal tissue and peripheral blood cells in aspirin intolerant asthmatics. Acta Otolaryngol. 1999;119(2):277–80.
224. Sestini P, Armetti L, Gambaro G, Pieroni MG, Refini RM, Sala A, et al. Inhaled PGE2 prevents aspirin-induced bronchoconstriction and urinary LTE4 excretion in aspirin-sensitive asthma. Am J Respir Crit Care Med. 1996;153(2):572–5.
225. Sousa AR, Parikh A, Scadding G, Corrigan CJ, Lee TH. Leukotriene-receptor expression on nasal mucosal inflammatory cells in aspirin-sensitive rhinosinusitis. N Engl J Med. 2002;347(19):1493–9.
226. Corrigan C, Mallett K, Ying S, Roberts D, Parikh A, Scadding G, et al. Expression of the cysteinyl leukotriene receptors cysLT(1) and cysLT(2) in aspirin-sensitive and aspirin-tolerant chronic rhinosinusitis. J Allergy Clin Immunol. 2005;115(2):316–22.
227. Adamjee J, Suh YJ, Park HS, Choi JH, Penrose JF, Lam BK, et al. Expression of 5-lipoxygenase and cyclooxygenase pathway enzymes in nasal polyps of patients with aspirin-intolerant asthma. J Pathol. 2006;209(3):392–9.
228. Dahlén B, Nizankowska E, Szczeklik A, Zetterström O, Bochenek G, Kumlin M, et al. Benefits from adding the 5-lipoxygenase inhibitor zileuton to conventional therapy in aspirin-intolerant asthmatics. Am J Respir Crit Care Med. 1998;157(4 Pt 1):1187–94.
229. Szczeklik A, Nizankowska E. Clinical features and diagnosis of aspirin induced asthma. Thorax. 2000;55 Suppl 2:S42–4.
230. Nasser SM, Patel M, Bell GS, Lee TH. The effect of aspirin desensitization on urinary leukotriene E4 concentrations in aspirin-sensitive asthma. Am J Respir Crit Care Med. 1995;151(5):1326–30.

231. Stevenson DD, Hankammer MA, Mathison DA, Christiansen SC, Simon RA. Aspirin desensitization treatment of aspirin-sensitive patients with rhinosinusitis-asthma: long-term outcomes. J Allergy Clin Immunol. 1996;98(4):751–8.
232. Feldweg AM, Horan RF. Aspirin treatment of patients with aspirin intolerance, asthma, and nasal polyps. Allergy Asthma Proc. 2001;22(6):377–82.
233. Gosepath J, Schäfer D, Mann WJ. Aspirin sensitivity: long term follow-up after up to 3 years of adaptive desensitization using a maintenance dose of 100 mg of aspirin a day. Laryngorhinootologie. 2002;81(10):732–8.
234. Szczeklik A, Gryglewski RJ, Czerniawska-Mysik G. Clinical patterns of hypersensitivity to nonsteroidal anti-inflammatory drugs and their pathogenesis. J Allergy Clin Immunol. 1977;60(5):276–84.
235. Steinke JW, Payne SC, Chen PG, Negri J, Stelow EB, Borish L. Etiology of nasal polyps in cystic fibrosis: not a unimodal disease. Ann Otol Rhinol Laryngol. 2012;121(9):579–86.
236. Babinski D, Trawinska-Bartnicka M. Rhinosinusitis in cystic fibrosis: not a simple story. Int J Pediatr Otorhinolaryngol. 2008;72(5):619–24.
237. Davis PB, Drumm M, Konstan MW. Cystic fibrosis. Am J Respir Crit Care Med. 1996;154(5):1229–56.
238. Wang X, Moylan B, Leopold DA, Kim J, Rubenstein RC, Togias A, et al. Mutation in the gene responsible for cystic fibrosis and predisposition to chronic rhinosinusitis in the general population. JAMA. 2000;284(14):1814–9.
239. De Gaudemar I, Contencin P, Van den Abbeele T, Munck A, Navarro J, Narcy P. Is nasal polyposis in cystic fibrosis a direct manifestation of genetic mutation or a complication of chronic infection? Rhinology. 1996;34(4):194–7.
240. Brinkmann V, Reichard U, Goosmann C, Fauler B, Uhlemann Y, Weiss DS, et al. Neutrophil extracellular traps kill bacteria. Science. 2004;303(5663):1532–5.
241. Yousefi S, Gold JA, Andina N, Lee JJ, Kelly AM, Kozlowski E, et al. Catapult-like release of mitochondrial DNA by eosinophils contributes to antibacterial defense. Nat Med. 2008;14(9):949–53.
242. Vandivier RW, Fadok VA, Ogden CA, Hoffmann PR, Brain JD, Accurso FJ, et al. Impaired clearance of apoptotic cells from cystic fibrosis airways. Chest. 2002;121(3 Suppl):89S.
243. Raynor EM, Butler A, Guill M, Bent JP. Nasally inhaled dornase alfa in the postoperative management of chronic sinusitis due to cystic fibrosis. Arch Otolaryngol Head Neck Surg. 2000;126(5):581–3.
244. Cimmino M, Nardone M, Cavaliere M, Plantulli A, Sepe A, Esposito V, et al. Dornase alfa as postoperative therapy in cystic fibrosis sinonasal disease. Arch Otolaryngol Head Neck Surg. 2005;131(12):1097–101.
245. Balsamo R, Lanata L, Egan CG. Mucoactive drugs. Eur Respir Rev. 2010;19(116):127–33.
246. Mainz JG, Schiller I, Ritschel C, Mentzel HJ, Riethmüller J, Koitschev A, et al. Sinonasal inhalation of dornase alfa in CF: a double-blind placebo-controlled cross-over pilot trial. Auris Nasus Larynx. 2011;38(2):220–7.
247. Cho DY, Hwang PH. Results of endoscopic maxillary mega-antrostomy in recalcitrant maxillary sinusitis. Am J Rhinol. 2008;22(6):658–62.
248. Ryan MW. Diseases associated with chronic rhinosinusitis: what is the significance? Curr Opin Otolaryngol Head Neck Surg. 2008;16(3):231–6.
249. Cannady SB, Batra PS, Koening C, Lorenz RR, Citardi MJ, Langford C, et al. Sinonasal Wegener granulomatosis: a single-institution experience with 120 cases. Laryngoscope. 2009;119(4):757–61.
250. McDonald TJ, DeRemee RA. Head and neck involvement in Wegener's granulomatosis (WG). Adv Exp Med Biol. 1993;336:309–13.
251. Fauci AS, Haynes BF, Katz P, Wolff SM. Wegener's granulomatosis: prospective clinical and therapeutic experience with 85 patients for 21 years. Ann Intern Med. 1983;98(1):76–85.
252. Kallenberg CG. Antineutrophil cytoplasmic antibodies (ANCA) and vasculitis. Clin Rheumatol. 1990;9(1 Suppl 1):132–5.

253. Specks U, Wheatley CL, McDonald TJ, Rohrbach MS, DeRemee RA. Anticytoplasmic autoantibodies in the diagnosis and follow-up of Wegener's granulomatosis. Mayo Clin Proc. 1989;64(1):28–36.
254. Aubart FC, Ouayoun M, Brauner M, Attali P, Kambouchner M, Valeyre D, et al. Sinonasal involvement in sarcoidosis: a case-control study of 20 patients. Medicine (Baltimore). 2006;85(6):365–71.
255. Coffinet L, Chan KH, Abzug MJ, Simões EA, Cool C, Liu AH. Immunopathology of chronic rhinosinusitis in young children. J Pediatr. 2009;154(5):754–8.
256. Nguyen KL, Corbett ML, Garcia DP, Eberly SM, Massey EN, Le HT, et al. Chronic sinusitis among pediatric patients with chronic respiratory complaints. J Allergy Clin Immunol. 1993;92(6):824–30.
257. Cunningham JM, Chiu EJ, Landgraf JM, Gliklich RE. The health impact of chronic recurrent rhinosinusitis in children. Arch Otolaryngol Head Neck Surg. 2000;126(11):1363–8.
258. Bhattacharyya N, Jones DT, Hill M, Shapiro NL. The diagnostic accuracy of computed tomography in pediatric chronic rhinosinusitis. Arch Otolaryngol Head Neck Surg. 2004;130(9):1029–32.
259. Hill M, Bhattacharyya N, Hall TR, Lufkin R, Shapiro NL. Incidental paranasal sinus imaging abnormalities and the normal Lund score in children. Otolaryngol Head Neck Surg. 2004;130(2):171–5.
260. Wald ER. Management of sinusitis in infants and children. Pediatr Infect Dis J. 1988;7(6):449–52.
261. Furukawa CT. The role of allergy in sinusitis in children. J Allergy Clin Immunol. 1992;90(3 Pt 2):515–7.
262. Leo G, Piacentini E, Incorvaia C, Consonni D, Frati F. Chronic rhinosinusitis and allergy. Pediatr Allergy Immunol. 2007;18 Suppl 18:19–21.
263. Di Domenicantonio R, De Sario M, Sammarro S, Compagnucci P, Forastiere F, Pistelli R, et al. Asthma and allergies in childhood in Rome: Italian contribution to the ISAAC II. Epidemiol Prev. 2003;27(4):226–33.
264. Barbero GJ. Gastroesophageal reflux and upper airway disease. Otolaryngol Clin North Am. 1996;29(1):27–38.
265. Bothwell MR, Parsons DS, Talbot A, Barbero GJ, Wilder B. Outcome of reflux therapy on pediatric chronic sinusitis. Otolaryngol Head Neck Surg. 1999;121(3):255–62.
266. Phipps CD, Wood WE, Gibson WS, Cochran WJ. Gastroesophageal reflux contributing to chronic sinus disease in children: a prospective analysis. Arch Otolaryngol Head Neck Surg. 2000;126(7):831–6.
267. Merck W. Pathogenic relationship between adenoid vegetations and maxillary sinusitis in children. HNO. 1974;22(6):198–9.
268. Fukuda K, Matsune S, Ushikai M, Imamura Y, Ohyama M. A study on the relationship between adenoid vegetation and rhinosinusitis. Am J Otolaryngol. 1989;10(3):214–6.
269. Tuncer U, Aydogan B, Soylu L, Simsek M, Akcali C, Kucukcan A. Chronic rhinosinusitis and adenoid hypertrophy in children. Am J Otolaryngol. 2004;25(1):5–10.
270. Berçin AS, Ural A, Kutluhan A, Yurttaş V. Relationship between sinusitis and adenoid size in pediatric age group. Ann Otol Rhinol Laryngol. 2007;116(7):550–3.
271. Bernstein JM, Dryja D, Murphy TF. Molecular typing of paired bacterial isolates from the adenoid and lateral wall of the nose in children undergoing adenoidectomy: implications in acute rhinosinusitis. Otolaryngol Head Neck Surg. 2001;125(6):593–7.
272. Lee D, Rosenfeld RM. Adenoid bacteriology and sinonasal symptoms in children. Otolaryngol Head Neck Surg. 1997;116(3):301–7.
273. Shin KS, Cho SH, Kim KR, Tae K, Lee SH, Park CW, et al. The role of adenoids in pediatric rhinosinusitis. Int J Pediatr Otorhinolaryngol. 2008;72(11):1643–50.
274. Chan KH, Winslow CP, Levin MJ, Abzug MJ, Shira JE, Liu AH, et al. Clinical practice guidelines for the management of chronic sinusitis in children. Otolaryngol Head Neck Surg. 1999;120(3):328–34.

275. Fiocchi A, Sarratud T, Bouygue GR, Ghiglioni D, Bernardo L, Terracciano L. Topical treatment of rhinosinusitis. Pediatr Allergy Immunol. 2007;18 Suppl 18:62–7.
276. Schenkel EJ, Skoner DP, Bronsky EA, Miller SD, Pearlman DS, Rooklin A, et al. Absence of growth retardation in children with perennial allergic rhinitis after one year of treatment with mometasone furoate aqueous nasal spray. Pediatrics. 2000;105(2):E22.
277. Brannan MD, Herron JM, Affrime MB. Safety and tolerability of once-daily mometasone furoate aqueous nasal spray in children. Clin Ther. 1997;19(6):1330–9.
278. Desrosiers MY, Kilty SJ. Treatment alternatives for chronic rhinosinusitis persisting after ESS: what to do when antibiotics, steroids and surgery fail. Rhinology. 2008;46(1):3–14.
279. Ramadan HH. Adenoidectomy vs endoscopic sinus surgery for the treatment of pediatric sinusitis. Arch Otolaryngol Head Neck Surg. 1999;125(11):1208–11.
280. Takahashi H, Honjo I, Fujita A, Kurata K. Effects of adenoidectomy on sinusitis. Acta Otorhinolaryngol Belg. 1997;51(2):85–7.
281. Vandenberg SJ, Heatley DG. Efficacy of adenoidectomy in relieving symptoms of chronic sinusitis in children. Arch Otolaryngol Head Neck Surg. 1997;123(7):675–8.
282. Ramadan HH. Surgical management of chronic sinusitis in children. Laryngoscope. 2004;114(12):2103–9.
283. Sobol SE, Samadi DS, Kazahaya K, Tom LW. Trends in the management of pediatric chronic sinusitis: survey of the American Society of Pediatric Otolaryngology. Laryngoscope. 2005;115(1):78–80.
284. Lusk RP, Muntz HR. Endoscopic sinus surgery in children with chronic sinusitis: a pilot study. Laryngoscope. 1990;100(6):654–8.
285. Hebert RL, Bent JP. Meta-analysis of outcomes of pediatric functional endoscopic sinus surgery. Laryngoscope. 1998;108(6):796–9.
286. Senior B, Wirtschafter A, Mai C, Becker C, Belenky W. Quantitative impact of pediatric sinus surgery on facial growth. Laryngoscope. 2000;110(11):1866–70.
287. Bothwell MR, Piccirillo JF, Lusk RP, Ridenour BD. Long-term outcome of facial growth after functional endoscopic sinus surgery. Otolaryngol Head Neck Surg. 2002;126(6):628–34.
288. Lusk RP, Stankiewicz JA. Pediatric rhinosinusitis. Otolaryngol Head Neck Surg. 1997;117(3 Pt 2):S53–7.
289. Younis RT, Lazar RH. Criteria for success in pediatric functional endonasal sinus surgery. Laryngoscope. 1996;106(7):869–73.
290. Younis RT. The pros and cons of second-look sinonasal endoscopy after endoscopic sinus surgery in children. Arch Otolaryngol Head Neck Surg. 2005;131(3):267–9.

Nasal Polyposis

6

Neville W.Y. Teo and Peter H. Hwang

Key Take Home Points

- Nasal polyposis may be a manifestation of certain underlying conditions, such as aspirin-exacerbated respiratory disease, allergic fungal sinusitis, or autoimmune vasculitis. These should be considered especially in recurrent polyposis.
- Surgery for nasal polyposis not only clears the airway to relieve nasal obstruction but also serves to open up the paranasal sinuses for optimal topical drug delivery as well as decrease the inflammatory burden.
- Advances in medical therapy, such as aspirin desensitization for aspirin-exacerbated respiratory disease, leukotriene modifiers, and topical steroid irrigations, have significantly contributed to controlling the inflammatory response and recurrence of nasal polyposis.

Nasal Polyposis

Nasal polyposis is a challenging clinical condition for the practicing otolaryngologist. While the presentation of polyps in the nasal cavity is the phenotypic expression of chronic inflammation, the underlying etiologies are much more varied. There is a

N.W.Y. Teo, MBBS, MRCS
Department of Otolaryngology, Singapore General Hospital,
The Academia, Level 5, 20 College Road, Singapore 169856, Singapore
e-mail: neville.teo.w.y@sgh.com.sg

P.H. Hwang, MD (✉)
Division of Rhinology and Endoscopic Skull Base Surgery, Department
of Otolaryngology – Head and Neck Surgery, Stanford University School of Medicine,
801 Welch Road, Stanford, CA 94305-5739, USA
e-mail: phwang@ohns.stanford.edu

P.S. Batra, J.K. Han (eds.), *Practical Medical and Surgical Management of Chronic Rhinosinusitis*, DOI 10.1007/978-3-319-16724-4_6

growing understanding that the diagnosis of nasal polyposis in and of itself is sometimes insufficient and that identifying the factors responsible for the individual's presentation can lead to not only directed treatment but also better outcomes.

Nasal polyps are pale edematous growths arising from the underlying nasal mucosa and can be either sessile or pedunculated. They are commonly noted endoscopically in the middle meatus and sphenoethmoid recess, but may also originate from deeper within the paranasal sinuses. Their presence indicates mucosal inflammation, most typically signifying underlying chronic rhinosinusitis (CRS). Nasal polyps may be the hallmark examination finding in certain comorbid conditions associated with CRS, such as aspirin-exacerbated respiratory disease (AERD), allergic fungal sinusitis (AFS), cystic fibrosis, autoimmune vasculitis, and primary ciliary dyskinesia. Choanal polyps, most commonly emanating from the maxillary sinus (antrochoanal), are a distinct clinical entity from typical nasal polyps, as evidenced by a reduced inflammatory profile, a unilateral presentation, and cystic composition.

Epidemiology

Most epidemiological studies focus on asthma, allergic rhinitis, and chronic rhinosinusitis, and there is relatively lesser information pertaining to nasal polyposis specifically. Hospital records from the United States in 1977 revealed a prevalence of nasal polyposis to be 4.2 %, with a higher prevalence of nasal polyposis of 6.7 % among asthmatics [1]. Worldwide figures range from 0.5 % in Korea to 4.3 % in Finland [2, 3]. The average age of onset of nasal polyposis is 42 years, which is older than that for allergic rhinitis or asthma. This later age of diagnosis may reflect in part that some patients may elude diagnosis for some time if they have small, asymptomatic polyps or are quiet sufferers; larger polyps tend to produce more dramatic symptoms that prompt patients to seek medical attention.

Patients with nasal polyposis may present primarily or as recurrent polyps. Studies have found differences in symptom presentations of nonpolyp patients compared with primary polyp and recurrent polyp cases, although overall symptom scores are similar across all three groups. Among these three groups, recurrent nasal polyposis significantly adds to the burden of disease in patients with CRS [4].

Nasal polyposis is not common in pediatric populations, and if found in a child, an underlying comorbid condition such as cystic fibrosis should be sought. Men tend to be more afflicted by the disease than women, although this gender predisposition is reversed in AERD [5].

Histopathological Subtypes

With the increasing awareness of the variety of conditions that may present with nasal polyps, greater focus has shifted to trying to identify the underlying cause for nasal polyposis. Different histopathological subtypes have been found over the years and may be reflected by variances in response to treatment in the different forms of polypoid disease.

Allergic Fungal Sinusitis

Nasal polyposis is one of the hallmark features of allergic fungal sinusitis (AFS). The Bent-Kuhn criteria for the diagnosis of AFS include nasal polyposis, eosinophilic mucin, presence of fungal elements therein, and type I hypersensitivity to fungi, with characteristic CT features of AFS. The initiation of the inflammatory cascade is likely multipronged, requiring the simultaneous occurrence of IgE-mediated sensitivity, specific T-cell HLA receptor expression, and exposure to specific fungi [6, 7]. Fungal allergens trigger IgE-mediated allergic and possibly type III immune complex-mediated mucosal inflammation in the atopic host. Once sensitized, the host demonstrates increased upper and/or lower airway hyperresponsiveness when exposed to an environment with high fungal content [8]. Bacterial superantigens and genetic predisposition may also contribute to the development of AFS, with the nasal polyps manifesting as the final end point of chronic inflammation. The link between fungi and nasal polyps in the absence of AFS is more tenuous, as fungal cultures have also been positive in as large a proportion of healthy controls as patients [9]. However, the presence of local IgE specific to *Alternaria* within nasal polyps, independent of systemic IgE levels or atopic status, suggests a potential role for fungi in the pathophysiology of some forms of nasal polyps, even in nonatopic patients [10].

Aspirin-Exacerbated Respiratory Disease

Aspirin-exacerbated respiratory disease (AERD), also known as Samter's triad, is another important clinical condition presenting with nasal polyps. Patients with AERD present with asthma, chronic rhinosinusitis with nasal polyposis, and anaphylactoid reaction to aspirin or other nonsteroidal anti-inflammatory drugs (NSAIDs). The underlying mechanism of AERD is a dysregulation of the arachidonic acid (AA) metabolism pathway. Arachidonic acid can be metabolized via either the 5-lipoxygenase or cyclooxygenase pathways. The metabolites of either pathway may have either proinflammatory or anti-inflammatory properties and may have stimulatory or inhibitory effects on the other pathway. In AERD, there is a constitutively decreased inhibition of the 5-lipoxygenase pathway, resulting in an overproduction of leukotrienes. This baseline decreased inhibition is likely to be due to decreased production of prostaglandin E_2 (PGE_2), which is an inhibitor of the production of these leukotrienes. The proinflammatory cysteinyl leukotrienes LTC4, LTD4, and LTE4 cause mucosal edema, bronchoconstriction, and mucus secretion as well as induce eosinophil chemotaxis. In addition, there is relative increase in PGD_2, which also acts as a chemoattractant to eosinophils and TH2 cells. Furthermore, AERD patients have been found to have greater expression of cysteinyl leukotrienes type 1 (CysLT1) receptors in nasal inflammatory leukocytes, aggravating their proinflammatory state [11]. Ingestion of aspirin by the patient with AERD causes irreversible inhibition of the cyclooxygenase pathway, further exacerbating the enhanced production of leukotrienes and typically leading to an anaphylactoid reaction marked by acute asthma, nasal congestion, and rhinorrhea.

Chronic Rhinosinusitis with Nasal Polyposis

Recent interest has also focused on identifying the histopathological characteristics of nasal polyps in an attempt to delineate disease endotypes. Hellquist had described four histopathological types of nasal polyps: type 1 is the edematous, eosinophilic allergic polyp; type 2 is the fibroinflammatory polyp with chronic inflammation and epithelial metaplasia; type 3 is similar to type 1, but with pronounced hyperplasia of the seromucinous glands; and type 4 with atypical stroma [12]. The classic "allergic" nasal polyp is found most commonly and, among Western populations, is the predominant form that has been reported in studies. However, while these polyps are associated with an eosinophilic infiltrate, the term "allergic" should be called into question, given the lack of evidence to show that polyps are associated with atopy. In comparison, tissue from Asians with CRSwNP appears to be more biased towards neutrophilic inflammation, although this characteristic may be shifting towards eosinophilic disease [13–16]. Zhang et al. compared nasal polyps from a southern Chinese population with a Belgian population and found that Chinese patients had a lower eosinophil cationic protein/myeloperoxidase ratio of 0.25, with a Th1/Th17 cell pattern instead of the classic Th2 pattern seen in eosinophilic polyps. A separate Chinese study found that 80 % of polyp tissue did not express IL-5, a key cytokine found in eosinophilic inflammation [16]. IL-5-positive polyps produced mediators promoting eosinophilic inflammation, whereas IL-5-negative polyps produced mediators promoting neutrophilic inflammation. In addition, these neutrophilic polyps were associated with a greater Gram-negative bacterial load compared with controls, while eosinophilic polyps were associated with greater Gram-positive bacterial colonization compared with controls and neutrophilic polyps. These differences are clinically significant as they can impact treatment options. One study found that after a 7-day course of prednisone, patients with neutrophil-positive nasal polyps had significantly less reductions in bilateral nasal polyp size scores, nasal congestion scores, total nasal symptom scores, and nasal resistance, compared with patients with neutrophil-negative polyps [13].

Antrochoanal Polyps

Antrochoanal polyps account for 4–6 % of all nasal polyps, but are clinically distinct from typical inflammatory polyposis [17]. Antrochoanal polyps usually present as an isolated unilateral polyp arising from the maxillary sinus. Endoscopically they can be seen to protrude from the maxillary antrum through the posterior fontanelle and extending towards the posterior choana, hence their name. Other types of choanal polyps have been described in the literature, based on their origin, such as sphenochoanal and ethmochoanal polyps [18]. The underlying pathophysiology of antrochoanal polyps remains unclear, although they are thought to arise from an expanding intramural cyst in the maxillary sinus. Clinically they appear distinct from CRSwNP in that they are large, unilateral, and singular and have a prominent cystic component within the maxillary sinus, while CRSwNP patients have multiple smaller polyps that are commonly bilateral. Antrochoanal polyps have a strong predisposition for recurrence if resection of the mass is incomplete. Surgical extirpation of the antrochoanal polyp therefore requires removal of the nasal component as well as meticulous dissection of the attachment site within the sinus cavity to reduce recurrence.

Cystic Fibrosis

Cystic fibrosis (CF) is an autosomal recessive disorder that affects the respiratory and gastrointestinal tracts and is more commonly found in the Caucasian population. The underlying genetic cause is a dysfunction or deficiency of the cystic fibrosis transmembrane conductance regulator (CFTR), which is involved in anionic transport across respiratory and exocrine glandular epithelial membranes. Disturbance of chloride and bicarbonate transport across respiratory membranes results in a much higher viscosity of mucus than normal and impairs mucociliary clearance [19]. CF patients have also been found to have increased proinflammatory cytokine, leukotriene, and prostaglandin production, as well as being more prone to *Pseudomonas* colonization, all of which may further contribute to having CRS. Beyond having CRS, a higher proportion of CF patients also have nasal polyposis compared with the non-CF population [20]. Nasal polyps in CF also typically show neutrophilic Th1-mediated inflammation rather than the eosinophilic Th2-mediated inflammation that is more commonly seen in CRSwNP [21, 22].

Etiology

Numerous factors have been identified that may contribute to the development of nasal polyposis. Factors such as allergy, bacterial superantigen stimulation, leukotriene metabolism, and fungi have all been implicated in the predominantly Th2-mediated inflammation that is seen in Western populations. Mechanical factors, such as defects in the mucosal barrier, ciliary dysfunction, and even the Bernoulli phenomenon, also can play a role in the pathogenesis of nasal polyps.

Inflammation

Regardless of other contributory factors or possible etiologies, inflammation plays a predominant role in the development of nasal polyposis. Nasal polyps, when noted in the nasal cavity, indicate the presence of chronic sinonasal inflammation. The majority of CRSwNP in the Western population is eosinophilic with Th2-mediated inflammation. Eosinophilic polyps are associated with raised interleukin (IL)-5 levels and elevated eosinophilic cationic protein (ECP) to myeloperoxidase (MPO) ratio of more than 1 [21, 23]. Recent studies have also implicated IL-25 and IL-33 as a link between the response from epithelial cells and Th2-mediated inflammation [24]. In contrast to the classic Th2-mediated inflammation, Th1-/Th17-mediated inflammation has been reported in Asian polyps, with either intermediate eosinophilic or neutrophilic infiltrates [13, 14]. Among Chinese with CRSwNP, studies have shown enhanced IL-17 in both eosinophilic and noneosinophilic inflammation [15, 25]. Further studies are indicated to further elucidate the inflammatory processes involved in the pathogenesis of various polyp subtypes, which will hopefully lead to the identification of novel therapeutic targets.

Bacterial Superantigen

Increasing interest has arisen regarding the role of bacterial superantigens in CRS with and without nasal polyps. Superantigens link directly with the major histocompatibility II complex (MHC II), bypassing the antigen-presenting cells (APCs), and cause non-specific polyclonal activation of T cells containing the specific Vβ region, resulting in massive cytokine release that further attracts more inflammatory cells [26]. Numerous studies have examined the association between *Staphylococcus aureus* enterotoxin superantigens and CRSwNP, with varying results. A recent meta-analysis collated 12 studies with 340 cases and 178 controls and found that the culture-positive rate of *Staphylococcus aureus*, detection rate of *Staphylococcus* superantigens, and titers of *Staphylococcus*-specific IgE were significantly higher in patients with CRSwNP than controls. They concluded that the presence of *Staphylococcus aureus* superantigens is related to disease severity and may be a risk factor for CRSwNP [27].

Atopy

There has been much interest in the role of allergy in CRSwNP, with mixed and sometimes conflicting evidence regarding an association between the two conditions. The striking tissue eosinophilia found in a majority of nasal polyps suggests that allergy may be implicated, but the significance of atopy remains controversial. A recent evidence-based review by Wilson et al. identified 18 studies examining this relationship, with 10 supporting an association, 7 showing no association, and 1 showing a possible association [28]. The 10 affirmative studies examined allergic reactions to aeroallergens, food allergies, and bacterial pathogens and suggested certain allergens, like perennial allergens, milk sensitivity, and *Staphylococcus aureus* colonization, being more responsible than others. On the other hand, the nonconfirmatory studies suggested that other sources of inflammation than allergy may play a role in nasal polyposis. The evidence linking asthma with CRSwNP is much stronger, with several studies showing that patients with CRSwNP had higher rates of asthma versus controls.

Ciliary Dysfunction

Abnormalities in ciliary function can result in stasis of mucus and lead to CRS. This dysfunction can be either primary or secondary. The former is epitomized by primary ciliary dyskinesia and Kartagener's syndrome, where structural defects in the cilia result in ineffective or discoordinated ciliary movement and abnormal mucociliary clearance. This leads to recurrent and chronic infections of the entire respiratory tract. Impaired mucociliary clearance is also partially responsible for the pathophysiology of CRS in CF patients. Secondary ciliary dysfunction can be found in patients with CRS, as well as postoperative patients, although this can possibly be reversed with time.

Epithelial Defects/Toll-Like Receptors

In the setting of similar exposure to potential triggers, what makes one individual develop CRSwNP and another not? Disorders in local host immunity and integrity of the epithelial barrier can possibly explain for this in part. Nasal polyps have been found to have decreased trans-tissue resistance, decreased expressions of tight junction proteins, epithelial adherens junction protein E-cadherin, and desmoglein-2 and desmoglein-3, which are postulated to be secondary to tissue inflammation. These changes contribute to a defective epithelial barrier found in patients with nasal polyposis [29–31].

Disorders of mucosal immunity can also contribute to inflammation. Decreased expression of toll-like receptors, markers of innate immunity, was found in postsurgical patients with recurrent polyposis [32]. Decreased expression of innate immune proteins of the palate, lung and nasal epithelium clone (PLUNC) family, specifically SPLUNC1 and LPLUNC2, was found in nasal polyps versus controls, with a corresponding reduced number of submucosal glands, further suggesting the role of local host immune dysfunction contributing to polyp formation [33, 34].

Bernoulli Phenomenon

Earlier work on the possible causes of CRS and nasal polyps suggested the possibility of Bernoulli's phenomenon contributing to the formation of polyps. Observations of mucosal edema at anatomic points of narrowing, such as the middle meatus, maxillary sinus ostium, and a deviated septum, led to the thinking that the negative pressure caused by airflow through these areas may lead to edema and polyp enlargement [35]. While no studies have been conducted to assess the veracity of this relationship, surgical principles in dealing with nasal polyposis are aimed at creating wide access to the paranasal sinuses to allow for improved drainage and clearance and topical drug delivery. A retrospective study had also found that resection of the middle turbinate helped in delaying return to revision surgery in patients with nasal polyposis, further suggesting a possible link [36].

Clinical Presentation

The typical presentation of patients with nasal polyposis is that of nasal obstruction or congestion, rhinorrhea, postnasal drainage, decreased or loss of sense of smell, and facial pain or pressure. Patients with CRS without polyps are more likely to present with facial pain or pressure and headaches, while patients with nasal polyps are more likely to present with nasal obstruction and hyposmia [4, 37, 38]. In addition, patient with advanced polyposis may have noticeable widening of the nasal bridge, and patients may sometimes present due to self-visualization of the polyps from the anterior nares.

Examination

Beyond an external nasal examination and anterior rhinoscopy, performing a detailed endoscopic examination of the nasal cavity provides the greatest diagnostic information. Notes should be made regarding the distribution, character, and appearance of polyps as well as their laterality and site of attachment if observable. The extent of nasal polyps can be endoscopically staged into the following: no polyps (0), restricted to middle meatus (1), extending below the middle turbinate (2), and massive polyposis (3). Differential diagnoses for unilateral nasal polyps vary from bilateral polyps; conditions that should be considered in unilateral polyposis include antrochoanal polyp, inverted papilloma, juvenile nasopharyngeal angiofibroma, olfactory neuroblastoma, and other sinonasal tumors. The character of the polyps may help differentiate between inflammatory polyps and sinonasal tumors. While the former appears pale and edematous, the latter conditions may appear more fleshy and hyperemic, with an irregular surface. Inverted papilloma may also be found within inflammatory polyps, and so vigilance should be practiced in noting any difference in the character of the polyps encountered (see Fig. 6.1a-c). Meningoceles and encephaloceles may also present as a unilateral mass without CSF rhinorrhea, especially with a history of previous sinus surgery or significant head trauma (see Fig. 6.2a, b). An isolated unilateral polyp is best assessed by imaging prior to obtaining pathology biopsy, unless the attachment is clearly visualized and is not attached to the skull base. In addition, any associated mucopurulence should be noted and cultured to guide antibiotic selection.

Imaging

Computed tomography (CT) of the paranasal sinuses remains the primary imaging modality for evaluating patients with nasal polyposis. Signal heterogeneity within the sinuses, best observed on soft tissue windows, may indicate underlying fungal sinusitis, secondary to the presence of metals such as iron or manganese, or calcium precipitates within the mucin. CT is excellent at detailing bony anatomy, and in the paranasal sinuses, bony changes of the skull base or lamina papyracea may differentiate polyps from other polyp-like masses. For example, focal hyperostosis seen adjacent to the edge of the polypoid mass may suggest the diagnosis of an inverted papilloma. Conversely, skull base erosion may indicate extrasinus expansion of a nasal polyp or mass, or the possibility of an encephalocele. In the setting of an isolated polyp-like mass with CT evidence of skull base erosion, magnetic resonance

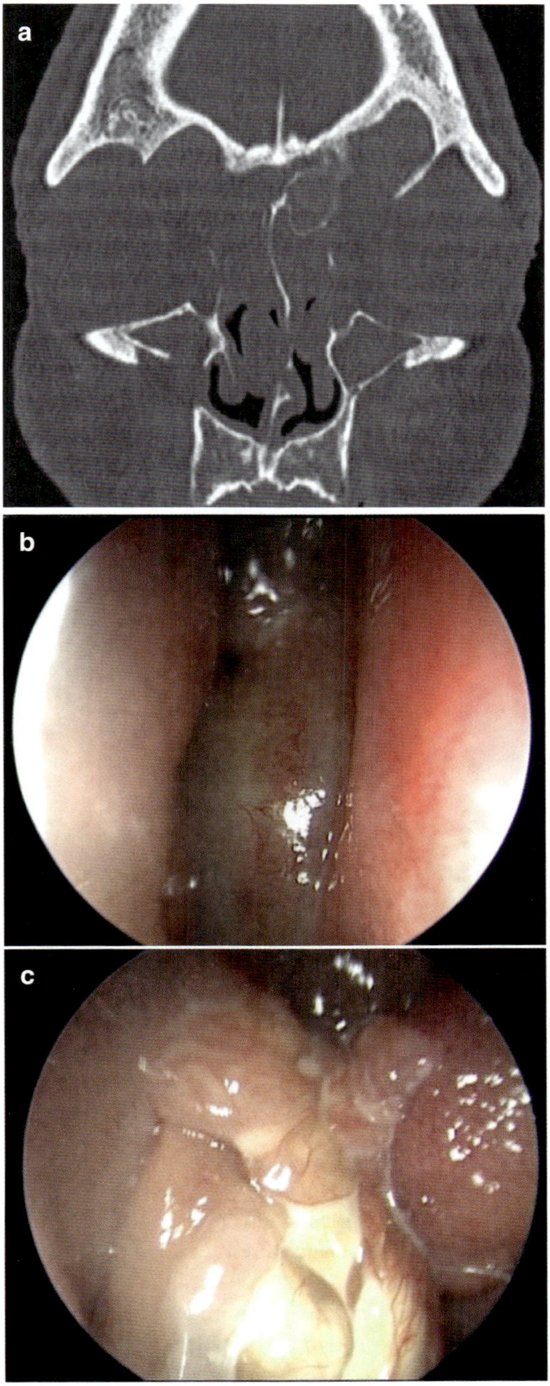

Fig. 6.1 (**a**-**b**) Coexistent nasal polyposis, frontal mucoceles, and inverted papilloma (IP). Note the fleshy looking appearance of the IP that is different from the edematous pale nasal polyps

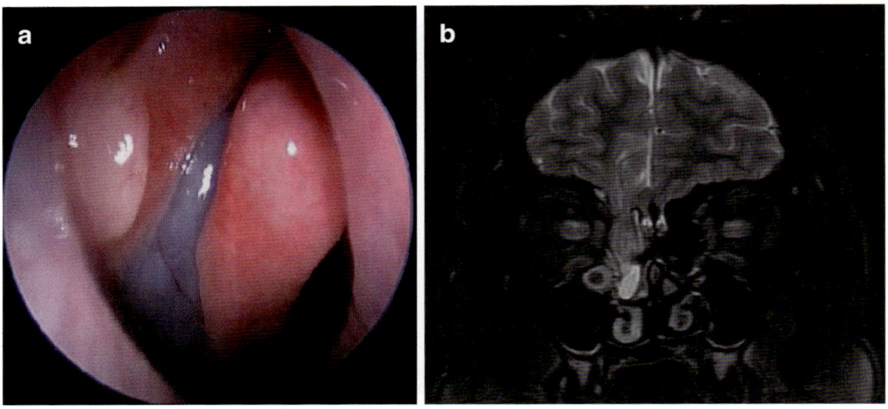

Fig. 6.2 (**a**) A meningoencephalocele can mimic the endoscopic appearance of a middle meatal polyp. (**b**) MRI revealing the presence of the meningoencephalocele

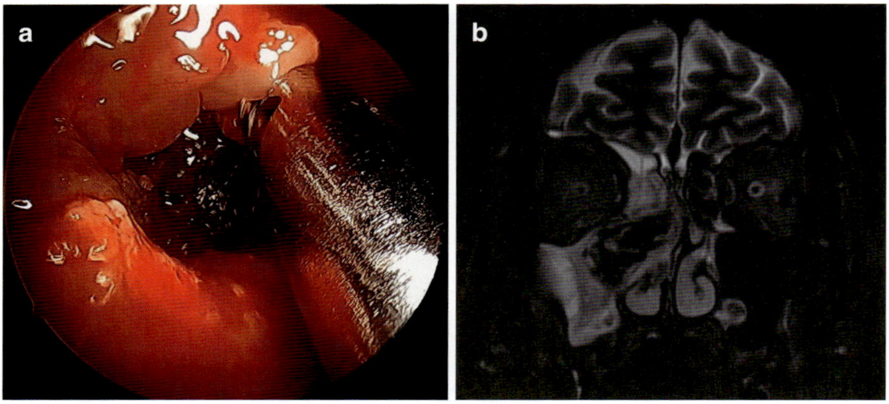

Fig. 6.3 (**a**) Allergic fungal sinusitis with polyps and fungal mucin obliterating the maxillary sinus. (**b**) T2-weighted MRI showing central hypointensity and signal void with peripheral hyperintensity in the inflamed mucosal lining

imaging is indicated to differentiate polyp from meningoencephalocele. CT scans can also be used for intraoperative navigation, especially in the setting of massive polyposis or revision surgery, where anatomy may be distorted.

Magnetic resonance imaging (MRI) is generally not performed in the workup of nasal polyposis, unless there are specific concerns of a meningoencephalocele or suspicion of a sinonasal tumor. MRI findings in allergic fungal sinusitis are characteristic, with a low T2 signal or signal void due to high concentration of various metals such as iron, magnesium, and manganese concentrated by fungal organisms as well as high protein and low free water content in allergic mucin. The inflamed mucosal lining will be hyperintense on T2-weighted imaging and demonstrate contrast enhancement (see Fig. 6.3a, b).

Allergy and Immune Workup

Allergy evaluation by skin or blood testing is indicated to rule out comorbid atopic disease that may play a role in some patients with CRSwNP. NSAID intolerance should also be specifically queried to rule out AERD. In patients with nasal polyposis who have had multiple recurring infections of the upper and lower respiratory tracts, a workup for selective immunodeficiency or common variable immunodeficiency may be considered, including measurements of serum immunoglobulin (Ig) levels and pre- and postpneumococcal vaccine titers. The possibility of Churg-Strauss syndrome should also be considered, especially in patients with preexisting asthma and allergic rhinitis with unexplained worsening of asthma and subsequent development of hypereosinophilia that may occur together with vasculitis. Cystic fibrosis (CF) testing should also be considered, either by sweat chloride test or genetic testing. Less commonly, primary ciliary dyskinesia may be present, and diagnosis will require obtaining nasal biopsy to examine ciliary ultrastructure by electron microscopy.

Treatment

The treatment of nasal polyposis has evolved, as an improved understanding of the underlying pathophysiological mechanisms has led to the development of newer therapies. In patients where surgery is contraindicated or not elected, medical therapy can be used to try to control or alleviate symptoms and polyp growth. Anti-inflammatory medications are playing a more important role now as there is a greater appreciation of the need to control inflammation and prevent polyp recurrence.

Surgical

Surgical treatment of nasal polyposis should not be viewed with an expectation to cure the disease, but rather as an important adjunctive therapy to ongoing medical treatment. Surgery can range from simple polypectomy to comprehensive endoscopic sinus surgery (ESS). Although the former may suffice in less severe disease as a temporizing measure, ESS with complete polyp removal and opening all paranasal sinuses should be considered the standard surgical therapy for symptomatic, medically refractory nasal polyposis. This not only reduces the inflammatory load and allows ventilation of the sinuses, but it also facilitates delivery of topical medications into the sinuses. Cadaveric and in vivo studies have shown that topical delivery of medications into the sinuses is improved post-ESS. Furthermore, a meta-analysis on topical steroid therapy for nasal polyps showed that the patients who underwent sinus surgery had a greater response to topical steroid treatments than those without surgery [39].

Certain surgical techniques may be employed to better optimize the surgical sinusotomies for delivery of topical medication. For example, partial resection of the middle turbinate has been shown to prolong the interval to revision surgery for nasal polyposis, although a retrospective study showed the time difference to be only 6 months [36]. The endoscopic maxillary mega-antrostomy, also known as modified endoscopic medial maxillectomy, can be helpful in the treatment of recalcitrant maxillary sinusitis [40]. This procedure involves removing the posterior half of the inferior turbinate and a portion of the medial wall of the maxillary sinus, so as to facilitate sinus hygiene and to improve delivery of topical medications and irrigations. This effect was possibly due to the increased air space which reduces polyp regrowth and allows better access for drug delivery.

Due to the propensity for recurrence of polyps, continued postoperative surveillance of the sinonasal cavities with serial endoscopy is important. For focal polyp recurrences, in-office polypectomies may help to maintain patency of sinus ostia for drug delivery without needing to bring the patient back to the operating room.

Medical

With newer methods of drug delivery, medical therapy has come to play an increased role in the management of nasal polyps. Whereas oral medications are useful to treat systemic conditions, for inflammatory disease restricted to the nose and paranasal sinuses, topical therapies can be directed to the target tissue while sparing systemic side effects.

Oral Steroids

Systemic corticosteroids can effectively reduce the size of nasal polyps, and while the benefits of relieving nasal obstruction and improving olfaction often outlast the duration of therapy, the therapeutic effects are relatively short-lived. For management of acute exacerbations and for pulsed steroid therapy, there is no evidence-based consensus on optimal dosing, although the upper limit in most studies has been 60 mg of prednisone daily for 20 days. Gastrointestinal upset, insomnia, and transient adrenal suppression are among the potential side effects of orally administered corticosteroids. When given preoperatively, oral steroids improve visualization of surgical field and potentially decrease blood loss and operative time. The literature suggests that a daily dose of 30 mg of prednisone started 5–7 days preoperatively is a safe and effective starting point [41]. Postoperatively, systemic steroids can help to reduce postsurgical edema and inflammation and prevent early synechiae formation [42].

While oral corticosteroids have been found to be effective in treating patients with classic eosinophilic polyps, patients with neutrophilic polyps seem to respond less favorably. Wen et al. found that oral steroid therapy reduces eosinophil counts but not neutrophil counts in nasal polyps, and patients with eosinophilic polyps had significantly better oral steroid responses than those with neutrophilic polyps, in terms of reduction of polyp size, nasal congestion and total nasal symptom scores, and nasal resistance [13]. Understanding the histopathology of nasal polyps may thus help to individualize therapy and improve treatment responses.

Topical Steroids: Sprays and Rinses

In contrast to the short-term efficacy of systemic steroids, the role of topical steroids is to maintain long-term control of nasal polyps. There are a variety of drug delivery mechanisms, ranging from low-volume low-pressure systems (nasal drops and sprays) to high-volume high-pressure systems (nasal irrigation). There is general agreement that topical steroid therapy helps to alleviate symptoms, reduces polyp size, and prevents recurrence of polyps postoperatively [43]. Intranasal corticosteroid sprays have been the most well studied and have proven to be efficacious for nasal polyposis.

Intranasal steroid irrigations have become popularized but are less well studied. The potential benefit of delivering a higher dose of corticosteroids locally while minimizing systemic side effects is attractive, although there are few randomized trials to date that specifically look at this therapy. Safety studies have found no negative effect on the hypothalamus-pituitary-adrenal (HPA) axis after 6–8 weeks of continuous irrigations with budesonide [44, 45].

Oral Antibiotics

Despite nasal polyposis being largely an inflammatory condition, infectious sinusitis may be an associated condition. Antibiotics can play a role in treating the infectious portion of the disease, although there are few randomized trials looking at this. Short-term courses of antibiotics should be considered, particularly when pus is present and can be cultured, as an adjunct to maximal medical therapy and in acute exacerbations. Antibiotic therapy longer than 3 weeks is generally not recommended for infectious indications.

Doxycycline and macrolide antibiotics have been used in the treatment of nasal polyposis for their intrinsic anti-inflammatory properties, which are thought to be more effective for neutrophil-associated inflammation than eosinophilic inflammation. Treatment duration is often longer than for infectious indications, even up to 1 year. One study compared doxycycline with methylprednisolone and placebo and found significant reduction in polyp size and postnasal drainage associated with doxycycline, although there was no other symptom improvement or improvement in peak nasal inspiratory flow (PNIF) [46].

Studies of macrolides have been characterized by heterogeneous inclusion criteria and treatment outcome measures. The number of high-quality studies is limited, with the majority being prospective observational studies. One controlled study showed improved patient symptoms and endoscopic findings using roxithromycin 150 mg daily for 3 months in refractory CRS patients, especially in the subgroup with low IgE levels [47], while another controlled study using low-dose azithromycin did not show any difference from placebo [48]. Overall data from observational studies however show general improvements in patient symptoms, endoscopic findings, imaging findings, and reduction of inflammatory markers within nasal mucus secretions [49]. Macrolides are thus a therapeutic option in the treatment of CRSwNP. Whether the beneficial effects are truly due to the anti-inflammatory properties or the antimicrobial effects of macrolide antibiotics, or a combination of both, bears further study. The optimal subgroup of patients who may benefit most from this therapy also remains to be determined.

Topical Antibiotics: Rinses

In contrast to topical corticosteroid therapy, topical antibiotic use in the management of nasal polyps is a lot more controversial. Theoretical benefits of topical antibiotics include eradication of biofilm and reduction of *Staphylococcus* superantigen load, although one small randomized trial showed only short-term improvement with mupirocin nasal rinses in recalcitrant Staphylococcal CRS which was not sustained in the longer term [50]. Studies have mostly focused on CRS and not specifically on nasal polyposis, so that it is not recommended for routine use in patients with CRSwNP.

Aspirin Desensitization

Aspirin desensitization is a key treatment modality in managing nasal polyposis in patients with AERD, as an adjunct to surgery and medical therapy. The exact mechanism of action is unknown, although rapid induction of oral tolerance is associated with a decrease in serum cysteinyl leukotrienes and improvement in the dysregulation of arachidonic acid metabolism [51, 52]. Aspirin desensitization has been shown to improve symptoms and quality of life, prevent polyp regrowth, and reduce the need for oral corticosteroids and revision surgery and is optimally initiated within 4–8 weeks after sinus surgery [53–56]. Desensitization protocols vary, although most can be executed in an ambulatory setting, in contrast to earlier years in which desensitization was performed in the intensive care unit. Once desensitization has been achieved, maintenance doses are typically from 650 mg to 1,300 mg daily for life, with repeat desensitization needed if more than 96 hours has elapsed between doses. Our experience with aspirin desensitization is that the majority of patients are able to tolerate and complete it, with sustained endoscopic and symptom improvement over a prolonged period [57].

Antifungal Therapy

Given the possible link between fungi and CRS, people have studied using antifungal therapy in the treatment of CRS and its subtypes. The results so far have not shown benefit for antifungal therapy in either CRSwNP or AFS. Two clinical trials evaluating nasal amphotericin B sprays in patients with nasal polyps did not show benefit in symptom scores [58, 59]. A more recent systematic review looking at antifungal therapy for AFS also showed no overall benefit in topical or oral antifungal therapy on endoscopic scores or patient reported outcomes, with no significant differences between treatment and control groups [60].

Immunotherapy

Immunotherapy should be considered in atopic patients with CRSwNP, as this can help with symptomatic outcomes postoperatively [61]. Fungal immunotherapy is also an option in treating patients with AFS specifically, since the disease is characterized by an excessive immune response to fungi. Studies are limited to using dilute antigen concentrations in patients who have been operated upon to decrease the inflammatory load, although recent practice parameters have advocated higher allergen concentrations [62]. Recommendations have also been made to initiate fungal immunotherapy 4–6 weeks after surgery, to avoid exacerbation of symptoms in patients with active AFS [63]. The overall role of immunotherapy can thus be seen as adjunctive in the treatment of nasal polyposis.

Leukotriene Modifiers

Leukotrienes are mediators in the inflammatory cascade, and so it is unsurprising that increased levels of leukotrienes and its receptors have been shown in nasal polyps. Leukotriene antagonists have been shown to be effective in chronic inflammatory conditions of the airway such as allergic rhinitis and asthma, conditions which are commonly coexistent with nasal polyposis. Examples of CysLT1 receptor antagonists include montelukast and zafirlukast, while zileuton is an inhibitor of 5-lipoxygenase. Randomized controlled trials have shown that montelukast is effective in symptom reduction of nasal polyposis compared with placebo and equally effective compared with intranasal corticosteroid sprays in this respect [64]. Combination therapy of montelukast with budesonide sprays showed significant improvement in headache, facial pain, and sneezing, compared to monotherapy with budesonide sprays [65]. Lower evidence studies have also shown zafirlukast and zileuton to provide similar symptom improvement in CRSwNP [66, 67].

When considering AERD where the underlying mechanism is due to dysregulation of arachidonic acid metabolism with decreased inhibition of the 5-lipoxygenase pathway, drugs such as the 5-lipoxygenase inhibitor zileuton should theoretically be effective in treating the disease. Ulualp et al. looked at zileuton and zafirlukast in AERD patients and found significant improvement in symptom scores, subjective reports, and endoscopic examination [66]. Montelukast was also found to have improvement in both aspirin-tolerant and aspirin-sensitive patients with nasal polyps and asthma, with improvements in polyp score only present in aspirin-tolerant patients [68]. Based on current literature, while we know that leukotriene antagonists can help in the management of nasal polyposis, finding the optimal use in the correct patient population and setting still requires further investigation.

Biologic Agents

The newest anti-inflammatory agents being investigated in the treatment of nasal polyposis are antibodies targeting parts of the inflammatory cascade. Anti-IL5 agents – mepolizumab and reslizumab – are humanized monoclonal antibodies that target eosinophilic inflammation. One trial evaluating reslizumab showed a decrease in total nasal polyp score and decrease in blood eosinophil counts compared to placebo, although there was rebound hypereosinophilia posttreatment [69]. There was however no significant difference in symptom scores or nasal peak inspiratory flow (nPIF) between treatment and placebo groups. Another trial compared mepolizumab against placebo and similarly showed improved nasal polyp score, blood eosinophil counts, and computed tomographic score [70]. These improvements were seen in 60 % of treated patients, and there were no markers to suggest possible responders to anti-IL5 therapy. There were also improvements in some symptom scores, namely hyposmia, congestion, and postnasal drip, although these did not reach significance.

Omalizumab is a recombinant DNA-derived humanized IgG monoclonal antibody that selectively binds to IgE. It has been studied in the treatment of asthma and allergic rhinitis and more recently in CRS. One trial specifically looked at the effect of omalizumab in treating patients with nasal polyps and comorbid asthma and found that there was significant reduction in total nasal polyp score with corresponding improvements in Lund-Mackay scores on CT [71]. There was also significant improvement in symptom scores and the Short-Form Health Questionnaire SF-36 on physical health, although no difference was found in mental health. No differences were found in treatment outcomes between allergic and nonallergic patients. There are however concerns with prescribing omalizumab, such as the risk of anaphylaxis in 1 patient per 1,000 as well as potential cardiac effects and thrombocytopenia. There is also the potential of higher than expected arterial thrombotic events. Earlier concerns regarding malignancies related to omalizumab seem unfounded, as recent studies do not suggest an association between omalizumab therapy and an increased risk of malignancy [72].

Conclusion

Nasal polyps remain a challenging entity to treat, with a great variation in clinical presentation and treatment responses. Such differences may be related to varied endotypes of polyposis, whose discernment is an emerging focus of current research. Indeed, nasal polyposis is a heterogeneous entity, with different phenotypic presentations, histological variations, and etiological factors contributing to its formation. Surgery and steroid medications remain the mainstays of treatment, but with the identification of novel therapeutic targets, more varied treatment options can be expected to emerge, with hope for improving outcomes for patients in the years ahead.

References

1. Settipane GA, Chafee FH. Nasal polyps in asthma and rhinitis. A review of 6,037 patients. J Allergy Clin Immunol. 1977;59(1):17–21.
2. Min YG, Jung HW, Kim HS, Park SK, Yoo KY. Prevalence and risk factors of chronic sinusitis in Korea: results of a nationwide survey. Eur Arch Otorhinolaryngol. 1996;253(7):435–9.
3. Hedman K, Kaprio J, Poussa T, Nieminen MM. Prevalence of asthma, aspirin intolerance, nasal polyposis and chronic obstructive pulmonary disease in a population-based study. Int J Epidemiol. 1999;28(4):717–22.
4. Bhattacharyya N. Assessing the additional disease burden of polyps in chronic rhinosinusitis. Ann Otol Rhinol Laryngol. 2009;118(3):185–9.
5. Chaaban MR, Walsh EM, Woodworth BA. Epidemiology and differential diagnosis of nasal polyps. Am J Rhinol Allergy. 2013;27(6):473–8.
6. Milroy CM, Blanshard JD, Lucas S, Michaels L. Aspergillosis of the nose and paranasal sinuses. J Clin Pathol. 1989;42:123–7.

7. Horst M, Hejjaoni A, Horst V, Michel FB, Bosquet J. Double-blind, placebo controlled rush immunotherapy with a standardized Alternaria extract. J Allergy Clin Immunol. 1990;85:460–72.
8. Downs S, Mitkakis T, Marks G, et al. Clinical importance of Alternaria exposure in children. Am J Respir Crit Care Med. 2001;164:455–9.
9. Ponikau JU, Sherris DA, Kern EB, Homburger HA, Frigas E, Gaffey TA, et al. The diagnosis and incidence of allergic fungal sinusitis. Mayo Clin Proc. 1999;74:877–84.
10. Sabirov A, Hamilton RG, Jacobs JB, Hillman DE, Lebowitz RA, Watts JD. Role of local immunoglobulin E specific for Alternaria alternata in the pathogenesis of nasal polyposis. Laryngoscope. 2008;118:4–9.
11. Ozen Z, Mumbuc S, Sari I, Baglam T, Karatas E, Kanlikama M. Cysteinyl leukotriene receptor expression in aspirin-sensitive nasal polyposis patients. ORL J Otorhinolaryngol Relat Spec. 2007;69:176–80.
12. Hellquist HB. Nasal polyps update. Histopathology. Allergy Asthma Proc. 1996;17(5):237–42.
13. Wen W, Liu W, Zhang L, et al. Increased neutrophilia in nasal polyps reduces the response to oral corticosteroid therapy. J Allergy Clin Immunol. 2012;129(6):1522–8.
14. Kirtsreesakul V. Update on nasal polyps: etiopathogenesis. J Med Assoc Thai. 2005;88(12):1966–72.
15. Zhang N, Van Zele T, Perez-Novo C, et al. Different types of T-effector cells orchestrate mucosal inflammation in chronic sinus disease. J Allergy Clin Immunol. 2008;122(5):961–8.
16. Ba L, Zhang N, Meng J, et al. The association between bacterial colonization and inflammatory pattern in Chinese chronic rhinosinusitis patients with nasal polyps. Allergy. 2011;66:1296–303.
17. Yaman H, Yilmaz S, Karali E, et al. Evaluation and management of antrochoanal polyps. Clin Exp Otorhinolaryngol. 2010;3:110–4.
18. Kizil Y, Aydil U, Ceylan A, et al. Analysis of choanal polyps. J Craniofac Surg. 2014;25(3): 1082–84.
19. Regnis JA, Robinson M, Bailey DL, et al. Mucociliary clearance in patients with cystic fibrosis and in normal subjects. Am J Respir Crit Care Med. 1994;150(1):66–71.
20. Robertson JM, Friedman EM, Rubin BK. Nasal and sinus disease in cystic fibrosis. Paediatr Respir Rev. 2008;9(3):213–9.
21. Van Zele T, Claeys S, Gevaert P, Van Maele G, Holtappels G, Van Cauwenberge P, et al. Differentiation of chronic sinus diseases by measurement of inflammatory mediators. Allergy. 2006;61(11):1280–9.
22. Claeys S, Van Hoecke H, Holtappels G, et al. Nasal polyps in patients with and without cystic fibrosis: a differentiation by innate markers and inflammatory mediators. Clin Exp Allergy. 2005;35(4):467–72.
23. Bachert C, Zhang N, Holtappels G, et al. Presence of IL-5 protein and IgE antibodies to staphylococcal enterotoxins in nasal polyps is associated with comorbid asthma. J Allergy Clin Immunol. 2010;126:962–8, 968.e1–6.
24. Lam M, Hull L, McLachlan R, Snidvongs K, et al. Clinical severity and epithelial endotypes in chronic rhinosinusitis. Int Forum Allergy Rhinol. 2013;3(2):121–8.
25. Jiang XD, Li GY, Li L, et al. The characterization of IL-17A expression in patients with chronic rhinosinusitis with nasal polyps. Am J Rhinol Allergy. 2011;25:e171–5.
26. Conley DB, Tripathi A, Seiberling KA, et al. Superantigens and chronic rhinosinusitis: skewing of T-cell receptor V beta-distributions in polyp-derived CD4+ and CD8+ T cells. Am J Rhinol. 2006;20(5):534–9.
27. Ou J, Wang J, Xu Y, et al. Staphylococcus aureus superantigens are associated with chronic rhinosinusitis with polyps: a meta-analysis. Eur Arch Otorhinolaryngol. 2014;271(10):2729–36.
28. Wilson KF, McMains KC, Orlandi RR. The association between allergy and chronic rhinosinusitis with and without nasal polyps: an evidence-based review with recommendations. Int Forum Allergy Rhinol. 2014;4:93–103.
29. Soyka MB, Wawrzyniak P, Eiwegger T, Holzmann D, Treis A, Wanke K, et al. Defective epithelial barrier in chronic rhinosinusitis: the regulation of tight junctions by IFN-gamma and IL-4. J Allergy Clin Immunol. 2012;130:1087–96.e10.

30. Shin HW, Cho K, Kim DW, Han DH, Khalmuratova R, Kim SW, et al. Hypoxia-inducible factor 1 mediates nasal polypogenesis by inducing epithelial-to-mesenchymal transition. Am J Respir Crit Care Med. 2012;185:944–54.
31. Zuckerman JD, Lee WY, DelGaudio JM, Moore CE, Nava P, Nusrat A, et al. Pathophysiology of nasal polyposis: the role of desmosomal junctions. Am J Rhinol. 2008;22:589–97.
32. Lane AP, Truong-Tran QA, Schleimer RP. Altered expression of genes associated with innate immunity and inflammation in recalcitrant rhinosinusitis with polyps. Am J Rhinol. 2006;20(2):138–44.
33. Seshadri S, Lin DC, Rosati M, et al. Reduced expression of antimicrobial PLUNC proteins in nasal polyp tissues of patient with chronic rhinosinusitis. Allergy. 2012;67(7):920–8.
34. Wei Y, Xia W, Ye X, et al. The antimicrobial protein short palate, lung, and nasal epithelium clone 1 (SPLUNC1) is differentially modulated in eosinophilic and noneosinophilic chronic rhinosinusitis with nasal polyps. J Allergy Clin Immunol. 2014;133(2):420–8.
35. Gray L. Deviated nasal septum. III. Its influence on the physiology and disease of the nose and ear. J Laryngol Otal. 1967;81:953–86.
36. Wu AW, Ting JY, Platt MP, et al. Factors affecting time to revision sinus surgery for nasal polyps: a 25-year experience. Laryngoscope. 2014;124(1):29–33.
37. Johansson L, Bramerson A, Holmberg K, Melen I, Akerlund A, Bende M. Clinical relevance of nasal polyps in individuals recruited from a general population based study. Acta Otolaryngol. 2004;124(1):77–81.
38. Banerji A, Piccirillo JF, Thawley SE, et al. Chronic rhinosinusitis patients with polyps or polypoid mucosa have a greater burden of illness. Am J Rhinol. 2007;21:19–26.
39. Kalish L, Snidvongs K, Sivasubramaniam R, Cope D, Harvey RJ. Topical steroids for nasal polyps. Cochrane Database Syst Rev. 2012;(12):CD006549.
40. Costa ML, Psaltis AJ, Nayak JV, Hwang PH. Long-term outcomes of endoscopic maxillary mega-antrostomy for refractory chronic maxillary sinusitis. Int Forum Allergy Rhinol. 2015;5(1):60–5.
41. Poetker DM, Jakubowski LA, Lal D, Hwang PH, Wright ED, Smith TL. Oral corticosteroids in the management of adult chronic rhinosinusitis with and without nasal polyps: an evidence-based review with recommendations. Int Forum Allergy Rhinol. 2013;3:104–20.
42. Wright ED, Agrawal S. Impact of perioperative systemic steroids on surgical outcomes in patients with chronic rhinosinusitis with polyposis: evaluation with the novel Perioperative Sinus Endoscopy (POSE) scoring system. Laryngoscope. 2007;117:1–28.
43. Fokkens WJ, Lund VJ, Mullol J, et al. European position paper on rhinosinusitis and nasal polyps 2012. Rhinol Suppl. 2012;23:1–298.
44. Bhalla RK, Payton K, Wright ED. Safety of budesonide in saline sinonasal irrigations in the management of chronic rhinosinusitis with polyposis: lack of significant adrenal suppression. J Otolaryngol Head Neck Surg. 2008;37(6):821–5.
45. Welch KC, Thaler ER, Dogrhamji LL, Palmer JN, Chiu AG. The effects of serum and urinary cortisol levels of topical intranasal irrigations with budesonide added to saline in patients with recurrent polyposis after endoscopic sinus surgery. Am J Rhinol Allergy. 2010;24(1):26–8.
46. Van Zele T, Gevaert P, Holtappels G, et al. Oral steroids and doxycycline: two different approaches to treat nasal polyps. J Allergy Clin Immunol. 2010;125:1069–76.
47. Wallwork B, Coman W, Mackay-Sim A, et al. A double-blind, randomized, placebo-controlled trial of macrolide in the treatment of chronic rhinosinusitis. Laryngoscope. 2006;116:189–93.
48. Videler WJ, Badia L, Harvey RJ, et al. Lack of efficacy of long-term, low-dose azithromycin in chronic rhinosinusitis: a randomized controlled trial. Allergy. 2011;66:1457–68.
49. Soler ZM, Oyer SL, Kern RC, et al. Antimicrobials and chronic rhinosinusitis with or without polyposis in adults: an evidenced-based review with recommendations. Int Forum Allergy Rhinol. 2013;3:31–47.
50. Jervis-Bardy J, Boase S, Psaltis A, Foreman A, Wormald PJ. A randomized trial of mupirocin sinonasal rinses versus saline in surgically recalcitrant staphylococcal chronic rhinosinusitis. Laryngoscope. 2012;122(10):2148–53.

51. Sousa AR, Parikh A, Scadding G, Corrigan CJ, Lee TH. Leukotriene-receptor expression on nasal mucosal inflammatory cells in aspirin-sensitive rhinosinusitis. N Engl J Med. 2002;347:1493–9.
52. Katial RK, Strand M, Prasertsuntarasai T, Leung R, Zheng W, Alam R. The effect of aspirin desensitization on novel biomarkers in aspirin-exacerbated respiratory diseases. J Allergy Clin Immunol. 2010;126:738–44.
53. Berges-Gimeno MP, Simon RA, Stevenson DD. Long-term treatment with aspirin desensitization in asthmatic patients with aspirin-exacerbated respiratory disease. J Allergy Clin Immunol. 2003;111:180–6.
54. Stevenson DD, Hankammer MA, Mathison DA, Christiansen SC, Simon RA. Aspirin desensitization treatment of aspirin-sensitive patients with rhinosinusitis-asthma: long-term outcomes. J Allergy Clin Immunol. 1996;98:751–8.
55. Kowalski ML, Grzelewska-Rzymowska I, Szmidt M, Rozniecki J. Clinical efficacy of aspirin in "desensitized" aspirin-sensitive asthmatics. Eur J Respir Dis. 1986;69:219–25.
56. Woessner KM, White AA. Evidence-based approach to aspirin desensitization in aspirin-exacerbated respiratory disease. J Allergy Clin Immunol. 2014;133(1):286–7.e1–9.
57. Cho KS, Soudry E, Psaltis AJ, et al. Long-term sinonasal outcomes of aspirin desensitization in aspirin exacerbated respiratory disease. Otolaryngol Head Neck Surg. 2014;151(4):575–81.
58. Weschta M, Rimek D, Formanek M, et al. Topical antifungal treatment of chronic rhinosinusitis with nasal polyps: a randomized, double-blind clinical trial. J Allergy Clin Immunol. 2004;113(6):1122–8.
59. Gerlinger I, Fittler A, Fonai F, et al. Postoperative application of amphotericin B nasal spray in chronic rhinosinusitis with nasal polyposis, with a review of the antifungal therapy. Eur Arch Otorhinolaryngol. 2009;266(6):847–55.
60. Mistry SG, Kumar BN. The value of antifungal therapy in allergic fungal rhinosinusitis. Rhinology. 2014;52(1):9–18.
61. Nishioka GJ, Cook PR, Davis WE, McKinsey JP. Immunotherapy in patients undergoing functional endoscopic sinus surgery. Otolaryngol Head Neck Surg. 1994;110(4):406–12.
62. Cox L, Nelson H, Lockey R, et al. Allergen immunotherapy: a practice parameter third update. J Allergy Clin Immunol. 2011;127:S1–55.
63. Hall AG, deShazo RD. Immunotherapy for allergic fungal sinusitis. Curr Opin Allergy Clin Immunol. 2012;12(6):629–34.
64. Wentzel JL, Soler ZM, DeYoung K, et al. Leukotriene antagonists in nasal polyposis: a meta-analysis and systematic review. Am J Rhinol Allergy. 2013;27(6):482–9.
65. Stewart R, Ram B, Hamilton G, et al. Montelukast as an adjunct to oral and inhaled steroid therapy in chronic nasal polyposis. Otolaryngol Head Neck Surg. 2008;139:682–7.
66. Ulualp S, Sterman BM, Toohill RJ. Antileukotriene therapy for the relief of sinus symptoms in aspirin triad disease. Ear Nose Throat J. 1999;78:604–10.
67. Parnes S, Chuma AV. Acute effects of antileukotrienes on sinonasal polyposis and sinusitis. Ear Nose Throat J. 2000;79:18–21.
68. Ragab S, Parikh A, Darby C, et al. An open audit of montelukast, a leukotriene receptor antagonist, in nasal polyposis associated with asthma. Clin Exp Allergy. 2001;31:1385–91.
69. Gevaert P, Lang-Loidolt D, Lackner A, et al. Nasal IL-5 levels determine the response to anti-IL-5 treatment in patients with nasal polyps. J Allergy Clin Immunol. 2006;118(5):1133–41.
70. Gevaert P, Van Bruaene N, Cattaert T, et al. Mepolizumab, a humanized anti-IL-5 mAb, as a treatment option for severe nasal polyposis. J Allergy Clin Immunol. 2011;128(5):989–95.
71. Gevaert P, Calus L, Van Zele T, et al. Omalizumab is effective in allergic and nonallergic patients with nasal polyps and asthma. J Allergy Clin Immunol. 2013;131(1):110–6.
72. Long A, Rahmaoui A, Rothman KJ, et al. Incidence of malignancy in patients with moderate-to-severe asthma treated with or without omalizumab. J Allergy Clin Immunol. 2014;134(3):560–7.

Fungal Rhinosinusitis

7

Drew P. Plonk, Amber Luong, and Martin J. Citardi

Key Take-Home Points

- Fungal rhinosinusitis is best characterized into noninvasive and invasive forms defined by the absence or presence of fungal invasion into tissues respectively.
- The noninvasive forms include saprophytic fungal infestation, fungus ball, and allergic fungal rhinosinusitis.
- The invasive forms include acute invasive fungal rhinosinusitis, chronic invasive fungal rhinosinusitis, and granulomatous invasive fungal rhinosinusitis.
- Saprophytic fungal infestation refers to the visible growth of fungus on a crust or other debris within the sinonasal cavities of an asymptomatic, immunocompetent individual. Treatment is removal of the crust and fungal elements.
- A fungal ball refers to a dense conglomeration of noninvasive fungal hyphae, most commonly in an isolated sinus cavity. Treatment is removal of all fungal elements and associated debris.
- Allergic fungal rhinosinusitis is characterized by (1) presence of nasal drainage, nasal obstruction, decreased sense of smell, and/or facial pressure for 12 weeks, (2) mucin within the sinus cavity containing fungal

D.P. Plonk, MD
Department of Otolaryngology, Wake Forest University School of Medicine, Medical Center Boulevard, Winston-Salem, NC 27157, USA
e-mail: dplonk@wakehealth.edu

A. Luong, MD, PhD • M.J. Citardi, MD (✉)
Department of Otorhinolaryngology – Head and Neck Surgery, University of Texas Medical School at Houston, 6431 Fannin Street, MSB 5.036, Houston, TX 77030, USA
e-mail: amber.u.luong@uth.tmc.edu; martin.j.citardi@uth.tmc.edu

P.S. Batra, J.K. Han (eds.), *Practical Medical and Surgical Management of Chronic Rhinosinusitis*, DOI 10.1007/978-3-319-16724-4_7

hyphae and degranulating eosinophils, (3) endoscopic evidence of inflammation within the sinus cavity, (4) CT or MRI findings consistent with chronic rhinosinusitis, (5) evidence of fungal-specific IgE by skin prick or serum IgE testing, and (6) no evidence of invasive fungal disease. Treatment consists of surgery for removal of all fungal elements and eosinophilic mucin combined with corticosteroid anti-inflammatory therapy.

- Acute invasive fungal rhinosinusitis involves invasion of fungi (most commonly *Aspergillus*, *Mucor*, and *Rhizopus*) into sinonasal mucosa and adjacent tissues of patients with immunocompromise (specifically with defects in neutrophil function). Treatment includes reversal of underlying immunodeficiency (to the extent that this is possible), extensive surgical debridement, and systemic antifungal treatments.
- Chronic invasive fungal rhinosinusitis represents a similar but less fulminant form of acute invasive fungal sinusitis. Patients have subtle immunological defects, and pathology shows fungal invasion with a sparse inflammatory response. Treatment is surgical debridement and systemic antifungal medications.
- Granulomatous invasive fungal rhinosinusitis is defined by granuloma formation in response to fungi. Treatment is surgical debridement coupled with systemic antifungal medications.

Introduction

Over the past 30 years, otorhinolaryngologists have developed a better appreciation of fungal rhinosinusitis (FRS), whose appearance is the end-state manifestation of a complex interaction of many host-specific and fungus-specific factors. Advances in immunology have fostered a better appreciation of the importance of host immunological function on FRS disease presentation. FRS diagnosis in years past was imprecise, but today, diagnostic criteria and methods are better established. Endoscopy affords a platform for both diagnosis and treatment, while contemporary imaging modalities facilitate both diagnosis and staging. Nonetheless, understanding of the underlying pathophysiology – and hence the role of fungi in rhinosinusitis – continues to evolve.

Principles of Mycology

The kingdom Fungi, which is separate from plants, animals, protista, and bacteria, consists of a large group of eukaryotic microorganisms that includes yeasts and molds. Fungi are ubiquitous in the environment, and it is thought that there are up to five million species, with only approximately 5 % formally classified [1]. Historically, fungi have been categorized into different taxa based on morphology;

however these classifications are evolving rapidly as DNA analysis is incorporated into taxonomy methods.

Mold fungi characteristically grow by producing hyphae, which are tubular, elongated, filamentous structures that can grow up to several centimeters in length. The growth occurs through the emergence of new tips along the length of the hyphae, a process also known as “branching” [2]. Additionally, septations may exist within the hyphae. Branching patterns and the presence or absence of septations are useful in classifying fungi. Yeast fungi, such as *Candida*, are unicellular and reproduce asexually through budding as opposed to forming hyphae. Multiple buds that fail to detach from each other are known as pseudohyphae. Both mold and yeast can form spores when conditions are not favorable for the survival and growth of the fungus. It is the spore, specifically through its inhalation, that is likely responsible for fungal entry into the human nasal cavity.

It is now appreciated that fungi are ubiquitously found within normal healthy human nasal cavity. Previously, limitations of fungal culture failed to detect the uniform presence of fungi within healthy individuals, leading to the notion that the presence of fungus in and of itself was the key pathogenic event in human fungal disease. However, polymerase chain reaction analysis showed nearly 100 % of individuals, regardless of whether or not sinusitis was present, had fungi within their sinonasal cavities [3]. Based on this study (and many others), it can be surmised that the presence of fungus in the sinonasal cavity is ubiquitous and most commonly commensal. The pathogenic potential is determined by not yet fully understood host-pathogen interactions and heavily influenced by the nature of the host’s immune system.

Classification and Terminology

FRS is classified broadly into two categories based on the absence or presence of fungal invasion into the soft tissues of the nasal cavity and paranasal sinuses and adjacent structures [4]. Noninvasive forms of FRS are saprophytic fungal infestation, fungus ball, and allergic fungal rhinosinusitis (AFRS). Invasive forms are acute invasive fungal rhinosinusitis (AIFRS) (previously known as fulminant or necrotizing fungal rhinosinusitis), granulomatous invasive fungal rhinosinusitis (GIFRS), and chronic invasive fungal rhinosinusitis (CIFS).

Eosinophilic mucin, which is characterized by the presence of eosinophils and eosinophil degradation products, is a hallmark of AFRS but may also be found in other forms of chronic rhinosinusitis (CRS), including aspirin-exacerbated respiratory disease (AERD). Identification of fungal elements in sinus secretions is problematic, since it may be influenced by concomitant treatments, tissue handling, and identification methods. Nonetheless, fungal elements are commonly seen in eosinophilic mucin from AFRS patients and less commonly identified in eosinophilic mucin from patients with other forms of CRS. For this reason, it may be more appropriate to speak of “eosinophil-related fungal rhinosinusitis, including AFRS,” which is a much broader category that alludes to recent data suggesting that fungi may play a role in other forms of CRS and not just limited to AFRS [5, 6].

Currently, chronic rhinosinusitis is categorized based upon the presence or absence of polyps into chronic rhinosinusitis with nasal polyps (CRSwNP) and chronic rhinosinusitis without nasal polyps (CRSsNP). In this categorization, both AERD and AFRS are subtypes of CRSwNP.

Traditionally FRS has been classified according to the presumed fungal etiologic agent. Thus, terms, such as "aspergillosis," "mucormycosis," and "zygomycosis," among many other terms, have been reported. These descriptive terms do not accurately categorize the underlying disease process, and their use should be discouraged. In reading the older published literature, it is quite common to encounter this terminology, and thus, it is important to look for actual descriptions of clinical and pathologic features in these older reports.

Noninvasive Fungal Sinusitis

Saprophytic Fungal Infestation

Saprophytic fungal infestation refers to the visible growth of fungus within the sinonasal cavities of an asymptomatic, immunocompetent individual [7]. In this disease entity, fungal growth commonly occurs on mucus and/or crusts in the postoperative nasal and sinus cavity and does not cause any visible adjacent inflammatory response. Histology of this material demonstrates viable hyphae, and mycology culture may grow a variety of different fungal species. It has been hypothesized that these saprophytic fungal infections may represent the initial stages of certain types of FRS, including fungus ball and even AFRS; however, no data have conclusively demonstrated this point.

Under most circumstances, the saprophytic fungal infestation should be addressed by removing all visible fungal elements, mucus, and crusts through endoscopic debridement. Saline irrigations, which also serve as a form of patient-administered debridement, may also be useful. After complete removal, recurrence is rare.

For patients who are immunocompromised, a more aggressive management strategy seems warranted to prevent progression to FRS forms that are potentially fatal, as saprophytic and opportunistic fungi are known causes of highly lethal invasive fungal disease in such hosts [8]. It should be remembered that fungal colonization exists in the sinonasal cavity regardless of whether saprophytic fungus is present, so removal of a saprophytic crust may not alter the risk of developing an opportunistic fungal infection in an immunocompromised patient.

Fungal Ball

A fungal ball refers to a dense conglomeration of noninvasive fungal hyphae, most commonly in an isolated sinus cavity although more than one sinus can be involved [5]. The maxillary sinus is the most commonly affected sinus; however, this phenomenon also frequently occurs in the sphenoid sinus and can occur in any sinus.

Diagnostic Criteria

Criteria for diagnosis of a fungal ball, as defined by deShazo, include (1) radiologic opacification of a sinus, often of a dual-density nature with adjacent boney thickening; (2) endoscopic findings of gritty clay-like and/or mucopurulent cheesy debris in the sinus cavity; and (3) histologic evidence of a dense matted conglomeration of fungal hyphae without evidence of tissue invasion but with nonspecific chronic mucosal inflammation without a predominance of eosinophils, granuloma, or eosinophilic mucin [9]. While aspergillus is classically thought to be a common cause, this can only be surmised from histology as up to 70 % of cultures are negative [5].

Clinical Presentation

Often, patients with a fungus ball have no sinonasal symptoms; rather, characteristic imaging findings are noted on imaging studies done for other purposes. Alternatively, a fungus ball may cause symptoms of pressure and fullness in the involved sinus. For the maxillary sinus, the discomfort will manifest itself in the cheek, while a sphenoid sinus fungus ball may cause pressure between the eyes or at the vertex of the skull. Rarely, a fungus ball may occur in the frontal sinus, with the potential to cause frontal pressure. If the fungus ball has a bacterial superinfection, purulent secretions may leak from the involved sinus, causing symptoms related to purulent rhinorrhea.

In many instances, the CT scan will provide strong evidence for the diagnosis of a fungus ball. On CT, the involved sinus will be partially or completely opacified, with areas of hyperdensity within the opacified sinus ("dual densities") (Figs. 7.1a, b and 7.2) [10]. The bone around the affected sinus may often be hyperostotic.

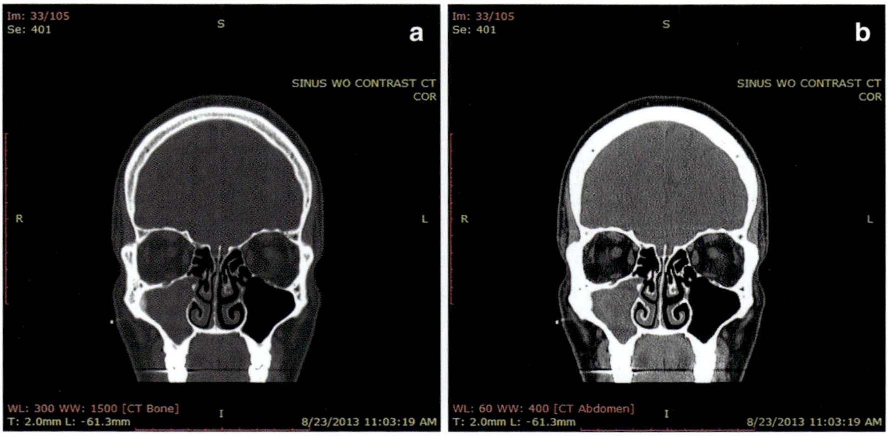

Fig. 7.1 (**a**) An isolated fungus ball may appear as nonspecific sinus opacification on a CT scan with bone window settings. Close inspection of the right maxillary sinus suggests some hyperdensities, but the finding is not dramatic. (**b**) This CT scan (now at soft tissue windows) of the same patient seen in (**a**) demonstrates hyperdensities that are characteristic of an isolated fungus ball. Intraoperative findings confirmed the diagnosis of a right maxillary fungus ball

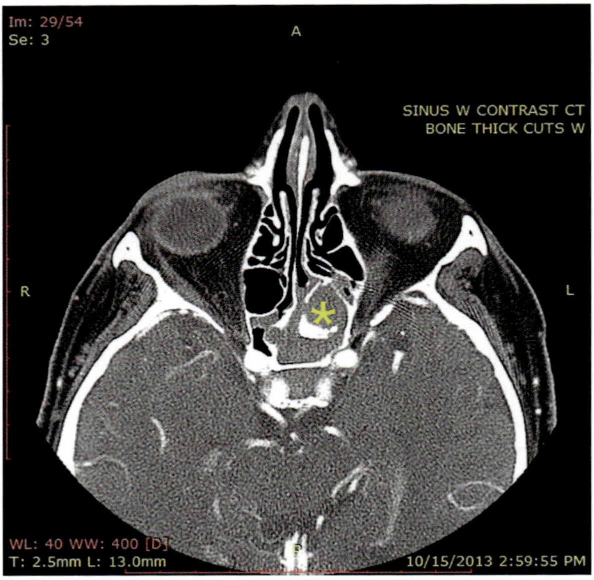

Fig. 7.2 Sinus CT angiogram demonstrates hyperdensity within an opacified left sphenoid sinus. This appearance is consistent with isolated sphenoid fungus ball

MRI findings of a fungus ball are somewhat less specific than CT findings. On MRI, a fungus ball may produce various signal intensities that reflect the extent of hydration of the sinus contents. At its extreme, a fungus ball will produce loss of signal on both T1 and T2 MRI modalities, and thus, in this circumstance, a long-standing fungus ball will produce no signal on MRI and will mimic the appearance of a normally aerated sinus.

Treatment

Treatment primarily consists of surgical debridement of the affected sinus cavity (Fig. 7.3), with relatively low rates of recurrence thereafter. Postoperative sinus cavity fungal balls may be amenable to in-office debridement or treatment with conservative nasal irrigation measures, although frequently more aggressive debridement measures under sedation are required. Medical therapy targeting this disease entity is largely ineffective.

Although it is a relatively straightforward decision to operate on a symptomatic fungal ball, an incidentally found, clinically quiescent fungal ball might give the clinician pause, especially in a patient with severe comorbidities and anesthesia risks. While observation is always a viable option, it should be noted that, in the immunocompromised host, progression of fungal ball to invasive fungal sinonasal disease has been reported [11]. This suggests the need for aggressive management when this entity is identified in someone with or at risk for immunosuppression. This potential for progression also justifies surgically treating the asymptomatic

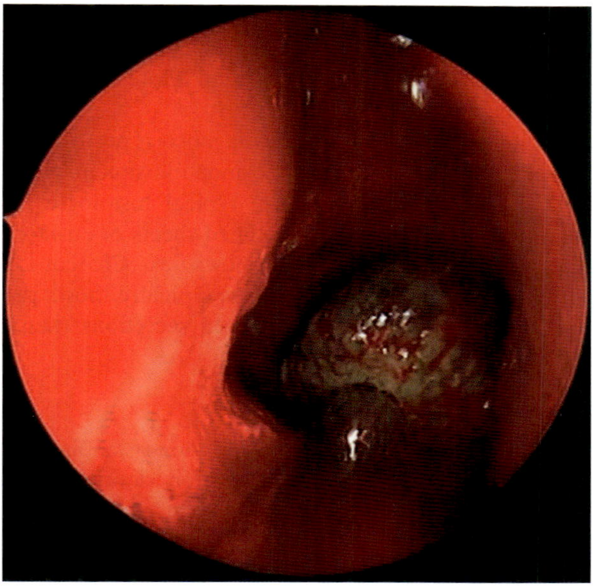

Fig. 7.3 During surgical removal, fungus balls appear as dense discrete balls of fungal elements and related debris, as seen in this endoscopic view of a right maxillary fungus ball that has been displaced into the middle meatus for removal

healthy individual, as the disease is likely to persist indefinitely over the course of one's lifetime and the risk for immunocompromising illness always exists. Furthermore, an opacified sinus may also harbor an occult neoplasm. Thus, surgical intervention is warranted for both asymptomatic and symptomatic fungal balls that are noted on imaging.

Allergic Fungal Rhinosinusitis

Allergic fungal rhinosinusitis (AFRS), originally described in 1983 by Katzenstein et al. [12], represents a subclass of CRS that accounts for up to 10 % of CRS cases in the United States [12, 13]. It most commonly affects young, immunocompetent individuals with fungal atopy, is mostly unilateral, and has a geographic predilection to both humid and arid environments, such as those seen in the southern United States, Middle East, Australia, and Africa [13–15].

Diagnostic Criteria

Consensus clinical guidelines, based on widely accepted criteria proposed by Bent and Kuhn, define AFRS by the following characteristics: (1) presence of nasal drainage, nasal obstruction, decreased sense of smell, and/or facial pressure for 12 weeks, (2) mucin within the sinus cavity containing fungal hyphae and degranulating eosinophils, (3) endoscopic evidence of inflammation within the sinus cavity, (4) CT or MRI findings consistent with chronic rhinosinusitis, (5) evidence of fungal-specific IgE by skin prick or serum IgE testing, and (6) no evidence of invasive fungal disease [16, 17].

Fungal culture, though contributory to the diagnosis if positive, is variably sensitive; therefore, the histologic appearance of eosinophilic mucin with fungus remains the more reliable indicator of AFRS [18]. Typical histologic findings include branching, noninvasive fungal hyphae, lamellated sheets of eosinophils, and elongated eosinophilic breakdown products known as Charcot-Leyden crystals (Fig. 7.4). Endoscopic evidence of inflammation typically shows polypoid mucosa in proximity to thick, highly viscous discolored secretions (tan, brown, and/or green) (Fig. 7.5).

Presentation

Patients with AFRS present with symptoms of long-standing, difficult-to-treat CRS. Major sinonasal symptoms include congestion, drainage, nasal obstruction, etc. Often patients with AFRS will report nonspecific symptom of congestion with

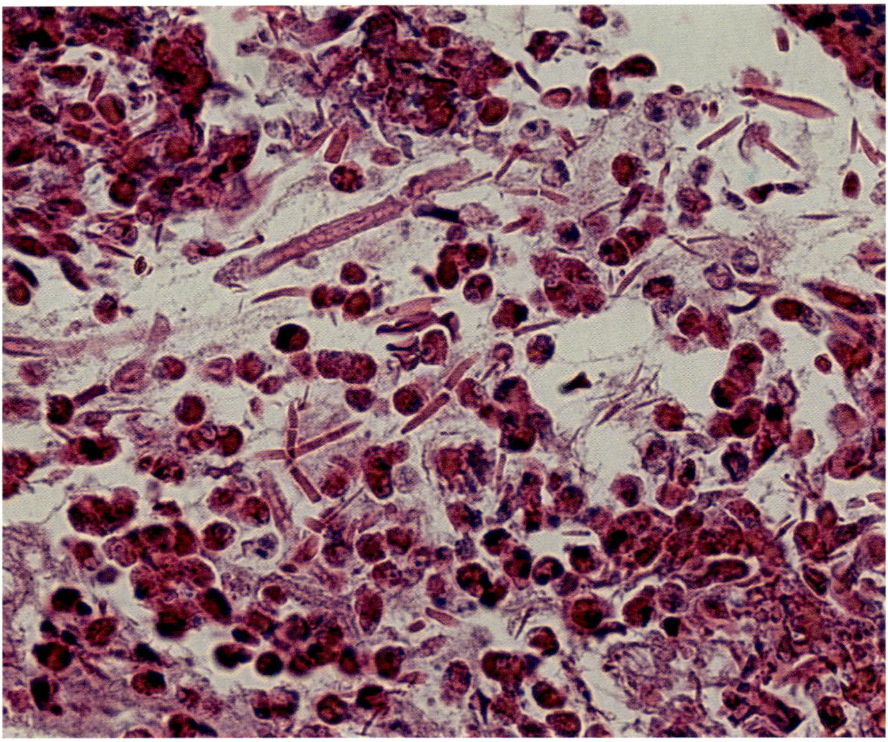

Fig. 7.4 Allergic fungal rhinosinusitis is characterized by eosinophils, fungal hyphae, and Charcot-Leyden crystals, as seen here (hematoxylin and eosin, 400×)

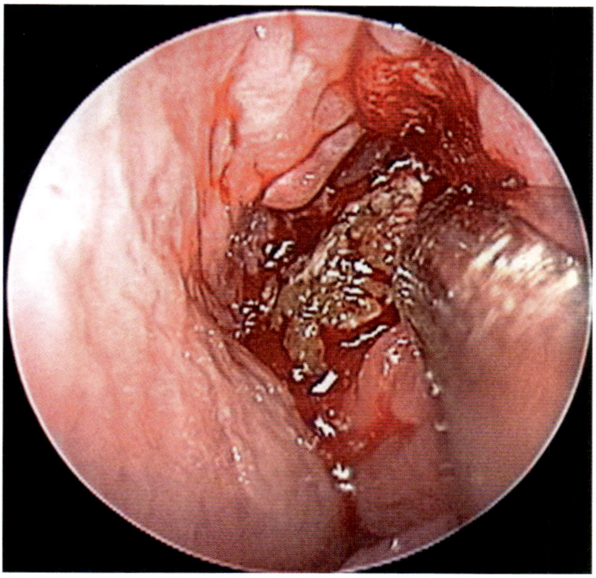

Fig. 7.5 Allergic fungal rhinosinusitis is characterized by the presence of eosinophilic debris, demonstrated in this endoscopic image

minimal quality of life impact. In rare instances, a patient with AFRS will present from proptosis due to otherwise asymptomatic expansion of adjacent sinus cavities with eosinophilic debris. Patients tend to be young adults and adolescents, and aspirin-exacerbated respiratory disease is rare in the AFRS patient cohort. These patients are considered immunocompetent by conventional testing methods. In fact, there is often some evidence of exuberant inflammatory response, as indicated by an elevated total serum IgE, which is typically elevated between 500 and 4,000 kUA/l [19]. Some AFRS patients will also have asthma. AFRS not uncommonly occurs asymmetrically; although up to 50 % of cases may show bilateral disease at presentation, 80 % of cases have a strong unilateral predominance [20]. If the AFRS is advanced, it may expand the bone, leading to orbital deformities and proptosis. Advanced AFRS may also cause diplopia and visual loss, due to compression of critical structures from sinus expansion. Nasal endoscopic examination typically demonstrates nasal polyps, as well as thick, tenacious, light tan/brown or green secretions known as eosinophilic mucin (Fig. 7.5).

Characteristic CT findings include expansion of involved sinuses with demineralization of cortical bone. Dual-density secretions are seen on CT, which are related to the accumulation of heavy metals and calcium salt precipitate within the mucin (Fig. 7.6). MRI often shows isointense or hypointense secretions on T1-weighted imaging and hypointense secretions on T2-weighted imaging related to the dehydrated state of mucin; adjacent mucosa enhances on both modalities (Figs. 7.6 and 7.7) [20, 21].

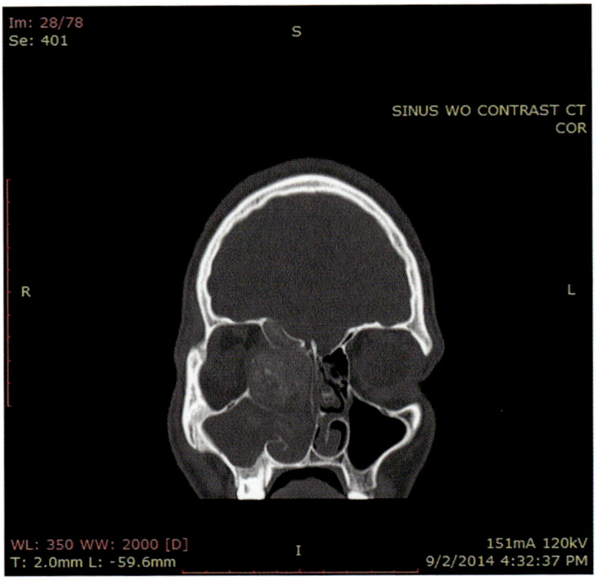

Fig. 7.6 In this CT scan, the right ethmoid sinuses contain an expansile process. Note the hyperdensities present in the right ethmoid sinuses and in the right maxillary sinus to a lesser extent. The orbital wall is eroded and the sinus process is compressing the orbital contents. The ethmoid roof has also been eroded. This CT scan illustrates the classic findings of allergic fungal rhinosinusitis

Etiology

The pathophysiology of AFRS remains unclear. Dysregulated T helper 2 (Th2) responses appear to be a major driver of the pathogenic pathway but the inciting actors and specific mechanisms eliciting the hyperactive Th2 immune cascade are still the subject of ongoing investigation.

Originally, AFRS was thought to represent purely an IgE-mediated type I hypersensitivity reaction to fungus in the sinonasal cavity. By definition, AFRS has a predominance of fungi within accumulated eosinophilic mucin in the affected sinuses; this association strongly suggested an etiologic role of fungi. Early observations on AFRS patients demonstrated a correlation between the presence of fungal allergy in patients with AFRS and CRS patients without AFRS. In one report, 8 patients with AFRS who had sinus cultures positive to *Bipolaris* also showed *Bipolaris*-specific IgE and IgG serum elevations and *Bipolaris* reactivity on skin prick testing; 80 % of CRS patients were negative on both serum and skin prick testing [18]. This fungal-specific IgE elevation suggests a pathologic contribution through the adaptive immune response which is further supported by elevated T helper 2 cytokines (i.e., IL-4, IL-5, and IL-13) and eosinophil levels within the sinonasal mucosa of AFRS patients [22]. Additionally, an in vitro challenge of peripheral blood mononuclear cells from patients with AFRS to common etiologic fungal antigens incited the secretion of Th2 cytokines from these cells; this response was not elicited in mononuclear cells from healthy controls exposed to the same

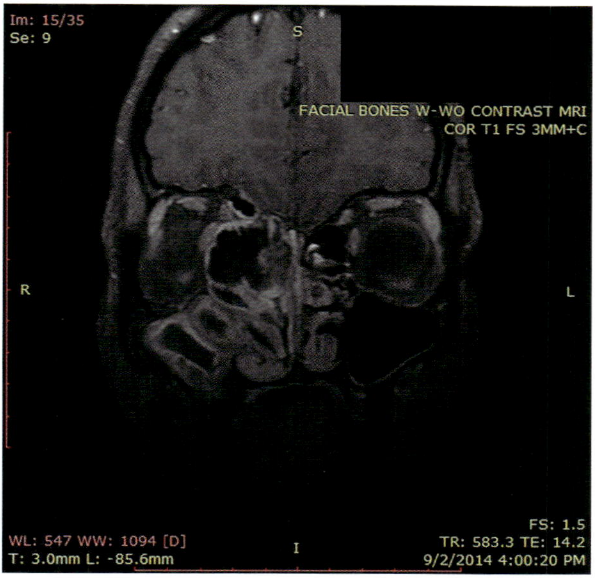

Fig. 7.7 This MRI image corresponds approximately to the same region as the CT scan in Fig. 7.6. The areas of signal dropout (which appear black in the image) correspond to the hyperdensities seen on the corresponding CT scan and represent areas of eosinophilic fungal debris. Imaging of adjacent orbital and intracranial structures confirm the absence of invasion by the sinus process. This MRI illustrates classic findings of allergic fungal rhinosinusitis

antigens [23]. These aforementioned studies support the conclusion that AFRS patients have fungal hypersensitivity and immunologic memory to fungi, but a causal relationship still has not been established.

Abnormalities in fungal-specific IgG have also been reported in AFRS patients. *Bipolaris*-specific IgG elevations have been identified in *Bipolaris*-positive AFRS patients [18]. Fungal-specific IgG elevation suggests a possible role of the Gel and Coombs type 3 hypersensitivity response, whose first step is immune complex formation between specific IgG to the target antigen. In support of presumed mechanism, fungal-specific IgG3 was the only marker that was distinctly elevated and thereby differentiated patients with eosinophilic CRS (including those that fit criteria for AFRS) from patients with other forms of CRS and from patients with allergic rhinitis only [24].

Defects in innate immunity have also been confirmed in AFRS. Fungal spores are ubiquitous in the environment and are considered immunologically inert; therefore, spores must breach the innate immune system and germinate into hyphae in order to incite an inflammatory reaction [25]. Structural abnormalities in airway epithelium may contribute to this process, with the subsequent defective clearance of spores fostering the germination of the fungal spore into hyphae [19]. This mechanism is the presumed cause of allergic bronchopulmonary aspergillosis, a pulmonary condition whose features are similar to AFRS. Additionally, it seems plausible that additional host factors such as a defect in innate immunity and/or mucosal structural abnormality must exist in order for the distinct pathology of AFRS to develop, since fungal atopy usually does not lead to the development of AFRS. The finding of an increased incidence of class II major histocompatibility complex (MHC) HLA-DQB1*0301 and *0302 in patients with AFRS implicates such defects in innate immunity playing a role in the disease process [26].

Once the innate immune defense system is infiltrated, allergic antigens such as fungi may utilize proteases to incite inflammation. Proteases have been shown to have activity that accompanies the antigenic activity of common allergens including mold [27, 28]. Additionally, protease exposure has been linked to allergic respiratory disease through occupational exposure studies [29]. The association of fungal protease activity and allergic airway disease is further supported by studies in which intranasal proteinase exposure in mice without prior sensitization was able to elicit pulmonary changes consistent with those seen in the classic model of allergic asthma [28]. The molecular signaling associated with fungal protease activity and allergic airway disease has been linked to at least two receptors: toll-like receptor 4 (TLR4) and protease-activated receptor 2 (PAR-2) [30, 31].

Another proposed etiologic factor in CRS (and AFRS) involves bacterial superantigen. Superantigen is known to have the ability to incite massive immune reactions through the nonspecific, polyclonal activation of T cells, and *Staphylococcus aureus*, recognized as a prodigious superantigen producer, is commonly found in the sinuses of individuals afflicted with AFRS [32, 33]. Recent work has shown that specific IgE to staphylococcal antigen enterotoxin (SE-IgE) is an independent risk factor for asthma in a concentration-dependent manner [34]. This same effect was not seen with specific IgE to aeroallergens. Additionally, the presence of SE-IgE was associated with elevated total IgE, representing possible polyclonal IgE production in response to the superantigen [34]. Interestingly, non-atopic asthmatics (negative skin prick testing and/or serum IgE testing against aeroallergens) were shown to be positive for SE-IgE [34, 35].

As in asthma, mechanisms of inflammation in AFRS may be similarly propagated through the staphylococcal enterotoxin. The Th2 immune response to fungus could foster the environment for *Staphylococcus aureus*, as inflammation hinders the ability of the innate immune system and the epithelial barrier to adequately defend against pathogens [36]. Subsequent polyclonal B- and T-cell activation induced by the superantigen would lead to ongoing inflammation [37]. In support of this, selective IgE was present in 16 of 17 patients with AFRS and there was a significant and strong correlation of SE-IgE to total IgE in these patients; this same effect on total IgE was not seen with specific IgE to fungal antigens [36]. However, co-expression of SE-IgE and selective IgE to fungal antigen did significantly elevate total IgE when compared to patients with CRSwNP. This suggests a possible synergistic relationship between fungus and *Staphylococcal aureus*. The recent detection of biofilms containing both fungi and *Staphylococcal aureus* on electron microscopy in the AFRS patients supports this hypothesis [36].

Recently, attention has been directed toward epithelial cell-derived cytokines driving the local Th2 response in both AFRS and CRSwNP. In addition to their barrier function, these pseudostratified epithelial cells of the sinus mucosa are able to incite a local Th2 immune reaction to various environmental triggers, including fungi [38]. Important mediators released by the epithelial cells include IL-25, IL-33, and thymic stromal lymphopoietin; recent studies have shown these actors to lead to increased IL-13 production and mast cell activation, thus propagating the Th2 pathway [38–40].

Treatment

AFRS treatment starts with appropriate diagnosis. Clinical symptoms, coupled with endoscopy and CT findings, will often yield a tentative AFRS diagnosis, but definitive diagnosis requires histopathologic analysis of mucin obtained at the time of surgery. In relatively rare instances, AFRS may only be detected during surgery for CRS refractory to medical treatments. As with other forms of FRS, endoscopic sinus surgery (ESS) provides platforms for diagnosis, treatment, and long-term management. It must be emphasized that surgery alone is rarely sufficient treatment; almost all patients will require ongoing treatment with oral or topical corticosteroids, which are potent ways to reduce the inflammatory burden in affected sinuses.

As previously stated, the first goal of ESS is to achieve a diagnosis. In addition, during ESS, the surgeon must remove all eosinophilic debris, which presumably contains inciting fungal antigens and other potential contributing triggers from all involved sinuses [15]. Failure to remove all debris leaves a focus that will drive persistent sinus inflammation and lead to surgical failure. The final goal of surgery is to create open sinus cavities so that patients can perform postoperative irrigations. Through irrigations, patients may deliver additional medications directly to the mucosa and space of the sinuses, and the irrigations themselves serve as debridement by washing out elements of fungus and mucin. After effective surgery, the surgeon may also easily visualize the state of the sinus mucosal health and perform additional office-based debridement of the open sinus cavities [15].

In preparation for surgery, many surgeons will institute systemic steroids (prednisone, at a dose 0.5/kg/day or more) for 3–5 days (or longer) preoperatively. The goal of this treatment is to reduce the inflammatory burden and thus reduce bleeding. It should be noted that the administration of preoperative systemic steroids may obscure an AFRS diagnosis, by reversing many of the findings of AFRS. In addition, some surgeons may treat with empiric or culture-directed systemic antibiotics, although the impact of such treatment has never been demonstrated.

Although the inflammatory burden is great, the surgeon must follow established principles of functional surgery, with care taken for preservation of normal structures. In advanced cases of AFRS, the eosinophilic debris will cause a massive expansion of the paranasal sinus volume, which may contain large amounts of thick, retained secretions that will often clog suctions easily. Thus, the surgeon must use meticulous techniques to remove all eosinophilic material. Intraoperative irrigation may help dislodge retained secretions. Clumps of eosinophilic material may often be found adjacent to areas of bony dehiscence; therefore, any surgical manipulation in these areas requires extra attention to avoid inadvertent injury to the skull base and orbit.

Destructive sinus procedures should be avoided, because in general, they are not necessary, and in some cases, they may complicate long-term care. In AFRS patients, the frontal recess access is typically expanded by the mucin, obviating need for extensive bone removal at the boundaries of the frontal recess. Frontal sinus obliteration procedures carry the risk of burying viable fungal elements in the obliterated cavity and thus may set up long-term complications. Even the presence of erosion of the bony sinus walls does not mandate sinus obliteration [41].

Comprehensive AFRS treatment includes a prolonged period of postoperative care. During the postoperative period, the surgeon will correlate symptoms against endoscopic findings and then use this information to guide ongoing medical treatment. The AFRS endoscopic staging system classifies the postoperative sinus cavities into 4 distinct stages: no evidence of disease (stage 0) (Fig. 7.8a), edematous mucosa with or without mucin (stage I) (Fig. 7.8b), polypoid mucosa with or without mucin (stage II) (Fig. 7.8c), and polyps with fungal debris (stage III) (Fig. 7.8d). The general principle of treatment is that medical treatments should only be reduced when the endoscopic examination is at stage 0 for at least 3–4 weeks. In addition, it is probably advisable to increase or at least maintain current treatment for patients with higher stages of postoperative disease, even if the patient is asymptomatic [42].

In addition to surgery, medical therapy targeted at the chronic inflammatory response is needed. Despite recent appreciation of activated immunologic pathways and the role of various environmental triggers in AFRS, steroids remain the cornerstone in medical treatment. Steroids, both topical and oral, are critical for treatment success. Multiple prior studies have shown improved symptom scores and lower polyp recurrences in postoperative AFRS patients who were treated with perioperative oral corticosteroids and/or prolonged topical steroids [43–49]. Despite this, chronic oral steroid use is limited by well-documented side effects, including but not limited to osteoporosis, osteonecrosis, diabetes, glaucoma, cataracts, weight gain, hypertension, and adrenal suppression. Fortunately, topical steroids, even when administered via irrigations, appear to have a positive safety profile in postoperative patients [48, 50].

Surgeons use many different protocols for postoperative corticosteroid treatment. Unfortunately, rigorous studies have not confirmed the benefits of one approach over another. In general, prednisone should be administered to AFRS in the immediate postoperative period at a dose 0.5 mg/kg/day; these steroids can be then tapered over 2–3 weeks or longer, depending on the endoscopic exam and symptoms. Many patients will require at least several weeks of systemic prednisone for stabilization of mucosal health. Before stopping the prednisone, most surgeons will also add in high-dose topical steroids, which are continued for longer periods. Standard formulations of nasal steroids delivered as nasal sprays can be used on BID-TID schedule (2–3 times the FDA-approved doses for allergic rhinitis). Other options include budesonide (0.25–0.5 mg BID-TID), fluticasone (3 mg BID-TID), and betamethasone (0.75 mg BID-TID), delivered via low-pressure/high-volume irrigations (200–250 ml of saline) or various commercially available sinonasal nebulizers (10–20 ml of saline). Budesonide is commercially available for nebulization for asthma treatment and thus may be purchased through large pharmacy chains and

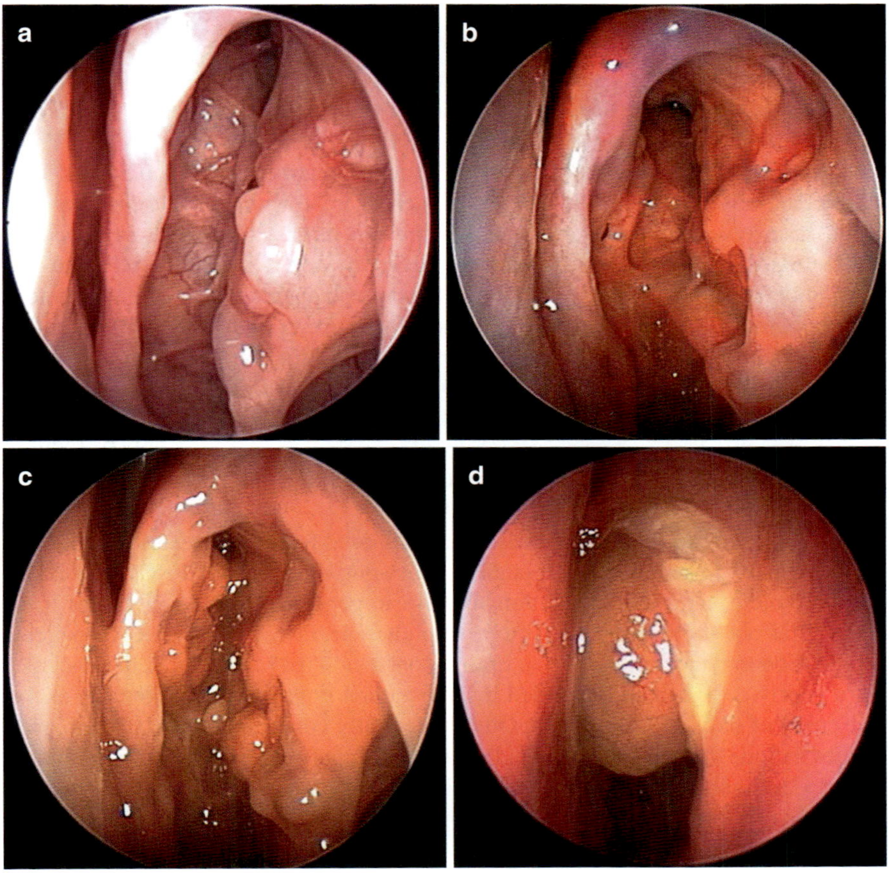

Fig. 7.8 (**a**) Stage 0 of the endoscopic staging system of allergic fungal rhinosinusitis is a normal exam, without any evidence of active mucosal inflammation. (**b**) In stage I of allergic fungal rhinosinusitis, the mucosa shows signs of edema with or without the presence of eosinophilic mucin. (**c**) In stage II of allergic fungal rhinosinusitis, the mucosa has become polypoid. Eosinophilic mucin may or may not be present. (**d**) In stage 4 of allergic fungal rhinosinusitis, the involved sinuses are filled with polyps and eosinophilic debris

neighborhood pharmacies. Both fluticasone and betamethasone may be available from compounding pharmacies. Of these three agents, betamethasone probably has the highest degree of systemic absorption.

Immunotherapy (IT) has also been recommended for AFRS treatment. Early studies, using relatively dilute concentrations of fungal antigen, showed improved outcomes over a 3–5-year period [51–54]. Benefit has also been shown when begun in the immediate postoperative period, with lower rates of disease recurrence and revision surgery in AFRS patients who received IT after surgery [55]. Concern over delayed local reactions and immune complex formation using fungal IT dampened initial enthusiasm, but recent studies have shown no evidence of this using high-dose fungal IT over prolonged follow-up periods, allowing future use and ongoing study of fungal IT in AFRS patients [56, 57].

AFRS exacerbations are often heralded by acute bacterial sinus infections, which, if untreated or undertreated, trigger the inflammatory cascade of AFRS. Thus, acute exacerbations require prompt evaluation. Treatment with culture-directed antibiotics, often coupled with increased steroid treatment (either topical or systemic), can reverse the exacerbation and prevent its progression to an advanced AFRS stage. AFRS has been associated with *Staphylococcus aureus*, and some otolaryngologists will empirically add topical anti-staph agents to the patient's postoperative regimen [33]. Mupirocin irrigations may be prescribed as a matter of routine or added later based upon culture results, since mupirocin nasal irrigation targets both planktonic and biofilm forms of *Staphylococcus aureus* [58]. Despite theoretical benefits, a recent review on topical therapy in CRS highlighted the need for further study of high-volume antimicrobial irrigations based on lack of currently available evidence [59]; however, formal studies of topical antibiotics for AFRS exacerbations have not been performed.

Topical antifungal agents have also been proposed for AFRS treatment, but studies are sparse. Several studies, though not focusing directly on AFRS, have examined the role of antifungal irrigations in CRS in general. A meta-analysis of these studies did not show any benefit from amphotericin B irrigations in CRS patients [60]. A Cochrane review came to a similar conclusion [61]. In general, these studies were poorly designed and included diverse patient populations without the exclusive study of only AFRS patients. Other potentially confounding variables in prior studies include the possibility of inadequate antifungal agent dosing and suboptimal delivery. In light of these deficiencies, it is conceivable that topical antifungal therapy could still prove to be efficacious in an appropriately selected patient population. Ultimately, further study is necessary before conclusions can be drawn regarding its use in AFRS.

Systemic antifungal therapy is also an appealing option for AFRS treatment, but no rigorous studies have been performed in this patient group. A systematic review of this treatment noted that both itraconazole and ketoconazole may have benefit in patients with CRS, but the vast majority of studies were poorly designed uncontrolled case series [61, 62]. A Cochrane review came to similar conclusion [62].

The use of advanced biologics in the treatment of AFRS have not been studied, although there have been a few reports of their use in the general CRS population. An underpowered study of anti-IgE therapy found no objective or symptomatic improvement in CRSwNP patients treated with this novel agent [63]. In another study, anti-IL-5 showed significantly decreased polyp size and less sinus opacification in CRSwNP patients 1 month after treatment compared to CRSwNP patients who did not receive anti-IL-5 therapy [64]. Based on recent findings regarding epithelial derived cytokines, future potential targets may also be directed at IL-25, IL-33, and thymic stromal lymphopoietin among others in the treatment of AFRS and CRS in general [65].

Invasive Fungal Sinusitis

Histologic Considerations for Invasive Fungal Rhinosinusitis Diagnosis

Because of its aggressive nature, early and accurate diagnosis of invasive fungal rhinosinusitis (IFRS) has important implications for treatment selection and eventual outcomes. The priority issue is determination of the presence or absence of fungal invasion into the tissue. Frozen section pathology is the only way to definitively assess for the fungal invasion at the time of surgery. Of course, clinical cues, including the absence of bleeding from affected tissue, also may guide the clinician to an accurate diagnosis. Culture, which is the gold standard for fungus speciation, does not always successfully yield fungal growth and requires days (or longer) for a definitive result.

Microscopic study of fungal morphology can be used to identify the fungus at genus or even supra-genus level. Among the causes of IFRS, fungi from the Mucoraceae family tend to be the most aggressive. As a result, its presence on frozen section strongly suggests the need for more aggressive surgical debridement, although intraoperative findings of tissue viability should primarily guide the extent of surgery.

A more important benefit of microscopic analysis is that antifungal therapy may be more effectively tailored to the specific offending genus [66]. Specifically, amphotericin B and posaconazole are both considered effective therapy for fungi from the Mucoraceae family, which includes *Absidia*, *Apophysomyces*, *Mucor*, *Rhizomucor*, and *Rhizopus*. In contrast, voriconazole, which is first-line therapy for IFRS due to *Aspergillus* species, has no anti-Mucoraceae activity. While amphotericin B is ideally avoided due to its side effect profile including nephrotoxicity and severe infusion reactions, it fortunately does have activity against both types of invasive fungi, and thus amphotericin B is often the ideal antifungal agent in all cases of IFRS, until fungal speciation is confirmed [67].

Important "buzzword" morphologic characteristics of Mucoraceae include "ribbonlike," "broad based, aseptate," and "90° (right-angle) branching hyphae." The *Rhizopus* species are the most common causes of acute, invasive fungal sinusitis; however, microscopic exam is sometimes the only indication of its presence, given that there is frequently a lack of growth in culture. Silver staining is often only slightly positive or negative in mucormycosis, so a specimen with poorly staining hyphae should alert the pathologist to the possibility of mucormycosis [68]. *Aspergillus* also has characteristic morphology; *Aspergillus* species are typically septated hyphae with acute-angle (45°) branching patterns.

In contrast to the fungal species associated with IFRS, various phaeohyphomycotic infections, including AFRS, are associated with dematiaceous fungi (including *Alternaria*, *Curvularia*, and *Bipolaris* species) [66]. An important histologic consideration of this fungal class is that hyphae may be enlarged and globose in shape and are sometimes misidentified as yeast or fungal spores. Nonetheless, it should be possible to distinguish these fungi from more aggressive fungi.

In regard to identification techniques, the primary aim of histopathologic analysis is to highlight the fungal cell wall. Doing so allows fungus to be differentiated from human tissue and its morphology can in turn be better evaluated. While both a pathology and a microbiology lab can perform direct examination of the specimen, one should not rely on gram stain analysis in a microbiology lab to rule out the presence of a fungus. Gram reagents stain fungal cytoplasm, but they do not stain the fungal cell wall. Rapidly growing mold often lacks concentrated areas of cytoplasm due to its transport out to growing tips; with sparse cytoplasmic staining and invisible cell walls, fungus can be missed [66]. More importantly, even if present, invasion cannot be assessed on mycology smears. Thus, formal histologic analysis is always important whenever IFRS is considered based upon clinical presentation.

Common methods used in the histology lab include the hematoxylin and eosin stain, which consists of basic and acidic dyes that stain nuclei dark and extracellular and cytoplasmic material pink. While this method is occasionally sufficient to identify *Rhizopus* and *Aspergillus*, other species may be missed as it usually does not highlight the fungal cell wall.

The most sensitive histologic stains to identify fungus are the calcofluor-white stain and the silver stain. The calcofluor-white stain is a fluorescent stain that is simpler, more sensitive, and more rapidly performed than the traditional potassium hydroxide (KOH) wet mounts that were classically used to identify fungi microscopically [19]. With the silver stain, silver is deposited into the fungal cell wall readily, allowing for identification of even one isolated fungal cell. Every specimen should undergo silver staining prior to definitively declaring an absence of fungus; without this stain, evaluation cannot be considered complete.

One final caution in histologic analysis is related to the ability of fungus to undergo sporulation, which can lead to an error in diagnosis. *Aspergillus* and *Scedosporium* are common spore formers, frequently in noninvasive fungus balls. Without a positive culture to guide results, *Candida* (yeast) may be incorrectly suspected; yeast is not currently thought to be a clinically significant actor in fungal sinusitis. However, recent findings have associated yeast with certain asthma symptoms [69].

A more clinically significant error can occur in the evaluation of *Aspergillus*. In addition to its typical acute-angle branching pattern of its septate hyphae, a second hyphal form, referred to as a conidiophore, can exist during the sporulation process. The conidiophore is broad and aseptate, similar to the often more aggressive *Zygomycetes*. Fortunately, the conidiophore always occurs in conjunction with the typical form of *Aspergillus*, so the presence of both aids in accurate identification. A diagnosis of zygomycosis in conjunction with either aspergillosis or yeast should alert the otorhinolaryngologist to this potential diagnostic pitfall.

Other techniques such as in situ hybridization and PCR analysis have several limitations, the most important being a lack of specificity compared to the traditional "gold standards" allowed for by pathologic analysis and culture [68]. For these reasons, these techniques are not commercially available at the current time.

Acute Invasive Fungal Rhinosinusitis

Acute invasive fungal rhinosinusitis (AIFRS) is an important disease entity, as early diagnosis is crucial if one hopes to alter its extremely grave prognosis. A recent retrospective review encompassing three decades of patients with AIFR revealed not only a relatively low disease clearance rate of 59 % but, more significantly, also showed only a 20 % all-cause survival rate at 6 months post diagnosis [70].

Clinical Presentation

This disease process, by definition, involves invasion of fungi into sinonasal mucosa and adjacent tissues. *Aspergillus*, *Mucor*, and *Rhizopus* species are the most commonly involved fungi [70, 71]. Patients are almost always immunocompromised, specifically with conditions causing neutropenia and/or neutrophil dysfunction, including hematologic malignancy, uncontrolled diabetes mellitus, aplastic anemia, etc. Patients receiving medical immunosuppressive treatments, including chemotherapeutic agents and corticosteroids, also are at risk for AIFRS. Interestingly, though described, HIV-associated AIFR is rare due to HIV's predilection for impacting T lymphocytes, sparing neutrophils and other granulocytes [19]. A recent case report demonstrating a case of AIFR in an apparently healthy male who was later found to be using anabolic steroids serves as reminder to maintain a broad differential diagnosis in working up patients with concerning sinonasal symptoms [72].

A typical presentation will involve fever of unknown origin in an immunocompromised individual who has sinonasal symptoms. Early symptoms include facial swelling, fever, nasal congestion, facial pain or dysesthesia, and ocular abnormalities [70, 73]. An early consistent finding is discoloration of the nasal mucosa, whether pale from ischemia or dark from thrombosis and necrosis [74]. These mucosal changes are most commonly identified on the middle turbinate (Fig. 7.9), nasal septum, palate, and inferior turbinate, in decreasing frequency [75]. Endoscopy in the operating room has been shown to be more sensitive than bedside endoscopy in diagnosing these changes, suggesting the need to proceed to the operating room even if bedside exam is negative in a patient with a concerning history and findings [76].

Imaging is nonspecific and cannot definitively rule out disease, but computed tomography (CT) (Fig. 7.10) and magnetic resonance imaging (MRI) (Fig. 7.11) still may provide clues regarding the presence or absence of the disease and also help in operative planning. The most consistent early CT finding is severe unilateral nasal edema, present in nearly all patients in one institutional review over a 15-year time period [77]. Other more specific findings on CT can include retro-maxillary fatty infiltration and focal bone erosion, although these findings are less often present or may occur later in the disease process. Contrast is typically only useful on CT if orbital or intracranial extension is suspected and, in the presence of MRI, is generally considered unnecessary. Compared to CT, MRI is more likely to demonstrate early changes in AIFRS, including extra-sinus invasion; this finding has a high specificity in the diagnosis of AIFRS [78]. Orbital and intracranial invasion can be readily assessed with MRI in addition to the status of the cavernous sinus in a patient

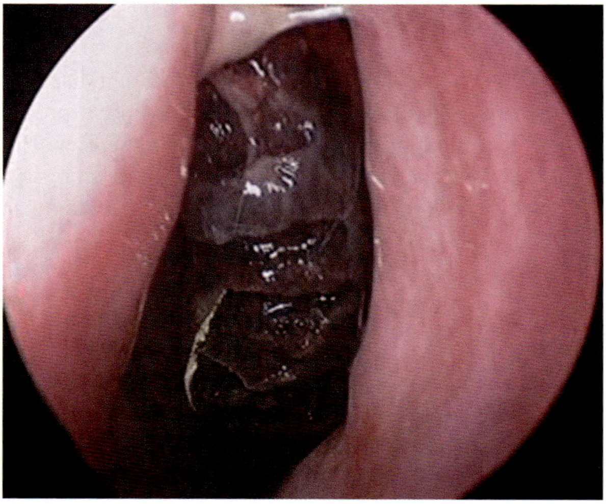

Fig. 7.9 The hallmark of acute invasive fungal rhinosinusitis is fungal tissue invasion that triggers infarction and death of normal structures, as seen in this example of an endoscopic view of a necrotic left middle turbinate in a patient with this condition

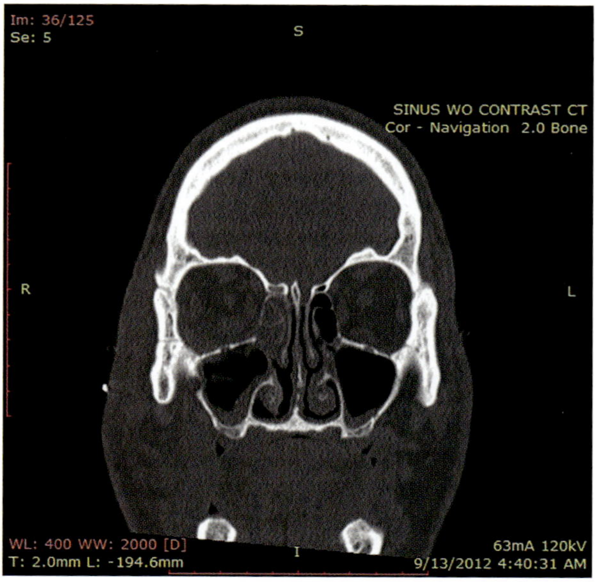

Fig. 7.10 CT scans of acute invasive fungal sinusitis often show nonspecific opacification of the involved paranasal sinuses. In this instance, there is some suggestion of destruction of the right medial orbital wall, but that finding alone is not pathognomonic of acute invasive fungal rhinosinusitis

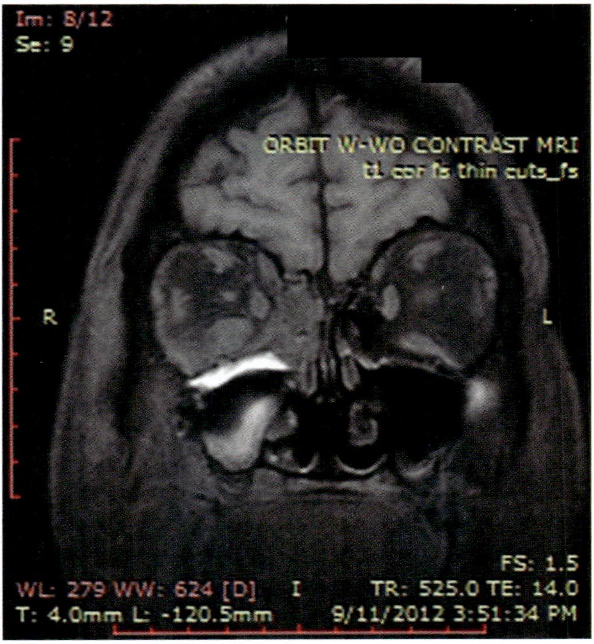

Fig. 7.11 This MRI of the same patient whose CT scan is presented in Fig. 7.10 shows abnormal signal in the right ethmoid with subtle signs of orbital involvement. Since MRI gives better soft tissue detail, it may be more sensitive in staging the extent of acute invasive fungal rhinosinusitis

with cranial nerve symptoms; even a finding as seemingly subtle as enlargement of the superior ophthalmic vein can indicate vascular occlusion caused by cavernous sinus thrombosis [74, 79].

Despite the utility of imaging, the gold standard for diagnosis involves proceeding to the operating room for biopsy. The pathologist is critical in assessing for the presence of fungal invasion within tissue and vasculature on frozen section and ultimately helps to guide the extent of debridement. Additionally, fungal culture should also be pursued to help guide medical therapy, but several days may be required for that workup to be complete.

Treatment

The three cornerstones of AIFR treatment are (1) surgical debridement of involved necrotic tissue, (2) rapid initiation of systemic antifungal therapy, and (3) reversal of immunosuppression [19].

Surgical debridement should involve endoscopic resection, as multiple reviews have shown that endoscopic sinus surgery has better survival outcomes than open surgery in the management of AIFR [73, 80, 81]. Additionally, extended open approaches and more aggressive resections, including orbital exenteration, have not been shown to improve survival [73, 82]. Even in the presence of ocular findings such as ophthalmoplegia and ptosis, orbital preservation can be achieved without affecting the likelihood of survival [83]. After surgery is performed, a "second-look" endoscopy should be performed 48–72 h after initial debridement to assess for residual disease, and subsequent nasal endoscopies should be performed on a routine basis thereafter, especially with persisting or recurrent neutropenic status [74].

Like surgery, antifungal therapy has to be expeditiously utilized in the treatment of AIFR. It should not, however, be relied upon without prior surgical debridement, as the combination of antifungal therapy with surgical debridement has dramatically higher survival rates than does antifungal therapy alone. In choosing the appropriate antifungal agent, amphotericin B, despite its side effect profile, is the antifungal of choice. Voriconazole, which is effective against *Aspergillus* and typically better tolerated, is ineffective against mucormycosis [79]. The liposomal formulation of amphotericin B, better tolerated from a side effect standpoint, has been shown to improve survival compared to the non-liposomal formulation; its use is unfortunately limited by its expense and is utilized only in patients with renal limitations or intolerance [79]. Although frozen section is limited in determining the specific causative fungal pathogen, culture results may allow the transition from amphotericin B to voriconazole several days into therapy.

Reversal of immunosuppression, while a key to therapy, is not always possible. In diabetics, treatment of hyperglycemia is of utmost importance and is readily achievable through the use of insulin. Mucormycosis is often associated with diabetes-related AIFRS and classically has been described as highly lethal when compared to other causes of AIFRS; however a recent systematic review of 398 cases by Turner et al. actually showed diabetes mellitus and surgery to be the only two independent predictors of survival [73]. It is theorized that relative ease of reversing hyperglycemia compared to other types of immunosuppression may increase survival. Yet, with mucormycosis, early identification is still paramount. In patients with medically induced neutropenia, such as solid-organ transplant recipients, immunosuppression should be withheld as soon as AIFRS is suspected. In those with hematologic malignancy, white blood cell transfusions and the administration of granulocyte colony-stimulating factor to increase absolute neutrophil count above 1,000/mm^3 are strategies to reverse the immunocompromised state [74]. Importantly, even in the setting of recovery of apparently normal immune system function and disease clearance, patients remain at risk for disease relapse if they become immunosuppressed in the future [84]. For this reason, antifungal prophylaxis in previously afflicted immunocompromised patients should be strongly considered.

Chronic Invasive Fungal Rhinosinusitis

Chronic invasive fungal rhinosinusitis may be classified into two categories: non-granulomatous chronic invasive fungal rhinosinusitis and granulomatous invasive fungal rhinosinusitis (GIFRS). As its name suggests, GIFRS is characterized by granuloma formation in response to fungi, while the non-granulomatous variant does not exhibit this feature.

Granulomatous Invasive Fungal Rhinosinusitis

GIFRS is rare in the United States and more commonly seen in immunocompetent individuals living in arid Middle Eastern, South Asian, and African countries such as Saudi Arabia, Pakistan, India, and Sudan [85]. GIFRS is the only type of invasive fungal sinusitis that readily affects healthy, immunocompetent individuals [86]. *Aspergillus flavus* and *Aspergillus fumigatus* (when occurring in North America) are the most common causative pathogens [86]. The most common presenting symptom is unilateral proptosis occurring on the order of weeks to months, in contrast to its acute invasive counterpart, AIFRS [86]. Commonly, a patient with GIFR will be taken to the OR for biopsy of a suspected tumor, and frozen section will instead reveal non-caseating granulomas with foreign body reaction and multinucleated giant cells in a background of considerable fibrosis, vascular proliferation, and vasculitis [5] (Fig. 7.12a, b). This should alert the pathologist to begin fungal analysis with appropriate staining.

Because GIFRS is a rare clinical entity, evidence regarding appropriate therapy is lacking. Classically, a treatment strategy mimicking that seen in AIFR is chosen; thus GIFRS patients receive comprehensive treatment, including aggressive surgical debridement of all involved tissue followed by prolonged use of antifungal therapy [87]. However, this treatment strategy can be problematic because GIFR, at least in part due to its relatively chronic indolent nature, is often beyond the confines of the sinus cavity at diagnosis with extensive intra-orbital and/or intracranial spread.

Recent trends in management, as supported by case reports, have shown dramatic success with a more conservative approach. One such example involved a 36-year-old immunocompetent African American male, who had symptoms present for greater than 1 year and was found by imaging to have extensive frontal and temporal lobe and orbital involvement. He was treated with endoscopic resection of involved sinuses with sparing of adjacent critical structures, followed by prolonged antifungal therapy. At 8 months post diagnosis, the patient had full resolution of symptoms and complete clearance of disease by MRI [87].

Non-granulomatous Chronic Invasive Fungal Rhinosinusitis

In contrast to GIFR, which occurs in immunocompetent individuals, the non-granulomatous form of CIFRS occurs in individuals with subtle immune abnormalities such as those associated with diabetes mellitus or those subjected to chronic corticosteroid treatment [19]. This disease entity likely represents a similar but less fulminant form of AIFRS, given its tendency to occur in a chronic indolent fashion in patients who still maintain some immune function compared to those patients who develop AIFRS. As in AIFRS, the common causative pathogens are *Aspergillus* species and *Mucorales* [88]. Orbital and/or intracranial invasion is common at the time of diagnosis and imaging often mimics a tumor, showing a soft tissue mass [19].

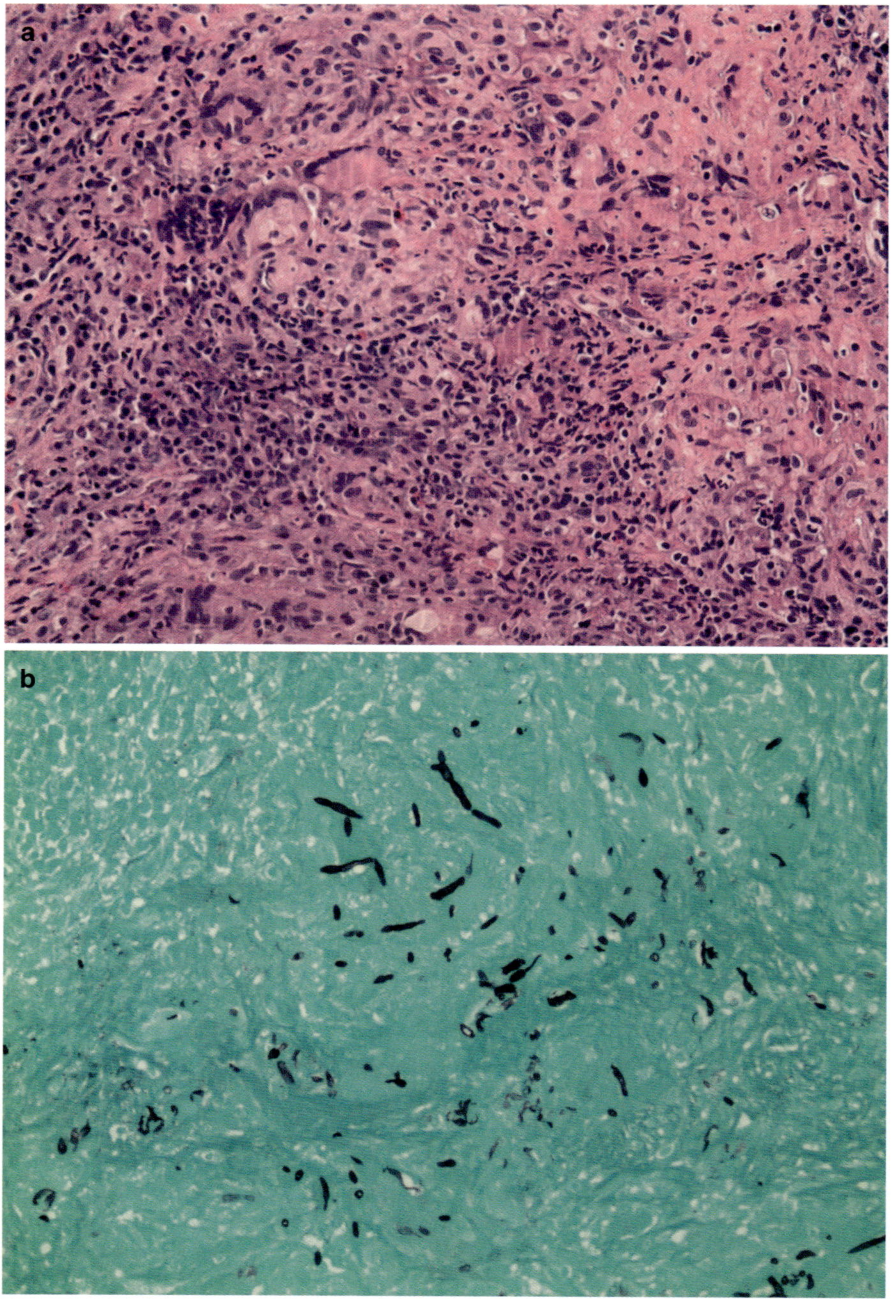

Fig. 7.12 (**a**) Granulomatous fungal rhinosinusitis is characterized by the presence of chronic inflammatory infiltrate with granuloma formation (as seen here (hematoxylin and eosin, 400×)). Fungal elements are typically difficult to identify. (**b**) In this fungal stain of the same specimen presented in (**a**), fungal elements are clearly demonstrated. The diagnosis of granulomatous fungal rhinosinusitis requires the findings seen in both (**a**) and this figure

In considering the diagnosis, the time course and the patient's immune status allow one to rule out AIFRS, and histopathologic differences distinguish non-granulomatous CIFRS from GIFR. Biopsy reveals dense accumulations of hyphae that resemble the pathology of a fungal ball [19]. The associated inflammatory reaction is considered sparse, and multinucleated giant cells and non-caseating granulomas will not be present. Though pathology is similar between fungal ball and CIFRS, clinical distinction between the two entities is straightforward; CIFR patients have symptoms seen in those with invasive processes and imaging that shows extra-sinus invasion and bone erosion; fungal ball will commonly show dual-density secretions surrounded by thick, osteitic bone without extra-sinus invasion.

Treatment of non-granulomatous CIFRS is similar to its AIFRS counterpart, relying on the reversal of the cause of relative immunosuppression, surgical debridement of involved tissue, and long-term use of antifungal agents. As in AIFR, recurrence of CIFRS can occur in accordance with a return to an immunocompromised state [88].

Conclusion

Fungal rhinosinusitis is best categorized into noninvasive and invasive forms, based upon the absence or presence of fungal invasion. Clinical criteria have grown more sophisticated over the past 20 years, and thus, it is easier for a clinician to provide an early and accurate diagnosis; however, clinical presentation of each disease type may be nonspecific, and the clinician must remain alert to subtle variations in presentation. Endoscopic sinus surgery techniques provide a method both for diagnosis confirmation and treatment. An isolated fungus ball is unlikely to recur after surgical removal with mucosal preservation; in contrast, treatment of allergic fungal rhinosinusitis will often require more extensive endoscopic surgery and postoperative treatment with systemic and topical corticosteroids. Systemic antifungal treatments are strongly indicated only for invasive fungal rhinosinusitis, which is best treated through extensive surgical debridements and antifungal medications.

References

1. Blackwell M. The fungi: 1, 2, 3 … 5.1 million species? Am J Bot. 2011;98(3):426–38.
2. Harris SD. Branching of fungal hyphae: regulation, mechanisms and comparison with other branching systems. Mycologia. 2008;100(6):823–32.
3. Kim ST, Choi JH, Jeon HG, Cha HE, Hwang YJ, Chung YS. Comparison between polymerase chain reaction and fungal culture for the detection of fungi in patients with chronic sinusitis and normal controls. Acta Otolaryngol. 2005;125(1):72–5.
4. deShazo RD, Chapin K, Swain RE. Fungal sinusitis. N Engl J Med. 1997;337(4):254–9.
5. Chakrabarti A, Denning DW, Ferguson BJ, Ponikau J, Buzina W, Kita H, et al. Fungal rhinosinusitis: a categorization and definitional schema addressing current controversies. Laryngoscope. 2009;119(9):1809–18.
6. Porter PC, Lim DJ, Maskatia ZK, Mak G, Tsai CL, Citardi MJ, et al. Airway surface mycosis in chronic T2-associated airway disease. J Allergy Clin Immunol. 2014;134(2):325–31.
7. Ferguson BJ. Definitions of fungal rhinosinusitis. Otolaryngol Clin North Am. 2000;33(2):227–35.

8. Cheng P, Meng F, Zhang D. Fatal fusarium solani infection after stem cell transplant for aplastic anemia. Exp Clin Transplant. 2014;12(4):384–7.
9. deShazo RD, O'Brien M, Chapin K, Soto-Aguilar M, Swain R, Lyons M, et al. Criteria for the diagnosis of sinus mycetoma. J Allergy Clin Immunol. 1997;99(4):475–85.
10. Ferreiro JA, Carlson BA, Cody 3rd DT. Paranasal sinus fungus balls. Head Neck. 1997;19(6):481–6.
11. Gungor A, Adusumilli V, Corey JP. Fungal sinusitis: progression of disease in immunosuppression – a case report. Ear Nose Throat J. 1998;77(3):207–10, 15.
12. Katzenstein AL, Sale SR, Greenberger PA. Allergic Aspergillus sinusitis: a newly recognized form of sinusitis. J Allergy Clin Immunol. 1983;72(1):89–93.
13. Schubert MS. Allergic fungal sinusitis: pathophysiology, diagnosis and management. Med Mycol. 2009;47 Suppl 1:S324–30.
14. Ferguson BJ, Barnes L, Bernstein JM, Brown D, Clark 3rd CE, Cook PR, et al. Geographic variation in allergic fungal rhinosinusitis. Otolaryngol Clin North Am. 2000;33(2):441–9.
15. Marple BF. Allergic fungal rhinosinusitis: current theories and management strategies. Laryngoscope. 2001;111(6):1006–19.
16. Bent 3rd JP, Kuhn FA. Diagnosis of allergic fungal sinusitis. Otolaryngol Head Neck Surg. 1994;111(5):580–8.
17. Meltzer EO, Hamilos DL, Hadley JA, Lanza DC, Marple BF, Nicklas RA, et al. Rhinosinusitis: developing guidance for clinical trials. J Allergy Clin Immunol. 2006;118(5 Suppl): S17–61.
18. Manning SC, Holman M. Further evidence for allergic pathophysiology in allergic fungal sinusitis. Laryngoscope. 1998;108(10):1485–96.
19. Callejas CA, Douglas RG. Fungal rhinosinusitis: what every allergist should know. Clin Exp Allergy. 2013;43(8):835–49.
20. Meltzer EO, Hamilos DL, Hadley JA, Lanza DC, Marple BF, Nicklas RA, et al. Rhinosinusitis: establishing definitions for clinical research and patient care. J Allergy Clin Immunol. 2004;114(6 Suppl):155–212.
21. Houser SM, Corey JP. Allergic fungal rhinosinusitis: pathophysiology, epidemiology, and diagnosis. Otolaryngol Clin North Am. 2000;33(2):399–409.
22. Bachert C, Gevaert P, Holtappels G, Cuvelier C, van Cauwenberge P. Nasal polyposis: from cytokines to growth. Am J Rhinol. 2000;14(5):279–90.
23. Luong A, Davis LS, Marple BF. Peripheral blood mononuclear cells from allergic fungal rhinosinusitis adults express a Th2 cytokine response to fungal antigens. Am J Rhinol Allergy. 2009;23(3):281–7.
24. Pant H, Kette FE, Smith WB, Wormald PJ, Macardle PJ. Fungal-specific humoral response in eosinophilic mucus chronic rhinosinusitis. Laryngoscope. 2005;115(4):601–6.
25. Aimanianda V, Bayry J, Bozza S, Kniemeyer O, Perruccio K, Elluru SR, et al. Surface hydrophobin prevents immune recognition of airborne fungal spores. Nature. 2009;460(7259): 1117–21.
26. Schubert MS, Hutcheson PS, Graff RJ, Santiago L, Slavin RG. HLA-DQB1 *03 in allergic fungal sinusitis and other chronic hypertrophic rhinosinusitis disorders. J Allergy Clin Immunol. 2004;114(6):1376–83.
27. Kheradmand F, Kiss A, Xu J, Lee SH, Kolattukudy PE, Corry DB. A protease-activated pathway underlying Th cell type 2 activation and allergic lung disease. J Immunol (Baltimore, MD: 1950). 2002;169(10):5904–11.
28. Porter P, Susarla SC, Polikepahad S, Qian Y, Hampton J, Kiss A, et al. Link between allergic asthma and airway mucosal infection suggested by proteinase-secreting household fungi. Mucosal Immunol. 2009;2(6):504–17.
29. Brant A, Upchurch S, van Tongeren M, Zekveld C, Helm J, Barnes F, et al. Detergent protease exposure and respiratory disease: case-referent analysis of a retrospective cohort. Occup Environ Med. 2009;66(11):754–8.
30. Millien VO, Lu W, Shaw J, Yuan X, Mak G, Roberts L, et al. Cleavage of fibrinogen by proteinases elicits allergic responses through Toll-like receptor 4. Science. 2013;341(6147): 792–6.

31. Kouzaki H, Tojima I, Kita H, Shimizu T. Transcription of interleukin-25 and extracellular release of the protein is regulated by allergen proteases in airway epithelial cells. Am J Respir Cell Mol Biol. 2013;49(5):741–50.
32. Ferguson BJ, Seethala R, Wood WA. Eosinophilic bacterial chronic rhinosinusitis. Laryngoscope. 2007;117(11):2036–40.
33. Clark DW, Wenaas A, Luong A, Citardi MJ, Fakhri S. Staphylococcus aureus prevalence in allergic fungal rhinosinusitis vs other subsets of chronic rhinosinusitis with nasal polyps. Int Forum Allergy Rhinol. 2013;3(2):89–93.
34. Bachert C, van Steen K, Zhang N, Holtappels G, Cattaert T, Maus B, et al. Specific IgE against Staphylococcus aureus enterotoxins: an independent risk factor for asthma. J Allergy Clin Immunol. 2012;130(2):376–81 e8.
35. Tomassen P, Jarvis D, Newson R, Van Ree R, Forsberg B, Howarth P, et al. Staphylococcus aureus enterotoxin-specific IgE is associated with asthma in the general population: a GA(2) LEN study. Allergy. 2013;68(10):1289–97.
36. Dutre T, Al Dousary S, Zhang N, Bachert C. Allergic fungal rhinosinusitis-more than a fungal disease? J Allergy Clin Immunol. 2013;132(2):487–9 e1.
37. Krysko O, Holtappels G, Zhang N, Kubica M, Deswarte K, Derycke L, et al. Alternatively activated macrophages and impaired phagocytosis of S aureus in chronic rhinosinusitis. Allergy. 2011;66(3):396–403.
38. Shaw JL, Fakhri S, Citardi MJ, Porter PC, Corry DB, Kheradmand F, et al. IL-33-responsive innate lymphoid cells are an important source of IL-13 in chronic rhinosinusitis with nasal polyps. Am J Respir Crit Care Med. 2013;188(4):432–9.
39. Mjosberg JM, Trifari S, Crellin NK, Peters CP, van Drunen CM, Piet B, et al. Human IL-25- and IL-33-responsive type 2 innate lymphoid cells are defined by expression of CRTH2 and CD161. Nat Immunol. 2011;12(11):1055–62.
40. Nagarkar DR, Poposki JA, Tan BK, Comeau MR, Peters AT, Hulse KE, et al. Thymic stromal lymphopoietin activity is increased in nasal polyps of patients with chronic rhinosinusitis. J Allergy Clin Immunol. 2013;132(3):593–600 e12.
41. Sautter NB, Citardi MJ, Perry J, Batra PS. Paranasal sinus mucoceles with skull-base and/or orbital erosion: is the endoscopic approach sufficient? Otolaryngol Head Neck Surg. 2008;139(4):570–4.
42. Kupferberg SB, Bent 3rd JP, Kuhn FA. Prognosis for allergic fungal sinusitis. Otolaryngol Head Neck Surg. 1997;117(1):35–41.
43. Bent 3rd JP, Kuhn FA. Allergic fungal sinusitis/polyposis. Allergy Asthma Proc. 1996;17(5):259–68.
44. Schubert MS, Goetz DW. Evaluation and treatment of allergic fungal sinusitis. II. Treatment and follow-up. J Allergy Clin Immunol. 1998;102(3):395–402.
45. Kuhn FA, Javer AR. Allergic fungal rhinosinusitis: perioperative management, prevention of recurrence, and role of steroids and antifungal agents. Otolaryngol Clin North Am. 2000;33(2):419–33.
46. Rupa V, Jacob M, Mathews MS, Seshadri MS. A prospective, randomised, placebo-controlled trial of postoperative oral steroid in allergic fungal sinusitis. Eur Arch Otorhinolaryngol. 2010;267(2):233–8.
47. Ikram M, Abbas A, Suhail A, Onali MA, Akhtar S, Iqbal M. Management of allergic fungal sinusitis with postoperative oral and nasal steroids: a controlled study. Ear Nose Throat J. 2009;88(4):E8–11.
48. Sachanandani NS, Piccirillo JF, Kramper MA, Thawley SE, Vlahiotis A. The effect of nasally administered budesonide respules on adrenal cortex function in patients with chronic rhinosinusitis. Arch Otolaryngol Head Neck Surg. 2009;135(3):303–7.
49. Kalish L, Snidvongs K, Sivasubramaniam R, Cope D, Harvey RJ. Topical steroids for nasal polyps. Cochrane Database Syst Rev. 2012;(12):CD006549.
50. Man LX, Farhood Z, Luong A, Fakhri S, Feldman RM, Orlander PR, et al. The effect of intranasal fluticasone propionate irrigations on salivary cortisol, intraocular pressure, and posterior subcapsular cataracts in postsurgical chronic rhinosinusitis patients. Int Forum Allergy Rhinol. 2013;3(12):953–7.

51. Mabry RL, Mabry CS. Immunotherapy for allergic fungal sinusitis: the second year. Otolaryngol Head Neck Surg. 1997;117(4):367–71.
52. Mabry RL, Marple BF, Folker RJ, Mabry CS. Immunotherapy for allergic fungal sinusitis: three years' experience. Otolaryngol Head Neck Surg. 1998;119(6):648–51.
53. Mabry RL, Marple BF, Mabry CS. Outcomes after discontinuing immunotherapy for allergic fungal sinusitis. Otolaryngol Head Neck Surg. 2000;122(1):104–6.
54. Mabry RL, Mabry CS. Allergic fungal sinusitis: the role of immunotherapy. Otolaryngol Clin North Am. 2000;33(2):433–40.
55. Bassichis BA, Marple BF, Mabry RL, Newcomer MT, Schwade ND. Use of immunotherapy in previously treated patients with allergic fungal sinusitis. Otolaryngol Head Neck Surg. 2001;125(5):487–90.
56. Greenhaw B, deShazo RD, Arnold J, Wright L. Fungal immunotherapy in patients with allergic fungal sinusitis. Ann Allergy Asthma Immunol. 2011;107(5):432–6.
57. Hall AG, deShazo RD. Immunotherapy for allergic fungal sinusitis. Curr Opin Allergy Clin Immunol. 2012;12(6):629–34.
58. Le T, Psaltis A, Tan LW, Wormald PJ. The efficacy of topical antibiofilm agents in a sheep model of rhinosinusitis. Am J Rhinol. 2008;22(6):560–7.
59. Rudmik L, Hoy M, Schlosser RJ, Harvey RJ, Welch KC, Lund V, et al. Topical therapies in the management of chronic rhinosinusitis: an evidence-based review with recommendations. Otolaryngol Head Neck Surg. 2013;3(4):281–98.
60. Isaacs S, Fakhri S, Luong A, Citardi MJ. A meta-analysis of topical amphotericin B for the treatment of chronic rhinosinusitis. Otolaryngol Head Neck Surg. 2011;1(4):250–4.
61. Sacks PL, Harvey RJ, Rimmer J, Gallagher RM, Sacks R. Topical and systemic antifungal therapy for the symptomatic treatment of chronic rhinosinusitis. Cochrane Database Systematic Reviews. 2011;(8):CD008263.
62. Thanasumpun T, Batra PS. Oral antifungal therapy for chronic rhinosinusitis and its subtypes: a systematic review. Int Forum Allergy Rhinol. 2011;1(5):382–9.
63. Pinto JM, Mehta N, DiTineo M, Wang J, Baroody FM, Naclerio RM. A randomized, double-blind, placebo-controlled trial of anti-IgE for chronic rhinosinusitis. Rhinology. 2010;48(3):318–24.
64. Gevaert P, Van Bruaene N, Cattaert T, Van Steen K, Van Zele T, Acke F, et al. Mepolizumab, a humanized anti-IL-5 mAb, as a treatment option for severe nasal polyposis. J Allergy Clin Immunol. 2011;128(5):989–95.e1-8.
65. Plonk DP, Luong A. Current understanding of allergic fungal rhinosinusitis and treatment implications. Curr Opin Otolaryngol Head Neck Surg. 2014;22(3):221–6.
66. Schell WA. Histopathology of fungal rhinosinusitis. Otolaryngol Clin North Am. 2000;33(2):251–76.
67. Lass-Florl C, Mayr A, Perkhofer S, Hinterberger G, Hausdorfer J, Speth C, et al. Activities of antifungal agents against yeasts and filamentous fungi: assessment according to the methodology of the European Committee on Antimicrobial Susceptibility Testing. Antimicrob Agents Chemother. 2008;52(10):3637–41.
68. Guarner J, Brandt ME. Histopathologic diagnosis of fungal infections in the 21st century. Clin Microbiol Rev. 2011;24(2):247–80.
69. Mak G, Porter PC, Bandi V, Kheradmand F, Corry DB. Tracheobronchial mycosis in a retrospective case-series study of five status asthmaticus patients. Clin Immunol. 2013;146(2):77–83.
70. Monroe MM, McLean M, Sautter N, Wax MK, Andersen PE, Smith TL, et al. Invasive fungal rhinosinusitis: a 15-year experience with 29 patients. Laryngoscope. 2013;123(7):1583–7.
71. Montone KT, Livolsi VA, Feldman MD, Palmer J, Chiu AG, Lanza DC, et al. Fungal rhinosinusitis: a retrospective microbiologic and pathologic review of 400 patients at a single university medical center. Int J Otolaryngol. 2012;2012:684835.
72. Kim IA, Thompson CF, Kedeshian PA, Palma-Diaz F, Suh JD. Invasive fungal sinusitis in a healthy athlete due to long-term anabolic steroid use. Laryngoscope. 2014;124(8):1756–9.

73. Turner JH, Soudry E, Nayak JV, Hwang PH. Survival outcomes in acute invasive fungal sinusitis: a systematic review and quantitative synthesis of published evidence. Laryngoscope. 2013;123(5):1112–8.
74. Epstein VA, Kern RC. Invasive fungal sinusitis and complications of rhinosinusitis. Otolaryngol Clin North Am. 2008;41(3):497–524, viii.
75. Gillespie MB, O'Malley Jr BW, Francis HW. An approach to fulminant invasive fungal rhinosinusitis in the immunocompromised host. Arch Otolaryngol Head Neck Surg. 1998;124(5):520–6.
76. Park AH, Muntz HR, Smith ME, Afify Z, Pysher T, Pavia A. Pediatric invasive fungal rhinosinusitis in immunocompromised children with cancer. Otolaryngol Head Neck Surg. 2005;133(3):411–6.
77. DelGaudio JM, Swain Jr RE, Kingdom TT, Muller S, Hudgins PA. Computed tomographic findings in patients with invasive fungal sinusitis. Arch Otolaryngol Head Neck Surg. 2003;129(2):236–40.
78. Groppo ER, El-Sayed IH, Aiken AH, Glastonbury CM. Computed tomography and magnetic resonance imaging characteristics of acute invasive fungal sinusitis. Arch Otolaryngol Head Neck Surg. 2011;137(10):1005–10.
79. Zuniga MG, Turner JH. Treatment outcomes in acute invasive fungal rhinosinusitis. Curr Opin Otolaryngol Head Neck Surg. 2014;22(3):242–8.
80. Chen CY, Sheng WH, Cheng A, Chen YC, Tsay W, Tang JL, et al. Invasive fungal sinusitis in patients with hematological malignancy: 15 years experience in a single university hospital in Taiwan. BMJ. Infect Dis. 2011;11:250.
81. Kasapoglu F, Coskun H, Ozmen OA, Akalin H, Ener B. Acute invasive fungal rhinosinusitis: evaluation of 26 patients treated with endonasal or open surgical procedures. Otolaryngol Head Neck Surg. 2010;143(5):614–20.
82. Hargrove RN, Wesley RE, Klippenstein KA, Fleming JC, Haik BG. Indications for orbital exenteration in mucormycosis. Ophthal Plast Reconst Surg. 2006;22(4):286–91.
83. Avet PP, Kline LB, Sillers MJ. Endoscopic sinus surgery in the management of mucormycosis. J Neuroophthalmol. 1999;19(1):56–61.
84. Parikh SL, Venkatraman G, DelGaudio JM. Invasive fungal sinusitis: a 15-year review from a single institution. Am J Rhinol. 2004;18(2):75–81.
85. Deshazo RD. Syndromes of invasive fungal sinusitis. Med Mycol. 2009;47 Suppl 1:S309–14.
86. Stringer SP, Ryan MW. Chronic invasive fungal rhinosinusitis. Otolaryngol Clin North Am. 2000;33(2):375–87.
87. Halderman A, Shrestha R, Sindwani R. Chronic granulomatous invasive fungal sinusitis: an evolving approach to management. Int Forum Allergy Rhinol. 2014;4(4):280–3.
88. Li Y, Li Y, Li P, Zhang G. Diagnosis and endoscopic surgery of chronic invasive fungal rhinosinusitis. Am J Rhinol Allergy. 2009;23(6):622–5.

Management of Functional Endoscopic Sinus Surgery (FESS) Failures

8

Ashleigh A. Halderman, Janalee Stokken, and Raj Sindwani

Key Take Home Points

- Some patients with chronic rhinosinusitis will fail standard medical and surgical therapy. This disease process is known as recalcitrant chronic rhinosinusitis.
- Anatomy, certain concurrent disease processes, and failure of the delivery of topical therapies can all contribute to unsuccessful management of recalcitrant sinusitis.
- The differential diagnosis for recalcitrant CRS includes underlying allergic rhinitis, aspirin-exacerbated respiratory disease (AERD), gastroesophageal reflux disease (GERD), mucociliary dysfunction, biofilms, autoimmune disease, and immunodeficiency.
- Some of the most common anatomic factors leading to revision surgery include lateralization of the middle turbinate, incomplete ethmoidectomy, scarring of the frontal recess, and middle meatal antrostomy stenosis.
- Multiple topical therapies and delivery mechanisms exist without clear evidence that one drug or one method of delivery is more effective than the others.

A.A. Halderman, MD • J. Stokken, MD • R. Sindwani, MD (✉)
Section of Rhinology, Sinus and Skull Base Surgery, Head and Neck Institute, Cleveland Clinic Foundation, 9500 Euclid Avenue, A71, Cleveland, OH 44195, USA
e-mail: haldera3@ccf.org; stokkej@ccf.org; sindwar@ccf.org

P.S. Batra, J.K. Han (eds.), *Practical Medical and Surgical Management of Chronic Rhinosinusitis*, DOI 10.1007/978-3-319-16724-4_8

Introduction

Chronic rhinosinusitis (CRS) is defined as a group of disorders characterized by inflammation of the mucosa of the nose and paranasal sinuses of at least 12 consecutive weeks' duration [1]. Further, CRS is often subdivided into chronic rhinosinusitis with nasal polyposis (CRSwNP) and chronic rhinosinusitis without polyposis (CRSsNP). The pathogenesis of CRS is multifactorial; thus the treatment can be challenging. The primary management of CRS includes systemic medical and topical therapies. When these fail, surgical management is considered in appropriate cases.

Recalcitrant CRS occurs when the disease process does not respond to maximal medical and surgical therapy. In this setting, it is important to reevaluate the patient, repeat computed tomography (CT) imaging, and obtain endoscopic cultures. Recalcitrant disease can occur if the primary surgical approach was insufficient, in the setting of certain systemic diseases (immunodeficiency or cystic fibrosis), or both as medical treatments can be refractory if there are predisposing anatomic factors. Obtaining more information will help guide further management decisions. Both revision surgery and optimization of systemic and topical medical therapies can be utilized to improve the patient's disease burden.

When endoscopic sinus surgery (ESS) results in an unsatisfactory outcome, the presence of an underlying disease process which may have been previously undiagnosed should definitely be considered. The differential diagnosis for recalcitrant CRS includes underlying allergic rhinitis, aspirin-exacerbated respiratory disease (AERD), gastroesophageal reflux disease (GERD), mucociliary dysfunction, biofilms, autoimmune disease, and immunodeficiency, to mention a few. A thorough history and physical exam, including rigorous evaluation with angled endoscopes, will help the clinician assess previous surgical completeness as well as guide further medical workup for the aforementioned disease processes.

Allergic Rhinitis/Inhalant Allergy

The relationship between allergic rhinitis and CRS is controversial. The association of allergy and CRS has been reported from 25 to 50 %, which is greater than the prevalence in the general population [1]. Batra et al. found an overall prevalence of inhalant allergy in 38.7 % of the patients undergoing revision ESS for refractory CRS [2]. Both allergic rhinitis and CRS with nasal polyposis have been shown to have a similar underlying pathophysiology driven by a shift in the immune system with a skewed T-helper 2 cell cytokine profile. Allergy could potentially lead to or exacerbate CRS by causing generalized inflammation of the mucosa and obstruction of the sinus ostia. It therefore stands to reason that targeting the allergies and improving any component of inflammation for which allergies may be responsible for could help in the overall management of CRS. Of note, there is large overlap in the symptoms of allergic rhinitis and CRS; this can complicate the assessment of patients for subjective improvement following treatment of sinus disease.

In a case of recalcitrant CRS where the history suggests a possible allergic component, allergy testing is recommended. Allergy should be considered when patients have seasonal symptoms, itching of the nose and eyes, conjunctivitis, nasal congestion, sneezing, or established environmental triggers. Allergy testing can be conducted by skin testing (intradermal, skin prick, or scratch) or by in vitro serologic testing such as modified radioallergosorbent (mRAST). In appropriate cases, immunotherapy (IT) should be initiated by an otolaryngologist or allergist. IT has been shown to improve both clinical measures (radiographic and endoscopic scores, fewer revision surgeries, fewer office visits) and symptoms of CRS when used in addition to traditional therapies [3]. The evidence-based literature up to this point is weak, however, and more data in the form of randomized controlled trials is required.

Aspirin-Exacerbated Respiratory Disease (AERD)

AERD is a disease process with a constellation of clinical symptoms including aspirin (ASA) sensitivity, nasal polyposis, and asthma, also known as "Samter's triad." Patients with AERD have abnormal arachidonic acid metabolism resulting in an overproduction of proinflammatory leukotrienes through the 5-lipoxygenase pathway [4, 5]. Aspirin inhibits cyclooxygenase, thereby decreasing prostaglandin-E2, which normally inhibits leukotriene production and also prevents mast cell degranulation [4, 5]. The inhibition of cyclooxygenase by aspirin thus triggers exacerbations.

In general, the CRSwNP component of AERD (Fig. 8.1) is treated with topical and systemic steroids with a large portion of patients failing purely medical therapy and requiring ESS. Surgery is rarely curative as this disease process represents one of the most recalcitrant forms of CRS with 37 % of the patients requiring revision surgery at 5 years and 89 % at 10 years [6]. This is compared to CRSwNP without ASA triad or asthma in which 10 % of the patients required revision surgery at 5 years and 17 % at 10 years [6].

Postoperative care for this subset of patients is a controversial topic. Many otolaryngologists utilize high-dose topical steroid irrigations in controlling the recurrence of this disease. However, one study has demonstrated that budesonide nasal irrigations have not been shown to alter postoperative recurrence of the disease at 1 year [7]. More research is needed to establish what effect, if any, high-dose nasal steroid irrigations have on disease progression and the need for revision surgery.

More recently, ASA desensitization has shown promise for patients with CRS and AERD. Aspirin desensitization and daily aspirin maintenance have been established as beneficial in the management of CRSwNP in patients with AERD [5, 8]. ASA desensitization has been shown to have a positive impact on endoscopic polyp scores and is associated with both a decreased frequency of sinus surgeries and sinus infections [5]. The process of ASA desensitization is conducted as an inpatient, medical day unit or outpatient setting. Patients undergo a pretreatment regimen including optimization of pulmonary status, daily montelukast, and treatment of other concomitant conditions. ESS if needed should be timed 4–6 weeks prior to desensitization, as the therapy is more effective at preventing the regrowth of polyps

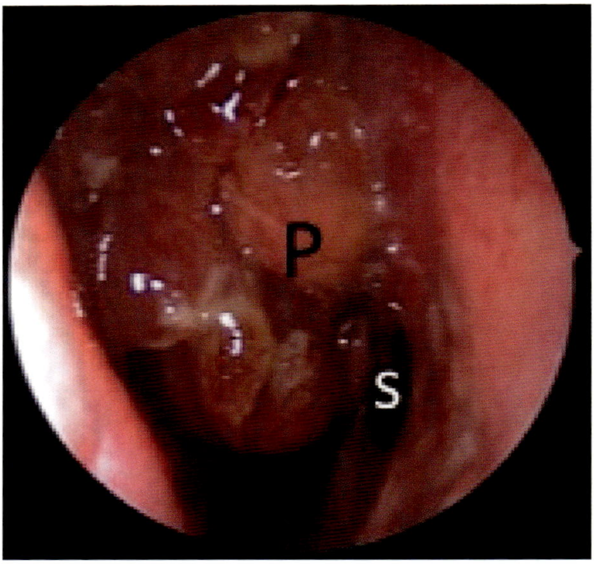

Fig. 8.1 Recurrent nasal polyposis (*P*) in the right nasal cavity in a patient with AERD and CRS. Septal perforation (*s*) secondary to previous surgery

than at reducing polyp size. A challenge is given by increasing doses of ASA until a target dose (usually 325 mg) is reached. The patient is then maintained on a maintenance dose (650 mg twice a day) indefinitely or risk re-sensitization. This dose can then often be weaned after a month if there is adequate symptom response, and systemic corticosteroids are reduced or eliminated [8].

Overall, ASA desensitization and ongoing maintenance therapy is tolerated in the majority of patients with only 8–23 % of the patients experiencing mild adverse events. Side effects including gastritis, dyspepsia, or epistaxis can be barriers to success. ASA desensitization has also shown a significant reduction of oral corticosteroid use by AERD patients and a significant improvement in subjective symptoms; however, double-blind randomized placebo-controlled studies are still necessary to prove causation [5].

Postoperative management in AERD and CRS should include twice-daily nasal saline irrigations with the addition of high-dose topical steroids at the discretion of the clinician. ASA desensitization should be considered in all AERD patients with severe or intractable symptoms or aggressive nasal polyp formation.

Gastroesophageal Reflux (GERD)

GERD has not been shown to cause or at least contribute to CRS. It is known to coexist in nearly half of the patients with postnasal drainage as a complaint, which can be misinterpreted by both patients and general practitioners as ongoing sinus disease [9]. However, GERD has been shown to be more prevalent in patients with refractive CRS than in patients with treatment responsive CRS and in healthy controls [10]. In addition, a few small studies have shown modest improvement of CRS symptoms in patients on once- or twice-daily proton pump inhibitor (PPI) therapy [10]. This suggests a possible causative effect that many feel represents contribution of reflux to underlying inflammation in the sinonasal tract. As such, in the setting of known GERD, symptoms suggestive of GERD, and/or findings on physical exam suggestive of GERD (flexible laryngoscopy findings), a referral for pH probe testing or initiation of PPI therapy should be considered.

Mucociliary Dysfunction

Most inherited forms of ciliary dysfunction, including Kartagener syndrome and cystic fibrosis (CF), are typically diagnosed in childhood. A detailed history and physical exam including past medical history and family history may heighten suspicion for these syndromes in patients with recalcitrant CRS. In the event of elevated suspicion, further testing for evaluation of Kartagener syndrome or CF should be considered. A referral to genetics for further genetic testing and counseling is necessary for any positive or equivocal test results.

Kartagener syndrome is a primary form of ciliary dyskinesia due to an abnormality in the dynein arm and is diagnosed by the saccharine mucociliary transport test or nasal biopsy with electron microscopy. It is associated with recurrent lung, ear, and sinonasal infections in children as well as hyposmia, infertility, and the findings of situs inversus and dextrocardia.

CF, an autosomal recessively inherited disease, results in secondary ciliary dysmotility by altering the viscosity of mucous through the disruption of transmembrane transport of chloride ions. The body's mucociliary transport mechanisms are not efficient with this more viscous form of mucous. Recurrent *Pseudomonas aeruginosa* and *Staphylococcus aureus* colonization and infections are common. CF is typically diagnosed in childhood in the setting of bronchiectasis, recurrent pulmonary infections, CRS, malabsorption, and stunted growth. CF should be ruled out in any child that presents with nasal polyps. Diagnosis is made through newborn screening, sweat testing, and/or genetic testing. CT imaging in CF will often reveal hypoplastic sinus cavities with mucosal thickening and sclerosis and thickening of the adjacent bony framework (Fig. 8.2). Some less severe phenotypes of CF may not be diagnosed until adulthood and should be in the differential diagnosis in refractory CRS.

The management of CF is difficult and requires a multidisciplinary approach. As the pathophysiology of this disease results in a chronic process, the management of CRS is primarily medical. However, many patients fail medical management and require a surgical approach. In general, the indications for ESS are sinus disease that is contributing to pulmonary exacerbations and declining pulmonary function, medically refractory polyposis with nasal obstruction, and lung transplant candidacy [11, 12]. As the survival of cystic fibrosis patients continues to increase, this number will likely increase. Larger surgical openings are generally advocated for the refractory CF patient with significant CRS.

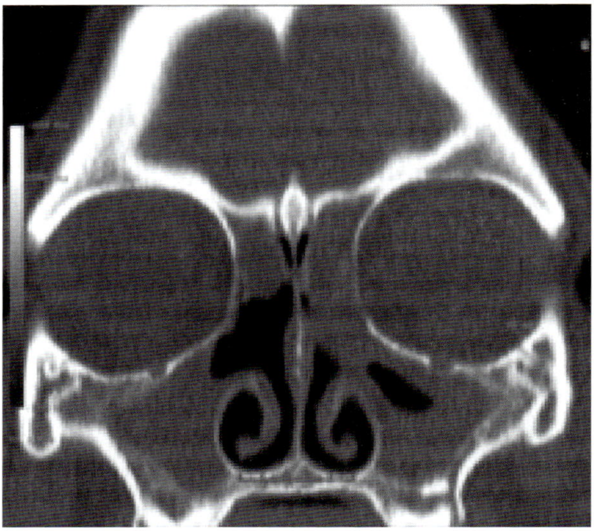

Fig. 8.2 Mucosal thickening and opacification of the bilateral maxillary, frontal, and ethmoid sinuses with characteristic hypoplastic maxillary sinuses as seen in CF

Biofilms

Certain common bacterial species including *Staphylococcus aureus* and *Pseudomonas aeruginosa* are capable of forming biofilms. Bacterial biofilms are defined as an assemblage of microbial cells enclosed in a self-produced polymeric matrix that is irreversibly associated with an inert or living surface [13]. The organized communities of bacteria attached to the sinonasal mucosa can then release planktonic bacteria that create acute exacerbations. The adherent and organized nature of the biofilm imparts a resistance to standard oral antibiotics.

The confirmation of the presence of biofilms depends on identification by scanning electron microscopy, confocal laser microscopy, or transmission electron microscopy, which are not accessible in the clinical setting. As such, the diagnosis is more often made with positive cultures for typical biofilm forming species in the setting of recalcitrant disease. CRS patients with biofilms have been shown to have more severe disease both preoperatively and postoperatively suggesting a role in recalcitrant disease [14].

Studies looking at topical antibiotic therapies have shown mixed results in patients with CRS. Various surfactants including 1 % baby shampoo in normal saline and manuka honey have shown some promising results in overall symptom control and antibiofilm activity; however, more research is necessary to establish evidence-based recommendations [15].

Immunodeficiency

Patients with immunodeficiency have recalcitrant disease because of their underlying immune disorder. Recurrent sinopulmonary infections are the most prevalent infections among primary immunodeficiency patients. CRS can be seen in common variable immunodeficiency (CVID), selective IgA deficiency, IgG subclass deficiency, and specific polysaccharide antibody deficiency [16]. CVID is the most common symptomatic primary immunodeficiency in adults and has been observed in up to 10 % of patients with refractory CRS [16, 17]. Further, more than 20 % of patients with CRS have lower than normal levels of one or more immunoglobulins [18].

Evaluation for immunodeficiency should be considered in patients with frequently recurrent, persistent, and/or severe infections or recalcitrant rhinosinusitis with rare organisms. These patients may also have associated atopy, autoimmune disease, or gastrointestinal disease. The importance of identifying an underlying immunodeficiency cannot be stressed enough as the management changes drastically. More judicious use of antibiotics, both prophylactic and culture directed, should be used, and IVIG may be indicated in certain situations. Once identified, these patients should be monitored in coordination with an immunologist.

Revision Surgery

As mentioned, sometimes more surgery can offer an advantage in the management of the refractory CRS patient who is not doing well after a prior surgical intervention. Both the endoscopic exam and repeat CT imaging will characterize when the etiology for failure is anatomic. The decision to proceed with revision surgery should be made on an individual basis depending on the underlying contributing factors. Symptomatic patients with obstruction on imaging or symptomatic patients with a significant disease burden are likely to be good candidates. The role of revision surgery in CRS is to improve medical management by reducing disease load and improving access for irrigations and topical therapies.

It has been estimated that 8–20 % of patients undergoing ESS will require revision surgery [19, 20]. Multiple studies have reviewed the common anatomic reasons for revision surgery. Musy reported the most common anatomic factors leading to revision surgery were lateralization of the middle turbinate (78 %), incomplete anterior ethmoidectomy (64 %), scarred frontal recess (50 %), incomplete posterior ethmoidectomy (41 %), and middle meatal antrostomy stenosis (39 %) [21]. Gore et al. noted residual anterior and posterior ethmoid cells or septations (75 %), a residual uncinate process (64 %), residual agger nasi cells (64 %), unopened sphenoid sinuses (53 %), and frontal cells (45 %) on preoperative imaging of patients undergoing revision surgery [22]. Bassiouni identified the most common location for polyp recurrence to be in the frontal sinus or frontal recess (55 %) followed by the ethmoid cavity (38 %) [23].

Revision surgery of the maxillary sinus is most often required when there is a residual uncinate process or a surgically created opening into the sinus not confluent with the natural ostium. The latter predisposes to recirculation of mucus from the natural opening back into the sinus via the "false" surgical opening, predisposing the patient to recurrent infections. A remnant uncinate can result in a bridge of tissue between the natural os and the surgical antrostomy causing recirculation (Fig. 8.3). Recirculation can also occur secondary to scarring or incomplete initial antrostomy. Another cause of maxillary sinus obstruction is persistent infraorbital ethmoid cells (Haller cells). These cells can be overlooked due to a more anterior position than expected. A 30° scope can be utilized to both ensure the natural os is included in the antrostomy and that there is not a residual Haller cell.

Although total ethmoidectomy is not indicated in all patients undergoing primary endoscopic sinus surgery, most will undergo uncinectomy, anterior ethmoidectomy, and maxillary antrostomy if they have severe enough disease to necessitate surgery. In revision ethmoid surgery, the entire ethmoid labyrinth should be opened in a posterior to anterior fashion. Surgical navigation can be helpful to identify unopened cells and the location of the skull base and lamina papyracea. The strut of the horizontal segment of the basal lamella should remain intact to prevent lateralization of the middle turbinate. A curette should be used to ensure the medial bulla has been removed, and all of the bony partitions along the lamina should be removed to reduce the mucosal surface area for recurrent polyp growth. Mucosal

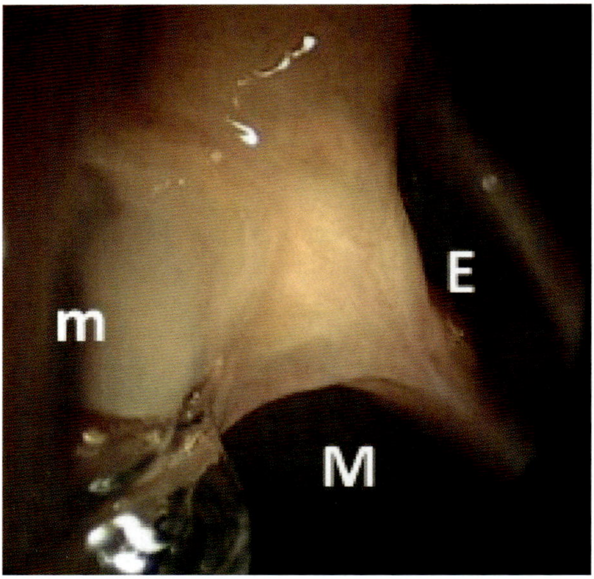

Fig. 8.3 Recirculation of mucous from the natural maxillary os (*m*) on the right into the maxillary antrostomy (*M*). Adjacent ethmoid (*E*) cells are also visible

preservation will reduce scarring and antrostomy stenosis; therefore, sharp dissection should be used to prevent mucosal stripping.

Patients with chronic frontal sinusitis should at minimum undergo resection of the agger nasi cell and complete excision of the superior uncinate process. Preoperative analysis of the frontal recess anatomy on imaging (especially using sagittal CT reconstructions) is particularly important to identify the drainage pathway and to identify reasons for failure. If the frontal recess is not obvious intraoperatively, an image-guided probe can be invaluable. Once identified, synechiae and bone fragments can be cut and removed. Curettes can be used to take down the beak anteriorly. A lateralized middle turbinate (Fig. 8.4) can often be an iatrogenic cause for frontal sinusitis; this can be addressed by medialization with a stitch (pexy),

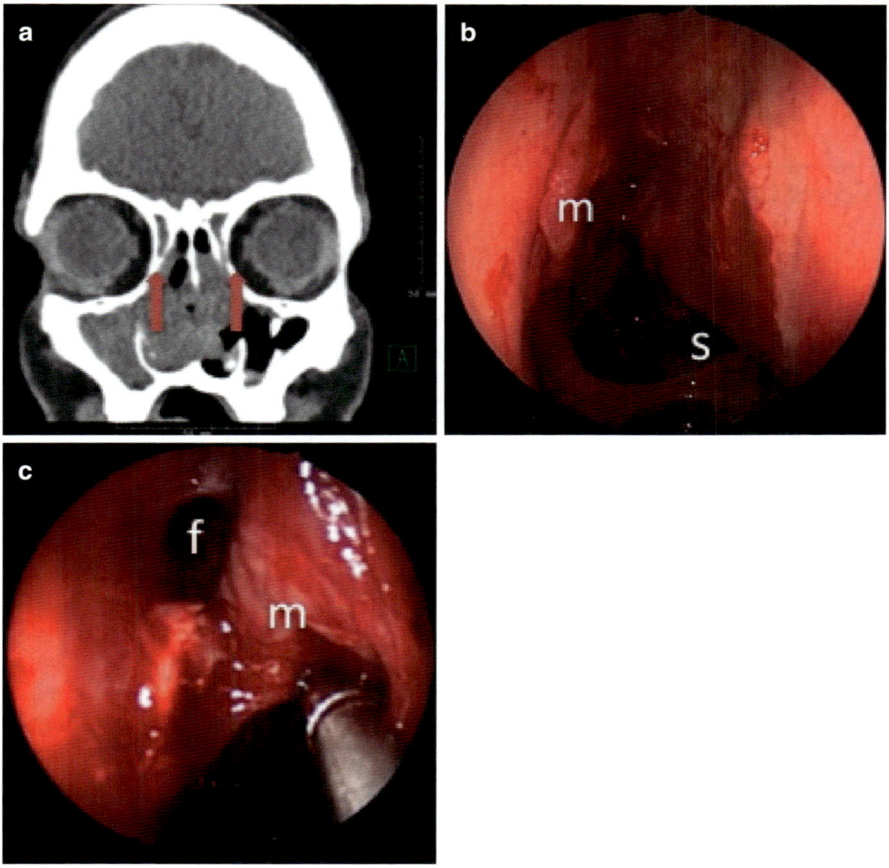

Fig. 8.4 (**a**) Lateralized middle turbinate remnant (*arrows*) obstructing the frontal recess bilaterally in the setting of AERD with recurrent polyps. (**b**) Lateralized middle turbinate remnant (*m*) obstructing the right frontal sinus. Posterior septal defect (*s*) and synechiae (*arrow*) secondary to previous surgery. (**c**) Right frontal recess (*f*) after medialization of the middle turbinate (*m*) and balloon dilation

spacer, or middle turbinate resection. The frontal sinus rescue procedure has also been described as a method to prevent recurrent stenosis [24]. More recently, aggressive management of the frontal recess by Draf 3/modified Lothrop/frontal drillout procedure has been shown to reduce long-term (>12 months) polyp recurrence, especially in more complicated patients with asthma and AERD [23].

The sphenoid sinus may be obstructed from stenosis and scarring. The location of the natural os can be identified medial to the superior turbinate or turbinate remnant. Image guidance may be helpful. A large sphenoidotomy should be created in revision surgery to reduce the risk of restenosis and to allow for adequate topical drug delivery. This should be accomplished in a medial and inferior direction using through-cutting instruments and good visualization to avoid vascular injury and to cut through the thick sphenoid bone.

Overall, the goals of revision surgery are to widely open obstructed sinus cavities, decrease disease burden by removing bulky polypoid tissue, remove residual cells and partitions that are acting as a nidus for infection or polyposis, and improve access for irrigations and topical therapies.

Topical Drug Delivery

Arguably, medical therapies for CRS are the strongest weapons in the veritable armamentarium of each physician and represent the true "workhorse" in the management of this chronic disease. Irrigations act by removing antigens, mucus, bacteria, and pollutants from the sinonasal mucosa. Topical therapies allow for direct application of medication to the diseased tissue at an increased concentration with decreased systemic absorption and associated side effects than systemic therapies. Topical therapy does however have limitations including variable penetration into the sinuses, adverse effects such as discomfort and epistaxis, and a need for education on the appropriate technique for mixing and using each therapy. All of which can limit compliance.

Delivery of irrigant into unoperated paranasal sinuses has been shown to be quite limited; the frontal and sphenoid sinuses are essentially not accessible, and high-flow devices provide some infiltration to the maxillary and ethmoid sinuses [25]. ESS allows for improvement in access for topical drug delivery, though the degree depends on the extent of surgery. Multiple types of therapies have been proposed as means to topically treat CRS including corticosteroids, antibiotics, and antifungals. The more commonly used medications and doses are listed in Table 8.1. Multiple delivery devices exist as well and are described below.

Nasal Saline

Nasal saline irrigations both preoperatively and postoperatively have become a standard of care. Evidence has established that irrigating with saline can improve symptoms and quality of life both before and after surgery [15]. High-volume (≥200 mL)

Table 8.1 Topical therapies [26–29]

Steroid
Budesonide (0.5 mg/2 ml Respules mixed in 240 cc bottle) [26]
Gram-positive antibiotic
Mupirocin 0.05 % (22 g tube in 1 L NS) [27]
Betadine (10 cc in 1 l of NS)
Gram-negative antibiotic
Tobramycin (80 mg/2 ml, 1 vial in 1 L NS) [28]
Gentamycin (80 mcg/ml, 1 vial in 1 L NS)
Ceftazidime (4 g in 40 cc saline stock, mix 3 ml stock w/ 300 cc saline)
Antifungal
Amphotericin – 100–250 μg/mL [29]

low-pressure irrigations have been shown to be more effective than low-volume low-pressure delivery systems. Hypertonic and isotonic solutions have been shown to be fairly equivocal in regard to symptom management [30]. It is important to note that nasal saline irrigations are often used as an adjuvant to other medical therapies for CRS and not in isolation. Fortunately, nasal saline is well tolerated with few side effects and is inexpensive.

Intranasal Steroids

Numerous metered-dose topical steroid sprays exist and include triamcinolone acetonide, fluticasone propionate, mometasone furoate, fluticasone furoate budesonide, and beclomethasone dipropionate monohydrate. In both CRSsNP and CRSwNP, metered-dose nasal steroid sprays improve both subjective and objective outcomes in patients including better endoscopy scores and significant decrease in polyp size [15]. Further, patients with sinus surgery had significantly greater reduction in polyp size while on nasal steroid sprays than did patients without sinus surgery [31]. Overall, metered-dose nasal steroid sprays are well tolerated; however, they have been associated with epistaxis and headache which may limit their use. The well-established benefit from this medical therapy, which is relatively safe (limited systemic absorption) and inexpensive, has made it another standard in the management in CRSwNP.

In an attempt to increase both the volume and concentration of steroid delivered topically to the mucosa, some physicians advocate irrigation with steroids such as budesonide mixed with saline, particularly in the setting of more recalcitrant forms of CRS. Not as much evidence exists for steroid irrigations as does for metered-dose nasal sprays, but at least one large case series has shown that postoperative use of budesonide or betamethasone in high-volume irrigation provides improvement in quality of life, symptoms, and endoscopy scores [32]. Another retrospective review showed that patients experienced worsening symptoms and endoscopy findings when not using budesonide irrigations despite the use of metered-dose nasal steroid sprays [33]. Studies have shown that twice-daily budesonide irrigations do not cause an appreciable change in serum or urine cortisol or significantly suppress adrenal function [15]. As these therapies are "off label" and not approved by the FDA, they can be prohibitively expensive which is a major disadvantage.

Antibiotics

Systemic antibiotics are a mainstay of treatment for acute exacerbations of CRS. The idea of topical delivery of antibiotics for chronically infected sinuses is appealing as the systemic side effect of antibiotics can be avoided. The literature is fairly mixed however, on the efficacy and role of topical antibiotic therapies. In their systematic review, Rudmik et al. identified three randomized controlled trials which were heterogenous in the antibiotics used and the methods of delivery; all of the studies failed to show any benefit of a topical antibiotic over placebo [15]. Other studies have shown that irrigation with topical antibiotics is effective in CRS [34–36].

Certain patient populations appear to derive a clearer benefit from topical antibiotics. One such population is patients with CF and pseudomonal infections. These patients have improved outcome scores and a decreased need for revision surgery while on tobramycin irrigations [28, 35]. Another population is those with chronic *Staphylococcus aureus* infection in the setting of CRS. Irrigation with 0.05 % mupirocin mixed in saline has been shown to decrease biofilm burden and improve endoscopic and symptoms scores [37, 38]. Despite these promising results, reinfection rates remain high in this subgroup [27].

Antifungals

It has been hypothesized that fungal elements contribute to mucosal inflammation in a subset of patients with CRS. Certainly, fungus plays a role in allergic fungal sinusitis, but a contribution to other types of chronic sinus disease has not been established and largely fallen out of favor.

While one study has shown improvement in endoscopy scores and CT scores in patients irrigating with amphotericin B versus placebo, four separate randomized controlled trials and two meta-analyses have shown no statistically significant difference between topical amphotericin B over placebo in regard to clinical outcomes [15]. Further, a Cochrane Review failed to show any benefit with either topical or systemic antifungals in CRS [39]. Topically delivered antifungals can cause adverse events such as nasal burning, epistaxis, and even exacerbation of CRS; therefore, the use of this therapy is not recommended as the risks appear to outweigh any benefits.

Delivery Devices

As stated above, ESS is a necessary prerequisite to allow for delivery of topical substances into the sinuses. Multiple delivery devices exist and can be classified by low-volume and high-volume delivery.

Low-Volume Devices and Properties

Low-volume delivery devices include metered-dose/nasal pump sprays and nebulizers. Each delivers a small volume of substance to the nasal cavities in either a spray or mist form. Numerous factors influence the delivery of particles to the paranasal sinuses and include a smaller particle size between 3 and 10 μm, higher flow rates, and ostial size (greater than 3.95 mm is necessary for maxillary penetration) [26]. Nasal sprays typically produce droplets 50–100 μm in size, and therefore, the vast majority of these particles are deposited in the anterior nasal cavity [26]. Nebulizers can produce particles of various sizes, and studies have shown improved particle deposition in the posterior nasal cavity and at the ostiomeatal complex when compared to metered-dose/nasal pump sprays [26].

High-Volume Devices and Properties

High-volume delivery devices include the squeeze bottle and the neti pot. The major difference between the two is that the volume is delivered by high pressure versus low pressure, respectively. In several studies, high-volume delivery devices have outperformed low-volume delivery devices in penetration into postoperative sinus cavities [26]. However, when comparing the neti pot to the squeeze bottle, or the low-pressure system to the high-pressure system, outcomes have been mixed with one outperforming the other in one study and in another study showing the reverse [40].

Other Delivery Devices

Topical drug delivery is an evolving field with many new up and coming products. These include drug-eluding stents (Fig. 8.5), dissolvable drug-saturated packing, and dissolvable drug-concentrated foam to name a few. As these products are

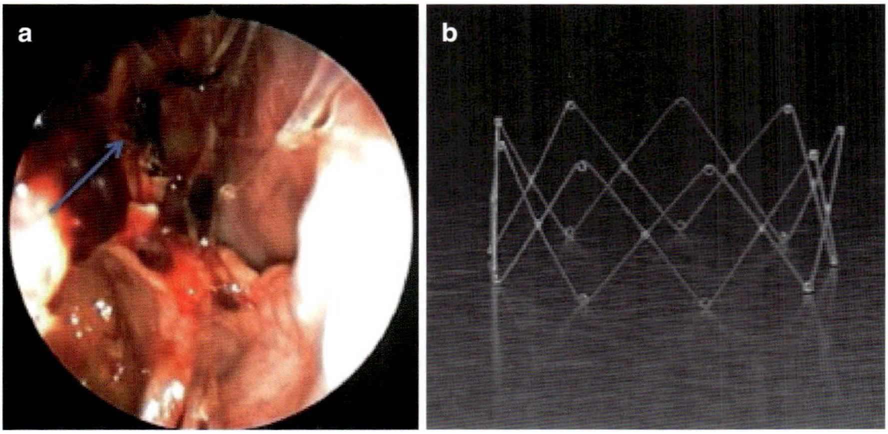

Fig. 8.5 (**a**) Steroid-eluting stent at 1-week post-op (*arrow*). (**b**) Propel steroid-eluting stent (Intersect ENT, Menlo Park, CA)

fairly recent innovations, ultimately more study is required to determine their efficacy in CRS.

A key point that should be underscored on the use of topical therapy is that up until now, investigations in this field have revolved around delivery into the sinus cavities. Little study has been done on the delivery of the active agent into the diseased tissues themselves (mucosa, polyps, etc.). As some recent studies have highlighted, any irrigant which enters into a sinus cavity stays for a very brief period of time before most of the solution flows out. A solution simply entering the sinus cavity is therefore likely a poor proxy for mucosal drug delivery [25]. Simply put, how much active drug is getting into the diseased tissue in the setting of polyposis, infection, etc. is the central question. A more sophisticated approach to study and practice of topical sinus drug delivery is desperately needed.

Conclusion

When faced with a patient who is not responding to maximal medical and surgical therapy, it is important to take a step back and approach them with a number of considerations. If the patient had surgery, it is essential to closely examine the sinonasal cavity for anatomic factors contributing to failure. The value of a thorough past medical history, family history, and review of systems with the goal of identifying underlying undiagnosed medical comorbidities cannot be overstated. Finally, consideration of the different topical therapies and an understanding of how various delivery mechanisms can impact sinus drug distribution are essential in these patients. Exploring factors related to therapeutic reasons for failure provides a deeper understanding of the patient's condition and can uncover opportunities to more effectively manage recalcitrant disease.

References

1. Benninger MS, Ferguson BJ, Hadley JA, et al. Adult chronic rhinosinusitis: definitions, diagnosis, epidemiology, and pathophysiology. Otolaryngol Head Neck Surg. 2003;129:S1–32.
2. Batra PS, Tong L, Citardi JL. Analysis of comorbidities and objective parameters in refractory chronic rhinosinusitis. Laryngoscope. 2013;123:S1–11.
3. DeYoung K, Wentzel JL, Schlosser RJ, Nguyen SA, et al. Systematic review of immunotherapy for chronic rhinosinusitis. Am J Rhino Allergy. 2014;28:145–50.
4. White AA, Stevenson DD. Aspirin-exacerbated respiratory disease: update on pathogenesis and desensitization. Semin Respir Crit Care Med. 2012;33:588–94.
5. Xu JJ, Sowerby L, Rotenberg BW. Aspirin desensitization for aspirin-exacerbated respiratory disease (Samter's Triad): a systematic review of the literature. Int Forum All Rhinol. 2013;3:915–20.
6. Mendelsohn D, Jeremic G, Wright ED, Rotenberg BW. Revision rates after endoscopic sinus surgery: a recurrence analysis. Ann Otol Rhinol Laryngol. 2011;120:162–6.
7. Rotenberg BW, Zhang I, Arra I, Payton KB. Postoperative care for Samter's triad patients undergoing endoscopic sinus surgery: a double-blinded, randomized controlled trial. Laryngoscope. 2011;121:2702–5.
8. Williams AN, Woessner KM. The clinical effectiveness of aspirin desensitization in chronic rhinosinusitis. Curr Allergy Asthma Rep. 2008;8:245–52.
9. Pawar S, Lim HJ, Gill M, et al. Treatment of postnasal drip with proton pump inhibitors: a prospective, randomized, placebo-controlled study. Am J Rhinol. 2007;21:695–701.

10. Lupa M, DelGaudio JM. Evidence-based practice: reflux in sinusitis. Otolaryngol Clin North Am. 2012;45:983–92.
11. Nishioka GJ, Cook PR. Paranasal sinus disease in patients with cystic fibrosis. Otolaryngol Clin North Am. 1996;29:193–205.
12. Shatz A. Management of recurrent sinus disease in children with cystic fibrosis: a combined approach. Otolaryngol Head Neck Surg. 2006;135:248–52.
13. Sanclement JA, Webster P, Thomas J, et al. Bacterial biofilms in surgical specimens of patients with chronic rhinosinusitis. Laryngoscope. 2005;115:578–82.
14. Singhal D, Psaltis AJ, Foreman A, Wormald PJ. The impact of biofilms on outcomes after endoscopic sinus surgery. Am J Rhinol All. 2010;24:169–74.
15. Rudmik L, Hoy M, Schlosser RJ, et al. Topical therapies in the management of chronic rhinosinusitis: an evidence-based review with recommendations. Int Forum Allergy Rhinol. 2013;3:281–98.
16. Ocampo CJ, Peters AT. Antibody deficiency in chronic rhinosinusitis: epidemiology and burden of illness. Am J Rhinol Allergy. 2013;27:34–8.
17. Chee L, Graham SM, Carothers DG, et al. Immune dysfunction in refractory sinusitis in a tertiary care setting. Laryngoscope. 2001;111:233–5.
18. Vanlerberghe L, Joniau S, Jorissen M. The prevalence of humoral immunodeficiency in refractory rhinosinusitis: a retrospective analysis. B-ENT. 2006;2:161–6.
19. Marchioni D, Alicandri-Ciufelli M, Mattioli F, et al. Middle turbinate preservation versus middle turbinate resection in endoscopic surgical treatment of nasal polyposis. Acta Otolaryngol. 2008;128:1019–26.
20. McMains KC, Kountakis SE. Revision functional endoscopic sinus surgery: objective and subjective surgical outcomes. Am J Rhinol. 2005;19:344–7.
21. Musy PY, Kountakis SE. Anatomic findings in patients undergoing revision endoscopic sinus surgery. Am J Otolaryngol. 2004;25(6):418–22.
22. Gore MR, Ebert Jr CS, Zanation AM, Senior BA. Beyond the "central sinus": radiographic findings in patients undergoing revision functional endoscopic sinus surgery. Int Forum Allergy Rhinol. 2013;3(2):139–46.
23. Bassiouni A, Wormald PJ. Role of frontal sinus surgery in nasal polyp recurrence. Laryngoscope. 2013;123(1):36–41.
24. Citardi MJ, Javer AF, Kuhn FA. Revision frontal sinusotomy with mucoperiosteal flap advancement: the frontal sinus rescue procedure. Otolaryngol Clin North Am. 2001;34(1):123–32.
25. Harvey RJ, Goddard JC, Wise SK, Schlosser RJ. Effects of endoscopic sinus surgery and delivery device on cadaver sinus irrigation. Otolaryngol Head Neck Surg. 2008;139:137–42.
26. Liang L, Lane AP. Topical drug delivery for chronic rhinosinusitis. Curr Otorhinolaryngol Rep. 2013;1:51–60.
27. Jervis-Bardy J, Wormald PJ. Microbiological outcomes following mupirocin nasal washes for symptomatic, *Staphylococcus aureus* with mupirocin irrigations. Int Forum Allergy Rhinol. 2012;2:111–5.
28. Desrosiers MY, Salas-Prato M. Treatment of chronic rhinosinusitis refractory to other treatments with topical antibiotic therapy delivered by means of a large-particle nebulizer: results of a controlled trial. Otolaryngol Head Neck Surg. 2001;125(3):265–9.
29. Sacks 4th PL, Harvey RJ, Rimmer J, Gallagher RM, et al. Antifungal therapy in the treatment of chronic rhinosinusitis: a meta-analysis. Am J Rhinol Allergy. 2012;26(2):141–7.
30. Pynnonen MA, Mukerji SS, Kim HM, et al. Nasal saline for chronic sinonasal symptoms: a randomized controlled trial. Arch Otolaryngol Head Neck Surg. 2007;133:1115–20.
31. Snidvongs K, Kalish L, Sacks R, et al. Topical steroid for chronic rhinosinusitis without polyps. Cochrane Database Sys Rev. 2011;10(8):CD009274.
32. Snidvongs K, Pratt E, Chin D, et al. Corticosteroid nasal irrigations after endoscopic sinus surgery in the management of chronic rhinosinusitis. Int Forum Allergy Rhinol. 2012;2:415–21.
33. Jang DW, Lachanas VA, Segel J, Kountakis SE. Budesonide nasal irrigations in the postoperative management of chronic rhinosinusitis. Int Forum Allergy Rhinol. 2013;3:708–11.

34. Lim M, Citardi MJ, Leong JL. Topical antimicrobials in the management of chronic rhinosinusitis: a systematic review. Am J Rhinol. 2008;22(4):381–9.
35. Moss RB, King VV. Management of sinusitis in cystic fibrosis by endoscopic surgery and serial antimicrobial lavage. Reduction in recurrence requiring surgery. Arch Otolaryngol Head Neck Surg. 1995;121(5):566–72.
36. Vaughan WC, Carvalho G. Use of nebulized antibiotics for acute infections in chronic sinusitis. Otolaryngol Head Neck Surg. 2002;127(6):558–68.
37. Le T, Psaltis A, Tan LW, Wormald PJ. The efficacy of topical antibiofilm agents in a sheep model of rhinosinusitis. Am J Rhinol. 2008;22:560–7.
38. Uren B, Psaltis A, Wormald PJ. Nasal lavage with mupirocin for the treatment of surgically recalcitrant chronic rhinosinusitis. Laryngoscope. 2008;118:1677–80.
39. Sacks PL, Harvey RJ, Rimmer J, Gallagher RM, Sacks R. Topical and systemic antifungal therapy for the symptomatic treatment of chronic rhinosinusitis. Cochrane Database Syst Rev. 2011;(8):CD008263.
40. Abadie WM, McMains KC, Weitzel EK. Irrigation penetration of nasal delivery systems: a cadaver study. Int Forum Allergy Rhinol. 2011;1:46–9.

Pediatric Rhinosinusitis

9

Michael C. Kao and Sanjay R. Parikh

Key Take Home Points

- Diagnosis of pediatric rhinosinusitis is primarily based on clinical signs. Imaging is not recommended for uncomplicated acute bacterial sinusitis.
- The paranasal sinuses commence development at different ages and have different rates of progression to adult size. In pediatric rhinosinusitis, the maxillary and ethmoid sinuses are most commonly involved.
- In children with chronic rhinosinusitis or complications of acute sinusitis, surgery can be a safe and effective treatment. Surgical considerations include adenoidectomy and functional endoscopic sinus surgery (FESS).
- Patients can have a number of underlying comorbidities which manifest with rhinosinusitis: allergic rhinitis, immune deficiency, cystic fibrosis, and others.

Introduction

Pediatric rhinosinusitis can be challenging to diagnose given the similarity of its presentation to many other childhood diseases. On average, a child will have 6–8 upper respiratory tract infections in any given year with approximately 5–10 % of these episodes being complicated by acute bacterial sinusitis [1, 2]. While the

M.C. Kao, MD
Department of Otolaryngology – Head and Neck Surgery, University of Washington, 1959 NE Pacific Street, Box 356515, Seattle, WA 98195-6515, USA
e-mail: mikekao@uw.edu

S.R. Parikh, MD, FACS (✉)
Department of Otolaryngology – Head and Neck Surgery, Seattle Children's Hospital, University of Washington, 4800 Sand Point Way NE, OA.9329, Seattle, WA 98105, USA
e-mail: sanjay.parikh@seattlechildrens.org

P.S. Batra, J.K. Han (eds.), *Practical Medical and Surgical Management of Chronic Rhinosinusitis*, DOI 10.1007/978-3-319-16724-4_9

workup and treatment of pediatric rhinosinusitis has many similarities to the adult population, the pediatric primary care provider and otolaryngologist should focus on the important subtle differences to the diagnosis, treatment, and complications of pediatric sinus disease.

Prevalence

The exact prevalence of pediatric rhinosinusitis is difficult to estimate. However, it is estimated that $1.8 billion in health care expenditure and $20 million in antibiotic prescriptions is attributed to rhinosinusitis. About 80 % of acute bacterial rhinosinusitis cases have a history of viral upper respiratory infection and is twice as likely to affect children who attend daycare than those who do not [3].

Anatomy and Etiology

Each of the paranasal sinuses commence development at different ages and have different rates of progression to adult size. At birth, only the maxillary and ethmoid sinuses are present which increase in size to full maturity at approximately age 14. The sphenoid sinus typically commences development at age 2, demonstrates pneumatization by age 5, and reaches its permanent size at age 12. The frontal sinuses are noted at age 6–8 and achieve full adult size at approximately age 16.

In children with the clinical diagnosis of rhinosinusitis, the most commonly involved sinus is the maxillary sinus (99 %) followed by the ethmoid sinus (91 %) [4].

Obstruction of the drainage pathway at the ostiomeatal complex is thought to predispose these two sinuses to disease. The function of the ostiomeatal complex is to drain the confluence of the anterior ethmoid, frontal, and maxillary sinuses. The narrow anatomical region of the ostiomeatal complex is such that the two mucosal surfaces are very close together. Edema or inflammation of those mucosal surfaces is often culpable in sinus obstruction and sinus disease.

Additional anatomical variations may exist unique to the pediatric sinuses. Sivalsi et al. studied the anatomical variations of the paranasal sinuses in pediatric patients with chronic rhinosinusitis [5]. A pneumatized middle concha was the most common anatomical variation, followed by pneumatization of the superior concha, Haller cell, and Agger Nasi cell. These variations must be considered when considering surgical intervention as treatment.

One unique consideration in the pediatric population is the presence of adenoid hypertrophy which may play a role in rhinosinusitis and/or Eustachian tube dysfunction. Evaluating a child for middle ear effusions, recurrent sinusitis, and adenoid hypertrophy is important when considering surgical intervention [6, 7].

Other predisposing and underlying medical diagnoses that may contribute to sinusitis include allergies, gastrointestinal reflux, and asthma [8–10]. Less common conditions which are often present in the pediatric population include cystic fibrosis, primary ciliary dyskinesia, and immunodeficiency.

Microbial Patterns

In all age groups and in acute or subacute sinusitis, *Haemophilus influenzae* and *Streptococcus pneumoniae* are the principal pathogens in most cases. In young children, more than 90 % of all cases of sinusitis are caused by five organisms: *Haemophilus influenzae*, *Streptococcus pneumoniae*, *Moraxella catarrhalis*, *Staphylococcus aureus*, and *Streptococcus pyogenes*.

It is well known that one of the leading causes of medically refractory rhinosinusitis is the opportunistic gram-negative bacteria, *Pseudomonas aeruginosa*. Biofilm formation has been demonstrated by many other bacterial species including *Staphylococcus aureus*, *Streptococcus pneumoniae*, *Haemophilus influenzae*, and *Moraxella catarrhalis* [11, 12]. *Pseudomonas aeruginosa* and *Staphylococcus aureus* composed 71 % of the samples that showed biofilm growth [13].

Diagnosis

The diagnosis of rhinosinusitis is primarily based on clinical signs and characteristic symptoms. To distinguish sinusitis from common upper respiratory infections or even adenoiditis, it is helpful to keep in mind the duration, persistence, and acuity of the symptoms as well as the ensuing complications. Efforts have been made by international working groups to develop standard criteria and classification for pediatric rhinosinusitis; two recent consensus statements are the European position paper on rhinosinusitis and nasal polyps (EPOS 2012) and clinical practice guidelines from the American Academy of Pediatrics (AAP 2013) [14, 15].

The most common symptoms of rhinosinusitis include daytime cough, rhinorrhea, nasal congestion, fevers, otitis media, irritability, and headache. Accurate diagnosis of rhinosinusitis and the initiation of appropriate and timely treatment of the infection will help prevent complications (see Table 9.1).

EPOS 2012: European Position Paper on Rhinosinusitis and Nasal Polyps

In 2012, EPOS presented/published new and updated guidelines for sinusitis. The broad principles of the classification and treatment highlight the importance for the clinician to establish duration of symptoms and chronological relation of onset. Some of the important EPOS 2012 updates included adding diagnostic symptom of cough and eliminating the diagnostic symptom of reduction or loss of smell. EPOS 2012 also defines a new category for acute bacterial rhinosinusitis and subcategory for post-viral acute rhinosinusitis.

Acute rhinosinusitis is defined by the presence of two or more of the following symptoms: nasal blockage, nasal discharge, facial pain, or cough with a duration of less than 12 weeks.

Table 9.1 International classification of sinusitis by time and symptoms

	EPOS 2012	AAP 2013
Acute rhinosinusitis	<12 weeks for complete resolution	
Acute viral rhinosinusitis	<10 days duration of symptoms	
Acute post-viral rhinosinusitis	Worsening symptoms after 5 days or persistent symptoms after 10 days	
Acute bacterial rhinosinusitis	+additional symptoms of colored discharge, severe local pain, fever >38 C, elevated ESR/CRP, double sickening	>10 days of symptoms and/or worsening course and/or >3 days of severe onset, fever >39 C and purulent discharge
Subacute bacterial sinusitis		30–90 days of symptoms in which symptoms resolve completely
Recurrent acute bacterial sinusitis		Episodes lasting <30 days separated by at least 10 days with no symptoms
Chronic sinusitis	≥12 weeks without complete resolution of symptoms	>90 days of symptoms

Chronic rhinosinusitis in children is not as well studied as in adults. The classification is similar with two or more of the following symptoms: nasal blockage, nasal discharge, facial pain, and/or cough with a duration of greater than 12 weeks without complete resolution of symptoms. Adenoid tissue is recognized as a prominent contributor to this disease.

Acute bacterial rhinosinusitis is defined by the presence of at least three of the following symptoms: discolored unilateral and purulent secretion, severe localized pain, fever, elevated ESR/CRP, and worsening of symptoms after short improvement following viral infection.

The guidelines also use the visual analog scale to assist in diagnosis when possible, asking patient to self-assess where along a 10 cm line. The symptoms are scaled accordingly, mild for 0–3, moderate for >3–7, severe for >7–10.

AAP 2013: Clinical Practice Guidelines from the American Academy of Pediatrics

AAP defines and categorizes sinusitis according to the duration of symptoms. If the duration of symptoms persists beyond 7–10 days, the diagnosis is acute sinusitis. If the symptoms last up to 30 days but has asymptomatic intervals of 10 days in between, the diagnosis is recurrent sinusitis. Subacute sinusitis is diagnosed when symptoms last 30–90 days. Chronic sinusitis is diagnosed when symptoms persist for greater than 90 days, 6 or more recurrent exacerbations of sinusitis in 1 year, or acute exacerbations without intervals of complete resolution.

Indications for Diagnostic Nasopharyngeal Endoscopy

The use of flexible or rigid nasal endoscopy in children can be helpful in the diagnosis of sinusitis and the exclusion of nasal foreign bodies or polyposis as a potential cause of sinusitis. The benefits of this invasive examination must be weighed against the possible risks given the age and cooperativeness of the pediatric patient.

Diagnostic Imaging

Plain films have little diagnostic value for evaluation of rhinosinusitis and should not be routinely used. Computed tomography (CT) with contrast or magnetic resonance imaging (MRI) with contrast in children should be considered for signs of acute complicated rhinosinusitis. Concern for orbital extension with proptosis, reduced or painful eye movement (ophthalmoplegia), decreased visual acuity (initially manifesting itself with reduced green/red color discrimination), or lethargy should prompt an urgent CT scan with contrast. MRI may be used when concerns of intracranial extension of disease are present, such as with intracranial cerebritis, abscess, or cavernous sinus thrombosis.

An additional update in AAP 2013 is that there is no indication for imaging for uncomplicated acute bacterial sinusitis. The basis of this recommendation is that there can be abnormalities seen on imaging studies in normal healthy children such as mucosal thickening or sinus opacification that could falsely lead to the diagnosis of acute bacterial sinusitis [16].

Laboratory Investigations

Children with chronic rhinosinusitis should be judiciously tested for contributing underlying conditions such as asthma, cystic fibrosis, and immunodeficiency.

Treatment

The two classification schemes each contain subtle differences in their recommendations and treatment algorithms. The specific recommendations are highlighted below, the theme of each highlight the importance to establish the diagnosis of acute sinusitis, attempt medical management and address any underlying pathology, and proceed to surgery if the infection is refractory to aggressive management or when complications are imminent or present.

Medical Management

EPOS 2012

The recommendations for treatment will vary depending on the time course and severity of the symptoms as discussed previously. According to EPOS, there is evidence that antibiotics and topical steroids are useful in the treatment of rhinosinusitis; the selection of monotherapy or combination therapy is based on the presumptive diagnosis and the severity of the disease.

The presumptive diagnosis of viral upper respiratory infection is made if symptoms have been present for 5 days or are remitting at that time, for which purely symptomatic treatment with nasal saline and decongestants is recommended. If symptoms have persisted for 10 days or are worsening after 5 days, the working diagnosis is post-viral sinusitis or acute bacterial rhinosinusitis. Based on the severity of symptoms, the recommendation is to initiate only topical nasal steroids for moderate symptoms and both topical steroids with antibiotics for severe symptoms. If patient improves after 48 h, the recommendation is to complete a treatment course of 7–14 days. If a patient fails to improve despite initial medical management, the recommendation is referral to an otolaryngologist (see Fig. 9.1).

The recommendations for antibiotics are based on studies where a clinical diagnosis of acute bacterial rhinosinusitis was made according to the criteria previously discussed. One recent randomized, placebo-controlled trial evaluated the efficacy of amoxicillin (90 mg/kg) with potassium clavulanate (6.4 mg/kg) or placebo in children 1–10 years of age with a clinical presentation compatible with bacterial ARS (persistent symptoms, acutely worsening symptoms, or severe symptoms) [17]. Symptom scores were obtained at multiple time points, and the children were evaluated at day 14 from onset of treatment and their condition rated as cured, improved, or failed. Twenty-eight patients in each group completed the study, and their average age was around 5 years. Children receiving the antibiotic were more likely to be cured (50 % vs. 14 %, $p=0.01$) and less likely to experience treatment failure (14 % vs. 68 %, $p<0.001$) than children receiving placebo.

AAP 2013

The most significant areas of change from the 2001 guidelines are the addition of a clinical presentation designated as "worsening course," inclusion of new data on the effectiveness of antibiotics in children with acute sinusitis, and a review of evidence indicating that imaging is not necessary to identify those children who will benefit from antimicrobial therapy [4].

Antibiotic therapy is indicated in acute sinusitis when symptoms are severe or persistent or if a child appears toxic. The guidelines suggest treatment for 10–14 days or for 1 week beyond symptom resolution.

For patients with chronic sinusitis, the guidelines indicate a prolonged 4-week treatment with a broad-spectrum beta-lactamase-resistant second-line antibiotic. If there is no clinical response after 1 week of treatment, changing the antibiotic should be considered. Cultures may also be considered at the time of initiation to direct therapy.

The guidelines make no recommendations on adjuvant treatments including saline irrigation, nasal steroids, decongestants, and mucolytic therapy citing inadequate evidence. Smaller studies have demonstrated saline sinus irrigation with efficacy in the treatment of acute and chronic sinusitis. The authors propose irrigation

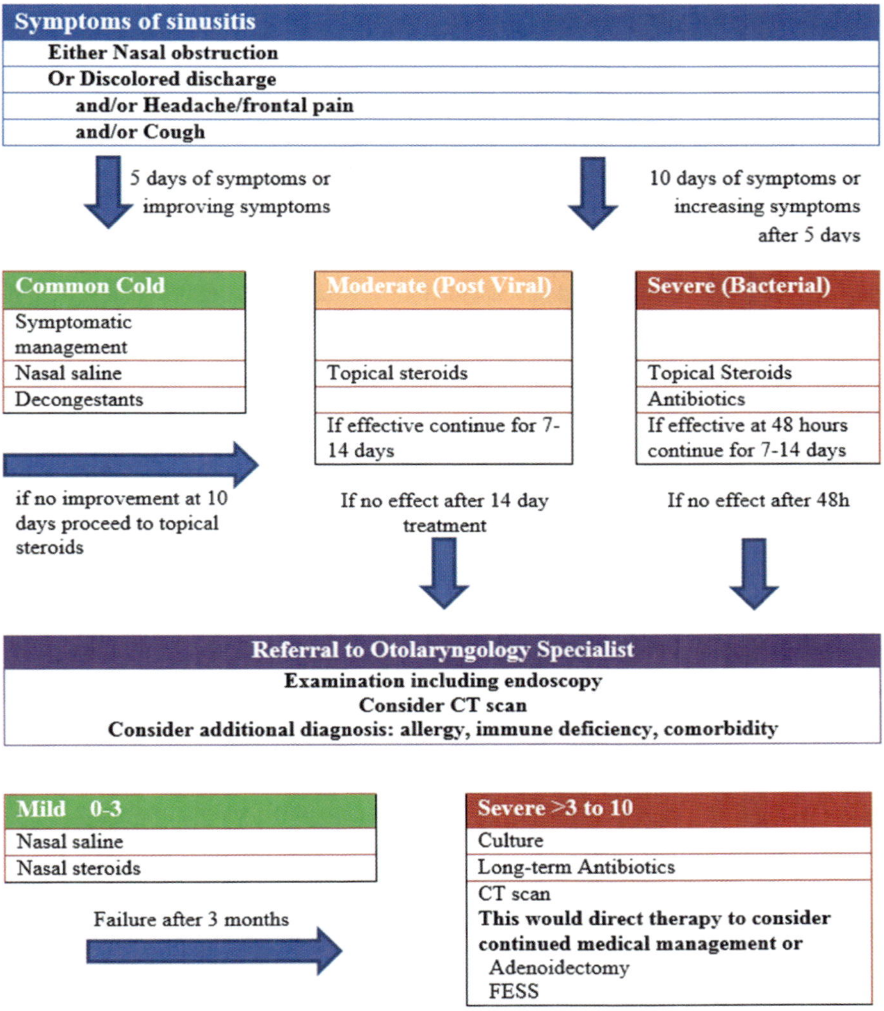

Fig. 9.1 EPOS 2012 guidelines

increases mucociliary flow, vasoconstriction, mechanically clears secretions, decreases bacterial counts, and clears allergens and environmental irritants from the nose [18, 19]. Cochrane reviews published on the use of saline irrigation in acute sinusitis in adults in 2010 and concluded that the trials were too small or too biased to be confident on benefits [20]. Intranasal steroids compared to placebo in children were shown to have modest reduction in symptoms although there are criticisms of the methodology for these studies [21]. There are several studies in acute sinusitis in adults which provide data supporting the use of intranasal steroid as either monotherapy or adjuvant therapy to antibiotics [22].

Antimicrobial Selection

The AAP Subcommittee of Sinusitis and Committee on Quality Improvement recommended amoxicillin as first-line therapy for children younger than 2 years of age suspected of having acute bacterial sinusitis of mild to moderate severity who do not attend daycare and who have not been treated recently with an antimicrobial agent. They recommend an amoxicillin dose of either 45 mg/kg/day in two divided doses or 90 mg/kg/day in two divided doses. The AAP committees further recommended that children who did not improve while receiving the lower amoxicillin dose, children with more severe illness, and children who attend daycare should be treated with high-dose amoxicillin-clavulanate 80–90 mg/kg/day of amoxicillin component in two divided doses [23].

Indications for Surgery

In pediatric rhinosinusitis, there is a significant overlap between adenoiditis and rhinosinusitis. In the setting of chronic sinus disease with adenoiditis, adenoidectomy resolves symptoms in 50 % of patients. A meta-analysis looking at the benefit of adenoidectomy alone in the treatment of children with CRS included nine studies that met the inclusion criteria. All studies showed that sinusitis symptoms or outcomes improved in half or more patients after adenoidectomy. Eight of nine studies were sufficiently similar to undergo meta-analysis, and in these, the summary estimate of the proportion of patients who significantly improved after adenoidectomy was 69.3 % [24]. Ramadan and Tiu reported on the refractory cases after adenoidectomy, reporting children younger than 7 years of age and those with asthma were more likely to fail after adenoidectomy and go on to require salvage functional endoscopic sinus surgery (FESS) [25].

In absence of adenoiditis or refractory sinus disease, FESS may be indicated to target uncinate removal, anterior ethmoidectomy, and maxillary antrostomy (see Fig. 9.2). A meta-analysis looking at outcomes of FESS in the pediatric population has shown that surgery is effective in reducing symptoms with an 88 % success rate and a low complication rate [26].

Image-guided surgery can be safely utilized in children with chronic rhinosinusitis, in those undergoing revision surgeries, and in any patient in whom the anatomy may be distorted, without increasing the rate of intraoperative complications [27]. The indications for image-guided surgery include patients with any distorted sinus anatomy; those with extensive sinonasal polyposis, pathologic processes in the frontal, posterior ethmoidal, or sphenoidal sinuses; and patients undergoing skull base surgery [28].

Concurrent Symptoms and Medical Conditions

Allergic Rhinitis

Allergic inflammation leads to nasal congestion and swelling of the mucous membrane, which may obstruct or impede normal sinus drainage. Subsequent inflammatory responses in the epithelium lead to an influx of granulocytes, with swelling and

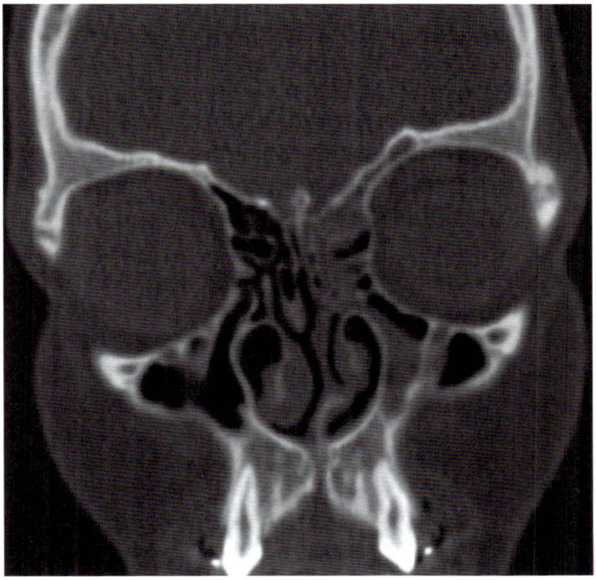

Fig. 9.2 Non-contrast coronal CT of an 11-year-old female undergoing FESS for symptomatic chronic unilateral rhinosinusitis. Note septal deviation and ipsilateral hypoplastic maxillary sinus

pain from the mucosa and thickened secretions. In children evidence of allergic rhinitis has been found in 36–60 % of patients with chronic rhinosinusitis [29–31].

Symptoms that can be associated with allergic rhinitis include sneezing, itching (of nose, eyes, ears, palate), rhinorrhea, postnasal drip, congestion, anosmia, headache, earache, tearing, red eyes, eye swelling, fatigue, drowsiness, and malaise [32].

The most commonly used methods of determining allergy to a particular substance are allergy skin testing (testing for immediate hypersensitivity reactions) and in vitro diagnostic tests, such as the radioallergosorbent test (RAST), which indirectly measures the quantity of antigen-specific IgE.

Immunodeficiency or Immunocompromised State

In the setting of a child with recurrent or chronic rhinosinusitis, immunodeficiency must be a part of the differential diagnosis. Patients with immunodeficiency may account for 8–20 % of patients with persistent or recurrent rhinosinusitis [33–35]. In patients with chronic rhinosinusitis, Chee et al. found an unexpectedly high incidence of immune dysfunction, the majority of which were common variable immunodeficiencies [36].

Cystic fibrosis should be suspected in any child demonstrating bilateral polyposis. The workup involves more specialized follow-up with a chloride sweat test for cystic fibrosis or by DNA analysis using a CFTR multi-mutation method looking at a panel of common mutations [37]. Nasal polyps are present in 20–50 % of patients with CF [38]. Although the role of endoscopic sinus surgery to improve lung function in CF is unclear, multiple studies have shown a significant improvement in the quality of life in CF patients following sinus surgery [39].

Primary ciliary dyskinesia has an incidence of 1:30,000 live births. In 50 % of such cases, this can be associated with situ inversus (Kartagener's syndrome). The diagnosis requires nasal brush biopsy of respiratory epithelium for electron microscopy to evaluate for ciliary microtubular structural abnormalities.

Asthma, Aspirin Sensitivity, and Chronic Rhinosinusitis

Patients with chronic rhinosinusitis have a 20 % prevalence of asthma [40]. Multiple studies demonstrate that medical treatment of rhinosinusitis and allergic rhinitis leads to better control of a patient's asthma and vice versa. The 2007 National Asthma Prevention Expert Panel Report 3 recognized sinusitis and allergies as comorbid conditions that aggravate asthma and impede its treatment [41]. Furthermore, Chen et al. describe aspirin sensitivity syndrome as an underdiagnosed entity in setting of non-cystic fibrosis patients with nasal polyposis [42].

Complications of Sinusitis

Orbital Infection

Orbital involvement from sinusitis presents with swelling, exophthalmos, impaired and painful extra-ocular eye movements, and diplopia which are features that distinguish it from preseptal cellulitis. Preseptal cellulitis occurs most frequently with upper respiratory infection and involvement of the eyelid without proptosis or limitations to extraocular movement to differentiate it from true orbital involvement [43, 44]. When concerned for orbital involvement from sinusitis, an ophthalmological consultation should always be sought to assess proptosis, ocular pressures, visual acuity, color vision, and movements.

The progression of ethmoiditis typically follows the path of preseptal cellulitis, orbital cellulitis, subperiosteal abscess, orbital abscess, and cavernous sinus thrombosis. Bacterial ethmoiditis may spread by direct orbit invasion through a thin and often dehiscent lamina papyracea or by venous thrombophlebitis.

Indications for surgical management of orbital infections include evidence of subperiosteal or intraorbital abscess by CT or MRI, reduced visual acuity/color/change to afferent pupillary reflex, worsening or non-improving symptoms after 48 h with IV antibiotics. The consensus is to perform not only an endoscopic drainage by taking down the lamina papyracea but also an ethmoidectomy to drain the paranasal sinuses. Recent studies in children with subperiosteal abscesses demonstrate that IV antibiotics can be trialed first prior to surgery in the setting of small volume abscess with no change that is responsive to systemic treatment [45–47].

Neurological Complications

Intracranial abscess, meningitis, and cavernous sinus thrombosis are intracranial complications of sinusitis with the mortality rate of 10–20 % [48]. Most infections arise by thrombophlebotic spread through the posterior table of the frontal sinus (see Fig. 9.3). Less commonly intracranial spread may occur from the ethmoid or sphenoid sinuses (see Fig. 9.4).

The signs and symptoms of intracranial infection include high fever, headache, nausea, vomiting, neck stiffness, altered mental status, increased intracranial pressures, and neurological deficits with attention to third, sixth, and seventh nerve palsy.

With infection tracking along valveless veins draining the paranasal sinus, cavernous sinus thrombophlebitis may ensue, resulting in lid drop, exophthalmos, ophthalmic neuralgia, retro-ocular headache with deep pain behind the orbit, complete ophthalmoplegia, papilledema, and signs of meningeal irritation associated with spiking fevers and prostration [49]. Urgent joint investigation by otolaryngology and neurosurgery with surgical drainage may be prudent.

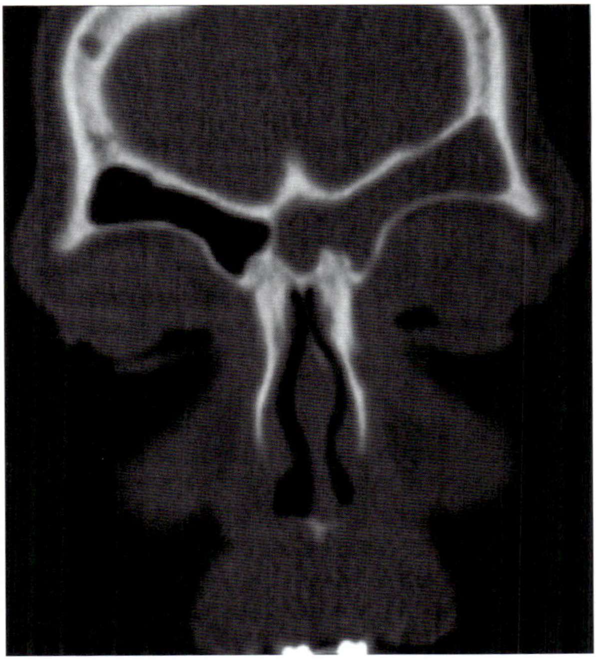

Fig. 9.3 Typical non-contrast coronal sinus CT scan of an adolescent male with unilateral frontal headache demonstrating isolated frontal sinusitis

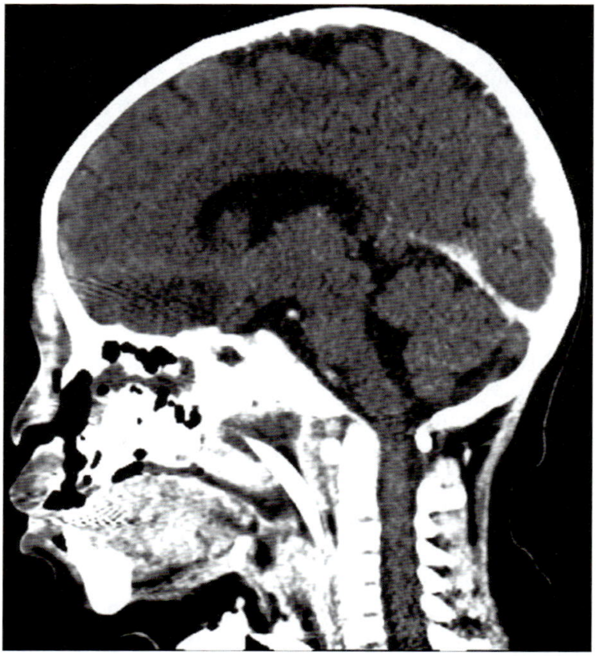

Fig. 9.4 Non-contrast sagittal brain CT scan of a 2-year-old immunocompromised female with acute leukemia and fungal frontal lobe brain abscess from mucormycosis

References

1. Aitken M, Taylor JA. Prevalence of clinical sinusitis in young children followed up by primary care pediatricians. Arch Pediatr Adolesc Med. 1998;152:244–8.
2. Wald ER, Guerra N, Byers C. Upper respiratory tract infections in young children: duration of and frequency of complications. Pediatrics. 1991;87:129–33.
3. Wald ER, Dashefsky B, Byers C, et al. Frequency and severity of infections in day care. J Pediatr. 1988;112:540–6.
4. Tatli MM, San I, Karaoglanoglu M. Paranasal sinus computed tomographic findings of children with chronic cough. Int J Pediatr Otorhinolaryngol. 2001;60(3):213–7.
5. Sivasli E, Sirikci A, Bayazyt YA, Gumusburun E, Erbagci H, Bayram M, et al. Anatomic variations of the paranasal sinus area in pediatric patients with chronic sinusitis. Surg Radiol Anat. 2003;24(6):400–5.
6. Takahashi H, Fujita A, Honjo I. Effect of adenoidectomy on otitis media with effusion, tubal function, and sinusitis. Am J Otolaryngol. 1989;10(3):208–13. PubMed.
7. Bernstein JM, Dryja D, Murphy TF. Molecular typing of paired bacterial isolates from the adenoid and lateral wall of the nose in children undergoing adenoidectomy: implications in acute rhinosinusitis. Otolaryngol Head Neck Surg. 2001;125(6):593–7. PubMed.
8. Huang SW. The risk of sinusitis in children with allergic rhinitis. Allergy Asthma Proc. 2000;21:85–8.
9. Bothwell MR, Parsons DS, Talbot A, et al. Outcome of reflux therapy on pediatric chronic sinusitis. Otolaryngol Head Neck Surg. 1999;121:255–62.

10. Dixon AE, Kaminsky DA, Holbrook JT, et al. Allergic rhinitis and sinusitis in asthma: differential effects on symptoms and pulmonary function. Chest. 2006;130:429–35.
11. Suh JD, Ramakrishnan V, Palmer JN. Biofilms. Otolaryngol Clin North Am. 2010;43:521–30.
12. Prince AA, Steiger JD, Khalid AN, et al. Prevalence of biofilm-forming bacteria in chronic rhinosinusitis. Am J Rhinol. 2008;22:239–45.
13. Smith A, Buchinsky FJ, Post JC. Eradicating chronic ear, nose, and throat infections: a systematically conducted literature review of advances in biofilm treatment. Otolaryngol Head Neck Surg. 2011;144(3):338–47. doi:10.1177/0194599810391620.
14. Fokkens WJ, Lund VJ, Mullol J, Bachert C, Alobid I, Baroody F, Cohen N, Cervin A, Douglas R, Gevaert P, Georgalas C, Goossens H, Harvey R, Hellings P, Hopkins C, Jones N, Joos G, Kalogjera L, Kern B, Kowalski M, Price D, Riechelmann H, Schlosser R, Senior B, Thomas M, Toskala E, Voegels R, de Wang Y, Wormald PJ. EPOS 2012: European position paper on rhinosinusitis and nasal polyps 2012. A summary for otorhinolaryngologists. Rhinology. 2012;50(1):1–12.
15. Wald ER, Applegate KE, Bordley C, Darrow DH, Glode MP, Marcy SM, Nelson CE, Rosenfeld RM, Shaikh N, Smith MJ, Williams PV, Weinberg ST. American Academy of Pediatrics: clinical practice guideline for the diagnosis and management of acute bacterial sinusitis in children aged 1 to 18 years. Pediatrics. 2013;132:e262–80.
16. Wald ER, Milmoe GJ, Bowen A, Ledesma-Medina J, Salamon N, Bluestone CD. Acute maxillary sinusitis in children. N Engl J Med. 1981;304(13):749–54.
17. Wald ER, Nash D, Eickhoff J. Effectiveness of amoxicillin/clavulanate potassium in the treatment of acute bacterial sinusitis in children. Pediatrics. 2009;124(1):9–15.
18. Jeffe JS, Bhushan B, Schroeder Jr JW. Nasal saline irrigation in children: a study of compliance and tolerance. Int J Pediatr Otorhinolaryngol. 2012;76(3):409–13.
19. Wei JL, Sykes KJ, Johnson P, He J, Mayo MS. Safety and efficacy of once-daily nasal irrigation for the treatment of pediatric chronic rhinosinusitis. Laryngoscope. 2011;121(9):1989–2000.
20. Kassel JC, King D, Spurling GK. Saline nasal irrigation for acute upper respiratory tract infections. Cochrane Database Syst Rev. 2010;3, CD006821.
21. Barlan IB, Erkan E, Bakir M, Berrak S, Basaran MM. Intranasal budesonide spray as an adjunct to oral antibiotic therapy for acute sinusitis in children. Ann Allergy Asthma Immunol. 1997;78(6):598–601.
22. Zalmanovici A, Yaphe J. Intranasal steroids for acute sinusitis. Cochrane Database Syst Rev. 2009;(4):CD005149.
23. American Academy of Pediatrics Subcommittee on Management of Sinusitis and Committee on Quality Improvement. Clinical practice guideline: management of sinusitis—subcommittee on management of sinusitis and committee on quality improvement. Pediatrics. 2001;108:798.
24. Brietzke SE, Brigger MT. Adenoidectomy outcomes in pediatric rhinosinusitis: a meta-analysis. Int J Pediatr Otorhinolaryngol. 2008;72(10):1541–5.
25. Ramadan HH, Tiu J. Failures of adenoidectomy for chronic rhinosinusitis in children: for whom and when do they fail? Laryngoscope. 2007;117(6):1080–3.
26. Herbert RL, Bent JP. Meta-analysis of outcomes of pediatric functional endoscopic sinus surgery. Laryngoscope. 1998;108(6):796–9.
27. Parikh SR, Cuellar H, Sadoughi B, et al. Indications for image-guidance in pediatric sinonasal surgery. Int J Pediatr Otorhinolaryngol. 2009;73:351–6.
28. American Academy of Otolaryngology—Head and Neck Surgery: policy on intra-operative use of computer-aided surgery.
29. Shapiro GG, Virant FS, Furukawa CT, Pierson WE, Bierman CW. Immunologic defects in patients with refractory sinusitis. Pediatrics. 1991;87:311–6. IIb.
30. Kogutt MS, Swischuk LE. Diagnosis of sinusitis in infants and young children. Pediatrics. 1973;52:121–4. IIb.
31. Rachelefsky GS, Siegel SC, Katz RM, Spector MD, Rohr AS. Chronic sinusitis in children. J Allergy Clin Immunol. 1991;87:219. IIb.

32. Druce HM. Allergic and nonallergic rhinitis. In: Middleton Jr EM, Reed CE, Ellis EF, Adkinson Jr NF, Yunginger JW, Busse WW, editors. Allergy: principles and practice. 5th ed. St. Louis: Mosby Year-Book; 1998. p. 1005–16.
33. Ferguson BJ, Otto BA, Pant H. When surgery, antibiotics, and steroids fail to resolve chronic rhinosinusitis. Immunol Allergy Clin North Am. 2009;29:719–32.
34. Carr TF, Koterba AP, Chandra R, et al. Characterization of specific antibody deficiency in adults with medically refractory chronic rhinosinusitis. Am J Rhinol Allergy. 2011;25:241–4.
35. Alqudah M, Graham SM, Ballas ZK. High prevalence of humoral immunodeficiency patients with refractory chronic rhinosinusitis. Am J Rhinol Allergy. 2010;24:409–12.
36. Chee L, Graham SM, Carothers DG, et al. Immune dysfunction in refractory sinusitis in a tertiary care setting. Laryngoscope. 2001;111:233–5.
37. De Boeck K, Wilschanski M, Castellani C, Taylor C, Cuppens H, Dodge J, Sinaasappel M. Cystic fibrosis: terminology and diagnostic algorithms. Thorax. 2006;61(7):627–35.
38. Mainz JG, Koitschev A. Management of chronic rhinosinusitis in CF. J Cyst Fibros. 2009;8:S10–4.
39. Jones JW, Parsons DS, Cuyler JP. The results of functional endoscopic sinus (FES) surgery on the symptoms of patients with cystic fibrosis. Int J Pediatr Otorhinolaryngol. 1993;28:25–32.
40. Jani AL, Hamilos DL. Current thinking on the relationship between rhinosinusitis and asthma. J Asthma. 2005;42:1–7.
41. National Asthma Education and Prevention Program. Expert Panel Report 3 (EPR-3): guidelines for the diagnosis and management of asthma-summary report 2007. J Allergy Clin Immunol. 2007;120:S94–138.
42. Chen BS, Virant FS, Parikh SR, Manning SC. Aspirin sensitivity syndrome (Samter's Triad): an unrecognized disorder in children with nasal polyposis. Int J Pediatr Otorhinolaryngol. 2013;77(2):281–3.
43. Sobol SE, Marchand J, Tewfik TL, Manoukian JJ, Schloss MD. Orbital complications of sinusitis in children. J Otolaryngol. 2002;31(3):131–6.
44. Wald ER. Sinusitis in children. N Engl J Med. 1992;326(5):319–23.
45. Ho CF, Huang YC, Wang CJ, Chiu CH, Lin TY. Clinical analysis of computed tomography-staged orbital cellulitis in children. J Microbiol Immunol Infect. 2007;40(6):518–24.
46. Jones NS, Walker JL, Bassi S, Jones T, Punt J. The intracranial complications of rhinosinusitis: can they be prevented? Laryngoscope. 2002;112(1):59–63.
47. Siedek V, Kremer A, Betz CS, Tschiesner U, Berghaus A, Leunig A. Management of orbital complications due to rhinosinusitis. Europ Arch Otorhinolaryngol. 2010;267(12):1881–6.
48. Broberg T, Murr A, Fischbein N. Devastating complications of acute pediatric bacterial sinusitis. Otolaryngol Head Neck Surg. 1999;120(4):575–9.
49. Josephson JS, Rosenberg SI. Sinusitis. Clin Symp. 1994;46(2):1–32.

Allergic Rhinitis

10

Rachel Georgopoulos and Elina Toskala

Key Take Home Points

- Allergic rhinitis is an IgE-mediated type 1 hypersensitivity response of the nasal mucosa to normally innocuous proteins.
- Reduced microbial exposure may result in a skewed predilection for the Th_2 cytokine response, referred to as the "hygiene hypothesis."
- Allergic rhinitis is not only associated with but is a risk factor for the development of asthma.
- Intranasal corticosteroids are the first-line treatment for allergic rhinitis and have also been shown to reduce bronchial hyperresponsiveness.
- Immunotherapy is efficacious in the management of allergic rhinitis and studies suggest that it may help prevent the development of asthma.

Background

Allergic rhinitis (AR) is more colloquially referred to as hay fever, although this is a misnomer as the disease is not associated with fever, but rather it is associated with catarrh symptoms similar to those experienced with viral colds. Originally, it was thought that the constellation of symptoms seen in AR was caused by some unknown component from hay. Incidentally, the season for hay harvest, being in the late spring and early summer, coincides with the seasons in which pollen concentrations are at their peak [19]. Dr. John Bostock, a physician from the 1800s, was personally afflicted with the disease and was the first to detail his symptoms for which he had suffered since childhood in "Case of a Periodical Affection of the Eyes and Chest

R. Georgopoulos, MD • E. Toskala, MD, PhD (✉)
Department of Otolaryngology – Head and Neck Surgery, Temple University Hospital, 3440 North Broad Street, Philadelphia, PA 19140, USA
e-mail: rachel.georgopoulos@tuhs.temple.edu; Elina.toskala@tuhs.temple.edu

P.S. Batra, J.K. Han (eds.), *Practical Medical and Surgical Management of Chronic Rhinosinusitis*, DOI 10.1007/978-3-319-16724-4_10

[20]." Referring to this disease as "catarrhus aestivus" or summer catarrh, although this name did not stick and the disease continues to be referred to as "hay fever" [20].

Epidemiology

The prevalence of AR in children aged 18 years and younger is higher than that of adults with 9–40 % of US children and 7.5–30 % of US adults affected [21–26]. Of the people who develop AR, 80 % will develop the disease prior to 20 years of age. That being said, AR rarely affects children younger than 2 years of age [23]. While boys are more likely than girls to be affected with AR, this changes into adulthood with women slightly more affected than men [22]. Black and Hispanic individuals are less commonly affected than white individuals, and the disease is more prevalent in high income homes [21, 22, 27].

Significant geographic variability exists regarding the prevalence of AR [28, 29]. Dahl et al. [28] performed a study looking at the prevalence of patient-reported allergic respiratory disorders in 10 European countries. Spain was found to have a significantly lower prevalence of allergic respiratory disorders, 11.7 % when compared to other European countries. Italy had a significantly higher prevalence at 33.6 % [28].

Risk Factors/Hygiene Hypothesis

The development of rhinitis is multifactorial with both environmental and genetic factors clearly playing a role [21, 23, 30]. In a study by Dold et al. [30] it was found that children with at least one parent with allergic rhinitis were more likely to have allergic rhinitis themselves OR 3.6. Furthermore, studies have shown that if both parents are atopic, the risk of the child having AR is even greater [23]. A series of genetic loci on a variety of chromosomes have been found to be responsible for T-cell differentiation; bronchial hyperresponsiveness and total serum IgE levels have been identified and are believed to contribute to development of atopy in certain individuals [2, 31–35].

Environmental exposures such as parental smoking, increase the risk of developing AR. Children exposed to tobacco smoke by a parent had a 2.7 fold increased risk of developing AR [36]. There is an inverse relationship between the number of siblings and the prevalence of AR [18]. It is believed that in large families children are exposed to microbial infection more frequently at an earlier age. Early microbial exposure serves as a stimulus for normal Th_1 maturation [37, 38]. Conversely, reduced microbial exposure in the postnatal period may result in a skewed predilection to the Th_2 cytokine response, referred to as the "hygiene hypothesis" [31, 39]. In a prospective birth cohort [40] it was found that after the age of 6, children with increased exposure to infection earlier in life were much less likely to wheeze. In addition, it has been shown that seropositivity to a variety of infections including hepatitis A, *Toxoplasma gondii*, and herpes simplex virus is associated with a lower probability of AR and asthma [37]. Differences in the bacterial content of dust may have implications in the development of atopy [39]. Widespread use of vaccination, strict public health measures, and high levels of cleanliness appear to be associated with increased Th_2 responses [18].

Comorbidities

There is an association between AR and a variety of comorbid conditions including malocclusion, chronic otitis media, conjunctivitis, sinusitis, and asthma. Chronic nasal obstruction in children can lead to chronic mouth breathing and dental malocclusion [41]. Among children with chronic otitis media with effusion, there is a significant association with allergic rhinitis [42]. There is a strong association with AR and allergic conjunctivitis. This is likely a result of both a direct interaction of the allergen with the conjunctival mucosa and a result of the nasal ocular reflex.

The "unified airway model" describes the nose and paranasal sinuses through the distal bronchioles as being one functional unit linked epidemiologically, biologically, and via a common therapeutic approach [43]. It is then not surprising that AR is associated with other inflammatory diseases of the respiratory system such as rhinosinusitis and asthma.

The association between rhinitis and asthma has been well described. Rhinitis is not only associated with, but is a risk factor for, the development of asthma [6–10]. Disease severity is linked. Individuals with more severe persistent forms of rhinitis are more likely to have symptomatic asthma than patients with intermittent forms of rhinitis [44]. Further support for the interrelationship between these two diseases comes from the fact that the treatment of AR has been found to improve asthma control [5]. In fact, it has been shown that management of AR at a young age with allergen directed immunotherapy may prevent the development of asthma in later life [15–17, 45].

Pathophysiology

AR is by definition an immunoglobulin E (IgE)-mediated type 1 hypersensitivity response of the nasal mucosa to normally innocuous proteins with resultant inflammation [46]. The allergic response is divided into an early and a late phase. In the early phase, antigens initially presented to the nasal mucosa are taken up and processed by antigen presenting cells (APCs) into short peptide fragments. These peptide fragments are exteriorized and then recognized by major histocompatibility complex (MHC) class II molecules. APCs in the draining lymph nodes attract naïve CD4+ T cells. In cases of allergic reaction, cytokines including IL-4 are released allowing for polarization and the differentiation of these naïve T cells into Th_2 cells. Activation of Th_2 result in the production of IL-4, IL-5, IL-10, and IL-13, which results in the recruitment of IgE producing B cells, mast cells, and eosinophils [47, 48]. Memory B cells maintain this antibody response. IgE molecules bind high affinity receptors, which "sensitize" the nasal mucosa [49, 50]. Re-exposure to the allergen results in cross-linking of adjacent IgE molecules on the surfaces of basophils and mast cells. This leads to the degranulation and release of preformed mediators such as histamine, proteases, kinins, and heparin. In addition, prostaglandin D_2 (PGD_2), cysteinyl leukotriene B_4 (LTB_4), leukotriene C_4 (LTC_4), leukotriene E_4 (LTE_4), and mediators of the arachidonic acid pathway are synthesized and secreted by mast cells. These mediators act locally on the surrounding vasculature and nerves located in the nasal mucosa resulting in increased vascular permeability, stimulation of glandular secretions, and peripheral vasodilation [50–59]. This results in an increase in nasal airway resistance, sneezing, rhinorrhea, and pruritus [51, 52, 58, 59]. Symptoms generally occur within minutes of exposure.

It has become evident that the nervous system plays an integral role in both the local and distal effects of allergen stimulation through neuronal reflexes [58–62]. Muscarinic receptors are located on the submucosal glands, blood vessels, and on the airway smooth muscle [63]. Inoculation of sensitized antigen to the unilateral nasal septum produces bilateral nasal symptoms, increased glandular markers, in particular lactoferrin, and upregulation of eosinophils in the bilateral maxillary sinuses and ocular symptoms [58–61]. In addition, sensory C nerve fibers are found innervating the walls of muscular arteries, arterioles, venules, venous sinusoids, and glands of both the upper and lower airways. They release a variety of neuropeptides, such as substance P (SP), tachykinin, neurokinin A (NKA), gastrin-releasing peptide, calcitonin gene-related peptide (CGRP), and vasoactive intestinal peptide (VIP) which are believed to augment the allergic inflammatory response [50, 59, 64–67].

Ocular symptoms are a result of a direct allergen reaction on the conjunctival mucosa nasal ocular reflex responses. This was demonstrated in a double-blind placebo-controlled crossover clinical trial conducted by Baroody et al. [68] in which allergen was administered topically to the unilateral nasal septum. This not only resulted in increased bilateral nasal symptoms of sneezing, rhinorrhea, and nasal congestion but ocular symptoms of itching and watery eyes as well. Both nasal and ocular symptoms were reduced by application of topical H1-receptor antagonist applied to the site of the nasal challenge.

Importantly, the allergic response is not confined to its acute symptoms; 30–40 % of people will have a delayed or late phase response (LPR) [2, 69–71]. The LPR occurs anywhere from 4 to 12 h after the initial exposure. The most prominent symptoms are nasal congestion with symptoms such as sneezing and rhinorrhea being less robust than in the early phase [51]. This is explained by an increase in the levels of histamine, tonsil-l-arginine methyl ester (TAME)-esterase, and to a lesser extent kinins. There is an influx in a variety of inflammatory cells and cellular mediators including Th2 lymphocytes, eosinophils, neutrophils, and basophils, which release chemokines and cytokines [2, 72, 73]. IL-4, IL-5, and IL-13 along with other inflammatory mediators and chemokines cause the transendothelial migration and activation of eosinophils [2, 74–76]. IL-5 plays an important role in eosinophil activation and functions to prevent eosinophil apoptosis [2, 75]. GM-CSF (granulocyte macrophage colony-stimulating factor) is another cytokine associated with eosinophil activation and survival and is increased during both early and late phase allergic inflammation [75]. Locally produced cytokine RANTES is chemotactic for and involved in eosinophil activation. RANTES and eotaxin are responsible for transendothelial migration of eosinophils and movement into the epithelium [76].

In addition, there is endothelial activation with enhanced expression of adhesion molecules, namely, ICAM-1 (intercellular adhesion molecule 1) and VCAM-1 (vascular adhesion molecule 1) [77]. These cells are important in the local recruitment of inflammatory cells during an allergic response. Late phase symptoms are most closely correlated with eosinophil levels [73]. Histamine levels correlate more closely with basophil levels suggesting that basophils and not mast cells are responsible for histamine release in the LPR [78].

Signs and Symptoms

Some of the commonly experienced symptoms experienced by patients with AR include nasal congestion, clear rhinorrhea, recurrent sneezing, and pruritus of the nose, palate, and posterior pharynx. An estimated 70 % of patients with AR experience both nasal and ocular symptoms [79]. Ocular symptoms are characterized by increased lacrimation, dryness, pruritus, and erythema. The ocular symptoms are a result of both local inflammatory response of the conjunctival mucosa to allergen exposure and nasal ocular reflexes [68, 80]. Although the offending allergen is not always apparent, symptoms generally occur within minutes of exposure [81]. Importantly, the allergic response is not confined to its acute symptoms; 30–40 % of people will have a delayed or late phase response (LPR) [2, 69–71]. These symptoms may present 4–12 h after the initial exposure. The predominant symptom in the late phase response is generally nasal congestion [51].

Traditionally, AR was subcategorized based on time of exposure into seasonal, perennial, or occupational. This method of categorization was not universally applicable as certain "seasonal" allergens may be present year round, depending on location, and many individuals were affected by both seasonal and perennial allergens. AR is now categorized based on duration of symptoms and level of impairment into "intermittent" or "persistent" [2].

History of the patient with suspected allergic rhinitis should include an inquiry as to the age of onset of symptoms, family history of atopic diseases, exposures to tobacco smoke or other irritants either at home, school or workplace, any seasonality of symptoms, food allergies, a history of asthma or dermatitis, and any prior treatments that may have been utilized. In addition, the patient should be asked about prior allergy or pulmonary function testing and the use of medications. It is important to ask about wheezing, chest tightness, shortness of breath during exercise, prolonged cough after viral infections, and/or nighttime cough which all may indicate asthmatic airway inflammation.

A thorough head and neck examination should be performed. Examination of the face may be significant for puffiness of the eyelids or over the cheeks. Darkening of the skin beneath the eyes is referred to as "allergic shiners" which results from prolonged venous congestion. A horizontal crease across the lower bridge of the nose may be present as a result of repeated upward rubbing of the nose and is referred to as the "allergic salute." Fine lines of the eyelids are referred to as "Dennie's lines" and result from spasm in the musculature of the eye [81]. Conjunctival erythema may also be appreciated. Rhinoscopy should be performed with attention to the quality of nasal drainage, presence of nasal polyps, and position of the nasal septum and appearance of the nasal mucosa. In patients with AR the nasal mucosa appears pale and boggy with a grayish white hue. Examination of the oropharynx in patients with AR may reveal a smooth irregular surface traditionally referred to as "cobblestoning" that is a result of the lymphoid follicles in the submucosa. In addition, otoscopic examination may reveal signs of effusion.

In light of the significant association of rhinitis with asthma, a pulmonary exam should be performed and pulmonary function tests should be considered if lower airway symptoms are present. Assess the skin for signs of eczema and/or dermatitis, as they commonly affect the atopic patient.

Allergy Testing

In order to confirm the diagnosis or identify causative allergens, IgE reactivity to various allergens either by skin prick test (SPT) or through allergen-specific IgE should be performed. Although test results take longer with antigen specific IgE, it is useful in patients with dermographism and dermatitis and in cases where antihistamines cannot be discontinued [46].

Treatment

Avoidance

It has been demonstrated that among patients with allergic rhinitis there is a dose-dependent increase in symptom severity with allergen exposure [6]. When possible, allergen avoidance is an important means of controlling symptoms [82] (see Table 10.1). For indoor allergens and, in particular, dust-mite, a variety of measures to decrease allergen burden have been suggested and include removal of carpets, cloth toys, linens and use of water vapor-permeable mattress covers, duvets, and pillows, in addition, at least weekly vacuuming. It is recommended that bedding be washed at least 60 °C [83]. While not robust, there have been some literature to support the use of acaricides (pesticide that kills dust mites) and extensive bedroom based control. There is little evidence to support the use of high efficiency particulate air (HEPA) filters alone, but they may be of use when combined with other methods of allergen avoidance although more studies need to be performed [84].

In patients who are allergic to animal dander, the animal should be removed, if possible, followed by subsequent vacuuming and cleaning of upholstery, bedding, and carpets. In situations where the animal cannot be removed from the house,

Table 10.1 Methods for allergen avoidance [82]

Allergen	Method for allergen avoidance
Pollen and outdoor molds	Limit outdoor activities during symptomatic period Avoid rubbing eyes and nose and wash hands when outdoors Close windows and use air-conditioning when in a vehicle and doors leading outside when in the home
Dust mite	Chemical Acaricidal Physical Use protective pillow, mattress, and duvet covers Regularly wash bedding at 60 °C Vacuum and damp dust house on a weekly basis Remove or regularly clean carpets, soft toys from the bedroom, upholstery curtains, and any other areas or objects that can gather dust Use a de-humidifier to reduce humidity in the home to between 35 and 50 %
Animal dander	Avoid contact with animals Keep pets outdoors or none at all Regularly vacuum the home and clean areas that gather animal dander Avoid rubbing eyes or nose after being in contact with animals Wash hands after clothes which have been in contact with animals

Modified with permission from Bilkhu et al. [82], with permission from Elsevier

frequent washings and prohibiting the animal from entering the bedroom may aid in decreasing the allergen burden.

In the cases of occupational rhinitis (OR), ensuring that there is adequate ventilation and wearing appropriate personal protective equipment may help decrease allergen burden. It has been suggested that OR is a precursor of occupational asthma. The risk of asthma has been shown to be as high as seven times that of controls, among farmers with occupational rhinitis [85]. Reduced exposure to known occupational triggers for rhinitis is important not only for symptom management but also for the potential prevention of occupational asthma.

Medical Treatment

Nasal Steroids

Intranasal corticosteroids (INS) are often a first-line agent used in the management of AR. In multiple randomized controlled trials, topical nasal steroids have been shown to be both safe and efficacious for use in both adults and children [78, 86, 87]. At the cellular level, nasal steroids have been found to inhibit cellular expression of mRNA for Th2 cytokines and subsequently decrease Th2 interleukins such as IL-4, IL5, and IL-13 [74, 75, 88]. Further, they decrease the number of Langerhans cells and decrease eosinophil infiltration and survival. At a gene level they work to decrease the expression of genes involved in the inflammatory response [89, 90]. They have found to improve symptoms of sneezing, rhinorrhea, nasal itching nasal congestion, and itchy watery eyes [80]. Subsequently, they have been found to improve sleep quality in patients with AR.

Not only has INS been found to be efficacious in the management of moderate-severe or persistent forms of rhinitis; they have also been shown to reduce BHR and improve asthma outcomes and should therefore be considered in the asthmatic patient [12, 13].

Some of the common side effects of topical corticosteroids include nasal crusting, dryness, and epistaxis. A variety of studies have not shown any increased risk of hypothalamic-pituitary axis suppression, or growth suppression with the use of INS, but additional studies need to be performed in children younger than 3 [88, 91, 92]. In addition, intranasal steroids have not been shown to lead to osteoporosis, ocular hypertension, or glaucoma [91, 93].

The onset of action of nasal steroids is around 6–12 h [94]. Moderate relief of symptoms is obtained within 72 h, but it may take over a week of regular use to obtain maximal benefit.

Systemic Steroids

Systemic corticosteroids have been found efficacious in the management of both rhinitis and asthma, but as a result of its side effect profile, systemic corticosteroid therapy is only used in severe refractory cases. They can be given in cases of rhinitis medicamentosa to provide some relief while discontinuing decongestants.

Oral Antihistamines

Oral antihistamines have proven to be efficacious in controlling symptoms of sneezing, itching, rhinorrhea, and ocular symptoms, while not having much affect on nasal congestion [95]. They function by inhibiting the release of preformed mediators from mast cells and basophils, as well as inhibiting the expression of cell adhesion molecules, recruitment and survival of eosinophils, and downregulation of transcription factors that are responsible for the production of pro-inflammatory cytokines and adhesion proteins [95–99]. Older H_1 antihistamines are referred to as first-generation antihistamines and are known for having more pronounced sedative and anticholinergic side effects, when compared to the newer second-generation antihistamines [95] (see Table 10.2).

Second-generation antihistamines are lipophobic and are recognized by P-glycoprotein efflux pump expressed on the luminal surface of the vascular endothelial cells, making for poor central nervous system penetration as compared to the first-generation antihistamines and subsequently less sedative side effects [95, 99]. In light of the decreased anticholinergic properties of the second-generation antihistamines, they are not as efficacious in the treatment of rhinorrhea [100]. Some H_1 antihistamines may cause QT prolongation, and in fact, astemizole and terfenadine have been taken off the market due to the risk of torsade de pointes [95, 101]. Antihistamines have proven efficacious in controlling the nasal and ocular symptoms of AR as well as aiding in asthma control [102]. The onset of action is between 1 and 3 h and the duration of action is at least 24 h.

Table 10.2 Antihistamines [95]

First-generation anti-histamines	Second-generation anti-histamines
Brompheniramine	Acrivastine
Chlorpheniramine	Cetirizine
Pheniramine[a]	Levocetirizine
Triprolidine	Desloratadine
Buclizine	Fexofenadine
Cyclizine	Levocabastine[a]
Hydroxyzine	Loratadine
Meclizine	Olopatadine[a]
Azatadine	Azelastine[a]
Cyproheptadine	Emedastine[a]
Diphenylpyraline	Epinastine[a]
Ketoifen[a]	
Carbinoxamine	
Clemastine	
Dimenhydrinate	
Diphenhydramine	
Doxylamine	
Antazoline	
Pyrilamine	
Tripelennamine	
Methdilazine	
Promethazine	
Doxepin	

Modified with permission from Simons[b] [95], with permission from *New England Journal of Medicine*
[a]Topical H1 antihistamine
[b]This medication is a tricyclic antidepressant with H1 and H2 antihistamine activities

Topical Antihistamines

H_1 antihistamines come in the form of a nasal spray and an ophthalmic solution as well. In light of the difference in the pharmacokinetics, these drugs are dosed twice a day as opposed to once daily. Nasal antihistamines such as azelastine significantly reduce rhinorrhea, but do have sedative properties.

Anticholinergics

Anticholinergic medications, such as ipratropium bromide, have been shown efficacious in the management of rhinorrhea but have no effect on nasal congestion or sneezing. They work by blocking the muscarinic receptors of the nasal seromucinous glands, effectively decreasing glandular secretion [83, 103].

Chromones

Chromones such as nedocromil are mast cell stabilizers with anti-inflammatory properties [83, 103]. Although chromones have been shown to improve symptoms in AR, studies comparing chromones to intranasal steroids have shown superior symptom control with intranasal steroids, and they are therefore not as commonly used [104, 105].

Decongestants

Decongestant is a broad term that refers to either oral or nasal medications that act on adrenergic receptors located on the precapillary and postcapillary blood vessels of the nasal mucosa with resultant vasoconstriction. This results in decreased blood flow and has been shown to significantly decrease nasal airway resistance (NAR) and significantly increase in peak nasal inspiratory flow (PNIF) [83, 106, 107]. They have a relatively quick onset of action. Decongestants when used in combination with nasal steroids or antihistamines have been shown to improve symptom control when compared with either treatment modality alone [108, 109]. Importantly, use of topical nasal decongestants are not recommended beyond 7–10 days as it may lead to rebound swelling of the nasal mucosa and worsening of nasal congestion, referred to as rhinitis medicamentosa. Decongestants should be avoided in children less than 1 year of age, elderly, and pregnancy. They should be avoided in hypertensive patients, patients with cardiac conditions, hyperthyroidism, prostate hypertrophy, glaucoma, and psychiatric disorders, and in patients on beta-blocker or MAO inhibitor [83].

Antileukotrienes

Leukotrienes are inflammatory mediators formed from the breakdown of arachidonic acid by mast cells, basophils, eosinophils, monocytes/macrophages, dendritic cells, and T lymphocytes [110]. Cysteinyl leukotrienes (CysLTs) refer to LTC_4, LTD_4, and LTE_4. Inhibitors of the 5-lipoxygenase pathways such as zileuton block the production of CysLTs, and leukotriene receptor antagonist, montelukast and zafirlukast, block the end organ effects of CysLTs. CysLTs have been shown to increase vascular permeability and nasal mucosal blood flow and significantly increase NAR [111, 112]. Montelukast has proven to be effective in the treatment of both nasal and ocular symptoms with comparable results to antihistamines [113]. When used in combination, montelukast and antihistamines have been shown to provide better symptom control than either used independently [114].

Anti-IgE

Omalizumab is a monoclonal anti-IgE antibody, which binds free circulating IgE. This reduces the amount of IgE available to bind to high affinity receptors on mast cells and therefore leads to a decrease in degranulation and the release of the preformed mediators responsible for the symptoms of AR [115].

Omalizumab has been shown to be efficacious in both the treatment of AR and allergic asthma, resulting in improvements in AR and asthma symptoms, as well as a decreased number of asthma exacerbations [116]. Omalizumab when used in combination with subcutaneous immunotherapy (SCIT) has shown to decrease the risk of anaphylaxis fivefold, allowing for a more rapid and higher regimen of immunotherapy to safely be administered and therefore decreased duration of treatment [117].

Immunotherapy

Immunotherapy is the only treatment modality that has been shown to alter the natural course of AR. In cases of severe persistent AR, not adequately controlled by pharmacologic means, or in patients with adverse reactions to allergy medications, allergen-specific immunotherapy may be indicated. Immunotherapy results in the production of allergen-specific T-regulatory cells. This suppresses the T-cell response to allergen and is referred to as T-cell tolerance [118, 119]. The Th2 polarized immune response is suppressed [120]. Allergen-specific IgG molecules are produced with a subsequent decrease in IgE. In addition, there is a decrease in the number of mast cells, basophils, and eosinophils [118].

Immunotherapy can be performed through subcutaneous injection and sublingual application. Treatment with subcutaneous immunotherapy requires repeat injections of allergen extract in an office or hospital setting. It has been estimated that there is a 0.1 % chance of developing a systemic reaction [46]. The risk is not insignificant, and immunotherapy should be administered by experienced personnel and in a properly equipped setting. Therapy lasts an average of 3–5 years and is marked by an initial "buildup phase" in which increasing doses of allergen are administered, followed by a "maintenance phase" [83].

Sublingual immunotherapy has been shown to be an effective and safe treatment option [121]. Unlike injection therapy only, the initial dose of sublingual immunotherapy needs to be administered in the office. The side effects are generally confined to gastrointestinal symptoms and respiratory symptoms such as wheezing.

Both SCIT and sublingual immunotherapy (SLIT) have shown to significantly improve symptoms, quality of life scores, and medication scores in multiple studies [122–126]. These improvements are sustained after therapy is discontinued. Durham et al. [126] performed a randomized, double-blind, placebo-controlled trial in which he was able to demonstrate that patients who had received 3–4 years of immunotherapy for grass pollen allergy had persistent improvements in symptoms and a decreased use of medications for 3 years after cessation of the immunotherapy. Use of immunotherapy in patients with AR may prevent the development of asthma. In a randomized controlled trial by Moller et al. [15], the use of immunotherapy to birch and/or timothy pollen in children with AR was shown to significantly prevent the development of asthma at 3 years.

Conclusion

Allergic rhinitis is one of the most common chronic diseases worldwide. While it is not a life-threatening condition, its impact on quality of life is substantial. AR is comorbid with a variety of other disease processes and is not only associated with but is a risk factor for the development of asthma [6–10]. Many treatment options exist and should be tailored to the individual. It has been shown that early and aggressive therapy of rhinitis may be preventative in development of asthma.

References

1. Bousquet J, Khaltaev N, Cruz AA, et al. Allergic rhinitis and its impact on asthma (ARIA). Allergy. 2008;63(86):8–160.
2. Bousquet J, Cauwenberge V, Khaltaev N, et al. Allergic rhinitis and its impact on asthma. J Allergy Clin Immunol. 2001;108(5):S147–334.
3. Wilken JA, Berkowitz R, Kane R. Decrements in vigilance and cognitive functioning associated with ragweed-induced allergic rhinitis. Ann Allergy Asthma Immunol. 2002;4:372–80.
4. Berrylin J, Ferguson MD. Influences of allergic rhinitis on sleep. Otolaryngol Head Neck Surg. 2004;130(5):617–29.
5. Bhattacharyya N. Incremental healthcare utilization and expenditures for allergic rhinitis in the United States. Laryngoscope. 2011;121:1830–3.
6. Guerra S, Sherrill DL, Martinez FD, et al. Rhinitis as an independent risk factor for adult-onset asthma. J Allergy Clin Immunol. 2002;109:419–25.
7. Corren J. Allergic rhinitis and asthma: how important is the link? J Allergy Clin Immunol. 1997;99:S781–6.
8. Settipane RJ, Hagy GY, Settipane GA. Long-term risk factors for developing asthma and allergic rhinitis: a 23-year follow-up of college students. Allergy Proc. 1994;15:21–5.
9. Leynaert B, Bousquet J, Neukirch C, Liar R, Neukirch F. Perennial rhinitis: an independent risk factor for asthma in nonatopic subjects: results from the European Community Respiratory Health Survey. J Allergy Clin Immunol. 1999;104(2):301–4.
10. Meltzer EO, Hamilos DL, Hadley JA, et al. Rhinosinusitis: establishing definitions for clinical research and patient care. Otolaryngol Head Neck Surg. 2004;131:1–62.
11. Jones C, Holt P. Immunopathology of allergy and asthma in childhood. Am J Respir Crit Care Med. 2000;162:S36–9.
12. Stelmach R, do Patrocinio T, Nunes M, et al. Effect of treating allergic rhinitis with corticosteroids in patients with mild-to-moderate persistent asthma. Chest. 2005;128:3140–7.
13. Watson WT, Becker AB, Simons FE. Treatment of allergic rhinitis with intranasal corticosteroids in patients with mild asthma: effect on lower airway responsiveness. J Allergy Clin Immunol. 1993;91:97–101.
14. Jani A, Hamilos D. Current thinking on the relationship between rhinosinusitis and asthma. J Asthma. 2005;42:1–7.
15. Möller C, Dreborg S, Ferdousi HA, et al. Pollen immunotherapy reduces the development of asthma in children with seasonal rhino- conjunctivitis (the PAT study). J Allergy Clin Immunol. 2002;109:251–6.
16. Johnstone DE, Dutton A. The value of hyposensitization therapy for bronchial asthma in children-a 14 year study. Pediatrics. 1968;42:793–802.
17. Jacobsen L, Nuchel PB, Wihl HA, et al. Immunotherapy with partially purified and standardized tree pollen extracts. IV: results from long-term (6 year) follow-up. Allergy. 1997;52:914–20.
18. Strachan DP. Hay fever, hygiene, and household size. BMJ. 1989;299(18):1259–60.

19. Crispen KL, Gillespie DN, Weiler EC. A comparison of 1978 and 2006 peak pollen seasons and sampling methods in Missoula, Montana. Grana. 2010;49:128–33.
20. Hurwitz SH. The lure of medical history John Bostock (1773-1846) author of the first clinical description of hay fever. Cal West Med. 1992;31(2):137–8.
21. Bloom B, Jones LI, Freeman G. Summary health statistics for U.S. children: National Health Interview Survey, 2012. National Center for Health Statistics. Vital Health Stat 10. 2013;(258):1–52.
22. Blackwell DL, Lucas JW, Clarke TC. Summary health statistics for U.S. adults: National Health Interview Survey, 2012. National Center for Health Statistics. Vital Health Stat 10. 2013;(260):4–122.
23. Kulig M, Klettke U, Wahn V, et al. Development of seasonal allergic rhinitis during the first 7 years of life. J Allergy Clin Immunol. 2000;106:832–9.
24. Blomme K, Tomassen P, Lapeere H. Prevalence of allergic sensitization versus allergic rhinitis symptoms in an unselected population. Int Arch Allergy Immunol. 2013;160(2):200–7.
25. Wright AL, Holberg CJ, Martinez FD, et al. Epidemiology of physician-diagnosed allergic rhinitis in childhood. Pediatrics. 1994;94(6 pt 1):895–901.
26. Dykewicz MS, Fineman F. Executive summary of joint task force practice parameters on diagnosis and management of rhinitis. Ann Allergy Asthma Immunol. 1998;81:463–8.
27. Jackson KD, Howie LD, Akinbami LJ. Trends in allergic conditions among children: United States, 1997–2011. NCHS data brief, no 121. Hyattsville: National Center for Health Statistics; 2013.
28. Dahl R, Andersen PS, Chivato T, et al. National prevalence of respiratory allergic disorders. Resp Med. 2004;98(5):398–403.
29. Pekkarinen PT, von Jertzen L, Laatikainen T, et al. A disparity in the association of asthma, rhinitis, and eczema with allergen-specific IgE between Finnish and Russian Karelia. Allergy. 2007;62:281–7.
30. Dold S, Wjst M, von Mutius E, et al. Genetic risk for asthma, allergic rhinitis and atopic dermatitis. Arch Dis Child. 1992;67:1018–22.
31. Romagnani S. Human TH1 and TH2 subsets: doubt no more. Immunol Today. 1991;12(8):256–7.
32. Baldini M, Lohman IC, Halonen M, Erickson RP, Holt PG, Martinez FD. A Polymorphism* in the 5′ flanking region of the CD14 gene is associated with circulating soluble CD14 levels and with total serum immunoglobulin E. Am J Respir Cell Mol Biol. 1999;20:976–83.
33. Hopkin JM, Cookson WO, Young RP. Asthma atopy and genetic linkage. Ann N Y Acad Sci. 1991;629:26–30.
34. Heinzmann A, Mao XQ, Akaiwa M, et al. Genetic variants of IL-13 signaling and human asthma and atopy. Hum Mol Genet. 2000;9(4):549–59.
35. Postma DS, Bleecher ER, Amelung PJ. Genetic susceptibility to asthma-bronchial hyperresponsiveness coinherited with a major gene for atopy. N Engl J Med. 1995;333:894–900.
36. Virkkula P, Liukkonen K, Suomalainen AK, et al. Parental smoking, nasal resistance and rhinitis in children. Acta Paediatr. 2011;100(9):1234–8.
37. Matricardi PM, Rosmini F, Panetta V, et al. Hay fever and asthma in relation to markers of infection. J Allergy Clin Immunol. 2002;110(3):381–7.
38. Holt PG, Macaubas C. Development of long-term tolerance versus sensitization to environmental allergens during the perinatal period. Curr Opin Immunol. 1997;9:782–7.
39. Pakarinen J, Hyvärinen A, Salkinoja-Salonen M. Predominance of gram-positive bacteria in house dust in the low-allergy risk Russian Karelia. Environ Microbiol. 2008;10(12):3317–25.
40. Ball TM, Castro-Rodriquez JA, Ka G, et al. Siblings, day-care attendance, and the risk of asthma and wheezing during childhood. N Engl J Med. 2000;343:538–43.
41. Spector SL. Overview of comorbid associations of allergic rhinitis. J Allergy Clin Immunol. 1997;99:773–8.
42. Alles R, Parikh A, Hawk L, et al. The prevalence of atopic disorders in children with chronic otitis media with effusion. Pediatr Allergy Immunol. 2001;12:102–6.

43. Krouse JH, Brown RW, Fineman SM, et al. Asthma and the unified airway. Otolaryngol Head Neck Surg. 2007;136:75–106.
44. Huse DM, Harte SC, Russel MW, et al. Allergic rhinitis may worse asthma symptoms in children: the international Asthma Outcomes registry. Am J Resp Crit Care Med. 1996;153:A860.
45. Hedin G, Graff-Lonnevig V, Heilborn H, et al. Immunotherapy with cat- and dog-dander extracts: V. Effects of 3 years of treatment. J Allergy Clin Immunol. 1991;87(5):955–64.
46. Greiner AN, Hellings PW, Rotiroti G. Allergic rhinitis. Lancet. 2012;378(9809):2112–22.
47. Romagnani S. The Th1/Th2 paradigm. Immunol Today. 1997;18(6):263–6.
48. Maggi E. The TH1/TH2 paradigm in allergy. Immunotechnology. 1997;3:233–44.
49. Çobanoğlu B, Toskala E, Ural A, et al. Role of leukotriene antagonists and antihistamines in the treatment of allergic rhinitis. Curr Allergy Asthma Rep. 2013;13:203–8.
50. Baroody FM, Naclerio RM. Immunology of the upper airway and pathophysiology and treatment of allergic rhinitis. In: Cummings otolaryngology: head & neck surgery, vol. 1. 5th ed. Philadelphia: Mobsy; 2010. p. 597–623.
51. Bousquet J, Vignola AM, Campbell AM, et al. Pathophysiology of the allergic response. Int Arch Allergy Immunol. 1996;110:207–18.
52. Castells M, Schwartz LB. Tryptase levels in nasal-lavage fluid as an indicator of the immediate allergic response. J Allergy Clin Immunol. 1988;82:348–55.
53. White MV, Kaliner MA. Mediators of allergic rhinitis. J Allergy Clin Immunol. 1992;90(4):699–704.
54. Baumgarten CR, Togias AG, Naclerio RM, et al. Influx of kininogens into nasal secretions following antigen challenge of allergic individuals. J Clin Invest. 1985;76:191.
55. Creticos PS, Peters SP, Adkinson Jr NF, et al. Peptide leukotriene release after antigen challenge in patients sensitive to ragweed. N Engl J Med. 1984;310:1626.
56. Bascom R, Pipkorn U, Proud D, et al. Major basic protein and eosinophil-derived neurotoxin concentrations in nasal lavage fluid after antigen challenge: effect of systemic corticosteroids and relationship to eosinophil influx. J Allergy Clin Immunol. 1989;84:338.
57. Min-Ho S, Averill FJ, Hubbard WC, et al. Nasal allergen challenge generates 1-0-Hexadecyl-2-lyso-sn-glycero-3-phosphocholine. Am J Respir Crit Care Med. 1994;149:660–6.
58. Wagenmann M, Baroody FM, Desrosiers M, et al. Unilateral nasal allergen challenge leads to bilateral release of prostaglandin D2. Clin Exp Allergy. 1996;26:371–8.
59. Raphael GD, Igarashi Y, White MV, et al. The pathophysiology of rhinitis: V. Sources of protein in allergen-induced nasal secretions. J Allergy Clin Immunol. 1991;88:33–42.
60. Baroody FM, Ford S, Lichtenstein LM, et al. Physiologic responses and histamine release after nasal antigen challenge: effect of atropine. Am J Respir Crit Care Med. 1994;149:1457–65.
61. Baroody FM, deTineo M, Naclerio RM. Unilateral nasal allergic reactions increase bilateral sinus eosinophil infiltration. J Appl Physiol. 2013;115:1262–7.
62. Canning BJ. Reflex regulation of airway smooth muscle tone. J Appl Physiol. 2006;101(3):971–85.
63. Ricci A, Mariotta S, Amenta F, et al. Changes in muscarinic cholinergic receptor expression in human peripheral blood lymphocytes in allergic rhinitis patients. Pulm Pharmacol Ther. 2008;21:79–87.
64. Baraniuk JN, Lundgren JD, Goff J, et al. Calcitonin gene-related peptide in human nasal mucosa. J Appl Physiol. 1990;258:L81–8.
65. Baraniuk JN, Lundgren JD, Okayama M, et al. Substance P and neurokinin A in human nasal mucosa. Am J Respir Cell Mol Biol. 1991;4:228.
66. Schierhorn K, Brunnée T, Schultz KD, et al. Substance-P-induced histamine release from human nasal mucosa in vitro. Int Arch Allergy Immunol. 1995;107:109.
67. Mosimann BL, White MV, Hohman RJ, et al. Substance P, calcitonin gene-related peptide, and vasoactive intestinal peptide increase in nasal secretions after allergen challenge in atopic patients. J Allergy Clin Immunol. 1993;92:95.

68. Baroody FM, Foster K, Markarian A, et al. Nasal ocular reflexes and eye symptoms in patients with allergic rhinitis. Ann Allergy Asthma Immunol. 2008;100(3):194–9.
69. Naclerio RM, Proud D, Togias AG, Adkinson N, et al. Inflammatory mediators in late antigen induced rhinitis. N Engl J Med. 1985;313(2):65–70.
70. Dvoracek JE, Yunginer JW, Kern EB, et al. Induction of nasal late-phase reactions by insufflation of ragweed-pollen extract. J Allergy Clin Immunol. 1984;73:363–8.
71. Taylor G, Shivalkar PR. "Arthus type" reactivity in the nasal airways and skin in pollen sensitive subjects. Clin Allergy. 1971;1:407–14.
72. Bentley AM, Jacobson MR, Cumberworth V, et al. Immunohistology of the nasal mucosa in seasonal allergic rhinitis: increases in activated eosinophils and epithelial mast cells. J Allergy Clin Immunol. 1992;89:877–83.
73. Pastorello EA, Galeazzo G, Riario-Sforza MD, et al. Comparison of rhinomanometry, symptom score and inflammatory cell counts in assessing the nasal late-phase reaction to allergen challenge. J Allergy Clin Immunol. 1994;93(1):85–92.
74. Masuyama K, Jacobson MR, Rak S, et al. Topical glucocorticosteroid (fluticasone propionate) inhibits cells expressing cytokine mRNA for interleukin-4 in the nasal mucosa in allergen- induced rhinitis. Immunology. 1994;82:192–9.
75. Nouri-Aria KT, Masuyama K, Jacobson MR, et al. Granulocyte/macrophage-colony stimulating factor in allergen-induced rhinitis: cellular localization relation to tissue eosinophilia and influence of topical corticosteroid. Int Arch Allergy Immunol. 1998;117:248–54.
76. Alam R, Stafford RA, Forsythe P, et al. RANTES is a chemotactic and activating factor for human eosinophils. J Immunol. 1993;150(8):3442–8.
77. Montefort S, Feather IH, Wilson SJ, et al. The expression of leukocyte-endothelial adhesion molecules is increased in perennial allergic rhinitis. Am J Respir Cell Mol Biol. 1992;7:393.
78. Bascom R, Wachs M, Naclerio RM, et al. Basophil influx occurs after nasal antigen challenge: effects of topical corticosteroid pretreatment. J Allergy Clin Immunol. 1988;81:580.
79. Canonica GW, Bousquet J, Mullol J, et al. A survey of the burden of allergic rhinitis in Europe. Allergy. 2007;62(85):17–25.
80. Baroody FM, Shenaq D, DeTineo M, et al. Fluticasone furoate nasal spray reduces the nasal-ocular reflex: a mechanism for the efficacy of topical steroids in controlling allergic eye symptoms. J Allergy Clin Immunol. 2009;123(6):1342–8.
81. Fornadley JA, Corey JP, Osguthorpe JD, Powell JP, et al. Allergic rhinitis: clinical practice guideline. Committee on practice standards. American Academy of Otolaryngic Allergy. Otolaryngol Head Neck Surg. 1996;115(1):115–22.
82. Bilkhu PS, Wolffohn JS, Naroo SA. A review of non-pharmacological and pharmacological management of seasonal and perennial allergic conjunctivitis. Cont Lens Anterior Eye. 2012;35(1):9–16.
83. Van Van Cauwenberge Bachert C, Passalacqua G, et al. Consensus statement on the treatment of allergic rhinitis. Allergy. 2000;55:116–34.
84. Sheikh A, Hurwitz B, Shehata Y. House dust mite avoidance measures for perennial allergic rhinitis. Cochrane Database Syst Rev. 2007;(1):CD001563.
85. Karjalainen A, Martikainen T, Klaukka T, et al. Risk of asthma among Finnish patients with occupational rhinitis. Occup Environ Lung Dis. 2003;123:283–8.
86. Yáñez A, Rodrigo GJ. Intranasal corticosteroids versus topical H1 receptor antagonists for the treatment of allergic rhinitis: a systematic review with meta-analysis. Ann Allergy Asthma Immunol. 2002;89:479–84.
87. Moller C, Ahlstrom H, Henricson KA. Safety of nasal budesonide in the long-term treatment of children with perennial rhinitis. Clin Exp Allergy. 2003;33:816–22.
88. Schenkel EJ, Skoner DP, Bronsky EA, et al. Absence of growth retardation in children with perennial allergic rhinitis after one year of treatment with mometasone furoate aqueous nasal spray. Pediatrics. 2000;105(2):E22.
89. Godhelp T, Holm AF, Blom H, et al. The effect of fluticasone propionate aqueous nasal spray on nasal mucosal inflammation in perennial allergic rhinitis. Allergy. 1995;50(23):21–4.

90. Mackle T, Gendy SS, Walsh M, et al. Role of sphingosine 1-phosphate receptor expression in eosinophils of patients with allergic rhinitis, and effect of topical nasal steroid treatment on this receptor expression. J Laryngol Otol. 2008;122:1309–17.
91. Wilson AM, Sims EJ, McFarlane LC, et al. Effects of intranasal corticosteroids on adrenal, bone, and blood markers of systemic activity in allergic rhinitis. J Allergy Clin Immunol. 1998;102:598–604.
92. Dibildox J. Safety and efficacy of mometasone furoate aqueous nasal spray in children with allergic rhinitis: results of recent clinical trials. J Allergy Clin Immunol. 2001;108:S54–8.
93. Garbe E, LeLorier J, Boivin JF, et al. Inhaled and nasal glucocorticoids and the risks of ocular hypertension or open-angle glaucoma. JAMA. 1997;277:722–7.
94. Berkowitz RB, Bernstein DI, LaForce C, et al. Onset of action of mometasone furoate nasal spray (NASONEX) in seasonal allergic rhinitis. Allergy. 1999;54(1):64–9.
95. Simons FE. Advances in H1-antihistamines. N Engl J Med. 2004;351(21):2203–17.
96. Schroeder JT, Schleimer RP, Lichtenstein LM, Kreutner W. Inhibition of cytokine generation and mediator release by human basophils treated with desloratadine. Clin Exp Allergy. 2001;31:1369–77.
97. Thomson L, Blaylock MG, Sexton DW, et al. Cetirizine and levocetirizine inhibit eotaxin-induced eosinophil transendothelial migration through human dermal or lung microvascular endothelial cells. Clin Exp Allergy. 2002;32:1187–92.
98. Ciprandi G, Passalacqua G, Canonica GW. Effects of H1 antihistamines on adhesion molecules: a possible rationale for long-term treatment. Clin Exp Allergy. 1999;29 Suppl 3:49–53.
99. Chishty M, Reichel A, Siva J, et al. Affinity of the p-glycoprotein efflux pump at the blood brain barrier may explain the lack of CNS side-effects of modern antihistamines. J Drug Target. 2001;9:223.
100. Van Steekelenburg J, Clement PAR, Beel MH. Comparison of five new antihistamines (H_1-receptor antagonists) in patients with allergic rhinitis using nasal provocation studies and skin tests. Allergy. 2002;53:346–50.
101. Tagialatela M, Timmerman H, Annunziato L. Cardiotoxic potential and CNS effects of first-generation antihistamines. Trends in pharmacological sciences. Trends Pharmacol Sci. 2000;21(2):52–6.
102. Aaronson DW. Evaluation of cetirizine in patients with allergic rhinitis and perennial asthma. Ann Allergy Asthma Immunol. 1996;76:440–6.
103. Kirkegaard J, Mygind N, Molgaard F, et al. Ordinary and high dose ipratropium in perennial nonallergic rhinitis. J Allergy Clin Immunol. 1987;79:585–90.
104. Bruijnzeel PL, Warringa RA, Kok PT, et al. Inhibition of neutrophil and eosinophil chemotaxis by nedocromil sodium and sodium cromoglycate. Br J Pharmacol. 1990;99:798–802.
105. Bousquet J, Chanal I, Alquie ME, et al. Prevention of pollen rhinitis symptoms: comparison of Fluticasone propionate aqueous nasal spray and disodium cromoglycate aqueous nasal spray. A multicenter, double-blind, double-dummy, parallel-group study. Allergy. 1993;48:327–33.
106. Vaidyanathan S, Williamson P, Lipworth B. Comparative evaluation of nasal blood flow and airflow in the decongestant response to oxymetazoline. Ann Allergy Asthma Immunol. 2012;108(2):77–80.
107. Calderon-Zapata MA, Davies RJ. Antiallergic and vasoactive drugs for rhinitis. In: Busse WW, Holgate ST, editors. Asthma and rhinitis. 2nd ed. Oxford: Blackwell Science Ltd; 2008. doi:10.1002/9780470694923.ch38.
108. Baroody FM, Brown D, Gavanescu L, et al. Oxymetazoline adds to the effectiveness of fluticasone furoate in the treatment of perennial allergic rhinitis. J Allergy Clin Immunol. 2011;127(4):927–34.
109. Storms WW, Bodman SF, Nathan RA, et al. A new antihistamine/decongestant for season allergic rhinitis. J Allergy Clin Immunol. 1989;83:1083–90.

110. Peters-Golden M, Gleason MM, Togias A. Cysteinyl leukotrienes: multi-functional mediators in allergic rhinitis. Clin Exp Allergy. 2006;36:689–703. doi:10.1111/j.1365-2222.2006.02498.x.
111. Bisgaard H, Olsson P, Bende M. Effect of leukotriene D_4 on nasal mucosal blood flow nasal airway resistance and nasal secretion in humans. Clin Allergy. 1986;16:289–97.
112. Maekawa A, Austen KF, Kanaoka Y. Targeted gene disruption reveals the role of cysteinyl leukotriene 1 receptor in the enhanced vascular permeability of mice undergoing acute inflammatory responses. J Biol Chem. 2002;277:20820–4.
113. van Adelsberg J, Philip G, LaForce CF, et al. Randomized controlled trial evaluating the clinical benefit of montelukast for treating spring seasonal allergic rhinitis. Ann Allergy Asthma Immunol. 2003;90(2):214–22.
114. Meltzer EO, Malmstrom K, Lu S, et al. Concomitant montelukast and loratadine as treatment for seasonal allergic rhinitis: a randomized, placebo-controlled clinical trial. J Allergy Clin Immunol. 2000;105(5):917–22.
115. Kaliner MA. Omalizumab and the treatment of allergic rhinitis. Curr Allergy Asthma Rep. 2004;4:237–44.
116. Vignola AM, Humbert M, Bousquet J, et al. Efficacy and tolerability of anti-immunoglobulin E therapy with omalizumab in patients with concomitant allergic asthma and persistent allergic rhinitis: SOLAR. Allergy. 2004;59:709–17.
117. Casale TB, Busse WW, Kline JN, et al. ; Immune Tolerance Network Group. Omalizumab pretreatment decreases acute reactions after rush immunotherapy for ragweed-induced seasonal allergic rhinitis. J Allergy Clin Immunol. 2007;117(1):134–40.
118. Akdis M, Akdis CA. Mechanisms of allergen-specific immunotherapy. J Allergy Clin Immunol. 2007;119:780–9.
119. Akdis CA, Akdis M, Blesken T, Wymann D, Müller U, et al. Epitope specific T cell tolerance to phospholipase A_2 in bee venom immunotherapy and recovery by IL-2 and IL-15 in vitro. J Clin Invest. 1996;98:1676–83.
120. Zhao CQ, Li TL, He SH, et al. Specific immunotherapy suppresses Th2 responses via modulating TIM1/TIM4 interaction on dendritic cells. Allergy. 2010;65:986–95.
121. Andre C, Vatrinet C, Galvain S, et al. Safety of sublingual-swallow immunotherapy in children and adults. Int Arch Allergy Immunol. 2000;121:229–34.
122. Calderon MA, Alves B, Jacobson M, et al. Allergen injection immunotherapy for seasonal allergic rhinitis. Cochrane Database Syst Rev. 2007;(1):CD001936.
123. Radulovic S, Calderon M, Wilson D, et al. Sublingual immunotherapy for allergic rhinitis. Cochrane Database Syst Rev. 2010;(12):CD002893.
124. Dretzke J, Meadows A, Novielli N, et al. Subcutaneous and sublingual immunotherapy for seasonal allergic rhinitis: a systematic review and indirect comparison. J Allergy Clin Immunol. 2013;131(5):1361–6.
125. Ross R, Nelson HS, Finegold I. Effectiveness of specific immunotherapy in the treatment of allergic rhinitis: an analysis of randomized, prospective, single or double-blind placebo-controlled studies. Clin Ther. 1999;22(3):342–9.
126. Durham SR, Walker SM, Varga EM, et al. Long-term clinical efficacy of grass-pollen immunotherapy. N Engl J Med. 1999;341:468.

Part II

Medical Therapy of Chronic Rhinosinusitis

Overview of the Medical Management of Chronic Rhinosinusitis

11

Dana L. Crosby and David W. Kennedy

Key Take-Home Points

- Chronic rhinosinusitis is a syndrome with multiple predisposing causes.
- Environmental factors, host factors, and local factors may all contribute to chronic rhinosinusitis.
- In developing a patient therapy, it is critical to consider the underlying causes.
- Anti-inflammatory therapy plays an important part in the management of chronic rhinosinusitis.
- Topical steroid therapy and nasal irrigations are mainstays of management in chronic rhinosinusitis.
- A variety of adjunctive therapies need to be considered in patients with refractive disease.

Introduction

In considering the medical management of chronic rhinosinusitis (CRS), it is important to understand that CRS is a term that refers to the common endpoint of a heterogenous group of disease processes. Despite recent advances, the etiology and

D.L. Crosby, MD
Division of Otolaryngology – Head and Neck Surgery, Southern Illinois University School of Medicine, 301 N. 8th Street, Springfield, IL 62704, USA
e-mail: dcrosby53@siumed.edu

D.W. Kennedy, FACS, FRCSI, MD (✉)
Department of Otorhinolaryngology – Head and Neck Surgery, Perelman School of Medicine, University of Pennsylvania, 3400 Spruce St., Ravdin 5, Philadelphia, PA 19104, USA
e-mail: kennedyd@uphs.upenn.edu

P.S. Batra, J.K. Han (eds.), *Practical Medical and Surgical Management of Chronic Rhinosinusitis*, DOI 10.1007/978-3-319-16724-4_11

pathophysiology of CRS remain poorly understood. In evaluating potential factors involved in the disease process, it is useful to consider potential general host factors, environmental factors, and local host factors that may contribute to the disease process (Table 11.1). Management of the environmental factors and underlying general host factors is obviously critical to long-term treatment success. Several different local host factors have also been proposed as being involved in CRS. These include biofilms, superantigens, and inflammation of the underlying bone. It has been hypothesized that these latter factors may lead to prolonged inflammation in patients who develop CRS. Most recently attention has been turned to evaluation of the microbiome in sinuses of patients with CRS. There is some evidence that patients with CRS are hyperresponsive to commensal organisms when compared to controls.

Over the years, various classification schemes based on clinical and pathologic findings have been used to attempt to delineate CRS into more discrete entities in order to convey information about etiology and to guide treatment. Commonly, CRS is subdivided into CRS with nasal polyps (CRSwNP) or CRS without nasal polyps (CRSsNP); however, there remains considerable variation within each of these groups. For instance, within the CRSwNP polyp group, there are aspirin-exacerbated respiratory disease (AERD), allergic fungal sinusitis, and cystic fibrosis-related sinusitis to

Table 11.1 General, local, and environmental host factors

General host factors
Genetic factors
Specific disorders (e.g., cystic fibrosis)
Genetic predispositions
Granulomatous diseases
Sarcoidosis
Granulomatosis with polyangiitis (GPA or Wegener's)
Immunologic disorders
Common variable immune deficiency (CVID)
IgA deficiency
Autoimmune disorders
Churg-Strauss (eosinophilic granulomatosis with polyangiitis or EGPA)
Ciliary dyskinesias
Atopy
Asthma
Local host factors
Chronic OMC inflammation
Obstruction (anatomic, polyps, neoplasia)
Local host immune deficiencies
Biofilms
Microbiota
Environmental
Pollution/chemical
Allergens
Tobacco (primary or secondary exposure)
Fungal exposure
Viruses/bacteria

name a few. Additionally, the presence and absence of polyps are not completely discrete entities. Instead, it may be more useful to use the classification of eosinophilic versus noneosinophilic CRS as a guide to treatment planning. Also factors such as asthma and allergic rhinitis may play a role in CRS with nasal polyps. This may also provide insight into expected outcomes as it has been shown that patients with increased tissue eosinophilia tend to have worse outcomes. As more is learned with regard to specific chemokine actions and pathways, additional and more precise classifications are likely.

Environmental Modification

Environmental exposure plays a significant role in sinonasal inflammation. When counseling patients with CRS, it is important to obtain a thorough social history including smoking, occupational exposure, and possible allergen exposure. It is well known that smoking, including secondhand smoke, can lead to impaired mucociliary clearance, making smoking cessation a necessity when trying to appropriately manage CRS. If patients are regularly exposed to noxious chemicals at work, they should be advised to use an appropriate respirator or even change their work environments when possible. Allergic rhinitis often plays an important role in mucosal inflammation and CRS. If there is a history suggestive of allergic rhinitis, allergy testing should be strongly considered, and the patient counseled regarding allergy therapy and the importance of making appropriate environmental changes. Lifestyle and environmental alterations are often a necessary first step for the successful long-term management of CRS.

In considering the medical management of CRS, the potential predisposing host factors should be carefully considered, especially in patients who have failed prior medical or surgical therapy and an appropriate evaluation performed for underlying immunologic or autoimmune problems. It should also be recognized that cystic fibrosis (CF) may present in adult patients with intractable CRS, and CF should be considered in any patient who has their first surgical procedure before the age of 18 years (Table 11.2).

Table 11.2 Evaluation considerations in the patient with difficult to treat disease

Immunologic evaluation
CBC with differential
Immunoglobulins and immunoglobulin subtypes
Active immunity (pneumococcus, etc.)
Autoimmune and granulomatous disease evaluation
CBC with differential
ESR, CRP
Rheumatoid factor
C-ANCA
ACE
Genetic disorders
Genetic evaluation for CF variants
Ciliary biopsy (coryna if patient has marked CRS)

Specific Therapeutic Options

Antibiotic Therapy

Systemic Antibiotics

Although bacterial infection likely plays a role in the inflammatory process, it is no longer believed to be the principal causative factor. However, antibiotics remain important in the management of exacerbations and in overall management [1]. Interestingly, it has been shown that selective pressure from antimicrobial agents can alter the bacterial composition seen in CRS [2]. The most common bacteria occurring in acute rhinosinusitis (ARS) have been well characterized; however, bacteria involved in CRS have been less clearly identified making it difficult to treat chronic bacterial infections empirically.

Antibiotic resistance is an increasingly common issue in the management of CRS. One study showed that resistance from erythromycin is increasing at a higher rate than for other antibiotics [3]. Another retrospective review of culture results from 324 CRS patients obtained over a 5-year period showed that *Pseudomonas* was resistant to levofloxacin in 13 % percent of cultures and ciprofloxacin in 5 % of cultures [4]. Methicillin-resistant *S. aureus* was seen in 21 % of cultures. Most importantly, it was reported that 62 % of cultures were resistant to at least one antibiotic. This highlights the dramatic prevalence of antibiotic resistance that we are facing. Because of the aforementioned issues, when possible endoscopic-directed culture should be obtained to decrease the use of broad-spectrum antibiotics [5].

There is a surprising lack of high level evidence supporting the use of antibiotics in the treatment of CRS, in fact there have been no randomized placebo-controlled studies evaluating the treatment of CRS with oral antibiotics. Currently, no antibiotic agents are approved for the use in CRS by the US Food and Drug Administration [6].

Macrolides

Because of their inherent anti-inflammatory properties, macrolides often receive special mention when discussing antibiotic management of CRS. This immunomodulatory effect was first noted during the treatment of diffuse panbronchiolitis in which profound neutrophilic inflammation is seen [7]. Macrolides exert their anti-inflammatory effect in multiple ways, all of which lead to the protection of the mucosa from the negative effects of prolonged neutrophil activity. Macrolide immunomodulatory effects stem from their ability to alter cytokine profiles and decrease damaging free radical production [8, 9]. Another important characteristic of macrolides is their ability to prevent biofilm adherence [10]. Unfortunately, studies evaluating the clinical benefit of these properties in CRS patients are mixed. Of note, a placebo-controlled study by Wallwork et al. evaluating the use of macrolide therapy showed improved symptomatic control in a subgroup with normal or low IgE levels [11]. Further studies should be done, especially in this subset of patients in order to evaluate the effectiveness of oral macrolide therapy in the management of CRS.

IV Antibiotics

There is very little in literature to support the use of intravenous antibiotics in the management of CRS. Indications for IV therapy include the presence of resistant organisms, intracranial or orbital complications, and intolerance to oral medications [12]. Although personal experience and several prior studies suggest that the underlying bone plays a significant part in making CRS resistant to therapy, there is currently no evidence for bacterial infection within the bone, and thus osteitis is not an indication for IV antibiotic therapy.

Topical Antibiotics

The goal of topical antibiotic therapy is to provide high concentrations of antimicrobials directly to the mucosa with the hope of eliminating the systemic absorption and side effects of traditional oral antibiotics. Although frequently utilized, currently little data exists to support efficacy in CRS. A recent meta-analysis of four randomized controlled clinical trials evaluated the use of topical antibacterial therapy [13]. Three of these studies showed no benefit of topical antibiotics; however, as pointed out by Cain and Lal [14], none of these studies utilized the high-volume low-pressure delivery technique that has been shown to be most beneficial in sinonasal topical delivery. Another study evaluated the use of topical mupirocin irrigation versus saline irrigation in post-endoscopic sinus surgery patients with positive *S. aureus* cultures [15]. At the 1-month time point, none of the patients treated with mupirocin irrigation had a positive culture, and endoscopic scores were improved, while 88.9 % of patients treated with saline irrigations had a positive culture. However, symptom scores were not statistically different. A 2007 review of the literature evaluated 14 studies with varying levels of evidence and suggested an overall low level of evidence for the use of topical antibacterials with the highest level of evidence existing in the postsurgical patients and in culture-directed therapy [16].

One hope is that topical delivery of antibiotic avoids systemic absorption; however, two studies utilizing gentamicin irrigation demonstrated mixed results [17, 18]. Taking these two studies into consideration, it appears that there may be a systemic accumulation of gentamicin over time. Further studies should be done in order to evaluate this topic and determine a safe duration of topical therapy especially in the case of gentamicin.

Systemic Antifungals

Fungi were originally proposed as the causative agent in CRS [19]. However, this has generally been discredited, and a placebo-controlled double-blind study using high-dose terbinafine showed no difference between active and placebo medication [20]. That said, personal clinical experience demonstrates that a small subset of patients with eosinophilic polypoid disease do appear to respond to oral itraconazole, although this may result from the antiangiogenesis effect of the medication rather than its antifungal effect. Given the hepatotoxic effects and potential cardiotoxic effects of the medication and its cost, as well as our inability to predict the small subset who will respond, itraconazole should be utilized sparingly and usually as a last resort. A review of the literature on oral antifungal therapy in the treatment of CRS was performed in 2011 and suggested some potential benefit from using itraconazole and ketoconazole, but the level of evidence was low [21].

Topical Antifungals

A variety of studies have evaluated the use of topical antifungal agents, and although an initial randomized controlled trial evaluating the use of topical amphotericin B appeared promising, this was not replicated in subsequent studies, and the use of topical antifungals is not recommended [22–26]. However, it should be noted that there have been no studies evaluating the use of oral or topical antifungals specifically in patients with allergic fungal sinusitis (AFS).

Anti-inflammatory Therapy

Systemic Steroids

The evidence supporting the use of systemic steroids varies among patients with CRSsNP, CRSwNP, and allergic fungal sinusitis (AFS). One literature review demonstrated that the level of evidence for the use of oral steroids in CRSsNP is low [27]. The use of systemic steroids in patients with CRSwNP is much more compelling both in clinical practice and in the literature, with evidence of improvement in nasal symptoms and airflow and reduction in polyp size [28–30]. Additionally, pretreatment with a short course of oral steroid followed by prolonged topical steroid therapy may be beneficial [31]. Similarly, the evidence is very strong for the use of oral steroids as an adjunct in the treatment of allergic fungal sinusitis (AFS) [31, 32]. However, since steroid use can occasionally induce fungal invasion in AFS, the prolonged use of steroids in the absence of surgical removal of bony partitions is not recommended.

It is important to keep in mind that side effects associated with systemic steroid use are common and include decrease in bone density, HPA axis suppression, hyperglycemia, weight gain, acne, cataract formation, mood alteration, insomnia, and gastric complications. The rare but devastating side effect of avascular necrosis should also be considered when weighing their use, and the use of oral steroids should be limited in patients with preexisting osteoporosis, diabetes, glaucoma, or a history of mental health issues. The risk to benefit ratio should be weighed on a patient to patient basis bearing in mind that the data are significantly more supportive of systemic steroid therapy in the setting of CRSwNP and AFS compared to CRSsNP.

Topical Steroids

Topical steroid preparations are the mainstay of treatment for allergic rhinitis, CRSwNP, and AFS but as with systemic steroids, their efficacy is less well documented in CRSsNP. FDA-approved, low-dose intranasal steroid sprays are known to be well tolerated with low bioavailability. An increased risk of epistaxis has been reported in patients who use steroid sprays improperly, live in dry climates, or use fluticasone propionate. Other side effects include nasal irritation and dryness, headache, and cough [33, 34].

For maximal effect, many rhinologists prefer the off-label use of topical steroids delivered in high-volume, high-dose method. It is believed that, in addition to the cleansing effect of the irrigation, this allows higher concentration of the topical steroid to be applied more diffusely throughout the sinonasal passages. However, at this point in time, there is little high-quality data to support the use of these medications and no long-term safety data. One 6-week study using 0.5 mg of budesonide mixed in 240 ml of saline over a 6-week period did not show any evidence of suppression of serum cortisol or urinary cortisol levels [35]. Similarly, a study of fluticasone propionate irrigation (3 mg in 240 ml of saline twice daily for 6 weeks) did not show evidence of suppression of salivary cortisol levels or ocular changes [36].

A recent retrospective review of prospectively collected data assessed the use of budesonide nasal irrigations (BNI) [37]. Subgroup analysis showed SNOT-20 scores were significantly improved with the use of BNI for patients with eosinophilic CRS (eCRS) and aspirin-exacerbated respiratory disease (AERD). Endoscopy scores were significantly improved only in the eCRS group. More prospective, randomized trials evaluating the efficacy and long-term safety of high-dose-high-volume steroid nasal irrigations are needed.

Steroid-Eluting Implants

It has been shown that topical steroid delivered is useful in treating patients with CRS; however, delivery of a drug in such a manner is fraught with uncertainty including the amount of drug reaching the mucosa, duration of contact with the mucosa, difficulty reaching areas such as ethmoid and frontal sinuses, as well as patient compliance issues. Bioabsorbable steroid-eluting implants (SEIs) are now available. SEIs deliver a known dose of steroid to the mucosa over a known period of time. With SEIs, there is minimal systemic absorption of steroid, and there is no reliance on patient compliance.

The currently FDA-approved SEIs are the Propel and Mini-Propel Steroid-Releasing Implants (IntersectENT, Menlo Park, CA). The Propel implant contains 370 µg of mometasone furoate embedded in a spring-like polylactide-co-glycolide polymer matrix [38]. This implant is bioabsorbable and lasts approximately 30 days if left in place. A recent meta-analysis by Han et al. pooled data from two previous studies [39]. A total of 143 patients at 11 centers were evaluated. There was found to be a significant decrease in adhesions on the treatment side, reduction in middle turbinate lateralization, and decreased need for postoperative interventions (lysis of adhesions and postoperative oral steroids). Currently, a multicenter study is evaluating outpatient placement of a 90-day SEI placed in patients with recurrent ethmoid sinusitis who would otherwise be candidates for revision surgical intervention [40].

Allergy

Immunotherapy

Allergic rhinitis and nonallergic rhinitis have been shown to be significant risk factors in the development of CRS [41]. In patients with refractory CRS, it was noted that the prevalence of allergy was approximately 60 %, while the prevalence was greater than 80 % in patients requiring endoscopic sinus surgery [42]. Nasal polyps are felt to be a result of a persistent inflammatory state. There is currently no data suggesting the benefit of immunotherapy in the treatment of patients with CRS, and the role of allergy in nasal polyp development is still unknown [43]. Because there is a theoretic benefit, low risk of severe side effects, and no negative long-term effects from the administration of immunotherapy, allergy testing and subsequent desensitization are often recommended for patients with eosinophilic chronic rhinosinusitis and allergic rhinitis [44].

Antihistamines

Although the use of antihistamines provides symptomatic relief in allergic rhinitis, there is limited data to support the use of antihistamines in the treatment of CRS. One randomized double-blind placebo-controlled trial placed patients with acute exacerbations of sinusitis into two groups. Both groups were treated with 2 weeks of antibiotics and 10 days of oral corticosteroids, while one group was given a placebo and the other loratadine. The loratadine group reported a significant decrease in sneezing at 14 days and nasal obstruction at 28 days. Physicians also reported subjective improvement in patients in the loratadine group [45]. Despite the lack of data, nonsedating antihistamines are often prescribed as a component of the medical management of CRS.

Leukotriene Modifiers

Leukotrienes have also been proposed as having a beneficial role in treating patients with chronic rhinosinusitis when a significant allergic component is present or in patients with aspirin triad. However, again, support for their use in CRS from the literature is limited [46–49].

Saline Irrigation

Saline irrigation as a primary or adjunct treatment in CRS is common practice as it has been shown to be efficacious with minimal risk. A 2007 meta-analysis evaluated eight studies in which saline irrigation was compared to no treatment, placebo, as an adjunct treatment, or against a topical nasal steroid spray [50]. This meta-analysis found evidence that saline irrigation as the sole modality of treatment as well as an adjunct treatment is beneficial. Nasal saline irrigation was found to be less effective than nasal steroid spray. Two studies compared the use of hypertonic saline to isotonic saline. The use of hypertonic saline showed no improvement in symptom control or radiologic scores when compared to isotonic saline. A randomized double-blind trial aimed to evaluate the mucociliary clearance and nasal patency in patients treated with isotonic versus hypertonic saline [45]. Both isotonic and hypertonic saline showed improvement in mucociliary clearance. It was demonstrated that isotonic saline irrigations improved nasal patency; however, this benefit was not observed in the hypertonic saline group.

Delivery methods of saline nasal irrigation have been evaluated as well. Wormald used a Technetium-99 m sulfur colloid labeling technique to evaluate the distribution of topical irrigation using different delivery methods [51]. This study evaluated nasal douching, metered nasal spray, and nebulization in patients who had previously undergone endoscopic sinus surgery. All three methods effectively delivered saline to the nasal cavity. Nasal douching proved better at delivery of irrigant to the maxillary sinus and frontal recess. The sphenoid sinus and frontal sinus were inadequately irrigated by all delivery methods. A later study using cadaveric specimens evaluated ostial size and head position in nasal irrigation delivery [52]. It was found that an ostium size of at least 4.7 mm was required for optimal delivery to the maxillary and sphenoid sinus, while anterior head tilt was required for optimal delivery to the frontal sinus.

Overall, the use of nasal saline irrigations has been shown to be beneficial in both the unoperated and operated patient. However, the overall improvement is greatest using large volume, low-pressure saline irrigation in patient who have had endoscopic sinus surgery [53, 54]. Indeed, it has been reported that 87 % of patients with sinonasal symptoms have used saline irrigation [55]. Side effects are typically mild and include nasal discomfort, drainage, epistaxis, headache, and otalgia.

Decongestants

Although decongestants are currently recommended during the first few days of an acute sinusitis, some patients report improvement in CRS. Decongestants, both oral and topical, may have significant side effects including tachycardia, hypertension, and insomnia and should be avoided in patients with hypertension and patients taking monoamine oxidase inhibitors. Topical decongestants such as oxymetazoline quickly develop tachyphylaxis and should not be used long term.

Mucolytics

Guaifenesin is the most commonly prescribed mucolytic; however, little data supporting its effectiveness in CRS is reported in the literature, and high doses are required for beneficial effect to be achieved. Erdosteine, a mucolytic, is known to have additional properties such as antibacterial, antioxidant, and anti-inflammatory effects [56]. A recent review of the literature showed that the application of various topical surfactants had some antibacterial properties in vitro as well as a modest inhibition of biofilm formation [57]. It was hypothesized that this was secondary to the mucolytic properties of surfactant. The review stated that the use of topical surfactant may be limited by nasal irritation as well as transient ciliotoxicity.

Anti-IgE Therapy

Omalizumab is a recombinant humanized monoclonal antibody that binds and reduces the level of IgE in tissue and serum. Treatment is very costly, and it is currently only FDA approved for patient with moderate to severe or severe allergic asthma and significantly elevated IgE. A small prospective uncontrolled trial looked at the efficacy of 16 weeks of omalizumab treatment in patients with eosinophilic chronic rhinosinusitis and severe atopic asthma [58]. This study showed improvement in rhinologic symptoms and sinus CT score in addition to improved asthma control. However, another randomized controlled trial showed no significant improvement [59]. Although personal experience has demonstrated that patients on omalizumab with asthma and markedly elevated IgE frequently demonstrate significant symptomatic improvement and decrease in polyps, larger-scale controlled trials are required.

Anti-IL-5

Most patients with CRSwNP have significant eosinophilia along with elevated levels of IL-5. IL-5 is known to be the main driver in eosinophilic proliferation. A double-blind randomized controlled trial enrolled 24 patients at two centers with bilateral nasal polyposis to receive one injection of 3 mg/kg of reslizumab, 1 mg/kg of reslizumab, or placebo. Nasal polyp score improved in only half of the treatment group; however, it was noted that responders tended to have higher levels of IL-5 in nasal secretions prior to treatment [60]. Another double-blinded randomized controlled trial evaluated 30 patients for the effectiveness of mepolizumab, a humanized monoclonal antibody that recognizes IL-5 [61]. Twenty patients were treated with two single injections of 750 mg of mepolizumab 28 days apart, while 10 patients were treated with placebo. At 8 weeks 12 out of 20 patients showed improvement in nasal polyp score and CT score, while only 1 out of 10 patients showed improvement in the placebo arm. Anti-IL-5 therapy shows promise in the treatment of eCRS; however, more studies are required to evaluate this.

IVIG

Immune deficiency is often undiagnosed in patients with CRS, and an immunologic evaluation should certainly be performed in patients who do not respond to routine medical and surgical therapy. An unexpectedly high incidence of humoral immunodeficiency has been identified in patients with at least three episodes of sinusitis in 1 year and those undergoing endoscopic sinus surgery [62]. Other studies have similarly shown unexpectedly high incidence of immune deficiency in patients with CRS. A study evaluating the result of intravenous immune globulin therapy showed significant initial improvements for these patients. Unfortunately, over time the disease process has a tendency to again progress.

Aspirin Desensitization

The use of aspirin desensitization in patients with aspirin triad or aspirin-exacerbated respiratory disease (AERD) has been evaluated extensively in the literature; however, most studies are of level 2 evidence. One uncontrolled open crossover trial with 65 patients with AERD underwent aspirin desensitization therapy with significant decrease in number of sinus infections per year, decrease in oral corticosteroid use, and decrease in number of sinus surgeries per year [63]. Another study evaluated the appropriate dose of aspirin to maintain therapeutic level as well as the long-term effects of symptom control [64]. Patients were maintained on either 100 mg per day or 300 mg of aspirin per day. All patients in the 100 mg per day group developed recurrence of nasal polyps within the first year of treatment, while those in the 300 mg per day group had decreased nasal polyps, improvement in sense of smell, and decreased need for revision surgery. Aspirin desensitization therapy remains a consideration in controlling symptoms in patients with AERD; however, patients should be treated with GI prophylaxis when taking daily aspirin therapy.

Conclusion

CRS is a syndrome resulting from a compilation of a variety of disease processes. Accordingly there is no one single medical management for all patients. That said, medical management is the cornerstone of the management of CRS, and surgery is largely an essential adjunct to the overall management of the syndrome. Careful patient assessment for environmental exacerbating factors, general host factors which may predispose to CRS as well as local factors leading to prolonged inflammation are essential parts of the assessment in determining appropriate medical management. In patients with a major environmental or allergy component, no management is likely to achieve long-term success without appropriate environmental control or allergy management, and ill-advised or premature surgical intervention may result in additional inflammation in a region not normally exposed to airflow. The combination of inflammation and surgical trauma can potentially lead to marked scarring, permanent reduction in quality of life, and even a nasal cripple. Similarly, inadequate or inappropriate postoperative medical management can also lead to a similar adverse end result.

Although disease classification into eosinophilic and noneosinophilic and polypoid and non-polypoid disease is helpful in guiding medical management of CRS, the appropriate role for topical and systemic steroids and antibiotic therapy needs to be individualized. Since patient symptoms are often not a reliable indicator of CRS and, in particular, are frequently a late indicator of recrudescence, the medical therapy of CRS, especially in the patient who has had prior surgical intervention, but has not yet achieved a stable mucosa.

In general, topical nasal steroids and nasal irrigations create the mainstay of therapy for CRS, supplemented by culture-based antibiotics and oral steroids, when necessary and not contraindicated. Antihistamines are helpful in patients with significant environmental allergies. However, given the complex nature of the syndrome, any of the adjunctive therapies may be required in individual patients, and in some much of the entire spectrum of therapies may be required in conjunction with meticulous surgery and postoperative debridement.

A solid understanding of the possible etiologies and presentations can help to tailor medical management to individual patients more effectively. It is important to try to elucidate the underlying environmental causes and attempt to eliminate them to improve the likelihood of medical therapy. Once this has been accomplished, attention should be shifted toward identification of the etiology of the patient's disease. If this can be accomplished, medical therapy can be better directed and will be more likely to be successful. The overall goal of management is to restore healthy mucosa and reduce inflammation. This can be quite a lengthy process and may require a broad spectrum of the various combinations of therapies that have been mentioned throughout this chapter.

References

1. Dubin MG, Liu C, Lin SY, Senior BA. American Rhinologic Society member survey on 'maximal medical therapy' for chronic rhinosinusitis. Am J Rhinol. 2007;21:483–8.
2. Brook I, Frazier ED, Foote PA. Microbiology of the transition from acute tochronic maxillary sinusitis. J Med Microbiol. 1996;45:372–5.
3. Bhattacharyya N, Kepnes LJ. Assessment of trends in antimicrobial resistance in chronic rhinosinusitis. Ann Otol Rhinol Laryngol. 2008;117(6):448–52.
4. Guss J, Abuzeid WM, Doghramji L, et al. Fluoroquinolone-resistant patterns in chronic rhinosinusitis. Am J Otolaryngol. 2004;25:323–8.
5. Kingdom TT, Swain Jr RE. The microbiology and antimicrobial resistance patterns in chronic rhinosinusitis. Am J Otolaryngol. 2004;25(5):323–8.
6. Suh JD, Kennedy DW. Treatment options for chronic rhinosinusitis. Proc Am Thorac Soc. 2011;8:132–40.
7. Kudoh S, Uetake T, Hagiwara M, et al. Clinical effect of low-dose long-term erythromycin chemotherapy on diffuse panbronchiolitis. Jpn J Thorac Dis. 1987;25:632–42.
8. Kanoh S, Rubin BK. Mechanisms of action and clinical application of macrolides as immunomodulatory medications. Clin Microbial Rev. 2010;23:590–615.
9. Harvey RJ, Wallwork BD, Lund VJ. Anti-inflammatory effects of macrolides: applications in chronic rhinosinusitis. Immunol Allergy Clin North Am. 2009;29:689–703.
10. Baumann U, Fischer JJ, Gudowius P, et al. Buccal adherence of Pseudomonas aeruginosa in patients with cystic fibrosis under long term therapy with azithromycin. Infection. 2001;29:7–11.
11. Wallwork B, Coman W, MacKay-Sim A, et al. A double-blind randomized, placebo controlled trial of macrolide in the treatment of chronic rhinosinusitis. Laryngoscope. 2006;116:189–93.
12. Gross ND, McInnes RJA, Hwang PH. Outpatient intravenous antibiotics for chronic rhinosinusitis. Laryngoscope. 2002;112:1758–61.
13. Woodhouse BM, Cleveland KW. Nebulized antibiotics for the treatment of refractory bacterial chronic rhinosinusitis. Ann Pharmacother. 2011;45:798–802.
14. Cain RB, Lal D. Update on the management of chronic rhinosinusitis. Infect Drug Resist. 2013;6:1–14.
15. Jervis-Bardy J, Boase S, Psaltis A, Foreman A, Wormald PJ. A randomized trial of mupirocin sinonasal rinses versus saline in surgically recalcitrant staphylococcal chronic rhinosinusitis. Laryngoscope. 2012;122(10):2148–53.
16. Lim M, Citardi MD, Jern-Lin L. Topical antimicrobials in the management of chronic rhinosinusitis: a systematic review. Am J Rhinol. 2008;22:381–9.
17. Whatley WS, Chandra RK, Macdonald CB. Systemic absorption of gentamicin nasal irrigation. Am J Rhinol. 2006;20:251–4.
18. Wong KK, Marglani O, Westerberg BD, Javer AR. Systemic absorption of topical gentamicin sinus irrigation. J Otolaryngol Head Neck Surg. 2008;37:395–8.
19. Ponikau JU, Sherris DA, Kern EB, et al. The diagnosis and incidence of allergic fungal sinusitis. Mayo Clin Proc. 1999;74(9):877–84.
20. Kennedy DW, Kuhn FA, Hamilos DL, et al. Treatment of chronic rhinosinusitis with high-dose oral terbinafine: a double-blind, placebo-controlled study. Laryngoscope. 2005;115:1793–9.
21. Thanasumpun T, Batra PS. Oral antifungal therapy for chronic rhinosinusitis and its subtypes: a systematic review. Int Forum Allergy Rhinol. 2011;1(5):382–9.
22. Ponikau JU, Sherris DA, Weaver A, Kita H. Treatment of chronic rhinosinusitis with intranasal amphotericin B: a randomized, placebo-controlled, double-blind pilot trial. J Allergy Clin Immunol. 2005;115(1):125–31.
23. Liang KL, Su MC, Shiao JY, et al. Amphotericin B irrigation for the treatment of chronic rhinosinusitis without nasal polyps: a randomized, placebo-controlled, double-blind study. Am J Rhinol. 2008;22(1):52–8.
24. Ebbens FA, Scadding GK, Badia L, et al. Amphotericin B nasal lavages: not a solution for patients with chronic rhinosinusitis. J Allergy Clin Immunol. 2006;118(5):1149–56.

25. Ebbens FA, Georgalas C, Luiten S, et al. The effect of topical amphotericin B on inflammatory markers in patients with chronic rhinosinusitis: a multicenter randomized controlled study. Laryngoscope. 2009;119(2):401–8.
26. Sacks 4th PL, Harvey RJ, Rimmer J, Gallagher RM, Sacks R. Antifungal therapy in the treatment of chronic rhinosinusitis: a meta-analysis. Am J Rhinol Allergy. 2012;26(2):141–7.
27. Lal D, Hwang PH. Oral corticosteroid therapy in chronic rhinosinusitis without polyposis: a systematic review. Int Forum Allergy Rhinol. 2011;1(2):136–43.
28. Poetker DM, Jakubowski LA, Lal D, Hwang PH, Wright ED, Smith TL. Oral corticosteroids in the management of adult chronic rhinosinusitis with and without nasal polyps: an evidence-based review with recommendations. Int Forum Allergy Rhinol. 2013;3(2):104–20.
29. Kirtsreesakul V, Wongsritrang K, Ruttanaphol S. Clinical efficacy of a short course of systemic steroids in nasal polyposis. Rhinology. 2011;49(5):525–32.
30. Vaidyanathan S, Barnes M, Williamson P, Hopkinson P, Donnan PT, Lipworth B. Treatment of chronic rhinosinusitis with nasal polyposis with oral steroids followed by topical steroids: a randomized trial. Ann Intern Med. 2011;154(5):293–302.
31. Rupa V, Jacob M, Mathews MS, Seshadri MS. A prospective, randomized, placebo-controlled trial of postoperative oral steroid in allergic fungal sinusitis. Eur Arch Otorhinolaryngol. 2010;267(2):233–8.
32. Landsberg R, Segev Y, DeRowe A, Landau T, Khafif A, Fliss DM. Systemic corticosteroids for allergic fungal rhinosinusitis and chronic rhinosinusitis with nasal polyposis: a comparative study. Otolaryngol Head Neck Surg. 2007;136(2):252–7.
33. Fokkens WJ, Lund VJ, Mullol J, et al. European position paper on rhinosinusitis and nasal polyps 2012. Rhinol Suppl. 2012;23:1–298.
34. Rudmik L, Hoy M, Schlosser RJ, et al. Topical therapies in the management of chronic rhinosinusitis: an evidence-based review with recommendations. Int Forum Allergy Rhinol. 2013;3(4):281–98.
35. Welch KC, Thaler ER, Doghramji LL, Palmer JN, Chiu AG. The effects of serum and urinary cortisol levels of topical intranasal irrigations with budesonide added to saline in patients with recurrent polyposis after endoscopic sinus surgery. Am J Rhinol Allergy. 2010;24(1):26–8.
36. Man LX, Farhood Z, Luong A, Fakhri S, et al. The effect of intranasal fluticasone propionate irrigations on salivary cortisol, intraocular pressure, and posterior subcapsular cataracts in postsurgical chronic rhinosinusitis patients. Int Forum Allergy Rhinol. 2013;3(12):953–7.
37. Jang DW, Lachanas VA, Kountakis SE. Budesonide nasal irrigations in the postoperative management of chronic rhinosinusitis. Int Forum Allergy Rhinol. 2013;3(9):708–11.
38. Intersect ENT. http://www.intersectent.com/advantage-how_it_works.html. Accessed 9 Feb 2014.
39. Han JK, Marple BF, Smith TL, et al. Effect of steroid-releasing sinus implants on postoperative medical and surgical interventions: an efficacy meta-analysis. Int Forum Allergy Rhinol. 2012;2:271–9.
40. Campbell RG, Kennedy DW. What is new and promising with drug-eluting stents in sinus surgery? Curr Opin Otolaryngol Head Neck Surg. 2014;22(1):2–7.
41. Gutman M, Torres A, Keen KJ, Houser SM. Prevalence of allergy in patients with chronic rhinosinusitis. Otolaryngol Head Neck Surg. 2004;130:545–52.
42. Benninger MS, Ferguson BJ, Hadley JA, et al. Adult chronic rhinosinusitis: definitions, diagnosis, epidemiology, and pathophysiology. Otolaryngol Head Neck Surg. 2003;129(Suppl): S1–32.
43. Rosenfeld RM, Andes D, Bhattacharyya N, et al. Clinical practice guideline: adult sinusitis. Otolaryngol Head Neck Surg. 2007;137 Suppl 3:S1–31.
44. Calderon MA, Alves B, Jacobson M, Hurwitz B, Sheikh A, Durham S. Allergen injection immunotherapy for seasonal allergic rhinitis. Cochrane Database Syst Rev. 2007;(1):CD001936.
45. Hauptmann G, Ryan MW. The effect of saline solutions on nasal patency and mucociliary clearance in rhinosinusitis patients. Otolaryngol Head Neck Surg. 2007;137:815–21.
46. Braun JJ, Alabert JP, Michel FB, et al. Adjunct effect of loratadine in the treatment of acute sinusitis in patients with allergic rhinitis. Allergy. 1997;52:650–5.

47. Parnes SM, Chuma AV. Acute effects of antileukotrienes on sinonasal polyposis and sinusitis. Ear Nose Throat J. 2000;79(1):18–20. 24–25.
48. Kieff DA, Busaba NY. Efficacy of montelukast in the treatment of nasal polyposis. Ann Otol Rhinol Laryngol. 2005;114(12):941–5.
49. Stewart RA, Ram B, Hamilton G, Weiner J, Kane KJ. Monteleukast as an adjunct to oral and inhaled steroid therapy in chronic nasal polyposis. Otolaryngol Head Neck Surg. 2008;139(5):682–7.
50. Harvey R, Hannan SA, Badia L, Scadding G. Nasal saline irrigations for the symptoms of chronic rhinosinusitis. Cochrane Database Syst Rev. 2007;(3):CD006394.
51. Wormald P, Cain T, Oates L, et al. A comparative study of three methods of nasal irrigation. Laryngoscope. 2004;114:2224–7.
52. Singhal D, Weitzel EK, Lan E, et al. Effect of head position and surgical dissection on sinus irrigant penetration in cadavers. Laryngoscope. 2010;120:2528–31.
53. Pinto JM, Elwany S, Baroody FM, Nacierio RM. Effects of saline sprays on symptoms after endoscopic sinus surgery. Am J Rhinol. 2006;20(2):191–6.
54. Pynnonen MA, Mukerji SS, Kim HM, Adams ME, Terrell JE. Nasal saline for chronic sinonasal symptoms: a randomized controlled trial. Arch Otolaryngol Head Neck Surg. 2007;133(11):1115–20.
55. Rabago D, Zgierska A, Mundt M, Barrett B, Bobula J, Maberry R. Efficacy of daily hypertonic saline nasal irrigation among patients with sinusitis: a randomized controlled trial. J Fam Pract. 2002;51(12):1049–55.
56. Hoza J, Salzman R, Starek I, Schalek P, Kellnerova R. Efficacy and safety of erdosteine in the treatment of chronic rhinosinusitis with nasal polyposis – a pilot study. Rhinology. 2013;51(4):323–7.
57. Rosen PL, Palmer JN, O'Malley Jr BW, Cohen NA. Surfactants in the management of rhinopathologies. Am J Rhinol Allergy. 2013;27(3):177–80.
58. Tajiri T, Matsumoto H, Hiraumi H, et al. Efficacy of omalizumab in eosinophilic chronic rhinosinusitis patients with asthma. Ann Allergy Asthma Immunol. 2013;110(5):387–8.
59. Pinto JM, Mehta N, DiTineo M, Wang J, Baroody FM, Naclerio RM. A randomized, double-blind, placebo-controlled trial of anti-IgE for chronic rhinosinusitis. Rhinology. 2010;48(3):318–24.
60. Gevaert P, Lang-Loidolt D, Lackner A, et al. Nasal IL-5 levels determine the response to anti-IL-5 treatment in patients with nasal polyps. J Allergy Clin Immunol. 2006;118(5):1133–41.
61. Gevaert P, Van Bruaene N, Cattaert T, et al. Mepolizumab, a humanized anti-IL-5 mAb, as a treatment option for severe nasal polyposis. J Allergy Clin Immunol. 2011;128(5):989–95.
62. Quinti I, Soresina A, Spadaro G, et al. Long-term follow-up and outcome of a large cohort of patients with common variable immunodeficiency. J Clin Immunol. 2007;27:308–16.
63. Stevenson DD, Pleskow WW, Simon RA, et al. Aspirin-sensitive rhinosinusitis asthma: a double-blind crossover study of treatment with aspirin. J Allergy Clin Immunol. 1984;73(4):500–7.
64. Rozsasi A, Polzehl D, Deutschle T, et al. Long-term treatment with aspirin desensitization: a prospective clinical trial comparing 100 and 300 mg aspirin daily. Allergy. 2008; 63(9):1228–34.

Oral Antibiotics as Anti-infectives

12

Justin T. Casey, Todd T. Kingdom, and Anne E. Getz

Key Take Home Points

- The indications for antibiotic use in CRS are ill-defined and supporting evidence for their use is sparse.
- Most of the data available pertains to the use of long-term macrolides, focusing on immune-modulatory rather than anti-infective properties.
- The most limited data lies in the use of long-term non-macrolide antibiotic treatment.
- Postoperative antibiotics are commonly used and have been frequently recommended; however, available data shows no clear benefit over placebo.
- *Staphylococcus aureus* is frequently present in CRS patients, and data suggests a potential role in treatment outcomes. There is no data, however, to support the sole use of oral antibiotics to treat nasal *S. aureus* colonization in patients with CRS.
- Side effects of oral antibiotics are not negligible and should always be strongly considered when prescribing.
- Resistance is a major and constantly evolving factor in oral antibiotics. Judicious use and culture-directed therapy may help control antibiotic resistance rates.

J.T. Casey, MD • T.T. Kingdom, MD • A.E. Getz, MD (✉)
Department of Otolaryngology – Head and Neck Surgery, University of Colorado School of Medicine, 12631 E. 17th Avenue, Mail Stop B-205, Aurora, CO 80045, USA
e-mail: Justin.casey@ucdenver.edu; todd.kingdom@ucdenver.edu; anne.getz@ucdenver.edu

P.S. Batra, J.K. Han (eds.), *Practical Medical and Surgical Management of Chronic Rhinosinusitis*, DOI 10.1007/978-3-319-16724-4_12

Introduction

Chronic rhinosinusitis (CRS) is a common condition that significantly impacts the lives of many patients. It has been estimated that up to 14 % of the adult population in the USA suffer from CRS, reporting significant changes in quality of life equal to or worse than those reported with COPD, CHF, and chronic back pain [1]. Our disease definitions and understanding of etiologic factors continues to evolve. Current consensus opinions define CRS as primarily a chronic inflammatory disorder, as opposed to a purely infectious condition. Most believe, however, that microbial infection plays an important role in the development of many forms of CRS. This is clearly reflected in prescribing patterns of practitioners who treat the disease. Two surveys, one of US otolaryngologists and another completed by members of the American Rhinologic Society, found that over 90 % of respondents routinely prescribe oral antibiotics in the medical treatment of CRS [2, 3].

Other available therapeutic options in the management of CRS include topical nasal steroids, topical antibiotics, systemic steroids, allergy therapy, and surgery. These, and other medical treatments, have been studied to varying degrees with a range of reported efficacy. The evaluation of the clinical efficacy of oral antibiotics in the management of CRS is problematic for a multitude of factors that prior authors have summarized [4]. Guidelines have historically fallen short in providing meaningful direction, as a paucity of well-designed trials exist. In this chapter the current understanding and utilization of oral antibiotics in the management of CRS will be discussed based on a thorough review of the relevant available literature.

Indications and Clinical Efficacy Data

The use of antibiotics in CRS can be broadly characterized into two clinical scenarios: short-term and long-term treatment. A third scenario is use as anti-inflammatory medications, and such use will be discussed in detail in a separate chapter. Although there are shortcomings to this and other classifications, viewing their utilization in this manner helps to better understand and explore treatment options.

Short-Term Antibiotic Treatment

Short-term antibiotics of 3 weeks or less comprise one of the most common treatment strategies for CRS among practitioners [2].

There are four randomized studies investigating short-term antibiotic therapy in CRS [5–8]. These studies, along with two observational studies, are well summarized in a recent article by Soler et al. [4]. Of the four randomized studies, only one had a placebo group. Regimens investigated in the four studies were doxycycline versus methylprednisolone versus placebo, cefotiam versus cefixime, amoxicillin/clavulanate versus ciprofloxacin, and cefaclor versus amoxicillin.

No statistically significant difference in symptom improvement was found between arms in the three studies comparing antibiotic regimens. One must also consider reports of symptom improvement carefully when no placebo or non-antibiotic group is available for comparison. In the placebo-controlled study (doxycycline versus methylprednisolone versus placebo), decrease in polyp size was noted in patients treated with doxycycline as compared to placebo. However, significant improvement in symptoms was not demonstrated when comparing the groups. Additionally, any clinical benefit was likely a function of anti-inflammatory properties, though this study could not absolutely establish this conclusion. While the aggregate quality of the available evidence is good, the relative paucity of data led to a recommendation of "optional" for the use of short-term antibiotic in CRS, per the review by Soler et al. [4].

The conclusion drawn in the comprehensive 2012 European Position Paper on Rhinosinusitis (EPOS) review of the aforementioned studies was that short-term (designated as less than 4 weeks) use of antibiotics in patients with CRS without nasal polyps (CRSsNP) is likely only appropriate for exacerbations with a positive culture [9]. In patients with CRS with nasal polyps (CRSwNP), the trials available showed only a small effect on polyp size and postnasal drip compared to placebo and only a trend towards effect [5, 10].

Long-Term Antibiotic Treatment

Extremely limited quality data exists on the efficacy of non-macrolide long-term antibiotic therapy in CRS. In an observational study by Dubin et al., 16 patients were treated with 6 weeks of clindamycin, amoxicillin/clavulanate, or doxycycline [11]. Response to therapy was measured by CT evaluation. Improvement was noted on sinus CT scores between baseline and 3 weeks, but further improvement at 6 weeks did not reach statistical significance. Although there may be certain subgroups that could benefit from prolonged therapy, there is insufficient evidence to support its use at this time. With only one study in this category, which focuses on radiographic changes rather than clinical outcomes, long-term non-macrolide antibiotic treatment in CRS should be further investigated and the risk-benefit ratio for the long-term use of non-macrolide antibiotic should be weighed on an individual basis.

Specific Therapy

Postoperative Antibiotics

The use of antibiotics in the postoperative period remains a common practice in otolaryngology and has long been discussed in the literature [12, 13]. This is based largely on the theoretical benefit of reducing the risk of infection during the healing phase postoperatively. Unfortunately, there is limited data on the use of postoperative antibiotic treatment in ESS in our current literature to adequately guide clinical decision making. Albu et al. performed a randomized, double-blind, placebo-controlled study looking at both subjective and objective symptoms after ESS [14]. Patients were treated with amoxicillin/clavulanate for 2 weeks following surgery, and symptom and endoscopic scores were measured at several intervals. They demonstrated improved nasal drainage and obstruction on postoperative day 5, as well as improved endoscopic scores on days 5 and 12 in the treatment group.

In contrast to this, three separate randomized, controlled trials demonstrated less convincing results. One of these studies, comparing postoperative cefuroxime to placebo found no significant differences in symptom or endoscopic scores [15]. However, the treatment course was limited to just 2 days of cefuroxime. In another study, amoxicillin/clavulanate was compared to a control group for 3 weeks following ESS [16]. No differences in rates of positive bacterial culture, symptom scores, or endoscopic scores were noted. Unfortunately, potential short-term benefits may have been missed as there was no follow-up until 3 weeks after surgery. Finally, in a prospective, randomized, placebo-controlled study, 4 weeks of amoxicillin was shown to be equivalent to placebo and 8 weeks of Chinese Herbal Medicine in subjective symptom scores of post-ESS patients [17]. Unfortunately, this study also had no short-term follow-up and did not evaluate patients until 8 weeks after surgery.

In a review of the evidence on postoperative care by Rudmik et al., the authors discussed the opportunity for bacterial infection during sinus surgery and potential implications, but also acknowledged the overall lack of clear evidence to support the routine use of antibiotics in this situation. Therefore, there is an "optional" recommendation for postoperative antibiotic following ESS [18].

Acute Exacerbations in CRS

Antibiotics are commonly prescribed for acute bacterial exacerbations of CRS (AECRS). Symptoms may include some or all of the following symptoms: acute worsening of nasal congestion, increased nasal drainage with the presence of mucopurulence, and decreased sense of taste and smell. By definition these symptoms generally return to baseline between episodes of exacerbation. The bacteriology for AECRS is believed to be similar to that of acute bacterial rhinosinusitis in many cases [19, 20]. Thus, common first-line antibiotics include amoxicillin/clavulanate, doxycycline, or a third-generation cephalosporin with clindamycin [21]. Similar to CRS, these exacerbations may commonly include anaerobes and polymicrobial infections. Culture-directed therapy continues to be recommended in the acute setting in order to most accurately target therapy, particularly in light of findings that baseline middle meatal cultures rarely reflect the bacteria isolated during an acute exacerbation [20, 22].

Staphylococcus Endotoxins

Staphylococcus aureus is commonly cultured in CRS and has become a focus of intense study in an attempt to better understand bacterial factors influencing treatment outcomes [19, 23]. Emerging research has shown *S. aureus* endotoxins may be important in the development of CRS. These endotoxins have been shown to act as superantigens in the immune response of the upper airway. They appear to have the ability to directly activate various populations of T lymphocytes, induce IgE production, and trigger T-helper-2 cytokine cascade, without the activation of the regulatory cytokines interleukin-10 and TFG-β1 [24, 25]. This may ultimately result to eosinophilic and lymphocytic tissue infiltration that is characteristic of CRS with nasal polyps [26]. There is currently no data on the effect of antibiotics on staphylococcus endotoxins, but it is possible that lowering the *S. aureus* bacterial load may also reduce the negative effects outlined above.

S. aureus has been associated with poor outcomes following ESS [27–31]. One of the most common treatments for positive culture in this patient group is topical mupirocin—which will be discussed in detail in another chapter. There are very few studies looking at treatment of sinonasal *S. aureus* with oral antibiotics. One double-blind, randomized, placebo-controlled study by Schalek et al. looked at patients with CRSwNP who were culture positive for endotoxin-producing *S. aureus* at the time of surgery [10]. These patients were given 3 weeks of either oral antibiotics based on sensitivity (MIC) data or placebo, in addition to nasal saline irrigations and topical steroids. There was no statistically significant difference noted in SNOT-22 scores, endoscopic scores, or symptoms scores between the two groups at 3 and 6 months.

Side Effects and Other Considerations

Side Effects

Potential side effects of antibiotic therapy should be carefully considered by the healthcare provider. Considering the frequency and duration of use of this therapeutic class in the management of CRS, their potential harmful impact ought to be recognized. Side effects can be broken down into patient-related side effects and the development of drug resistance.

Common antibiotic side effects experienced by patients are drug specific, but may include diarrhea, abdominal pain, nausea, vomiting, elevation in liver enzymes, and rash. The less common but more severe reactions include anaphylaxis, Stevens-Johnson syndrome (more commonly with penicillins and sulfa), tendonitis or tendon rupture (more commonly with quinolones), *C. difficile* infection (classically with clindamycin), and toxic megacolon. Additionally, adverse reactions can be confounded when patients are concomitantly using oral steroids, antihistamines, or other medications commonly used in CRS.

Development of Resistance

The development of bacterial resistance is another concern that stems from use of antimicrobials. In treating CRS, the clinician must consider a potentially more complicated antibiotic resistance profile among the offending bacteria, along with the potential to further drive changes in antibiotic sensitivity patterns by repeatedly treating a patient. As mentioned previously, methicillin-resistant *S. aureus* is one of the most common isolates found in cultures from CRS patients [19, 23]. In addition, postsurgical CRS patients have culture isolates with beta-lactamase resistance rates of 43 % or more [32, 33]. The use of culture-directed therapy through endoscopically guided cultures has been emphasized in treatment guidelines and by various authors to help prevent the development of these resistance patterns; however, the theoretical benefit and importance of this approach remains to be proven [34, 35]. One study found that endoscopically guided cultures changed the initial antibiotic management in over one-half of patients, but clinical efficacy could not be demonstrated [36]. It follows that culture-directed therapy is a reasonable approach that could aid in more targeted therapy, resulting in less resistance and improved outcomes. There are many factors, however, that influence the development of bacterial resistance and treatment response in CRS.

Another consideration affecting the potential for resistance is compliance. When looking at compliance across both acute and chronic disease medications, mean compliance was 79 % for once-daily dosage, 69 % for the twice-daily dosage, 65 % for the thrice-daily dosage, and 51 % for four-times daily dosage [37]. Intuitively it is hard to expect patients to reliably take a medication four times a day for weeks or even months, as is commonly the case in CRS. Suboptimal and/or incomplete antibiotic dosing has long been thought to promote antimicrobial resistance [38, 39].

Our understanding of the relationship between bacteria and the pathogenesis of CRS is changing rapidly with active research in the field of molecular diagnostic methods and the introduction of microbiome concepts [40]. Interestingly, these methods are able to show significant shifts in the host's microbiome with antibiotic use, which include a reduction in biodiversity richness and evenness of nasal flora, as well as changes in the abundance of pathogens (*S. aureus*) when compared to controls [41]. This area of research will likely trigger changes in how clinicians obtain and interpret bacterial culture data and subsequently reshape antibiotic utilization in the treatment of our patients. Although the significance is not yet known, this data points to the concept that factors beyond changes in bacterial resistance patterns are important predictors of treatment response and a potential undesirable consequence of antibiotic use in CRS.

Despite all of this, it should be noted that the safety of long-term use of macrolides in cystic fibrosis patients has been well documented [42–44]. Additionally, safe long-term use has been demonstrated with doxycycline in periodontitis and acne patients and trimethoprim-sulfamethoxazole for prophylaxis of urinary tract infections [45–47].

Other Considerations

A history of drug allergies should also be closely scrutinized, especially those that involve anaphylaxis. Recent antibiotic treatment should also be taken into account; if a patient has been treated with antibiotics recently and only realized a partial or temporary response, a longer course or new antibiotic regimen may be appropriate.

Lastly, cost is another important consideration. Antibiotics create a greater economic burden than many practitioners may realize. The cost of antibiotics alone was found to be up to $866 per patient per year in those suffering from CRS with nasal polyps [48]. Bhattacharyya et al. found that the average patient presenting to an otolaryngologist for sinus complaints had already received an average 2.6 courses of antibiotics in the past year. Additionally, they had been on oral antibiotics for an average of 5 weeks during that time [49].

Mechanism of Action

The most commonly used antibiotics in patients for CRS include amoxicillin/clavulanate, sulfamethoxazole/trimethoprim, clindamycin, azithromycin and other macrolides, and levofloxacin or ciprofloxacin. These are briefly summarized in Table 12.1 [50]. Other antibiotics and antibiotic classes are discussed in more detail below.

Beta-Lactams

Beta-lactams are one of the more commonly used antibiotics in rhinosinusitis. Amoxicillin with or without clavulanate and less commonly third-generation cephalosporins are often used in CRS. Depending on local resistance patterns that vary from region to region, amoxicillin has fair activity against common

Table 12.1 Commonly used antibiotics in CRS

Antibiotic	Mechanism of action
Amoxicillin/clavulanate	Binds penicillin-binding proteins, inhibiting final transpeptidation step of peptidoglycan synthesis in bacterial cell walls. Addition of clavulanate inhibits beta-lactamase, which renders antibiotic resistance by destroying the beta-lactam ring common to penicillins and other antibiotics. Bactericidal
Trimethoprim-sulfamethoxazole	Blocks consecutive steps in the synthesis of nucleic acids. Sulfamethoxazole inhibits bacterial synthesis of dihydrofolic acid, while trimethoprim inhibits the formation of tetrahydrofolic acid from dihydrofolic acid. Bacteriostatic
Clindamycin	Suppresses bacterial protein synthesis by binding the 50S ribosomal subunit. Bacteriostatic
Quinolones	Inhibits DNA gyrase, blocking DNA relaxation. Bactericidal
Macrolides	Suppresses bacterial protein synthesis by binding the 50S ribosomal subunit. Bacteriostatic
Doxycycline	Suppresses bacterial protein synthesis by binding the 30S ribosomal subunit. Primarily bacteriostatic

sinusitis pathogens such as *Streptococcus pneumoniae*, *Moraxella catarrhalis*, and *Haemophilus influenzae* [51]. Both beta-lactamase and penicillin-binding protein resistance patterns have been documented with amoxicillin, however, and the addition of a beta-lactamase inhibitor like clavulanate improves the coverage against agents such as *H. influenzae*, *M. catarrhalis*, and *S. aureus* [52]. In the case of *S. pneumoniae* resistance, which is based on penicillin-binding protein changes, resistance can be overcome by higher amoxicillin serum levels. The commonly used adult amoxicillin dosages are usually sufficient [53].

Second- and third-generation cephalosporins have increased activity against *H. influenza* and gram-negative aerobes. Third-generation cephalosporins generally have very good activity against *M. catarrhalis* and *H. influenzae*, with fair activity against *S. pneumoniae* [51]. No oral cephalosporins are active against *Pseudomonas aeruginosa*.

Macrolides

Macrolides are frequently prescribed in CRS due to the anti-infective and anti-inflammatory properties. Macrolides used in CRS include azithromycin, clarithromycin, and erythromycin. Their greatest antimicrobial property is against streptococci, staphylococci, and other gram-positive pathogens, but also against atypical microbes such as *Mycoplasma pneumoniae*. Similarly to beta-lactams, *S. pneumoniae* resistance is an increasing problem and has reached rates over 20 % in many European countries [54].

Fluoroquinolones

Fluoroquinolones have gained common use in CRS for their broad spectrum of activity, but more importantly for their coverage of *P. aeruginosa* and other gram-negative bacteria. This group covers many gram-positive agents well, specifically *H. influenzae*, *M. catarrhalis,* and *S. pneumoniae*. The agents in this group used for CRS most commonly are levofloxacin, ciprofloxacin, and moxifloxacin. Ciprofloxacin and levofloxacin generally have the best activity against *P. aeruginosa* and the least against gram-positives [55]. Therefore, ciprofloxacin and levofloxacin should be thoughtfully used and possibly reserved for *P. aeruginosa.*

Trimethoprim-Sulfamethoxazole

Used predominantly in acute sinusitis, trimethoprim-sulfamethoxazole has gained use in chronic sinusitis due to its activity against community-acquired methicillin-resistant *Staphylococcus aureus*. Due to its seldom use in chronic sinusitis, there is often less resistance to trimethoprim-sulfamethoxazole for bacterial organisms associated with chronic sinusitis.

Clindamycin

Clindamycin is known for its activity against anaerobic gram-negative organisms, but it also has fairly good coverage against gram-positive organisms, including *S. pneumonia* and several staphylococci species. It has also been commonly used to treat MRSA; however resistance rates vary widely in different areas of the country, so local resistance patterns should be considered.

Doxycycline

Doxycycline is an agent whose use can be helpful in CRS because of its activity against methicillin-resistant *S. aureus*. The effectiveness of this drug against MRSA depends on local resistance rates, but is generally over 80 % [56]. This drug also has good coverage of atypical microbes like *Mycoplasma pneumonia*.

References

1. Metson RB, Gliklich RE. Clinical outcomes in patients with chronic sinusitis. Laryngoscope. 2000;110:24–8.
2. Kaszuba S, Stewart M. Medical management and diagnosis of chronic rhinosinusitis: a survey of treatment patterns by United States otolaryngologists. Am J Rhinol. 2006;20(2):186–90.
3. Dubin M, Liu C, Lin S, Senior B. American Rhinologic Society member survey on "maximal medical therapy" for chronic rhinosinusitis. Am J Rhinol. 2007;21(4):483–8.
4. Soler ZM, Oyer SL, Kern RC, Senior BAM, Kountakis SE, Marple BF, et al. Antimicrobials and chronic rhinosinusitis with or without polyposis in adults: an evidenced-based review with recommendations. Int Forum Allergy Rhinol. 2013;3:31–47.
5. Van Zele T, Gevaert P, Holtappels G, Beule A, Wormald PJ, Mayr S, et al. Oral steroids and doxycycline: two different approaches to treat nasal polyps. J Allergy Clin Immunol. 2010;125:1069–1076.e4.
6. Dellamonica P, Choutet P, Lejeune JM, Lucht F, Morgon A, Pessey JJ, et al. Efficacy and tolerance of cefotiam hexetil in the super-infected chronic sinusitis. A randomized, double-blind study in comparison with cefixime. Ann Otolaryngol Chir Cervicofac Bull Soc Otolaryngol Hop Paris. 1994;111:217–22.
7. Legent F, Bordure P, Beauvillain C, Berche P. A double-blind comparison of ciprofloxacin and amoxycillin/clavulanic acid in the treatment of chronic sinusitis. Chemotherapy. 1994;40:8–15.
8. Huck W, Reed BD, Nielsen RW, Ferguson RT, Gray DW, Lund GK, et al. Cefaclor vs amoxicillin in the treatment of acute, recurrent, and chronic sinusitis. Arch Fam Med. 1993;2:497–503.
9. Fokkens W, Lund V, Mullol J. European position paper on rhinosinusitis and nasal polyps. Rhinol Suppl. 2007;2007:1–136.
10. Schalek P, Petras P, Klement V, Hahn A. Short-term antibiotics treatment in patients with nasal polyps and enterotoxins producing Staphylococcus aureus strains. Eur Arch Otorhinolaryngol. 2009;266:1909–13.
11. Dubin MG, Kuhn FA, Melroy CT. Radiographic resolution of chronic rhinosinusitis without polyposis after 6 weeks vs 3 weeks of oral antibiotics. Ann Allergy Asthma Immunol. 2007;98:32–5.

12. Kennedy DW. Prognostic factors, outcomes and staging in ethmoid sinus surgery. Laryngoscope. 1992;102:1–18.
13. Stammberger H, Posawetz W. Functional endoscopic sinus surgery. Concept, indications and results of the Messerklinger technique. Eur Arch Otorhinolaryngol. 1990;247:63–76.
14. Albu S, Lucaciu R. Prophylactic antibiotics in endoscopic sinus surgery: a short follow-up study. Am J Rhinol Allergy. 2010;24:306–9.
15. Annys E, Jorissen M. Short term effects of antibiotics (Zinnat) after endoscopic sinus surgery. Acta Otorhinolaryngol Belg. 2000;54:23–8.
16. Jiang R, Liang K, Yang K, Shiao J, Su M, Hsin C, et al. Postoperative antibiotic care after functional endoscopic sinus surgery. Am J Rhinol. 2008;22(6):608–12.
17. Liang K-L, Su Y-C, Tsai C-C, Lin J-S, Jiang R-S, Su M-C. Postoperative care with Chinese herbal medicine or amoxicillin after functional endoscopic sinus surgery: a randomized, double-blind, placebo-controlled study. Am J Rhinol Allergy. 2011;25:170–5.
18. Rudmik L, Soler ZM, Orlandi RR, Stewart MG, Bhattacharyya N, Kennedy DW, et al. Early postoperative care following endoscopic sinus surgery: an evidence-based review with recommendations. Int Forum Allergy Rhinol. 2011;1:417–30. Available from: http://www.ncbi.nlm.nih.gov/pubmed/22144050.
19. Brook I, Frazier EH, Foote PA. Microbiology of the transition from acute to chronic maxillary sinusitis. J Med Microbiol. 1996;45:372–5.
20. Brook I. Bacteriology of chronic sinusitis and acute exacerbation of chronic sinusitis. Arch Otolaryngol Head Neck Surg. 2006;132:1099–101.
21. Chow AW, Benninger MS, Brook I, Brozek JL, Goldstein EJC, Hicks LA, et al. IDSA clinical practice guideline for acute bacterial rhinosinusitis in children and adults. Clin Infect Dis. 2012;54:e72–112.
22. Bhattacharyya N, Gopal HV, Lee KH. Bacterial infection after endoscopic sinus surgery: a controlled prospective study. Laryngoscope. 2004;114:765–7.
23. Finegold SM, Flynn MJ, Rose FV, Jousimies-Somer H, Jakielaszek C, McTeague M, et al. Bacteriologic findings associated with chronic bacterial maxillary sinusitis in adults. Clin Infect Dis. 2002;35:428–33.
24. Bachert C, Zhang N, Patou J, van Zele T, Gevaert P. Role of staphylococcal superantigens in upper airway disease. Curr Opin Allergy Clin Immunol. 2008;8:34–8.
25. Conley D, Tripathi A, Seiberling K, Schleimer R, Suh L, Harris K, Paniagua M, Grammer LKR. Superantigens and chronic rhinosinusitis: Skewing of T-cell receptor Vβ-distributions in polyp-derived CD4+ and CD8+ T cells. Am J Rhinol. 2006;20(5):534–9.
26. Bernstein JM, Ballow M, Shlievert PM, Rich G, Allen CDD. A superantigen hypothesis for the pathogenesis of chronic hyperplastic sinusitis with massive nasal polyposis. Am J Rhinol. 2003;17(6):321–6.
27. Singhal D, Psaltis AJ, Foreman AWP. The impact of biofilms on outcomes after endoscopic sinus surgery. Am J Rhinol Allergy. 2010;24(3):169–74.
28. Singhal D, Foreman A, Bardy JJ, Wormald PJ. Staphylococcus aureus biofilms: Nemesis of endoscopic sinus surgery. Laryngoscope. 2011;121:1578–83.
29. Tan NC, Foreman A, Camille J, Richard D, Vreugde S, Wormwald PJ. Intracellular Staphylococcus aureus: the Trojan horse of recalcitrant chronic rhinosinusitis? Int Forum Allergy Rhinol. 2013;3(4):261–6.
30. Foreman A, Wormald PJ. Different biofilms, different disease? A clinical outcomes study. Laryngoscope. 2010;120:1701–6.
31. Bardy J, Foreman A, Field J, Wormald P. Impaired mucosal healing and infection associated with staphylococcus aureus after endoscopic sinus surgery. Am J Rhinol Allergy. 2009;23(5):549–52.
32. Brook IHJ. Microbiology of acute and chronic maxillary sinusitis in smokers and nonsmokers. Ann Otol Rhinol Laryngol. 2011;120(11):707–12.
33. Bhattacharyya N, Kepnes LJ. The microbiology of recurrent rhinosinusitis after endoscopic sinus surgery. Arch Otolaryngol Head Neck Surg. 1999;125:1117–20.
34. Bhattacharyya N, Kepnes LJ. The risk of development of antimicrobial resistance in individual patients with chronic rhinosinusitis. Arch Otolaryngol Head Neck Surg. 2004;130:1201–4.

35. Kingdom TT, Swain RE. The microbiology and antimicrobial resistance patterns in chronic rhinosinusitis. Am J Otolaryngol. 2004;25:323–8.
36. Cincik H, Ferguson BJ. The impact of endoscopic cultures on care in rhinosinusitis. Laryngoscope. 2006;116:1562–8.
37. Claxton AJ, Cramer J, Pierce C. A systematic review of the associations between dose regimens and medication compliance. Clin Ther. 2001;23:1296–310.
38. Thomas JK, Forrest A, Bhavnani SM, Hyatt JM, Cheng A, Ballow CH, et al. Pharmacodynamic evaluation of factors associated with the development of bacterial resistance in acutely ill patients during therapy. Antimicrob Agents Chemother. 1998;42:521–7.
39. Pradier C, Dunais B, Carsenti-Etesse H, Dellamonica P. Pneumococcal resistance patterns in Europe. Eur J Clin Microbiol Infect Dis. 1997;16:644–7.
40. Feazel LM, Frank DN, Ramakrishnan VR. Update on bacterial detection methods in chronic rhinosinusitis: implications for clinicians and research scientists. Int Forum Allergy Rhinol. 2011;1:451–9.
41. Feazel LM, Robertson CE, Ramakrishnan VR, Frank DN. Microbiome complexity and Staphylococcus aureus in chronic rhinosinusitis. Laryngoscope. 2012;122:467–72.
42. Shi ZL, Peng H, Hu XW, Hu JG. Effectiveness and safety of macrolides in bronchiectasis patients: a meta-analysis and systematic review. Pulm Pharmacol Ther. 2014;28(2):171–8.
43. Wu Q, Shen W, Cheng H, Zhou X. Long-term macrolides for non-cystic fibrosis bronchiectasis: a systematic review and meta-analysis. Respirology. 2014;19:321–9.
44. Yang M, Dong BR, Lin X, Wu HM. Macrolides for diffuse panbronchiolitis. Cochrane Database Syst Rev 2009, Issue 2. Art. No: CD007716. DOI: 10.1002/14651858.CD007716.pub3.
45. Ciancio S, Ashley R. Safety and efficacy of sub-antimicrobial-dose doxycycline therapy in patients with adult periodontitis. Adv Dent Res. 1998;12:27–31.
46. Baxter BT, Pearce WH, Waltke EA, Littooy FN, Hallett JW, Kent KC, et al. Prolonged administration of doxycycline in patients with small asymptomatic abdominal aortic aneurysms: report of a prospective (Phase II) multicenter study. J Vasc Surg. 2002;36:1–12.
47. Scherwin J, Holm P. Long-term treatment with sulphamethoxazole/trimethoprim (Bactrim) and nitrofurantoin in chronic urinary tract infections. A controlled clinical trial. Chemotherapy. 1977;23:282–8.
48. Bhattacharyya N. Assessing the additional disease burden of polyps in chronic rhinosinusitis. Ann Otol Rhinol Laryngol. 2009;118:185–9.
49. Bhattacharyya N. The economic burden and symptom manifestations of chronic rhinosinusitis. Am J Rhinol. 2003;17(1):27–32.
50. Katzung BG, Masters SB, Trevor AJ. Basic and clinical pharmacology. 11th ed. New York: McGraw-Hill Medical, New York, NY; 2009.
51. Harrison CJ, Woods C, Stout G, Martin B, Selvarangan R. Susceptibilities of Haemophilus influenzae, Streptococcus pneumoniae, including serotype 19A, and Moraxella catarrhalis paediatric isolates from 2005 to 2007 to commonly used antibiotics. J Antimicrob Chemother. 2009;63:511–9.
52. Finlay J, Miller L, Poupard JA. A review of the antimicrobial activity of clavulanate. J Antimicrob Chemother. 2003;52:18–23.
53. Weinstein MP, Klugman KP, Jones RN. Rationale for revised penicillin susceptibility breakpoints versus Streptococcus pneumoniae: coping with antimicrobial susceptibility in an era of resistance. Clin Infect Dis. 2009;48:1596–600.
54. Riedel S, Beekmann SE, Heilmann KP, Richter SS, Garcia-de-Lomas J, Ferech M, et al. Antimicrobial use in Europe and antimicrobial resistance in Streptococcus pneumoniae. Eur J Clin Microbiol Infect Dis. 2007;26:485–90.
55. Zhanel G, Palatnick L, Nichol K, Bellyou T, Low D, Hoban D. Antimicrobial resistance in respiratory tract streptococcus pneumoniae isolates: results of the Canadian Respiratory Organism Susceptibility study, 1997 to 2002. Antimicrob Agents Chemother. 2003;47(6):1867–74.
56. Bhambri S, Grace K. Use of oral doxycycline for community-acquired methicillin-resistant staphylococcus aureus infections. J Clin Aesthet Dermatol. 2009;2(4):45–50.

Oral Antibiotics as Anti-inflammatories 13

C. Carrie Liu, Timothy L. Smith, and Luke Rudmik

Key Take-Home Points

- The inflammatory process involved in chronic rhinosinusitis can be dominated by either eosinophils or neutrophils.
- There is increasing evidence that antibiotics have anti-inflammatory properties and that long-term antibiotic therapy may be therapeutic in patients with chronic rhinosinusitis that is refractory to conventional treatment regimens.
- Macrolide antibiotics may improve symptoms and endoscopic findings associated with chronic rhinosinusitis. They can be considered as adjunctive treatment, especially in patients who have low serum IgE levels.
- Tetracyclines may decrease the size of nasal polyps for a longer duration of benefit than systemic corticosteroids.
- Other antibiotics with anti-inflammatory properties are trimethoprim-sulfamethoxazole and dapsone.

C.C. Liu, MD • L. Rudmik, MD, MSc (✉)
Division of Otolaryngology – Head and Neck Surgery, Department of Surgery, Foothills Medical Centre, University of Calgary,
South Tower Room 602, 1403 29th Street NW, Calgary, AB T2N 2T9, Canada
e-mail: ccliu@ucalgary.ca; lukerudmik@gmail.com

T.L. Smith, MD, MPH
Division of Rhinology and Sinus Surgery, Department of Otolaryngology–Head and Neck Surgery, Oregon Sinus Center, Oregon Health and Science University,
3181 SW Sam Jackson Park Road, PV01, Portland, OR 97239, USA
e-mail: smithtim@ohsu.edu

P.S. Batra, J.K. Han (eds.), *Practical Medical and Surgical Management of Chronic Rhinosinusitis*, DOI 10.1007/978-3-319-16724-4_13

Inflammatory Pathophysiology of Chronic Rhinosinusitis

Chronic rhinosinusitis (CRS) is an inflammatory disease of the nasal and sinus mucosa which is often multifactorial with several different humoral and cellular dysfunctions. The accepted classification scheme for CRS is based on the presence or absence (CRSsNP) of nasal polyps (CRSwNP). Evidence increasingly elucidates, however, that this classification is not based purely on morphology, but rather there are distinct inflammatory mechanisms that drive the pathology in each group. With consideration of this, it is useful to conceptualize CRS based on the characteristics of the inflammation and the mediators and infiltrates that drive these processes. Specifically, CRS can also be classified based on whether the inflammation is eosinophil or neutrophil dominant.

The primary goal for managing CRS is to reduce mucosal inflammation and reconstitute normal physiologic function of the paranasal sinuses. In order to achieve this goal, it is important to first have an understanding of the underlying pathophysiologic mechanisms involved in CRS-related inflammation.

The objective of this chapter is to outline the inflammatory pathophysiology in CRS (summarized in Table 13.1) and the application of antibiotics as agents that interfere with these pathways to decrease inflammation. We will discuss the proposed anti-inflammatory mechanisms of antibiotics as well as review current literature investigating their use in this setting.

Eosinophil-Dominant Inflammation

Chronic rhinosinusitis with predominantly eosinophilic inflammation refers to a group of entities including allergic fungal rhinosinusitis, eosinophilic mucin rhinosinusitis, and nasal polyposis. In this group of patients, inflammation is predominantly driven by immunoglobulin E (IgE).

The inciting event is the exposure to an antigen, which can arise from the environment or be produced by organisms residing in the nasal mucosa.

Table 13.1 Characteristics of eosinophilic and neutrophilic inflammation in chronic rhinosinusitis

	Eosinophilic	Neutrophilic
Stimulus for inflammation	Allergen	Microorganism
Cell-mediated immunity	Th2 predominant	Th1 predominant
Key cytokines	IL-4, IL-5, IL-9, IL-13	IL-1β, IL-6, IL-8, TNF-α
Granulocyte-specific inflammatory products	Major basic protein → *epithelial desquamation, mucus-cell hyperplasia, and mucosal edema*	Proteases and superoxides → *mucociliary dysfunction and mucin hypersecretion*
Other pathogenic features	Superantigen production	Increased fibrosis

Antigen-processing cells process the allergen into a peptide, which is then presented to type 2 T-helper (Th2) cells within major histocompatibility complex II (MHC II). Antigen-processing cells include dendritic cells, mast cells, macrophages, eosinophils, and natural helper cells [1]. An activated Th2 cell produces the cytokines interleukin (IL)-4, IL-13, IL-5, and IL-9. IL-4 and IL-13 stimulate the production of IgE by B-cells. IL-13 also assists in eosinophil migration from blood vessels to the nasal mucosa [2]. IL-5 facilitates eosinophilic chemotaxis and prolongs their survival by reducing apoptosis, while IL-9 leads to the propagation of mast cells [3].

Ongoing allergen exposure leads to cross-linking of IgE, now bound to the surface of sensitized mast cells. Activated mast cells release their contents, including histamine, leukotrienes, tumor necrosis factor (TNF-α), and cytokines. The resultant effect is an inflammatory and edematous state with increased vascular permeability and mucus secretion, as well as mucociliary function impairment. In addition, the mediators released by mast cells are chemotactic for eosinophils, which are the dominant inflammatory cells in the late allergy phase. Eosinophils contain major basic protein (MBP), a granule that contains cytotoxic material that when deposited causes epithelial desquamation, thickening of the basement membrane, mucus-cell hyperplasia, and edema [4]. Repeated exposure to allergens perpetuates the above pathways, causing ongoing eosinophil deposition and the associated inflammation and injury of sinonasal epithelium. Figure 13.1 outlines the common features of the eosinophilic inflammatory response.

A subset of patients with eosinophilic disease has negative atopy testing. The working hypothesis is that inflammation in these patients may be driven by allergen exposure; however, IgE production occurs locally, and there is a lack of systemic symptoms and serum measures of atopy. This is supported by studies that have shown an increase in nasal lavage IgE levels following allergen provocation [5–7].

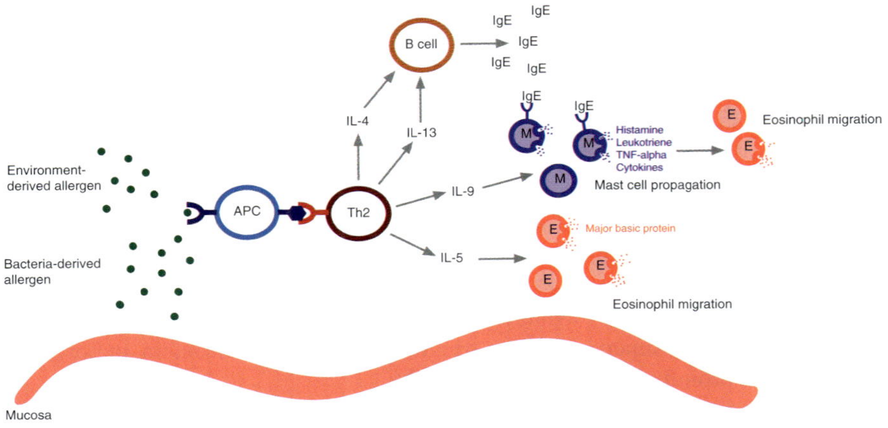

Fig. 13.1 Mechanism of eosinophilic inflammation. *APC* antigen-presenting cell, *Th2* type 2 helper T-cell, *IL interleukin, IgE immunoglobulin* E, *M* mast cell, *E* eosinophil, *TNF-α* tumor necrosis factor alpha

Therefore, the local allergic state plays an important role in CRS and may not be reflected at the systemic level. The presence of local allergy in the absence of corresponding systemic atopy is referred to as 'entopy' [8]. Another possible explanation for the eosinophilic sinus mucosal disease is leukotriene. This is further discussed in Chap. 18.

In some eosinophilic CRS, the mucosa is frequently colonized by *Staphylococcus aureus*, with carrier rates up to 63.6 % in CRS with nasal polyps (CRSwNP) [9]. This is compared to a carrier rate of 27.3 % in CRS without nasal polyps (CRSsNP). *Staphylococcus aureus* can produce pathogenic exotoxins, otherwise known as superantigens by their ability to mass activate T cells [10]. The superantigens bind to antigen-presenting cells as well as T lymphocytes. The activation of T lymphocytes leads to T-cell proliferation, the production of IL-5, and subsequent eosinophil infiltration and associated inflammation. Superantigens also stimulate B cells to produce superantigen-specific IgE [9]. Finally, superantigens are associated with the ongoing activation of mast cells. This amplification of the inflammatory response associated with bacterial colonization is becoming a recognized phenomenon in the pathogenesis of CRS.

Neutrophil-Dominant Inflammation

Neutrophil-dominant inflammation is commonly seen in CRSsNP. It is associated with bacteria, ciliary dyskinesis, cystic fibrosis, or a foreign body [11]. Once triggered, various inflammatory pathways can continue despite the removal of the pathogen from the mucosa, resulting in a chronic inflammatory state.

Initially, there is exposure of the nasal mucosa to microorganisms. In response, macrophages are stimulated to produce IL-1β and TNF-α. This subsequently stimulates epithelial cells to secrete the cytokines IL-6 and IL-8, as well as granulocyte macrophage colony-stimulating factor (GM-CSF). Mucosal epithelial cells can also be directly stimulated by bacteria to secrete IL-8 [12]. IL-8 stimulates transendothelial migration of neutrophils by increasing adhesion molecules on both the neutrophils as well as the vasculature [12, 13]. Neutrophils, once migrated to the nasal mucosa and sinus exudate, also secrete IL-8, as well as leukotriene B, thereby propagating the inflammatory response. It has been proposed that IL-8 may play a role in the formation of neutrophil-dominant polyps that are distinct from the typical eosinophil-dominant polyps seen in the case of allergy-associated CRS [13].

In addition to secreting IL-8, neutrophils also produce proteases and superoxides, leading to mucociliary dysfunction and the stagnation of sinus drainage [12]. These proteases and superoxides also trigger hypersecretion of mucin and ongoing production of proinflammatory cytokines [14].

An upregulation of transforming growth factor beta (TGF-β) is also seen in CRSsNP. TGF-β plays a key role in collagen deposition and fibrosis by stimulating extracellular matrix protein production as well as inhibiting the breakdown of these proteins. TGF-β contributes to the regulation of matrix metalloproteinases (MMPs). MMPs are a group of proteolytic peptidases that control tissue remodeling and help

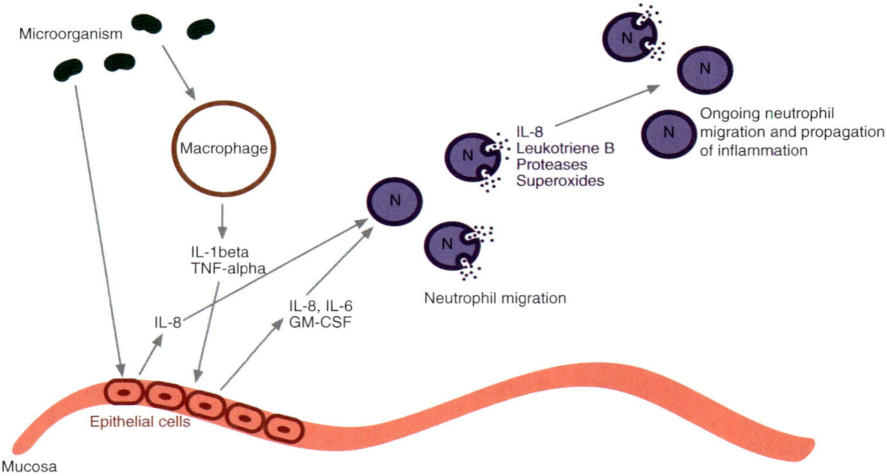

Fig. 13.2 Mechanism of neutrophilic inflammation. *IL interleukin, TNF-α* tumor necrosis factor alpha, *GM-CSF* granulocyte macrophage colony-stimulating factor, *N* neutrophil

recruit immune cells. Conversely, TGF-β is downregulated in CRSwNP. This increase in fibrosis is another differentiating feature of CRSsNP from CRSwNP [15, 16]. Figure 13.2 outlines the common features of the neutrophilic inflammatory response (see Table 13.1).

Antibiotics as Anti-inflammatories

The primary goal of CRS management is the reduction of sinonasal mucosal inflammation in order to promote normal physiologic functioning. Common first-line treatment options include high-volume sinonasal saline irrigations, topical corticosteroid therapies, and systemic therapies such as short-course oral corticosteroids and oral antibiotics. Endoscopic sinus surgery (ESS) is an important treatment modality for patients with refractory CRS as it provides open and accessible sinus cavities in order to facilitate the delivery of topical anti-inflammatory therapy [17]. In the setting where the above mainstay therapies fail to alleviate symptoms, second-line therapies can be considered. These therapies include prolonged anti-inflammatory antibiotics, antihistamines, anti-IgE monoclonal antibody (omalizumab), and anti-IL-5 monoclonal antibody (mepolizumab). However, the evidence for several of these second-line agents in the setting of CRS is still preliminary.

Antibiotics have been used liberally in CRS as bacteria are frequently cultured in these patients [18]. However, their exact therapeutic role is not well established. There is growing evidence that certain antibiotics have action beyond being bacteriostatic or bactericidal. Studies suggest that certain antibiotics may exert anti-inflammatory effects, thereby addressing the underlying pathologic state in CRS. For this reason, certain antibiotics can be added to the list of second-line agents when standard therapies fail. The following sections will discuss the antibiotics that have been used as anti-inflammatory agents in the management of CRS.

Macrolides

First discovered in 1952, macrolides are derivatives of polyketides, which are metabolites produced by bacteria, fungi, plants, and animals [19]. They exert their bacteriostatic effects through the disruption of bacterial ribosomal function. This class of antibiotics includes erythromycin, clarithromycin, roxithromycin, and azithromycin.

Macrolides are most effective against Gram-positive bacteria and are most commonly employed in upper respiratory tract infections. Having efficacy for *Streptococcus pneumoniae*, *Haemophilus* spp., *Moraxella catarrhalis, and Mycoplasma pneumoniae* , macrolides remain as the mainstay for the treatment of community-acquired pneumonia.

While conventionally they are used for their antibacterial effects, macrolides are increasingly being investigated for their anti-inflammatory and immunomodulatory effects [19–22]. Specifically, macrolides have been hypothesized to have a role in regulating cytokine production, neutrophil apoptosis, and mucociliary clearance.

Macrolides as Anti-inflammatories

In vitro studies have shown that a primary mechanism by which macrolides act as an anti-inflammatory is through its ability to inhibit nuclear factor kappa B (NFκB). NFκB facilitates the transcription of the inflammatory genes that when expressed leads to the production of IL-2, IL-6, IL-8, TNF-α, GM-CSF, and other inflammatory mediators [23]. Various viruses and bacteria can activate the NFκB pathway of inflammation, and exposure to macrolides leads to a decrease in the expression of these inflammatory genes. The downregulation of the expression of certain inflammatory genes has been confirmed in vivo, where several studies have demonstrated a decrease in local sinonasal mucosal levels of IL-8 following macrolide therapy [13, 24, 25].

Macrolides have several other beneficial effects in the setting of CRS. First, it improves mucociliary function of the sinonasal cavity. This was shown in two animal models, whereby 2 weeks of roxithromycin increased mucociliary clearance [26, 27]. Second, macrolides have been found to normalize mucus production and consistency [28, 29]. Third, macrolides decrease neutrophil accumulation and encourage their apoptosis, which reduces the damage caused by the release of cytotoxic substances [24, 30, 31]. Finally, macrolides interfere with TGF-β function by blocking its receptor [32]. This decreases collagen deposition and the subsequent fibrosis that is seen in TGF-β upregulation. Figure 13.3 outlines the mechanisms of action for macrolides as anti-inflammatories.

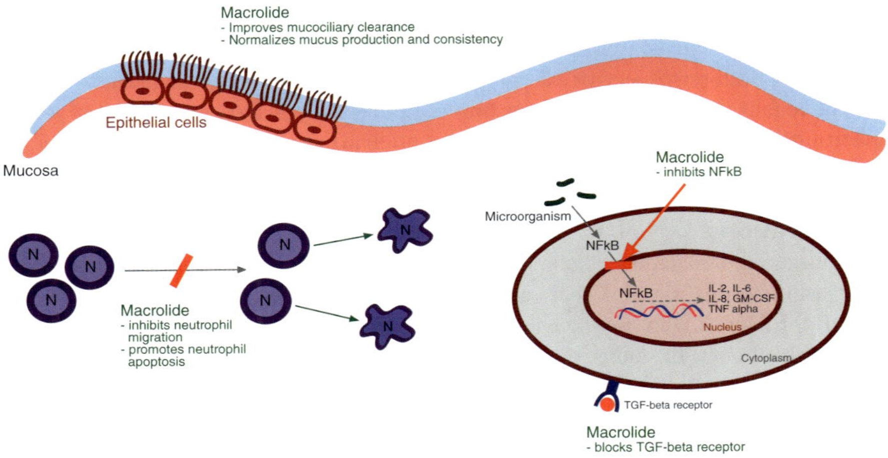

Fig. 13.3 Macrolide anti-inflammatory mechanism of action. *N* neutrophil, *NFκB* nuclear factor kappa B, *IL* interleukin, *GM-CSF* granulocyte macrophage colony-stimulating factor, *TNF-α* tumor necrosis factor alpha, *TGF-β* transforming growth factor beta

Clinical Efficacy

Various studies have investigated the utility of macrolide use in the management of CRS; however, there are only two randomized controlled trials evaluating the effectiveness of prolonged macrolide therapy in patients with CRS. In 2006, Wallwork performed a randomized, double-blind placebo-controlled trial evaluating oral roxithromycin 150 mg daily for 3 months in CRSsNP [20]. The results demonstrated that macrolide therapy provided significant improvements in both quality of life (QoL) and endoscopic findings at the end of the treatment period. Quality of life, however, was no longer significantly improved at 3-month follow-up after stopping macrolide treatment. Additionally, they identified that patients with decreased serum IgE levels experienced greater benefit from macrolide therapy. In 2011, Videler et al. performed a randomized, double-blind placebo-controlled trial evaluating oral azithromycin 500 mg daily for 3 days followed by 500 mg once a week for 11 weeks [21]. In contrast to the study by Wallwork et al., their results failed to demonstrate a significant improvement in both QoL and endoscopic findings [21]. A possible explanation for the lack of significant results obtained by Videler et al. is that 500 mg given once a week was an underdose of the amount that would be required to improve symptoms.

There are ten observational studies that have investigated symptom improvement with macrolide therapy [33–42]. All studies report symptom improvement in over 50 % and endoscopic improvement in 40–70 % of study subjects; however, none used a validated instrument to evaluate sinus symptomatology. There are two studies that retrospectively examined the role of macrolide antibiotics following endoscopic sinus surgery. In both studies, a significant improvement in symptoms was found in the group that was treated with long-term macrolides [38].

In 2013, an evidence-based review with recommendations by Soler et al. summarized the evidence on prolonged macrolide therapy in CRS [43]. They identified 17 studies, both retrospective and prospective. They concluded that because a consistent benefit was seen in numerous observational studies and one controlled study, macrolide antibiotics would be a reasonable option in patients with CRS. Furthermore, macrolides should be especially considered in patients with low serum IgE levels.

Complications

Complications of macrolide antibiotics include hypersensitivity reactions, hepatotoxicity, and gastrointestinal upset. Other reported complications include ototoxicity and prolonged QT interval with subsequent dysrhythmia. There is also a risk of adverse drug-to-drug interactions with statins, antidepressants, antiepileptics, and methotrexate. Finally, there is the theoretical risk of antibiotic resistance; however, none of the abovementioned studies reported cases of bacterial resistance as a result of prolonged macrolide use.

Summary: Macrolides

At this time, available evidence suggests that a long course of at least 12 weeks of low-dose macrolide antibiotics may help alleviate symptoms of CRS that are refractory to conventional therapy. The evidence suggests that macrolide therapy is most effective in patients who have nonallergic CRS with low serum IgE levels. Those who have allergic disease and predominantly eosinophilic inflammation are less likely to experience clinical improvement.

In patients with refractory CRS, it is reasonable to consider trial therapy with a macrolide [44]. Furthermore, it may be prudent to obtain a serum IgE level to identify those individuals who would most likely benefit from macrolide therapy. Table 13.2 summarizes the macrolide antibiotics that have been used in CRS, their dosages, and contraindications.

Tetracyclines

Tetracyclines are a group of mostly bacteriostatic antibiotics. They inhibit bacterial protein synthesis by binding to the 30S ribosomal subunit. The first tetracycline

Table 13.2 Summary of macrolide treatment options

Macrolide	Dose (mg)	Frequency	Duration (weeks)	Contraindications
Clarithromycin	250 or 500	QD	12	Hypersensitivity to macrolide antibiotics[a]
				Concurrent statin therapy
Azithromycin	500	Once a week dose after daily dose × 3	12	Previous hepatic dysfunction secondary to azithromycin use
Erythromycin	250	BID	12	Concurrent use of pimozide, cisapride, ergotamine, and statin
Roxithromycin	150	QD	12	Porphyria

[a]Applies as a contraindication to all macrolide antibiotics

discovered was chlortetracycline. Five more tetracyclines have been developed since that time, including doxycycline, tetracycline, minocycline, oxytetracycline, and demeclocycline.

They are broad-spectrum antibiotics with action against various organisms, including Gram-positive and Gram-negative bacteria, as well as atypical pathogens such as *Rickettsia* spp., *Chlamydia* spp., *Mycoplasma pneumoniae,* and *Treponema* spp.

Tetracyclines as Anti-inflammatories

There has been great interest in studying the non-antimicrobial properties of tetracyclines. One of the most well-known properties is its ability to inhibit matrix metalloproteinases (MMPs). Doxycycline decreases MMP activity by both direct inhibition of MMP molecules as well as the downregulation of their production [45]. MMPs mediate proteolysis of the extracellular matrix and play an important role in connective tissue remodeling. As such, MMPs are involved in the pathogenesis of wound healing, tumor invasion, and inflammation [46–50]; therefore, inhibiting MMPs may reduce the inflammatory response in the mucosa of patients with CRS.

Tetracyclines exert an anti-inflammatory effect through other mechanisms, including the stabilization of reactive oxygen specifies, inhibition of nitric oxide synthesis, and reduction of neutrophil chemotaxis [45, 51–53]. Additionally, tetracyclines have been implicated in decreasing IgE production, while levels of IgA, IgM, and IgG are unaffected [54, 55]. A possible explanation for this is that it interferes with terminal B lymphocyte differentiation and class switching [56]. By virtue of decreasing IgE, it also decreases IgE-mediated responses such as the mast cell-dominant late allergy phase [54]. Figure 13.4 outlines the mechanisms of action for tetracyclines as anti-inflammatories.

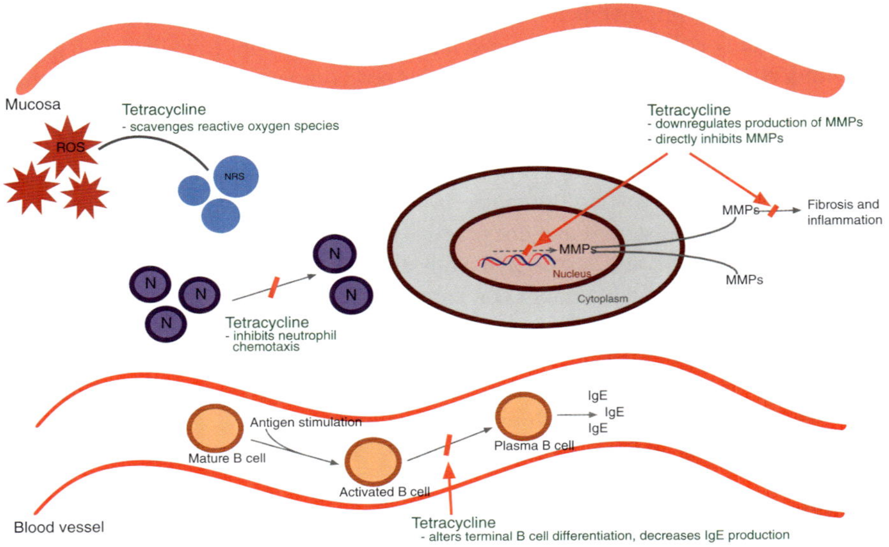

Fig. 13.4 Tetracycline anti-inflammatory mechanism of action. *ROS* reactive oxygen species, *NRS* nonreactive species, *N* neutrophil, *MMP* metalloproteinases, *IgE* immunoglobulin E

Clinical Efficacy

Two studies have investigated the anti-inflammatory effects of doxycycline applied to CRS. Sommer et al. examined the ability of doxycycline to alter the expression of various inflammatory markers in vitro, using tissues obtained from patients with CRSwNP and CRSsNP [57]. They did not find a significant decrease in the expression of IL-5, which, as mentioned previously, is an important cytokine in eosinophil activation and propagation. The matrix metalloproteinase MMP-9 was significantly elevated in tissues obtained from patients with CRS compared to the healthy group. Treatment with doxycycline led to a decrease in the expression of MMP-9 in both CRSsNP and CRSwNP; however, neither decrease was significant. Finally, the authors investigated the changes in eotaxin-3 expression, a beta-chemokine involved in eosinophil accumulation. Interestingly, they found an increase in eotaxin-3 expression associated with increased doses of doxycycline. A potential explanation for this finding was not provided.

Van Zele et al. performed a randomized, double-blind controlled trial which randomly assigned 47 patients with CRSwNP into one of three groups: (1) 20-day tapering course of methylprednisolone (32–8 mg daily), (2) 20-day course of doxycycline (loading dose of 200 mg once followed by 100 mg/day for 19 days), or placebo [58]. The steroid group had a significant decrease in polyp size compared to the placebo group at 2 weeks, after which point polyps began to recur. At 12-week follow-up, there was no longer any significant difference in polyp size. Subjects receiving doxycycline also had a significant reduction in polyp size compared with the placebo group. Unlike the steroid group, however, the reduction in polyp size was sustained at 12-week follow-up. Patients were also assessed with regard to CRS symptoms. There was a significant decrease in postnasal drip in the doxycycline group at week 2, which then trended to no longer be significant after 2 weeks. There was no significant improvement in nasal congestion, rhinorrhea, or sense of smell. While this study compared the doxycycline and steroid groups to the placebo group individually, the two treatment groups were not compared with each other with regard to endoscopic findings or symptomatology.

For inflammatory markers, Van Zele et al. found a decreased serum level of IL-5 receptor alpha (IL-5rα) in the doxycycline group at 4-week follow-up compared to the placebo group. There was no difference in actual IL-5 levels. IgE levels were also decreased in both the steroid and doxycycline groups compared to placebo. Finally, doxycycline treatment was associated with a significant decrease in MMP-9 and myeloperoxidase in nasal secretions compared to both the placebo and steroid groups.

The role for tetracyclines is better established in other disease processes. It is used frequently in dermatologic conditions based on its inhibition of neutrophil chemotaxis, proinflammatory cytokines, and MMPs (predominantly MMP-2 and MMP-9) [59]. Because of its inhibitory effect on MMPs, it is also being used in rheumatoid arthritis and periodontal disease [60–63].

Complications

The most common adverse effect of tetracycline antibiotics is gastrointestinal upset, including abdominal pain, nausea, and vomiting. There are also reports of esophageal ulcerations and strictures, which can be circumvented by washing the medication down with large volumes of water. Hypersensitivity reactions and hepatotoxicity can occur as well. Finally, tetracyclines are avoided in children due to teeth discoloration and bony deposition of the medication.

Summary: Tetracyclines

Tetracyclines are known to have effects beyond its antimicrobial properties. The precise mechanisms by which its anti-inflammatory effects occur are ongoing areas of investigation. While most of the literature on its clinical effectiveness is in the realm of dermatology and rheumatology, there is one well-designed, randomized controlled trial in patients with CRSwNP, whereby there was a significant and lasting decrease in nasal polyp size. With the exception of a temporary decrease in postnasal drip, there were no other significant improvements in CRS-related symptoms. It is possible that a longer course of tetracycline may have yielded more significant results.

Tetracyclines could potentially be good options for patients with eosinophilic-dominant inflammation, with CRSwNP and elevated IgE levels. However, further research is needed to confirm its therapeutic effects. Until there is stronger evidence, it is challenging to recommend the routine use of tetracyclines in the management of CRS, but it remains an option for patients with refractory disease.

Other Antibiotics with Anti-inflammatory Properties

Trimethoprim-Sulfamethoxazole

A sulfonamide derivative, trimethoprim-sulfamethoxazole (T-S) exerts its antibacterial effect by interfering with bacterial folic acid synthesis. Since the 1980s, it has been investigated for its role in treating granulomatosis with polyangiitis (GPA, previously known as Wegener granulomatosis).

Trimethoprim-sulfamethoxazole may be anti-inflammatory in the setting of GPA because it decreases the toxic metabolites produced by neutrophils and scavenges reactive oxygen species, both of which decrease tissue damage [64, 65]. However, the T-S antimicrobial properties are the most likely reason for its beneficial effects in patients with GPA since it decreases *Staphylococcus aureus,* which has been shown to increase relapse rates [66]. The most important indication for T-S in GPA is the prevention of *Pneumocystis jirovecii* pneumonia, in which patients are susceptible to a given long-term immunosuppressive therapy [67].

Currently, T-S is an adjunct in GPA maintenance therapy once remission is achieved with immunosuppressants [67]. The widely accepted rationale of T-S use is that it decreases microbial colonization, and the anti-inflammatory effects are often overlooked. Given that long-term, low-dose T-S therapy is generally well-tolerated with minimal side effects, this may be an antibiotic that is worthy of future investigations in the management of CRS.

Dapsone

Dapsone is a synthetic sulfone. Similar to sulfonamides, dapsone's antimicrobial effect is through the inhibition of folic acid synthesis. It has been used for decades in the treatment of leprosy and malaria [68]. It has been noted to have anti-inflammatory effects in conditions where there is neutrophilic infiltration. While the precise mechanism is unclear, the leading theory is that dapsone scavenges reactive oxygen species and minimizes neutrophil-driven oxidative damage as well as decreases neutrophil migration [68, 69].

Dapsone has also been used as an anti-inflammatory in bullous dermatologic diseases, vasculitides, connective tissue diseases, and neutrophilic dermatosis [68]. The greatest drawback is its side effect profile. The adverse effects are usually dose-dependent, and the most common side effect is mild hemolytic anemia secondary to the oxidative metabolites of dapsone. Other complaints include gastrointestinal upset, headache, poor appetite, tachycardia, and insomnia [68, 69].

Conclusion

Over the past three decades, antibiotics have been increasingly investigated for their non-antimicrobial properties – chief among these properties is an ability to act as anti-inflammatories. The antibiotics that have shown promise to exhibit clinically beneficial anti-inflammatory effects include macrolides, tetracyclines, trimethoprim-sulfamethoxazole, and dapsone. A summary of the anti-inflammatory mechanisms of these antibiotics is shown in Table 13.3. The only classes that have been used in the rhinologic setting, and specifically in CRS, are macrolides and tetracyclines.

A consistent trend is seen across observational studies as well as in one randomized controlled study to support macrolide use. Specifically, the patients that appear to experience the greatest benefit are those with low serum IgE levels. Therefore, it would be reasonable to undertake a prolonged trial of macrolide

Table 13.3 Summary of antibiotic anti-inflammatory effects

Antibiotic class	Anti-inflammatory effects
Macrolide	Inhibits nuclear factor kappa B (NFκB) → decreases the production of IL-2, IL-6, IL-8, TNF-α, GM-CSF
	Improves mucociliary clearance
	Normalizes mucus production
	Decreases neutrophil accumulation
	Blocks TGF-β function
Tetracyclines	Decreases MMP production
	Scavenges reactive oxygen species
	Inhibits nitric oxide synthesis
	Reduces neutrophil chemotaxis
	Decreases IgE production
Trimethoprim-sulfamethoxazole	Decreases neutrophil production of toxic metabolites
	Scavenges reactive oxygen species
Dapsone	Scavenges reactive oxygen species
	Decreases neutrophil migration

therapy (at least 12 weeks) in patients with recalcitrant nonallergic CRS and low serum IgE levels.

Tetracyclines have been shown in one study to significantly decrease nasal polyp size; however, this same study failed to show any lasting improvements in symptoms. This class of antibiotics has potential to be an effective treatment option for patients with CRSwNP but should be further investigated before any definitive conclusions can be made.

References

1. Barnes PJ. Pathophysiology of allergic inflammation. Immunol Rev. 2011;242(1):31–50.
2. Benninger MS, et al. Adult chronic rhinosinusitis: definitions, diagnosis, epidemiology, and pathophysiology. Otolaryngol Head Neck Surg. 2003;129(3 Suppl):S1–32.
3. Bachert C, et al. Important research questions in allergy and related diseases: 3-chronic rhinosinusitis and nasal polyposis – a GALEN study. Allergy. 2009;64(4):520–33.
4. Harlin SL, et al. A clinical and pathologic study of chronic sinusitis: the role of the eosinophil. J Allergy Clin Immunol. 1988;81(5 Pt 1):867–75.
5. Rondon C, et al. Local IgE production and positive nasal provocation test in patients with persistent nonallergic rhinitis. J Allergy Clin Immunol. 2007;119(4):899–905.
6. Carney AS, et al. Atypical nasal challenges in patients with idiopathic rhinitis: more evidence for the existence of allergy in the absence of atopy? Clin Exp Allergy. 2002;32(10):1436–40.
7. Wedback A, et al. Seasonal non-allergic rhinitis (SNAR)–a new disease entity? A clinical and immunological comparison between SNAR, seasonal allergic rhinitis and persistent non-allergic rhinitis. Rhinology. 2005;43(2):86–92.
8. Powe DG, Bonnin AJ, Jones NS. 'Entopy': local allergy paradigm. Clin Exp Allergy. 2010;40(7):987–97.
9. Van Zele T, et al. Staphylococcus aureus colonization and IgE antibody formation to enterotoxins is increased in nasal polyposis. J Allergy Clin Immunol. 2004;114(4):981–3.
10. Krakauer T. Immune response to staphylococcal superantigens. Immunol Res. 1999;20(2):163–73.
11. Hatipoglu U, Rubinstein I. Anti-inflammatory treatment of chronic rhinosinusitis: a shifting paradigm. Curr Allergy Asthma Rep. 2008;8(2):154–61.
12. Yoon BN, et al. Induction of interleukin-8 from nasal epithelial cells during bacterial infection: the role of IL-8 for neutrophil recruitment in chronic rhinosinusitis. Mediators Inflamm. 2010;2010:813610.
13. Yamada T, et al. Macrolide treatment decreased the size of nasal polyps and IL-8 levels in nasal lavage. Am J Rhinol. 2000;14(3):143–8.
14. Konstan MW, Davis PB. Pharmacological approaches for the discovery and development of new anti-inflammatory agents for the treatment of cystic fibrosis. Adv Drug Deliv Rev. 2002;54(11):1409–23.
15. Van Crombruggen K, et al. Pathogenesis of chronic rhinosinusitis: inflammation. J Allergy Clin Immunol. 2011;128(4):728–32.
16. Branton MH, Kopp JB. TGF-beta and fibrosis. Microbes Infect. 1999;1(15):1349–65.
17. Thomas WW 3rd, et al. Distribution of topical agents to the paranasal sinuses: an evidence-based review with recommendations. Int Forum Allergy Rhinol. 2013;3(9):691–703.
18. Dubin MG, et al. American Rhinologic Society member survey on "maximal medical therapy" for chronic rhinosinusitis. Am J Rhinol. 2007;21(4):483–8.
19. Harvey RJ, Wallwork BD, Lund VJ. Anti-inflammatory effects of macrolides: applications in chronic rhinosinusitis. Immunol Allergy Clin North Am. 2009;29(4):689–703.
20. Wallwork B, et al. A double-blind, randomized, placebo-controlled trial of macrolide in the treatment of chronic rhinosinusitis. Laryngoscope. 2006;116(2):189–93.

21. Videler WJ, et al. Lack of efficacy of long-term, low-dose azithromycin in chronic rhinosinusitis: a randomized controlled trial. Allergy. 2011;66(11):1457–68.
22. Shinkai M, Henke MO, Rubin BK. Macrolide antibiotics as immunomodulatory medications: proposed mechanisms of action. Pharmacol Ther. 2008;117(3):393–405.
23. Cervin A. The anti-inflammatory effect of erythromycin and its derivatives, with special reference to nasal polyposis and chronic sinusitis. Acta Otolaryngol. 2001;121(1):83–92.
24. MacLeod CM, et al. Anti-inflammatory activity of clarithromycin in adults with chronically inflamed sinus mucosa. Adv Ther. 2001;18(2):75–82.
25. Suzuki H, et al. Effects of long-term low-dose macrolide administration on neutrophil recruitment and IL-8 in the nasal discharge of chronic sinusitis patients. Tohoku J Exp Med. 1997;182(2):115–24.
26. Nakano T, et al. Roxithromycin reinforces epithelial defence function in rabbit trachea. Acta Otolaryngol Suppl. 1998;538:233–8.
27. Sugiura Y, Ohashi Y, Nakai Y. Roxithromycin stimulates the mucociliary activity of the Eustachian tube and modulates neutrophil activity in the healthy guinea pig. Acta Otolaryngol Suppl. 1997;531:34–8.
28. Ikeda K, Wu D, Takasaka T. Inhibition of acetylcholine-evoked Cl-currents by 14-membered macrolide antibiotics in isolated acinar cells of the guinea pig nasal gland. Am J Respir Cell Mol Biol. 1995;13(4):449–54.
29. Rhee CS, et al. Effects of clarithromycin on rheological properties of nasal mucus in patients with chronic sinusitis. Ann Otol Rhinol Laryngol. 2000;109(5):484–7.
30. Aoshiba K, Nagai A, Konno K. Erythromycin shortens neutrophil survival by accelerating apoptosis. Antimicrob Agents Chemother. 1995;39(4):872–7.
31. Chin AC, et al. Anti-inflammatory benefits of tilmicosin in calves with Pasteurella haemolytica-infected lungs. Am J Vet Res. 1998;59(6):765–71.
32. Wang T, Donahoe PK, Zervos AS. Specific interaction of type I receptors of the TGF-beta family with the immunophilin FKBP-12. Science. 1994;265(5172):674–6.
33. Haruna S, et al. A study of poor responders for long-term, low-dose macrolide administration for chronic sinusitis. Rhinology. 2009;47(1):66–71.
34. Song Y, Bai W, Ji W. An empirical study of treating chronic sinusitis with low dose Roxithromycin. Lin Chung Er Bi Yan Hou Tou Jing Wai Ke Za Zhi. 2009;23(8):357–8, 363.
35. Cervin A, et al. One-year low-dose erythromycin treatment of persistent chronic sinusitis after sinus surgery: clinical outcome and effects on mucociliary parameters and nasal nitric oxide. Otolaryngol Head Neck Surg. 2002;126(5):481–9.
36. Katsuta S, et al. Therapeutic effect of roxithromycin on chronic sinusitis with nasal – polyps clinical, computed tomography, and electron microscopy analysis. Nihon Jibiinkoka Gakkai Kaiho. 2002;105(12):1189–97.
37. Kimura N, et al. Clinical effect of low-dose, long-term roxithromycin chemotherapy in patients with chronic sinusitis. Acta Med Okayama. 1997;51(1):33–7.
38. Moriyama H, et al. Evaluation of endoscopic sinus surgery for chronic sinusitis: post-operative erythromycin therapy. Rhinology. 1995;33(3):166–70.
39. Kita H, Takezawa H. Long-term low dose erythromycin and roxithromycin therapy for chronic sinusitis. Practica Otologica Kyoto. 1995;84(Suppl):62–9.
40. Minami T, Kubo N, Kumazawa H, et al. Long-term low dose roxithromycin therapy for chronic sinusitis. Practica Otologica Kyoto. 1995;88:1229–36.
41. Hashiba M, Baba S. Efficacy of long-term administration of clarithromycin in the treatment of intractable chronic sinusitis. Acta Otolaryngol Suppl. 1996;525:73–8.
42. Kikuchi S, Suzaki H, Aoki A, et al. Clinical effect of long-term low-dose erythromycin therapy for chronic sinusitis. Practica Otologica Kyoto. 1991;84:41–7.
43. Soler ZM, et al. Antimicrobials and chronic rhinosinusitis with or without polyposis in adults: an evidenced-based review with recommendations. Int Forum Allergy Rhinol. 2013;3(1):31–47.
44. Fokkens, WJ, et al. European position paper on rhinosinusitis and nasal polyps 2012. Rhinol Suppl. 2012;(23): p. 3 p preceding table of contents, 1–298.

45. Griffin MO, Ceballos G, Villarreal FJ. Tetracycline compounds with non-antimicrobial organ protective properties: possible mechanisms of action. Pharmacol Res. 2011;63(2):102–7.
46. Spinale FG. Matrix metalloproteinases: regulation and dysregulation in the failing heart. Circ Res. 2002;90(5):520–30.
47. d'Ortho MP, et al. Membrane-type matrix metalloproteinases 1 and 2 exhibit broad-spectrum proteolytic capacities comparable to many matrix metalloproteinases. Eur J Biochem. 1997;250(3):751–7.
48. Peterson JT. Matrix metalloproteinase inhibitor development and the remodeling of drug discovery. Heart Fail Rev. 2004;9(1):63–79.
49. Rohde LE, et al. Matrix metalloproteinase inhibition attenuates early left ventricular enlargement after experimental myocardial infarction in mice. Circulation. 1999;99(23):3063–70.
50. Stetler-Stevenson WG, Liotta LA, Kleiner Jr DE. Extracellular matrix 6: role of matrix metalloproteinases in tumor invasion and metastasis. FASEB J. 1993;7(15):1434–41.
51. D'Agostino P, et al. Tetracycline inhibits the nitric oxide synthase activity induced by endotoxin in cultured murine macrophages. Eur J Pharmacol. 1998;346(2–3):283–90.
52. Esterly NB, Furey NL, Flanagan LE. The effect of antimicrobial agents on leukocyte chemotaxis. J Invest Dermatol. 1978;70(1):51–5.
53. Elewski BE, et al. In vivo suppression of neutrophil chemotaxis by systemically and topically administered tetracycline. J Am Acad Dermatol. 1983;8(6):807–12.
54. Joks R, Durkin HG. Non-antibiotic properties of tetracyclines as anti-allergy and asthma drugs. Pharmacol Res. 2011;64(6):602–9.
55. Joks R, et al. Tetracycline-mediated IgE isotype-specific suppression of ongoing human and murine IgE responses in vivo and murine memory IgE responses induced in vitro. Int Immunol. 2010;22(4):281–8.
56. Kuzin II, et al. Tetracyclines inhibit activated B cell function. Int Immunol. 2001;13(7):921–31.
57. Sommer JU, et al. In vitro effects of doxycycline on inflammatory cytokines and gelatinases in chronic rhinosinusitis. In Vivo. 2012;26(3):369–74.
58. Van Zele T, et al. Oral steroids and doxycycline: two different approaches to treat nasal polyps. J Allergy Clin Immunol. 2010;125(5):1069–76.e4.
59. Sapadin AN, Fleischmajer R. Tetracyclines: nonantibiotic properties and their clinical implications. J Am Acad Dermatol. 2006;54(2):258–65.
60. Kloppenburg M, et al. The influence of tetracyclines on T cell activation. Clin Exp Immunol. 1995;102(3):635–41.
61. Tilley BC, et al. Minocycline in rheumatoid arthritis. A 48-week, double-blind, placebo-controlled trial. MIRA Trial Group. Ann Intern Med. 1995;122(2):81–9.
62. O'Dell JR, et al. Treatment of early seropositive rheumatoid arthritis: a two-year, double-blind comparison of minocycline and hydroxychloroquine. Arthritis Rheum. 2001;44(10):2235–41.
63. Ciancio S, Ashley R. Safety and efficacy of sub-antimicrobial-dose doxycycline therapy in patients with adult periodontitis. Adv Dent Res. 1998;12(2):27–31.
64. Roberts DE, Curd JG. Sulfonamides as antiinflammatory agents in the treatment of Wegener's granulomatosis. Arthritis Rheum. 1990;33(10):1590–3.
65. Suematsu M, et al. Sulfasalazine and its metabolites attenuate respiratory burst of leukocytes–a possible mechanism of anti-inflammatory effects. J Clin Lab Immunol. 1987;23(1):31–3.
66. Stegeman CA, et al. Association of chronic nasal carriage of Staphylococcus aureus and higher relapse rates in Wegener granulomatosis. Ann Intern Med. 1994;120(1):12–7.
67. White ES, Lynch JP. Pharmacological therapy for Wegener's granulomatosis. Drugs. 2006;66(9):1209–28.
68. Grunwald MH, Amichai B. Dapsone - the treatment of infectious and inflammatory diseases in dermatology. Int J Antimicrob Agents. 1996;7(3):187–92.
69. Chang DJ, et al. Dapsone in rheumatoid arthritis. Semin Arthritis Rheum. 1996;25(6):390–403.

Topical and Intravenous Antibiotics

14

John Craig and Parul Goyal

Key Take-Home Points

- Topical antibiotic use may be appropriate in certain subsets of patients with acute exacerbations of recalcitrant CRS, with culture-proven *S. aureus*, MRSA, or *P. aeruginosa.*
- To achieve adequate sinus distribution, topical antibiotics should be delivered by high-volume irrigations rather than by nebulizers or sprays and should only be used in patients who have undergone sinus surgery.
- Topical antibiotic therapy should be culture directed whenever possible, either alone or with concurrent oral antibiotics.
  - *S. aureus* or MRSA: mupirocin
  - *P. aeruginosa*: tobramycin, gentamicin, ceftazidime
- Long-term outpatient IV antibiotics may be considered for CRS patients who fail oral antibiotics or develop orbital or intracranial complications.

Introduction

Antibiotic therapy is frequently used in the management of chronic rhinosinusitis (CRS). Bacteria are thought to play a role in the pathogenesis of CRS, although exact mechanisms remain unknown to date. Bacteria represent one group of inflammatory stimuli that can modulate the clinical course of CRS. Bacterial flora may colonize the sinonasal mucus layer or the mucosal

J. Craig, MD
Department of Otolaryngology, Henry Ford Hospital,
2799 W Grand Blvd, K-8, Detroit, MI 48203, USA
e-mail: johncraig2240@gmail.com

P. Goyal, MD, MBA (✉)
Syracuse Otolaryngology, 1101 Erie Boulevard East, Suite 200, Syracuse, NY 13210, USA
e-mail: syracuseoto@gmail.com

P.S. Batra, J.K. Han (eds.), *Practical Medical and Surgical Management of Chronic Rhinosinusitis*, DOI 10.1007/978-3-319-16724-4_14

surface. Pathogenic bacteria may invade the surface epithelium to reside within the mucosa or submucosa, with the rare potential for systemic vascular spread. Whether invasive or commensal, sinonasal bacteria have the potential to incite significant mucosal inflammation. The sinonasal mucosa is normally protected from damage and bacterial infection by mucociliary clearance and the host inflammatory response. Dysfunction in these protective mechanisms contributes to the manifestations of CRS. Examples of such dysfunction in CRS patients include dysfunctional mucociliary clearance [1], mucosal barrier disruption which leads to an augmented local inflammatory response [2], and a baseline hyperresponsive inflammatory response even to commensal bacteria [3]. Overall, a vicious cycle of mucociliary dysfunction, local infection, and chronic inflammation leads to the persistent symptoms and decreased quality of life experienced by patients with CRS [4].

Bacteria of the sinonasal cavities exist in either free-floating planktonic or biofilm forms. Biofilms are aggregates of bacteria encased in an exopolysaccharide matrix, which adhere to mucosal surfaces. Biofilms have been found on the mucosa of CRS patients and have been implicated in the development of recalcitrant CRS [5–7]. While the precise relationship between biofilms and CRS has yet to be determined, biofilms have the ability to stimulate both chronic mucosal inflammation and acute infectious exacerbations, through a variety of mechanisms [8]. Additionally, bacteria in biofilms are more resistant to antibiotics and the host immune response than those in planktonic form [9, 10].

Both medical and surgical interventions are often employed to treat the different pathologic components of CRS to achieve long-term symptom control. The mainstays of medical management for CRS have been topical and systemic steroids to decrease mucosal inflammation and systemic antibiotics to treat acute bacterial exacerbations. A recent systematic review of antimicrobial therapy for CRS indicated that moderate levels of evidence support the use of oral antibiotics for 3 weeks or less for acute exacerbations of CRS [11]. Patients with recalcitrant CRS often require multiple long-term courses of oral antibiotics, which may not be tolerated by patients due to side effects, thus increasing the risk of antibiotic resistance.

Topical and intravenous (IV) antibiotics for CRS have been explored as potential alternative routes of drug delivery. Topical antibiotics have been used either as an adjunct or alternative to oral antibiotic therapy. Topical agents can be delivered directly to diseased mucosa at higher local concentrations with less systemic absorption, minimizing the risk of systemic side effects. IV antibiotics have been considered for CRS patients who fail oral antibiotics, are poor surgical candidates, or have orbital or intracranial complications [12]. Topical and IV antibiotics have suffered from a general lack of evidence supporting their efficacy, and no clear guidelines have been established regarding their use in CRS. This chapter is an evidence-based review of the most commonly used topical and IV antibiotic regimens for recalcitrant CRS.

Topical Antibiotics: Concepts and Local Drug Delivery

Topical antibiotics are formulated at concentrations well above the planktonic organisms' minimum inhibitory concentration (MIC) when treating acute exacerbations of CRS [10, 13]. When possible, culture-directed therapy is implemented to maximize the killing of pathogenic bacteria and to minimize the risk of developing antibiotic resistance. *S. aureus* and *P. aeruginosa* are among the most commonly cultured bacteria from CRS patients in the postoperative setting [14, 15], and CRS patients harboring *S. aureus* or *P. aeruginosa* biofilms at the time of surgery have worse postoperative outcomes [16–18]. Patients with recalcitrant CRS have higher rates of resistant strains, with up to 54 % of *S. aureus* and 22 % of *P. aeruginosa* displaying antibiotic resistance [19].

The efficacy of topical antibiotic therapy is affected by microscopic and macroscopic factors that impact local drug absorption and local drug distribution [20]. Factors affecting sinus distribution of topical medication include the surgical patency of the sinuses, type of delivery device, and patient positioning. Large sinus openings are imperative for medication delivery, as delivery is minimal into sinuses prior to surgical intervention [21]. Endoscopic sinus surgery (ESS) has been shown to allow for effective sinonasal distribution of topical medications, especially for delivery to the frontal and sphenoid sinuses [22]. An ostial diameter of at least 4.7 mm has been shown to be the minimal size allowing adequate delivery of topical irrigation fluid to the sinuses [23]. In addition to adequate ostial diameter, irrigation volumes of at least 100 mL per side are necessary to ensure adequate topical medication delivery to the sinuses [24]. Topical nasal antibiotics have been delivered by a variety of delivery devices, including low-volume sprays [25] and nebulizers [26, 27], high-volume squeeze bottles [28, 29], or direct sinus cannulation [30]. While controlled studies have shown clinical improvements with high-volume topical antibiotic irrigations [29] or direct sinus cannulation [30], no clinical benefits have been found with low-volume devices in controlled studies [11, 31]. This evidence suggests that when topical antibiotics are administered, they should be delivered by high-volume irrigations, which leads to a larger amount of antibiotic being delivered directly to the diseased sinus mucosa.

Topical Antibiotics for CRS

Clear indications for topical antibiotic use in CRS have yet to be established due to a lack of high-quality evidence regarding their efficacy and optimal dosing regimens. Very few randomized controlled trials (RCTs) have been published comparing topical antibiotics with placebo for CRS. Studies to date exhibit significant heterogeneity with regard to topical antibiotic selection, dosage, regimen, delivery method, patient selection, outcome measures, and adverse effects. Additionally, data is generally lacking with regard to pharmacokinetics and systemic bioavailability of commonly used topical antibiotics.

Given the predominance of *S. aureus* and *P. aeruginosa* in recalcitrant CRS patients, the most commonly studied topical antibiotics have been topical mupirocin and aminoglycosides. In the next sections, topical mupirocin, aminoglycosides, and other less commonly used topical antibiotics will be discussed with respect to the highest levels of evidence for each. Table 14.1 shows the most common dosage regimens of the topical antibiotics utilized in refractory CRS.

Mupirocin

Mupirocin inhibits bacterial isoleucyl-tRNA synthetase, leading to disruption of protein synthesis. Mupirocin has bacteriostatic and bactericidal effects against most aerobic gram-positive bacteria in both planktonic and biofilm form, with less activity against gram-negative and anaerobic bacteria. With regard to the common bacteria in recalcitrant CRS, mupirocin displays high levels of activity against *S. aureus*, including MRSA, with low activity against *P. aeruginosa*. The MIC of mupirocin for *S. aureus* has been found to be 0.12–1.0 μg/mL, and the minimal bactericidal concentration (MBC) has been found to be 4–32 μg/mL [37]. The MIC for MRSA is 0.5–2 μg/mL [38]. It has been suggested that topical antibiotic regimens be formulated with anti-biofilm intent, requiring antibiotic concentrations well above the MIC of a given bacterium's planktonic form [33]. Ha et al. performed in vitro

Table 14.1 Various topical sinonasal antibiotic irrigation regimens reported in the literature [28–30, 32–36]

Topical antibiotics	Studies	Dosing regimens
Mupirocin	Uren et al. [28]	100 mL/nostril, twice daily × 3 weeks
		0.05 % solution (500 μg/mL)
		100 mg in 200 mL lactated ringers
	Jervis-Bardy et al. [29]	120 mL/nostril, twice daily × 4 weeks
		0.05 % solution (500 μg/mL)
		120 mg in 240 mL saline
	Solares et al. [32]	50 mL/nostril, twice daily × 4–6 weeks
		22 g/L solution
Tobramycin	Elliott and Stringer [33]	50 mL/nostril (40 mg), twice daily × variable duration
		80 mg/L solution
	Moss and King [30]	1 mL/irrigation (40 mg), three times daily × 7–10 days
		Via maxillary sinus catheters
Gentamicin	Wei et al. [34]	40 mL/nostril, daily × 6 weeks
		80 mg/L solution
	Whatley et al. [35]	40 mL/nostril, twice daily × 3–15 weeks
		80 mg/L solution
Ceftazidime	Leonard and Bolger [36]	150 mL/nostril, three times daily
		1 g/L solution

testing of mupirocin on *S. aureus* and showed that a concentration of 125 μg/mL was able to reduce the biofilm mass by over 90 % [13].

The pharmacokinetics and dynamics of mupirocin sinonasal irrigations have mostly been extrapolated from topical skin applications. Mupirocin undergoes rapid degradation to an inactive metabolite in serum, and studies using topical skin preparations of mupirocin have revealed no detectable levels of the drug in serum after standard therapeutic dosages for 3–5 days [39]. No studies have assessed mupirocin serum levels after sinonasal irrigations. Very few minor adverse effects have been reported with topical intranasal mupirocin use, such as local irritation [28]. There is a theoretical risk of mupirocin causing renal damage given its renal excretion and polyethylene glycol base. Patients with renal insufficiency could therefore be at higher theoretical risk. However, no studies to date have documented nephrotoxicity.

Antimicrobial resistance is another potential concern, and variable resistance rates have been reported with topical mupirocin use. A resistance rate of 2.4 % was shown after 1 month of topical mupirocin sinus irrigations [40], while higher resistance rates of 11–65 % have been reported in areas of widespread topical mupirocin use [41–44].

Topical mupirocin is available as either a 2 % ointment or cream, both being formulated with polyethylene glycol base. While the cream is more water soluble, the ointment will dissolve in saline if mixed vigorously (Fig. 14.1). Since the cream is significantly more expensive, the ointment is more commonly used. Mupirocin irrigations have been formulated most commonly as 0.05 % solutions. This can be achieved by dissolving 120 mg of mupirocin into 240 mL of saline, often in a positive-pressure squeeze bottle. It is usually administered twice daily, for about a month [28, 29]. The effective mupirocin concentration of 500 μg/mL is significantly greater than the MIC and MBC of both *S. aureus* and MRSA.

Mupirocin irrigations have shown promising results in several in vivo studies of CRS patients with *S. aureus* and MRSA-positive recalcitrant CRS. Solares et al. retrospectively reviewed their use of topical mupirocin irrigations to treat 42 MRSA-related CRS exacerbations in 24 patients. They used a 22 g/L (0.02 %) solution, administering 50 mL twice daily for 4–6 weeks, either alone or in combination with oral antibiotics. Although topical mupirocin resulted in symptomatic improvement for 67 % of cases, 50 % of patients experienced symptom recurrence during the mean follow-up period of 11.8 months. The authors concluded that while the benefit from topical mupirocin may be temporary, it may be a less morbid alternative than IV antibiotic therapy for MRSA-positive CRS exacerbations [32].

Uren et al. performed a small prospective, observational cohort pilot study of 16 recalcitrant CRS patients, evaluating the effects of 0.05 % mupirocin irrigations twice daily for 3 weeks in patients with *S. aureus*-positive refractory CRS. Fifteen patients demonstrated *S. aureus* culture negativity at the conclusion of treatment, implying mupirocin irrigations were effective at eradicating the planktonic forms of *S. aureus*. Patients also had improved endoscopic and overall symptom scores with minimal adverse effects. No long-term follow-up was performed [28].

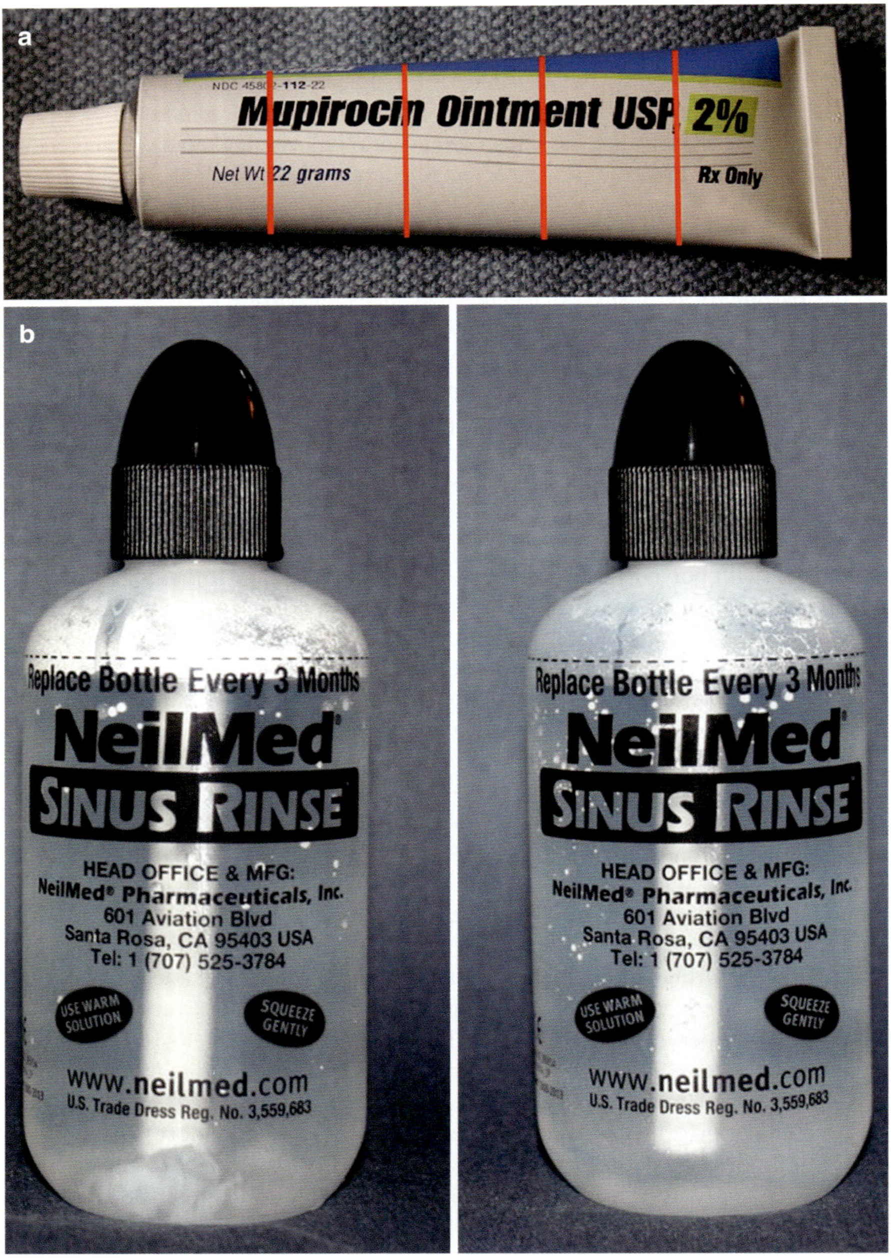

Fig. 14.1 (**a**) 22 g tube of mupirocin ointment. For each use, approximately one-fourth of a tube (110 mg) can be mixed into 240 mL of saline in a squeeze bottle to create nearly a 0.05 % solution. (**b**) Mupirocin ointment initially precipitates out in a saline squeeze bottle (*left*), but dissolves after vigorous mixing and can be used to perform sinus irrigations (*right*)

Jervis-Bardy et al. recently performed a retrospective review of 57 recalcitrant CRS patients treated with 0.05 % mupirocin nasal irrigations for 1 month and followed them long term. These patients had a 73.7 % rate of *S. aureus* positivity on repeat culture, with a mean relapse time of 144 days. Sensitivities from the repeat cultures revealed only 1 patient developed mupirocin resistance, for an overall resistance rate of 2.4 % [40].

Jervis-Bardy et al. also conducted a double-blinded RCT utilizing mupirocin irrigations. Twenty-five *S. aureus*-positive recalcitrant CRS patients with persistent symptoms after ESS were administered either 0.05 % topical mupirocin or placebo saline irrigations for 1 month. The mupirocin treatment group showed a culture negativity rate of 89 %, compared with 0 % of controls. They also showed both symptomatic and endoscopic improvement compared to controls. At a 3-month follow-up visit, while cultures remained negative in 85 % of patients, prior symptomatic and endoscopic improvement had deteriorated to baseline [29].

Although high-volume mupirocin irrigations have demonstrated promising results in *S. aureus*-positive recalcitrant CRS, reinfection is common and further research is needed to determine its role in managing CRS patients.

Aminoglycosides

Aminoglycosides demonstrate bacteriostatic and bactericidal activity against many aerobic gram-positive and gram-negative bacteria, due to both bacterial 30S ribosome inhibition and bacterial cell wall disruption. Aminoglycosides lack activity against anaerobes. Tobramycin and gentamicin have been employed most commonly in the treatment of CRS, although some earlier studies used neomycin. These topical agents have been used both empirically and for *P. aeruginosa*-positive CRS exacerbations and have been formulated as either nebulized sprays or high-volume irrigations.

An in vivo study in rabbits by Chiu et al. assessed the response of *P. aeruginosa* biofilms in rabbit maxillary sinuses to topical tobramycin irrigations through a maxillary sinus catheter. At standard therapeutic concentrations (80× MIC), topical tobramycin was effective against planktonic bacteria, but could not eradicate biofilms, even at significantly higher concentrations (400× MIC) [45].

Sykes et al. performed the first double-blinded RCT of intranasal topical antibiotics for CRS. Fifty CRS patients were randomized to receive one of three empiric treatment regimens by nasal spray delivery: dexamethasone and tramazoline with neomycin, dexamethasone and tramazoline without neomycin, or a placebo of propellant alone. Patients administered the medication as a metered-dose spray four times daily for 2 weeks. Both of the treatment groups showed improvement over placebo, but there was no significant difference in outcomes between the two treatment groups [25].

Moss and King performed a nonrandomized controlled trial with 51 cystic fibrosis patients with recalcitrant CRS and treated them with either a combination of surgery and postoperative tobramycin irrigations ($n=32$) or surgery alone ($n=19$).

Through maxillary sinus catheters placed intraoperatively, patients with positive *P. aeruginosa* cultures were administered 1 mL (40 mg) of tobramycin per side three times daily for the first 7–10 postoperative days. Thereafter the catheters were removed, but the patients still received 1 mL of tobramycin irrigations directly into the maxillary sinus by way of a curved suction under endoscopic guidance at monthly follow-up visits. A statistically significant decrease in nasal polyposis and the need for revision surgery were reported in the tobramycin surgery group (22 %) versus controls (72 %) [30].

Desrosiers et al. performed an RCT with 20 recalcitrant CRS patients who had failed medical and surgical intervention. Patients were randomized into one of two treatment groups: nebulized tobramycin (4 mL, three times daily for 4 weeks) or nebulized saline-quinine placebo. No differences in postoperative symptom or quality of life scores were found between the tobramycin and placebo groups [26].

Wei et al. evaluated 40 pediatric CRS patients, only evaluating patients who had not undergone sinus surgery. Patients received either gentamicin/saline irrigation or saline placebo irrigation (40 mL daily × 6 weeks). While both groups of patients improved symptomatically, no differences were noted between the groups [34].

Minor side effects from topical nasal aminoglycoside use have been reported. Vaughan and Carvalho reported sore throat and cough after nebulized tobramycin in 7–10 % of patients [27]. Desrosiers et al. also reported a significantly higher rate of nasal congestion with nebulized tobramycin compared with placebo [26]. There have also been concerns raised with topical aminoglycoside use and the potential for nephrotoxicity and ototoxicity. Two small pilot studies demonstrated that gentamicin was detectable in serum after nasal irrigations, though no otologic or renal complications occurred [35, 46]. While the serum levels in those studies were considered nontoxic, there have been reports of nontoxic serum levels still leading to ototoxicity and, therefore, remains a potential concern with these antibiotics.

Other Topical Antibiotics

Ceftazidime is a third-generation cephalosporin with broad-spectrum activity against *S. aureus* and *P. aeruginosa*. Leonard et al. reported retrospectively on 50 recalcitrant CRS patients treated with 0.1 % ceftazidime irrigations (300 mL, three times daily). Both symptomatic and endoscopic improvements were noted [36].

Videler et al. treated 14 patients with *S. aureus*-positive recalcitrant CRS with either nebulized bacitracin-colimycin or saline for 8 weeks, following 2 weeks of oral levofloxacin. While both the nebulized antibiotic and saline groups improved in symptom and quality of life scores, no significant difference was demonstrated between the two treatment groups [47].

Other antibiotics have been formulated into topical solutions, although in vitro studies have shown that *S. aureus* is less susceptible to many of these agents. For example, the MICs for vancomycin and ciprofloxacin were found to be >1,000 μg/mL [13], and moxifloxacin was found to be effective at lowering *S. aureus* counts only when formulated as a concentration 1,000× the MIC [10].

Reviews of Topical Antibiotic Used for CRS

Three systematic reviews have been conducted recently to assess the efficacy of topical antibiotics in the management of CRS. Lim et al. reviewed nine studies on topical antibiotic use, though only 1 RCT was available. Uncontrolled studies showed clinical improvements in CRS patients receiving topical antibiotics, with most benefit being noted for postsurgical patients, culture-directed therapy, and higher-volume delivery. The authors concluded that topical antibiotics should not be first-line management but may be attempted in patients refractory to oral antibiotics and traditional topical steroids [48].

Rudmik et al. reviewed 3 RCTs that assessed topical neomycin spray, nebulized tobramycin, or nebulized bacitracin-colimycin, and they also evaluated the review by Lim et al. [31]. Soler et al. reviewed nine studies on topical antibiotic use, of which three were RCTs. A wide variety of antibiotic classes were studied across the studies reviewed, as well as a wide variety of delivery methods [11]. This review was the only review that evaluated the study on mupirocin irrigations by Uren et al. [28], but did not review the mupirocin RCT by Jervis-Bardy et al. [29]. Both reviews by Rudmik et al. and Soler et al. reached similar conclusions that, based on current levels of evidence, topical antibiotics cannot be recommended for routine use in CRS. However, they may still play a role in certain subsets of recalcitrant CRS [11, 31].

Intravenous Antibiotics in CRS

Long-term broad-spectrum IV antibiotic therapy for select CRS patient populations became possible with the advent of peripherally inserted central catheter (PICC) lines. Benefits of outpatient IV antibiotics include improved patient convenience and decreased health care costs by avoiding inpatient hospital stays [49]. Outpatient IV antibiotic therapy has been considered by some authors as an alternative to surgery for specific populations of refractory CRS patients who have failed oral antibiotics and who do not meet criteria for inpatient hospitalization. Given the 100 % bioavailability of IV antibiotic therapy, higher local tissue concentrations of the antibiotic can be achieved within the sinuses, allowing for a more bactericidal effect. Gross et al. proposed the following indications be met before initiating outpatient IV antibiotic therapy for CRS: (1) resistance developed to oral antibiotics, (2) patient intolerance of oral antibiotics, (3) extrasinus complications of CRS, and (4) patients who either are poor surgical candidates or refuse to undergo surgery [12]. In addition to these indications, other authors have advocated for long-term IV antibiotic therapy for CRS patients with evidence of "osteitis" or hyperostosis due to bony sinus wall remodeling in CRS [50]. Given the image-based and histopathologic similarities between hyperostotic CRS and chronic osteomyelitis, these authors have advocated for 4–6 week courses of IV antibiotics, as would be prescribed commonly for osteomyelitis [51].

Anand et al. conducted a prospective uncontrolled cohort study of 52 recalcitrant CRS patients diagnosed with hyperostotic sinusitis or "osteitis" on CT scan. Patients were either not surgical candidates or refused to undergo sinus surgery. Patients were administered 6 weeks of IV antibiotics, and 21 different antibiotic combinations were utilized. For outcomes, they only measured pre- and posttreatment patient-reported subjective symptom scores. They did find a statistically significant improvement in all 15 symptoms evaluated 3 weeks after the completion of therapy. There was no control or other treatment group to which IV antibiotics were compared [50].

Fowler et al. conducted a retrospective review of 31 adult CRS patients treated with IV antibiotics. Twenty-four of the patients had undergone prior FESS. When available, IV antibiotic choice was culture directed. In the absence of a positive culture, ceftriaxone was administered. Only 29 % of patients (9/31) achieved resolution as defined by CT scan, nasal endoscopy, or both. Eighty-nine percent of patients (8/9) who achieved resolution relapsed within a mean of 11.5 weeks [52].

While only one uncontrolled study has supported the use of IV antibiotics for CRS, multiple studies have reported high rates of complications with outpatient IV antibiotics. Complications can be grouped into PICC line-related and antibiotic-related complications. PICC-related complications include thrombophlebitis, deep venous thrombosis, catheter occlusion, or catheter dislodgement. Antibiotic-related complications include pruritus, rash, fever, neutropenia, elevated liver enzymes, pseudomembranous colitis, and anaphylaxis. Anand et al. reported complications in 16 % of patients, including elevations in liver function enzymes, neutropenia/septicemia, bleeding, and rash [50]. Fowler et al. reported a 26 % incidence of complications that required discontinuing therapy, including PICC line-related infections, deep venous thrombosis, and acute drug reactions [52]. Lin et al. conducted the largest review of complication rates for outpatient IV antibiotic therapy for CRS. In this retrospective review of 177 patients, 18 % of patients developed a treatment-related complication, 16 % related to the antibiotic and 2 % due to the PICC line, the majority of which required a change in therapy [53].

A recent systematic review by Soler et al. reviewed all of the aforementioned studies on IV antibiotic use and concluded that, given the preponderance of harm over benefit, IV antibiotic use should not be recommended in CRS patients [11].

Conclusion

Topical antibiotics should not be considered a first-line treatment for routine CRS. Patients with recalcitrant CRS may benefit symptomatically from culture-directed topical antibiotic therapy, but such therapy should only be considered in postsurgical patients and should be delivered by high-volume irrigations rather than by nebulizers or sprays. Depending on the culture sensitivities in recalcitrant CRS cases, mupirocin should be considered the agent of choice for *S. aureus*-positive CRS, while tobramycin, gentamicin, or ceftazidime should be considered for *P. aeruginosa*-positive CRS. Larger RCTs comparing specific topical antibiotic regimens, delivery methods, and culture-directed versus empiric therapies in postoperative patients are still necessary to establish treatment regimens that yield the most consistent and optimal outcomes for recalcitrant CRS patients.

IV antibiotic use in CRS should be limited to acute exacerbations leading to intracranial or intraorbital complications, in patients with culture-proven resistance to appropriate alternative oral antibiotics, or in patients who are unable to or refuse to undergo surgery. Otherwise, given the paucity of supporting evidence and the high incidence of significant complications, routine use of IV antibiotic therapy in CRS is not recommended.

References

1. Cohen NA. Sinonasal mucociliary clearance in health and disease. Ann Otol Rhinol Laryngol. 2006;196:20–6.
2. Kern RC, Conley DB, Walsh W, Chandra R, Kato A, Tripathi-Peters A, et al. Perspectives on the etiology of chronic rhinosinusitis: an immune barrier hypothesis. Am J Rhinol. 2008;22:549–59.
3. Aurora R, Chatterjee D, Hentzleman J, Prasad G, Sindwani R, Sanford T. Contrasting the microbiomes from healthy volunteers and patients with chronic rhinosinusitis. JAMA Otolaryngol Head Neck Surg. 2013;139:1328–38.
4. Fokkens WJ, Lund VJ, Mullol J, Bachert C, Isam Alobid I, Baroody F, et al. European position paper on rhinosinusitis and nasal polyps. Rhinol Suppl. 2012;23:1–298.
5. Cryer J, Schipor I, Perloff JR, et al. Evidence of bacterial biofilms in human chronic sinusitis. ORL J Otorhinolaryngol Relat Spec. 2004;66:155–8.
6. Ferguson BJ, Stolz DB. Demonstration of biofilm in human bacterial chronic rhinosinusitis. Am J Rhinol. 2005;19:452–7.
7. Psaltis AJ, Ha KR, Beule AG, Tan LW, Wormald PJ. Confocal scanning laser microscopy evidence of biofilms in patients with chronic rhinosinusitis. Laryngoscope. 2007;117:1302–6.
8. Suh JD, Ramakrishnan V, Palmer JN. Biofilms. Otolaryngol Clin North Am. 2010;43:521–30.
9. Ceri H, Olson ME, Stremick C, Read R, Morck D, Buret A. The calgary biofilm device: new technology for rapid determination of antibiotic susceptibilities of bacterial biofilms. J Clin Microbiol. 1999;37:1771–6.
10. Desrosiers M, Bendouah Z, Barbeau J. Effectiveness of topical antibiotics on *Staphylococcus aureus* biofilm in vitro. Am J Rhinol. 2007;21:149–53.
11. Soler ZM, Oyer SL, Kern RC, Senior BA, Kountakis SE, Marple BF, et al. Antimicrobials and chronic rhinosinusitis with or without polyposis in adults: an evidenced-based review with recommendations. Int Forum Allergy Rhinol. 2013;3:31–47.
12. Gross ND, McInnes RJA, Hwang PH. Outpatient intravenous antibiotics for chronic rhinosinusitis. Laryngoscope. 2002;112:1758–61.
13. Ha KR, Psaltis AJ, Butcher AR, Wormald PJ, Tan LW. In vitro activity of mupirocin on clinical isolates of *Staphylococcus aureus* and its potential implications in chronic rhinosinusitis. Laryngoscope. 2008;118:535–40.
14. Bhattacharyya N, Kepnes LJ. The microbiology of recurrent rhinosinusitis after endoscopic sinus surgery. Arch Otolaryngol Head Neck Surg. 1999;125:1117–20.
15. Brook I, Frazier EH. Correlation between microbiology and previous sinus surgery in patients with chronic maxillary sinusitis. Ann Otol Rhinol Laryngol. 2001;110:148–51.
16. Bendouah Z, Barbeau J, Hamad WA, Desrosiers M. Biofilm formation by *Staphylococcus aureus* and *Pseudomonas aeruginosa* is associated with an unfavorable evolution after surgery for chronic sinusitis and nasal polyposis. Otolaryngol Head Neck Surg. 2006;134:991–6.
17. Jervis-Bardy J, Foreman A, Field J, Wormald PJ. Impaired mucosal healing and infection associated with *Staphylococcus aureus* after endoscopic sinus surgery. Am J Rhinol Allergy. 2009;23:549–52.

18. Singhal D, Psaltis AK, Foreman A, Wormald PJ. The impact of biofilms on outcomes after endoscopic sinus surgery. Am J Rhinol. 2010;24:169–74.
19. Desrosiers M. Refractory chronic rhinosinusitis: pathophysiology and management of chronic rhinosinusitis persisting after endoscopic sinus surgery. Curr Allergy Asthma Rep. 2004;4:200–7.
20. Harvey RJ, Schlosser RJ. Local drug delivery. Otolaryngol Clin North Am. 2009;42:829–45.
21. Snidvongs K, Chaowanapanja P, Aeumjaturapat S, Chusakul S, Praweswararat P. Does nasal irrigation enter paranasal sinuses in chronic rhinosinusitis? Am J Rhinol. 2008;22:483–6.
22. Harvey RJ, Goddard JC, Wise SK, Schlosser RJ. Effects of endoscopic sinus surgery and delivery device on cadaver sinus irrigation. Otolaryngol Head Neck Surg. 2008;139:137–42.
23. Singhal D, Weitzel EK, Lin E, Feldt B, Kriete B, McMains KC, et al. Effect of head position and surgical dissection on sinus irrigant penetration in cadavers. Laryngoscope. 2010;120:2528–31.
24. Beule A, Athanasiadis T, Athanasiadis E, Field J, Wormald PJ. Efficacy of different techniques of sinonasal irrigation after modified lothrop procedure. Am J Rhinol Allergy. 2009;23:85–90.
25. Sykes DA, Wilson R, Chan KL, et al. Relative importance of antibiotic and improved clearance in topical treatment of chronic mucopurulent rhinosinusitis. A controlled study. Lancet. 1986;2:359–60.
26. Desrosiers MY, Salas-Prato M. Treatment of chronic rhinosinusitis refractory to other treatments with topical antibiotic therapy delivered by means of a large-particle nebulizer: results of a controlled trial. Otolaryngol Head Neck Surg. 2001;125:265–9.
27. Vaughan WC, Carvalho G. Use of nebulized antibiotics for acute infections in chronic sinusitis. Otolaryngol Head Neck Surg. 2002;127:558–68.
28. Uren B, Psaltis A, Wormald PJ. Nasal lavage with mupirocin for the treatment of surgically recalcitrant chronic rhinosinusitis. Laryngoscope. 2008;118:1677–80.
29. Jervis-Bardy J, Boase S, Psaltis A, Foreman A, Wormald PJ. A randomized trial of mupirocin sinonasal rinses versus saline in surgically recalcitrant staphylococcal chronic rhinosinusitis. Laryngoscope. 2012;122:2148–53.
30. Moss RB, King VV. Management of sinusitis in cystic fibrosis by endoscopic surgery and serial antimicrobial lavage. Reduction in recurrence requiring surgery. Arch Otolaryngol Head Neck Surg. 1995;121:566–72.
31. Rudmik L, Hoy M, Schlosser RJ, Harvey RJ, Welch KC, Lund V, et al. Topical therapies in the management of chronic rhinosinusitis: an evidence-based review with recommendations. Int Forum Allergy Rhinol. 2013;3:281–98.
32. Solares CA, Batra PS, Hall GS, Citardi MJ. Treatment of chronic rhinosinusitis exacerbations due to methicillin-resistant *Staphylococcus aureus* with mupirocin irrigations. Am J Otolaryngol. 2006;27:161–5.
33. Elliott KA, Stringer SP. Evidence-based recommendations for antimicrobial nasal washes in chronic rhinosinusitis. Am J Rhinol. 2006;20:1–6.
34. Wei JL, Sykes KJ, Johnson P, He J, Mayo MS. Safety and efficacy of once-daily nasal irrigation for the treatment of pediatric chronic rhinosinusitis. Laryngoscope. 2011;121:1989–2000.
35. Whatley WS, Chandra RK, MacDonald CB. Systemic absorption of gentamicin nasal irrigations. Am J Rhinol. 2006;20:251–4.
36. Leonard DW, Bolger WE. Topical antibiotic therapy for recalcitrant sinusitis. Laryngoscope. 1999;109:668–70.
37. Sutherland R, Boon RJ, Griffin KE, Masters PJ, Slocombe B, White AR. Antibacterial activity of mupirocin (pseudomonic acid), a new antibiotic for topical use. Antimicrob Agents Chemother. 1985;27:495–8.
38. Chapnick EK, Gradon JD, Kreiswirth B, Lutwick LI, Schaffer BC, Schiano TD, et al. Comparative killing kinetics of methicillin-resistant *Staphylococcus aureus* by bacitracin or mupirocin. Infect Control Hosp Epidemiol. 1996;17:178–80.

39. Ward A, Campoli-Richards DM. Mupirocin: a review of its antibacterial activity, pharmacokinetic properties and therapeutic use. Drugs. 1986;32:425–44.
40. Jervis-Bardy J, Wormald PJ. Microbiological outcomes following mupirocin nasal washes for symptomatic, *Staphylococcus aureus* positive chronic rhinosinusitis following endoscopic sinus surgery. Int Forum Allergy Rhinol. 2012;2:111–5.
41. Miller MA, Dascal A, Portnoy J, Mendelson J. Development of mupirocin resistance among methicillin-resistant *Staphylococcus aureus* after widespread use of nasal mupirocin ointment. Infect Control Hosp Epidemiol. 1996;17:811–3.
42. Vivoni AM, Santos KR, de-Oliveira MP, Giambiagi-deMarval M, Ferreira AL, Riley LW, et al. Mupirocin for controlling methicillin-resistant Staphylococcus aureus: lessons from a decade of use at a university hospital. Infect Control Hosp Epidemiol. 2005;26:662–7.
43. Vasquez JE, Walker ES, Franzus BW, Overbay BK, Reagan DR, Sarubbi FA. The epidemiology of mupirocin resistance among methicillin-resistant *Staphylococcus aureus* at a Veterans' Affairs hospital. Infect Control Hosp Epidemiol. 2000;21:459–64.
44. Walker ES, Levy F, Shorman M, David G, Abdalla J, Sarubbi FA. A decline in mupirocin resistance in methicillin-resistant *Staphylococcus aureus* accompanied administrative control of prescriptions. J Clin Microbiol. 2004;42:2792–5.
45. Chiu AG, Antunes MB, Palmer JN, Cohen NA. Evaluation of the in vivo efficacy of topical tobramycin against *Pseudomonas* sinonasal biofilms. J Antimicrob Chemother. 2007;59:1130–4.
46. Wong KK, Marglani O, Westerberg BD, Javer AR. Systemic absorption of topical gentamicin sinus irrigation. J Otolaryngol. 2008;37:395–8.
47. Videler WJM, van Drunen CM, Reitsma JB, Fokkens WJ. Nebulized bacitracin/colimycin: a treatment option in recalcitrant chronic rhinosinusitis with *Staphylococcus aureus*? A double-blind, randomized, placebo-controlled, cross-over pilot study. Rhinology. 2008;46:92–8.
48. Lim M, Citardi MJ, Leong JL. Topical antimicrobials in the management of chronic rhinosinusitis: a systematic review. Am J Rhinol. 2008;22:381–9.
49. Balinsky W, Nesbitt S. Cost-effectiveness of outpatient parenteral antibiotics: a review of the literature. Am J Med. 1989;87:301–5.
50. Anand V, Levine H, Friedman M, et al. Intravenous antibiotics for refractory rhinosinusitis in nonsurgical patients: preliminary findings of a prospective study. Am J Rhinol. 2003;17:363–8.
51. Salvati E, Small R, Brause B, et al. Infections associated with orthopedic devices. In: Sugarman B, Young E, editors. Infections associated with prosthetic devices. Boca Raton: CRC Press; 1984. p. 181–218.
52. Fowler KC, Duncavage JA, Murray JJ, Tanner S. Chronic sinusitis and intravenous antibiotic therapy: resolution, recurrence, and adverse events. J Allergy Clin Immunol. 2003;111:S85.
53. Lin JW, Kacker A, Anand VK, Leviene H. Catheter and antibiotic-related complications of ambulatory intravenous antibiotic therapy for chronic refractory rhinosinusitis. Am J Rhinol. 2005;19:365–9.

Oral Corticosteroids

15

David M. Poetker

Key Take-Home Points

- Corticosteroids decrease inflammation by stabilizing lysosomal membranes, decreasing inflammatory mediator release, and decreasing the capillary permeability.
- Limited data exists to support the use of corticosteroids in CRS, though CRS with nasal polyps has been shown to provide short-term improvement both subjectively and objectively.
- Corticosteroids are associated with psychiatric, ophthalmic, endocrine, infectious, and orthopedic complications.
- Use of corticosteroids must balance the expected benefit with the potential harm.

Introduction

Corticosteroids, such as prednisone, cortisone, dexamethasone, prednisolone, and methylprednisolone, are commonly used in otolaryngology for their anti-inflammatory effects. They are all synthetic chemicals designed to mimic the effects of cortisol, a steroid hormone produced in the cortex of the adrenal gland.

Corticosteroids, particularly prednisone, are commonly used in the armamentarium of otolaryngologists for the management of chronic rhinosinusitis (CRS). Their use has been reported anecdotally and documented through various surveys. A survey of the American Academy of Otolaryngology – Head and Neck Surgery members reported on 80 respondents. Thirty-six percent

D.M. Poetker, MD, MA
Department of Otolaryngology, Zablocki VA Medical Center, Medical College of Wisconsin, 9200 W. Wisconsin Avenue, Milwaukee, WI 53226, USA
e-mail: dpoetker@mcw.edu

P.S. Batra, J.K. Han (eds.), *Practical Medical and Surgical Management of Chronic Rhinosinusitis*, DOI 10.1007/978-3-319-16724-4_15

considered oral steroids part of "maximal medical therapy" for CRS [1]. A follow-up survey of the American Rhinologic Society reported on their members' use of corticosteroids. Of the 308 respondents, 51.5 % used corticosteroids more than half the time to treat CRS and about 10 % "always" used corticosteroids for CRS. Doses started, on average, at 50 mg of prednisone per day and ranged from 10 to 120 mg of prednisone daily. The usual duration was between 6 and 14 days [2].

Corticosteroid Mechanism of Action

Inflammation can result from some sort of insult or trauma to the tissues. This can be in the form of direct injury such as physical trauma or insult as a response to a stimulus such as an infection. The basic tenets of inflammation include release of inflammatory mediators such as histamine, bradykinin, proteolytic enzymes, prostaglandins, and leukotrienes from the damaged tissue, increased blood flow to the involved area, increased capillary permeability causing leakage of plasma into the tissues, and infiltration of the area by white blood cells.

Corticosteroids address the inflammation by both preventing the early stages of inflammation and speeding the resolution of chronic inflammation [3]. Corticosteroids stabilize lysosomal membranes, thereby decreasing the quantity of the proteolytic enzymes and other inflammatory mediators. They reduce the capillary permeability, thus decreasing the plasma in tissues. The migration of leukocytes into the inflamed areas is decreased as is the overall number of eosinophils and lymphocytes. Corticosteroids also decrease prostaglandin and leukotriene formation. Finally, corticosteroids can reduce body temperature (fevers), resulting in reduced formation of interleukin-1 and reduced vasodilation in the inflamed areas.

When taken orally, prednisone has a bioavailability of 92 %. It is metabolized in the liver to its active metabolite, prednisolone. The half-life is about 3 h, with the duration of effect lasting about 12 h. The potency of oral corticosteroids is frequently compared to the natural corticosteroid, cortisol. Cortisone is slightly less potent than cortisol. Prednisone is about four times more potent, while methylprednisolone is about five times more potent than cortisol. Dexamethasone is a very potent drug, approximately 30 times more potent than cortisol and 7–8 times more potent than prednisone [3].

Side Effects of Corticosteroids

Corticosteroids are known to have extensive side effects. Many of these are dose and duration dependent, presenting with higher doses and prolonged courses of therapy. Thorough reviews of these effects exist in the literature; a cursory overview of the potential side effects of corticosteroids is presented here (Table 15.1) [4].

Table 15.1 Potential complications following oral corticosteroids [4]

Complication	Signs/symptoms	Notes
Psychiatric	Mild effects: agitation, anxiety, hypomania, insomnia, irritability, mood lability, and tearfulness	Incidence: 27.6 % (range 13–62 %)
	Severe reactions: mania, depression, mixed state	Incidence: 5.7 % (range 1.6–50 %)
		No correlation between psych history and a psych reaction
Ophthalmic	Cataracts	Usually requires months to years of use
	Glaucoma	Up to 5 % develop pressure increases within weeks
Hyperglycemia	Elevated blood sugars	Degree of elevation is variable
Infection	Bacterial, fungal, and viral infections	Multiple effects on leukocytes
		Usually requires prolonged courses
Gastrointestinal	Peptic ulceration	No conclusive evidence to support associations
		Gastritis symptoms common
Adrenal suppression	Multiple systemic effects, blood pressure changes, water retention, lack of stress response	Variability in the dose that can lead to suppression
		Incidence of clinically evident adrenal insufficiency is believed to be much lower than the incidence based on objective measures
Bone metabolism	Decrease bone density	Effect usually transient
	Avascular necrosis	Due to impaired perfusion of the bone
		Can present months after use

Psychiatric

The most common psychiatric manifestations include agitation, anxiety, hypomania, insomnia, irritability, mood lability, and tearfulness, reported to occur in 27.6 % (range 13–62 %) of individuals. Severe reactions include mania, depression, or a mixed state which have been reported in 5.7 % (range 1.6–50 %) [5, 6].

Corticosteroid dosage has been found to be the most significant risk factor associated with psychiatric reactions. When symptoms were analyzed based on dose, there was a 1.3 % incidence in those patients receiving a daily prednisone dose ≤40 mg, a 4.6 % incidence in those receiving 41–80 mg of prednisone, and a 18.4 % incidence in those receiving >80 mg [7]. Reduction of the dose resulted in resolution of symptoms in all cases. Past reactions are not predictive of a future reaction, nor is past tolerance predictive of future tolerance [5]. No correlation between a history of psychiatric illness and a psychiatric reaction to corticosteroids has been established [8].

Ophthalmic

Cataract formation and increased intraocular pressure (glaucoma) are the most commonly encountered ophthalmologic side effects. It has been proposed that steroid molecules bond covalently with the lysine residues of the lens, leading to opacities, or that corticosteroids inhibit the sodium-potassium pump in the lens, leading to coagulation of lens proteins. Most studies report doses of 10 mg or more daily for at least one year before the onset of cataract formation [9].

The exact mechanism by which corticosteroids cause glaucoma is unknown; corticosteroids may exert a negative impact on the trabecular meshwork, leading to fluid retention and elevated pressures. Between 18 and 36 % of the population will develop at least a moderate (5 mmHg or greater) increase in pressure with prolonged steroid treatment [10]. Risk factors include a history of open-angle glaucoma, diabetes mellitus, high myopia, rheumatoid arthritis, hypertension, migraine headaches, and first-degree relatives with open-angle glaucoma [9, 10].

Hyperglycemia

Corticosteroids increase blood sugars by increasing hepatic gluconeogenesis, decreasing glucose uptake in peripheral tissues, and decreasing the ability of adipocytes and hepatocytes to bind insulin. This effect can occur within hours of beginning therapy and tends to decrease with prolonged use [11]. Upon cessation of corticosteroids, the inhibition of glucose uptake and metabolism in peripheral tissues usually returns to normal [11].

Infection

The mechanism by which corticosteroids decrease inflammation may also lead to immunosuppressive effects. Although circulating neutrophils increase as a result of enhanced release from bone marrow and reduced migration from blood vessels, other leukocytes decrease due to migration from the vascular bed to the lymphoid tissue [12]. Corticosteroids impact neutrophil function by reducing their bactericidal activity as well as limit the function of macrophages and other antigen-presenting cells [12, 13].

A meta-analysis found that patients who received a daily dose of less than 10 mg per day or a cumulative dose of less than 700 mg of prednisone did not have an increased rate of infectious complications [14]. A second meta-analysis of over 8,700 patients reported bacterial sepsis occurred 1.5 times more frequently in patients using corticosteroids than in those using placebo ($P<0.01$). Mean daily dose was the equivalent of 35 mg of prednisone and the mean total dose was 2,200 mg of prednisone [15].

Gastrointestinal

Despite the commonly held perception that steroid use increases the risk of peptic ulcer disease, several large meta-analyses of randomized, placebo-controlled trials have failed to show this association [16], although the studies did find that patients using corticosteroids complained of peptic ulcer-type symptoms more frequently than control patients [15]. In addition to gastric issues, pancreatitis has been reported with the use of corticosteroids, though the exact incidence and the mechanism are unknown [17].

Adrenal Suppression

Exogenous steroids increase the circulating corticosteroid levels, which can lead to a negative feedback on the hypothalamic-pituitary-adrenal axis at the levels of both the hypothalamus and the pituitary gland. This effect can lead to a decrease production of both corticotropin-releasing hormone from the hypothalamus and corticotropin or adrenocorticotropic hormone from the pituitary gland [18]. Decreased production of adrenocorticotropic hormone then leads to decreased cortisol secretion from the adrenal cortex.

The dose of exogenous corticosteroids that can lead to adrenal suppression is highly variable. The incidence of clinically evident adrenal insufficiency is unknown, yet it is believed to be much lower than the incidence based on objective measures [17].

Bone Metabolism

The role of corticosteroids in bone loss is well described and may occur through several different mechanisms. They reduce intestinal calcium absorption and increase urinary calcium excretion. This stimulates parathyroid hormone which sacrifices bone mass, releasing calcium into the circulation [10, 19].

Corticosteroids also suppress the production of adrenal androgens and can cause apoptosis of osteoblasts and osteocytes. This effect can occur within 1 month of use; however it slows after 6–12 months and rapidly reverses with cessation of the corticosteroid [20, 21]. Several studies have demonstrated that supplemental calcium, vitamin D, and bisphosphonates can help reduce the steroid-induced bone loss [17].

Osteonecrosis

Corticosteroid use has been associated with avascular necrosis or osteonecrosis, usually in the head of the femur, although all bones may be affected [19]. The etiology is not completely understood but is due to impaired perfusion of the bone, either as a result of embolic events, hyperviscous blood, or increased pressure in the femoral head, resulting in decreased blood flow [19, 22, 23].

One review identified 15 patients treated with a single course of corticosteroids who developed osteonecrosis of the femoral head [24]. Ages ranged from 20 to 41 years (mean 32.2 years), mean cumulative dose was 850 mg of prednisone (range 290–3,300 mg), and the mean duration of therapy was 20.5 days (range 6–39 days). The mean time from treatment to symptoms in the study was 16.6 months (range

6–33). A second series of 1,352 patients treated with corticosteroids identified 4 cases of avascular necrosis, a risk of 0.3 % [25]. The mean age was 26 years (range 21–31), the mean cumulative dose was equivalent to 673 mg of prednisone (range 389–990 mg of prednisone equivalents), and the mean duration was 20 days (15–27 days). The time to onset of symptoms in this group ranged from 4 to 27 months, with a mean of 14.5 months.

Indications and Data on Use of Oral Corticosteroids

Despite the widespread use of corticosteroids in CRS, the data is remarkably lacking. Only four studies have evaluated the benefit of oral corticosteroids in patients with CRS without nasal polyps. Unfortunately, most include oral corticosteroids used in combination with other interventions such as antibiotics, topical steroids, and saline irrigations. Three of the four included CRS patients with and without nasal polyps.

The only study that evaluated the effect of oral corticosteroids alone on CRS symptoms was done by Ikeda et al. [26]. Twelve patients with CRS without nasal polyps, who had failed topical nasal steroids, underwent olfactory testing before and after a 10–14-day taper of prednisone. They found significant improvements in both detection and recognition thresholds following the prednisone course. Improved olfactory function occurred in ten patients with eight patients having persistent improvement for many months and only two reporting no improvement in olfactory function.

Lal and colleagues reported their series of 145 patients, 82 of whom had CRS without nasal polyps [27]. All patients received 4 weeks of antibiotics, a 12-day oral corticosteroid taper, nasal steroid sprays, topical decongestants, and saline irrigations. Fifty-five percent of the CRS without nasal polyp patients reported complete resolution of symptoms, while 45 % "failed" therapy, reporting persistent symptoms.

Subramanian et al. reported on 40 patients, 23 of whom had CRS without nasal polyps [28]. Patients reported significant improvements in symptom scores post-treatment and had significant improvements in the Lund-MacKay CT score post-treatment. The degree of benefit from each component of the therapy could not be identified.

A trend toward significant overall improvement in the SNOT-21 scores was found in 84 patients (50 CRS without nasal polyps) following a prednisone course for ≥11 days [29]. Patients received antibiotics, nasal steroids, antihistamines, anti-leukotrienes, herbal medications, and saline. They found no difference in the baseline or change in SNOT-21 scores in the patients with or without nasal polyps.

The data regarding the use of oral corticosteroids in CRS with nasal polyps is much stronger, with three randomized controlled trials. Hissaria and colleagues randomized 41 subjects to receive 50 mg of prednisolone or placebo daily for 14 days [30]. At the completion of the treatment, the steroid group showed a significant improvement over the placebo group in quality of life scores as well as nasal endoscopy and MRI.

A second study randomized 60 CRS with nasal polyp patients to receive 25 mg of prednisolone or placebo daily for 14 days [31]. The authors reported significant improvement in objective measures such as nasal endoscopy and subjective measures such as the mini Rhinoconjunctivitis Quality of Life Questionnaire following the oral corticosteroids.

The third study included 109 patients, randomized to receive 50 mg of prednisolone or placebo daily for 14 days [32]. Subjective symptoms significantly improved in the steroid group. The steroid group also had significant improvements in nasal endoscopy measures.

Many providers use oral corticosteroids perioperatively in patients with CRS. No data exists addressing the use of oral corticosteroids for CRS patients without nasal polyps, but there are two randomized controlled trials evaluating corticosteroids for CRS with nasal polyps in the perioperative period. The first study randomized 36 patients to receive prednisone or nothing for 5 days immediately preceding surgery. They found no significant difference in blood loss but significantly better visibility and shorter operative time in the steroid group [33]. The second study randomized 26 patients to either 30 mg of prednisone daily or placebo for 5 days immediately preoperative and 9 days postoperative [34]. They found no significant differences in operative time or blood loss. Postoperatively, they found a significant improvement in olfaction in the steroid group at 2 weeks and a clinically significant improvement in the endoscopic appearance of the sinus cavities after surgery.

Guideline Recommendations

The American Academy of Otolaryngology released a Clinical Practice Guidelines for Adult Sinusitis in 2007 [35]. They make no mention of the use of corticosteroids to treat CRS with or without polyps. The more recent European Position Paper on Rhinosinusitis and Nasal Polyps dedicated a section to the use of corticosteroids for both CRS and CRS with nasal polyps [36]. They highlight the lack of high-level data supporting the use of oral or systemic corticosteroids for CRS. They very nicely outline the existing data on systemic corticosteroids for the treatment of CRS with nasal polyps. The authors point out that the data supports the use of systemic corticosteroids in CRS with nasal polyps but denote the short-term benefit of steroids and suggest weighing the short-term benefits with the long-term potential for side effects.

A recent iterative review presented the data for the various indications for corticosteroids and CRS [37]. They presented the summation of the data and then gave recommendations based on the strength of that data. When evaluating the data for corticosteroids use in CRS without nasal polyps, they found the quality of the evidence was a “C” with four level 4 studies. The data showed subjective improvement in patient symptoms associated with CRS and objective improvement in imaging. Their recommendation for the use of oral corticosteroids in CRS without nasal polyps was “Optional” suggesting that patients with more severe disease may have a more favorable benefit to harm ratio than patients with mild disease.

The quality of evidence for the use of corticosteroids in CRS with nasal polyps was "A" with five level 2 studies and multiple additional level 3 and 4 studies. The data demonstrates significant short-term improvements in subjective and objective measures with relatively low risks. Their recommendation was a "Strong recommendation."

The review recommended providers consider the use of oral corticosteroids in the perioperative management of CRS patients with nasal polyps based on "B" evidence consisting of two level 2 studies and an additional level 3 study. Their review found the corticosteroids improved surgical visualization and may decrease operative time with a relatively low risk to patients. There was insufficient evidence to make a recommendation for corticosteroids in the perioperative period in CRS patients without nasal polyps.

Conclusion

Corticosteroids are commonly used to treat CRS despite the relatively limited data to support their use. They address inflammation by limiting inflammatory mediator release and decreasing capillary permeability. Many side effects and complications are associated with corticosteroid use. It is imperative that the practitioner be familiar with these to properly weigh the expected benefits to the potential risks.

References

1. Kaszuba SM, Stewart MG. Medical management and diagnosis of chronic rhinosinusitis: a survey of treatment patterns by United States otolaryngologists. Am J Rhinol. 2006;20:186–90.
2. Dubin MG, Liu C, Lin SY, Senior BA. American Rhinologic Society member survey on "maximal medical therapy" for chronic rhinosinusitis. Am J Rhinol. 2007;21:483–8.
3. Hall JE. Adrenocortical hormones. In: Hall JE, editor. Guyton and hall textbook of medical physiology. 12th ed. Philadelphia: Saunders Elsevier; 2011. p. 921–37.
4. Poetker DM, Reh DD. Complications in the use of systemic steroids for sinusitis. Otolaryngol Clin N Am. 2010;43:753–68.
5. Warrington TP, Bostwick JM. Psychiatric adverse effects of corticosteroids. Mayo Clin Proc. 2006;81:1361–7.
6. Lewis DA, Smith RE. Steroid-induced psychiatric syndromes. J Affect Disord. 1983;5:319–32.
7. The Boston Collaborative Drug Surveillance Program. Acute adverse reactions to prednisone in relation to dosage. Clin Pharmacol Ther. 1972;13:694–8.
8. Kershner P, Wang-Cheng R. Psychiatric side effects of steroid therapy. Psychosomatics. 1989;30:135–9.
9. Carnahan MC, Goldstein DA. Ocular complications of topical, peri-ocular, and systemic corticosteroids. Curr Opin Ophthalmol. 2000;11:478–83.
10. Allen DB, Bielory L, Derendorf H, Dluhy R, Colice GL, Szefler SJ. Inhaled corticosteroids: past lessons and future issues. J Allergy Clin Immunol. 2003;112:S1–40.
11. Hirsch IB, Paauw DS. Diabetes management in special situations. Endocrinol Metab Clin North Am. 1997;26:631–45.
12. Chrousos GP. Adrenocorticosteroids & adrenocortical antagonists. In: Katzung BG, editor. Basic & clinical pharmacology. 10th ed. New York: The McGraw-Hill Companies; 2007. p. 635–52.
13. Segal BH, Sneller MC. Infectious complications of immunosuppressive therapy in patients with rheumatic diseases. Rheum Dis Clin North Am. 1997;23:219–37.
14. Stuck AE, Minder CE, Frey FJ. Risk of infectious complications in patients taking glucocorticosteroids. Rev Infect Dis. 1989;11:954–63.

15. Conn HO, Poynard T. Corticosteroids and peptic ulcer: meta-analysis of adverse events during steroid therapy. J Intern Med. 1994;236:619–32.
16. McEvoy CE, Niewoehner DE. Adverse effects of corticosteroid therapy for COPD. Chest. 1997;111:732–43.
17. Fardet L, Kassar A, Cabane J, Flahault A. Corticosteroid-induced adverse events in adults. Drug Saf. 2007;30:861–81.
18. Ganong WF. The adrenal medulla & adrenal cortex. In: Ganong WF, editor. Review of medical physiology. 22nd ed. New York: The McGraw-Hill Companies; 2007. p. 356–81.
19. Keenan GF. Management of complications of glucocorticoid therapy. Clin Chest Med. 1997;18:507–20.
20. Ton FN, Gunawardene SC, Lee H, Neer RM. Effects of low-dose prednisone on bone metabolism. J Bone Miner Res. 2005;20:464–70.
21. van Staa TP, Leufkens HGM, Cooper C. The epidemiology of corticosteroid-induced osteoporosis: a meta-analysis. Osteoporos Int. 2002;13:777–87.
22. Cui Q, Wang G-J, Balian G. Steroid-induced adipogenesis in a pluripotential cell line from bone marrow. J Bone Joint Surg Am. 1997;79-A:1054–63.
23. Mirzai R, Chang C, Greenspan A, Gershwin ME. The pathogenesis of osteonecrosis and the relationship to corticosteroids. J Asthma. 1999;36:77–95.
24. McKee MD, Waddell JP, Kudo PA, Schemitsch EH, Richards RR. Osteonecrosis of the femoral head in men following short-course corticosteroid therapy: a report of 15 cases. CMAJ. 2001;164:205–6.
25. Wong GK, Poon WS, Chiu KH. Steroid-induced avascular necrosis of the hip in neurosurgical patients: epidemiological study. ANZ J Surg. 2005;75:409–10.
26. Ikeda K, Sakurada T, Suzaki Y, Takasaka T. Efficacy of systemic corticosteroid treatment for anosmia with nasal and paranasal sinus disease. Rhinology. 1995;33:162–5.
27. Lal D, Scianna JM, Stankiewicz JA. Efficacy of targeted medical therapy in chronic rhinosinusitis, and predictors of failure. Am J Rhinol Allergy. 2009;23:396–400.
28. Subramanian HN, Schechtman KB, Hamilos DL. A retrospective analysis of treatment outcomes and time to relapse after intensive medical treatment for chronic sinusitis. Am J Rhinol. 2002;16:303–12.
29. Hessler JL, Piccirillo JF, Fang D, et al. Clinical outcomes of chronic rhinosinusitis in response to medical therapy: results of a prospective study. Am J Rhinol. 2007;21:10–8.
30. Hissaria P, Smith W, Wormald PJ, et al. Short course of systemic corticosteroids in sinonasal polyposis: a double-blind, randomized, placebo-controlled trial with evaluation of outcome measures. J Allergy Clin Immunol. 2006;118:128–33.
31. Vaidyanathan S, Barnes M, Williamson P, Hopkinson P, Donnan PT, Lipworth B. Treatment of chronic rhinosinusitis with nasal polyposis with oral steroids followed by topical steroids: A randomized trial. Ann Intern Med. 2011;154:293–302.
32. Kirtsreesakul V, Wongsritrang K, Ruttanaphol S. Clinical efficacy of a short course of systemic steroids in nasal polyposis. Rhinology. 2011;49:525–32.
33. Sieskiewicz A, Olszewska E, Rogowski M, Grycz E. Preoperative corticosteroid oral therapy and intraoperative bleeding during functional endoscopic sinus surgery in patients with severe nasal polyposis: a preliminary investigation. Ann Otol Rhinol Laryngol. 2006;115:490–4.
34. Wright ED, Agrawal S. Impact of perioperative systemic steroids on surgical outcomes in patients with chronic rhinosinusitis with polyposis: evaluation with the novel Perioperative Sinus Endoscopy (POSE) scoring system. Laryngoscope. 2007;117(11 Pt 2 Suppl 115):1–28.
35. Rosenfeld RM, Andes D, Bhattacharyya N, Cheung D, Eisenberg S, et al. Clinical practice guideline: adult sinusitis. Otolarygol Head Neck Surg. 2007;137:S1–31.
36. Fokkens WJ, Lund VJ, Mullol J, Bachert C, Alobid I, Baroody F, et al. The european position paper on rhinosinusitis and nasal polyps 2012. Rhinol Suppl. 2012;23:1–299.
37. Poetker DM, Jakubowski LA, Lal D, Hwang PH, Wright ED, Smith TL. Oral corticosteroids in the management of adult chronic rhinosinusitis with and without nasal polyps: an evidence-based review with recommendations. Int Forum Allergy Rhinol. 2013;3:104–20.

Topical Steroids

16

Kevin C. Welch

Key Take-Home Points

- Steroids are potent anti-inflammatory medications that significantly improve subjective and objective findings in chronic sinusitis.
- Topical delivery systems provide an alternative means of delivering steroids to the sinuses, potentially without significant systemic side effects or reactions.
- There is strong evidence for the use of topical steroids in chronic sinusitis without polyps as well as chronic sinusitis with polyps.
- High-volume delivery systems (irrigations) appear to be more effective than low-volume systems (sprays, drops) in delivering topical steroids to the sinuses.
- Endoscopic sinus surgery can enhance delivery of topical steroids to the sinuses.

Introduction

The medical and surgical management of chronic rhinosinusitis (CRS) is ever evolving. Since the advent of endoscopic sinus surgery (ESS) [1] over 30 years ago, our capacity to manage medically refractory CRS has greatly expanded. An expanded understanding of the underlying pathophysiology of CRS has helped us recognize that some patients suffer from local and host factors that directly lead to mucosal inflammation that may not improve with appropriate medical and surgical

K.C. Welch, MD, FACS
Department of Otolaryngology – Head and Neck Surgery,
Feinberg School of Medicine, Northwestern University,
676 N. St. Clair Street, Suite 1325, Chicago, IL 60611, USA
e-mail: doctorkevinwelch@gmail.com

P.S. Batra, J.K. Han (eds.), *Practical Medical and Surgical Management of Chronic Rhinosinusitis*, DOI 10.1007/978-3-319-16724-4_16

management. These patients may suffer from persistent mucosal inflammation and inflammatory discharge or early recurrence when systemic therapy is ceased—despite widely patent sinus cavities.

The persistence of local inflammation has made the delivery of topical therapies an attractive therapeutic alternative to systemic medical therapy. With multiple options for delivery and decreased systemic side effects, topical therapy is now a hotbed for clinical research. In this chapter, the effectiveness of delivery devices will be explored as well as the data on outcomes of CRS treated with topical steroids.

Background

Synthetic steroids used in the treatment of CRS encompass a class of chemotherapeutic agents synthesized from animal or plant sources that are available in oral, intravenous, or topical preparations. When administered, steroids mediate their effects through endogenous cellular glucocorticoid receptors, which are bound to heat shock proteins. The heat shock proteins dissociate from the receptor, and the receptor complex is actively transported to the nucleus of the cell where it binds to glucocorticoid receptor elements on targeted genes where protein synthesis is ultimately modified by this action. Negative feedback through pituitary adrenocorticotropic hormone (ACTH) occurs to downregulate endogenous cortisol production.

Steroids reduce inflammation by mediating and downregulating leukocyte infiltration as well as their function, inhibiting cell-cell interaction via cell adhesion molecules, and while increasing neutrophil serum counts, lymphocyte movement from the vascular to the lymphatic compartment is reduced. The effect of steroids on gene transcription includes the increased production of IL-1 receptor antagonist and IL-1 decoy receptors, IL-10, annexin 1, and IκB-α (inhibits NF-κB) while simultaneously decreasing transcription of many interleukin cytokines, including IL-1, IL-2, IL-4, and IL-5; chemokines, such as RANTES, eotaxins, and IL-8; adhesion molecules, such as ICAM-1, VCAM-1, and E-selectin; and inflammatory mediators, such as iNOS and multiple other molecules [2].

Prevalence of Use

In a survey of the American Rhinologic Society members, Dubin et al. [3] reported on the use of steroids in the treatment of CRS. Over half of physicians surveyed reported using oral steroids in patients with CRS. Moreover, physicians reported using topical steroids in 97 % of cases. With such frequent usage, one would expect there to be overwhelming support for the use of topical steroids in CRS. Despite their frequent use, often in off-label uses, the efficacy of topical steroids in the management of CRS is not always unclear.

The American Academy of Allergy, Asthma and Immunology (AAAAI), and the American College of Allergy, Asthma, and Immunology (ACAAI) [4] have recommended that topical steroids be used in the treatment of CRS. Despite a lack of evidence at the time of this statement, given the overall improvement in symptoms and low side effect profile, their use was deemed "reasonable." A newer practice parameter guideline for CRS that is currently under review, however, gives a strong recommendation for the use of steroid nasal sprays in both CRS with nasal polyps (CRSwNP) and CRS without nasal polyps (CRSsNP).

The European Position Paper on Rhinosinusitis and Nasal Polyps in 2012 [5] provides an exhaustive review of the literature covering topical steroids for both CRSsNP and CRSwNP. Their statement includes level 1a evidence that topical steroids improve symptoms and patient-reported outcomes in CRSsNP, direct delivery to the sinuses effects greater change, and newer steroids are not superior to older steroids with respect to that effect. Other statements include level 2a evidence that topical steroids have a greater effect on patients who have undergone surgery and that side effects are minimal. The position on topical steroids for CRSwNP is essentially the same; however, the level of evidence for the use of topical steroids following surgery is 1a with a grade A recommendation.

While the Clinical Practice Guideline [6] released by the American Academy of Otolaryngology—Head and Neck Surgery Foundation discusses steroids at length for viral rhinosinusitis and acute bacterial rhinosinusitis, it offers no explicit recommendation for or against the use of topical steroids in CRSsNP or CRSwNP.

Methods of Delivery

There are five basic modes of delivery: pump sprays/metered-dose inhaler, nebulizer systems, drop delivery, high-volume/low-pressure bottle irrigation, and local delivery via biomaterials/implants. It is important to remember that the only FDA-approved methods for delivery are pump sprays/metered-dose inhalers or steroid-eluting implant.

Pump Sprays/Metered-Dose Inhaler

All FDA-approved steroids for routine topical administration to the nasal cavity and sinuses exist in aqueous or nonaqueous solutions delivered by either a pump spray or a metered-dose inhaler (See Table 16.1). These preparations provide daily to twice daily treatment in an easy-to-use and portable manner. Despite their frequent use in patients with CRS, none actually has an FDA-approved indication for use in initial medical management of CRS. Mometasone furoate monohydrate (Nasonex) is indicated, however, in the treatment of nasal polyps, and beclomethasone dipropionate (Beconase, Qnasl) is indicated in the treatment of recurrent polyps following surgical removal.

The ability to treat inflammation within the paranasal sinuses depends on the ability of the medication to reach the intended areas, and the distribution of medicated particles delivered by pump sprays or metered-dose inhalers has been

Table 16.1 Commonly prescribed nasal steroid spray preparations

Generic name	Trade name	Dose (mcg)	Delivery	FDA-approved indications
Beclomethasone dipropionate monohydrate	Beconase AQ	42	Aqueous spray	1. Seasonal and allergic rhinitis in adults 2. CRSwNP in adults
Beclomethasone dipropionate	Qnasl	80	Nonaqueous spray	Seasonal and perennial allergic rhinitis in adults and adolescents >12 year/o
Budesonide	Rhinocort AQ	32	Aqueous spray	Seasonal and perennial allergic rhinitis in patients >6 year/o
Ciclesonide	Omnaris	50	Aqueous spray	1. Seasonal allergic rhinitis in adults and children >6 year/o 2. Perennial allergic rhinitis in adults and children >12 year/o
Ciclesonide	Zetonna	37	Nonaqueous spray	Seasonal and perennial allergic rhinitis in adults and adolescents >12 year/o
Flunisolide	Nasalide	58	Aqueous spray	Seasonal and perennial allergic rhinitis
Fluticasone propionate	Flonase	50	Aqueous spray	1. Seasonal and perennial allergic rhinitis in patients >4 year/o 2. Non-allergic rhinitis in patients >4 year/o
Fluticasone furoate	Veramyst	27.5	Aqueous spray	Seasonal and perennial allergic rhinitis in patients >2 year/o
Mometasone furoate monohydrate	Nasonex	50	Aqueous spray	1. Seasonal and perennial allergic rhinitis in patients >2 year/o 2. Prophylaxis of seasonal allergic rhinitis in patients >12 year/o 3. CRSwNP in patients >18 year/o
Triamcinolone acetonide	Nasacort AQ	55	Aqueous spray	Seasonal and perennial allergic rhinitis in patients >2 year/o

extensively studied over the years. Several early studies [7–9] demonstrated that spray deposition occurred only in the anterior 1/3 of the nasal cavity, specifically regions of the vestibule, inferior turbinate, and nasal floor. These early studies imply that significant deposition to the middle meatus may not occur; thus standard pump delivery systems may be ineffective for CRS treatment. When volume of medication was increased to 50–100 μL [8], the likelihood of deposition beyond the anterior 1/3 of the nasal cavity was increased. Keyhani and colleagues [10] demonstrated that particle distribution into nasal airstreams depended on location of release with the most optimal delivery to the middle meatus occurring when the release point was anterior and lateral within the *naris*. This placement may facilitate flow into the middle meatus; however, whether particles deposited actually enter the sinuses themselves remained a question. Hyo et al. [11] determined that the optimal particle size varied with maxillary sinus ostium size. While 3–10 μm was found to be ideal for penetrating the sinus, only 3 % of those particles actually penetrated the sinus. Using a cast model study, Saijo and colleagues [12] demonstrated that both angle of release and particle size played significant roles in penetration of the ostiomeatal complex (OMC) and maxillary sinus following surgery. Computer simulations revealed a 45-degree angle improved deposition over a 30-degree angle and particles 5.63 μm in diameter were significantly more effective than particles 16.37 μm in diameter. Whether 5.63 μm or 16.37 μm, this particle diameter is notably smaller than the average droplet size (50–100 μm) [13] delivered with conventional pump release sprays, and this raises the question as to whether FDA-approved sprays for CRS deliver any significant medication to any of the paranasal sinuses.

Nebulizer Systems

Similar to nebulizer systems for managing asthma and other chronic pulmonary conditions, nebulizers deliver medications to the nose and paranasal sinuses in the form of an aerosolized mist or vapor. Nebulizers may be subdivided into passive-diffusion systems that produce smaller-sized particles that travel via lower velocity in a single direction and vortex-propelled systems that produce larger particles. Commercially available passive-diffusion systems include the SinuNeb™ (PARI Respiratory Equipment, Midlothian, VA), which generates particles <5 μm in diameter, relies on inspiration, and is subject to placement and the predicted pathways of nasal airflow. ViaNase™ (Kurve Technology, Inc, Lynnwood, WA) is an example of a vortex-propelled system that generates particles between 9 and 11 μm in diameter that are inhaled. Both passive-diffusion systems and vortex-propelled systems were studied by Hwang and coworkers [14] using radiolabeled saline. Sinus penetration was noted to be poor with both systems, although the vortex-propelled system showed greater frontal sinus (30 %) and sphenoid sinus (30 %) penetration. Endoscopic sinus surgery did not significantly enhance distribution.

As noted by Hyo and colleagues [11], particles between 3 and 10 μm were theorized to achieve maxillary sinus penetration, while Saijo and coworkers [12] demonstrated that smaller particles (5.63 μm v. 16.37 μm) *and* higher flow rate had improved maxillary sinus penetration; however, ostial size was noted to the biggest factor in sinus penetration. Therefore, a number of factors call into question the efficacy of many nebulizer systems as a method for treating CRS since particle size may be incompatible with significant sinus penetration and the method of particle generation may result in significant nasal cavity filtering.

Pulsating nebulizers such as RhinoFlow™ (Respironics, Inc., Cedar Grove, NJ) and NasoNeb™ (Medinvent, Medina, OH) generate large-sized particles (>10 μm, average 20–30 μm), which are large enough to be filtered by the nasal cavity and, based on previously mentioned studies, may be too large to penetrate the unoperated sinuses. Negley and coworkers [15] evaluated the effectiveness of the RhinoFlow™ system in a small sample of patients without CRS and found inconsistent delivery of Tc^{99m} into the sinuses. Whether surgery enhanced nebulizer delivery was tested by Manes and colleagues [16] who evaluated the NasoNeb nebulizer on five cadaver heads before and after ESS. This trial revealed consistent delivery of aerosolized saline with fluorescein to the middle meatus/ethmoid cavity and sphenoethmoidal recess. After cadavers underwent endoscopic sinus surgery, there was a significant improvement in delivery to middle meatus and to the maxillary sinus and ethmoid cavities. Delivery to the frontal sinus was enhanced by performing an endoscopic modified Lothrop.

Finally, Möller et al. [17] evaluated the distribution of ^{99m}Tc-DTPA in 11 patients with CRSsNP before and after endoscopic sinus surgery in patients using the Vibrent nebulizer (PARI Pharma GmbH, Starnberg, Germany), which generates 3.0 μm particles. Deposition in the nasal cavity as well as the paranasal sinuses was measured, and by at least 2 months following surgery, there was a significant decrease in total nasal deposition matched by a simultaneous significant increase in maxillary and sphenoid sinus deposition. An interesting and unexpected finding in their study was that the deposition of particles within the nasal cavity in healthy volunteers did not differ significantly from patients with CRSsNP, suggesting that in patients with CRSsNP, the nasal cavity is still an effective filter. They found evidence of deposition into the maxillary and sphenoid sinuses in patients with CRSsNP, which was also an unexpected finding.

Nebulizer devices vary in technology and delivery technique; however, it would seem that as a group, these devices do not consistently offer a reproducible and reliable means of delivering medications to the sinuses. Although a cadaveric study using the NasoNeb system appears promising, more studies on this device are required before definitive conclusions can be drawn.

Drop Delivery

Otologic or ophthalmic preparations of steroids have been used to treat CRS as well. Delivery of such low-volume drop medications to the sinuses depends heavily on technique, and a handful of studies have looked at the distribution of drops within the nasal cavity and sinuses. Kubba et al. [18] found that betamethasone delivery to the middle meatus was best achieved in the Mygind and "head down and forward position" positions and that the "head back" technique (See Fig. 16.1) resulted in nothing more than nasal floor and nasopharynx distribution. The Mygind position was recommended since it was generally viewed as more comfortable than the "head down and forward" position. The delivery of drops to the middle meatus may not be optimal, however, as evidenced by Homer and coworkers [19] who found that although the average amount of radiolabeled medication in middle meatus pledgets was higher in the patients using drops, it was not more significant than in those using a nasal spray device. In another study, Rudman and colleagues [20] utilized a cone beam scanner to evaluate the distribution of a radiopaque contrast solution via drop delivery when in the vertex-to-floor position. Contrast was not seen in areas superior to the middle turbinate; rather nasal cavity spaces such as the vestibule, inferior meatus, and anterior nasal cavity had the majority of distribution.

a
b
c
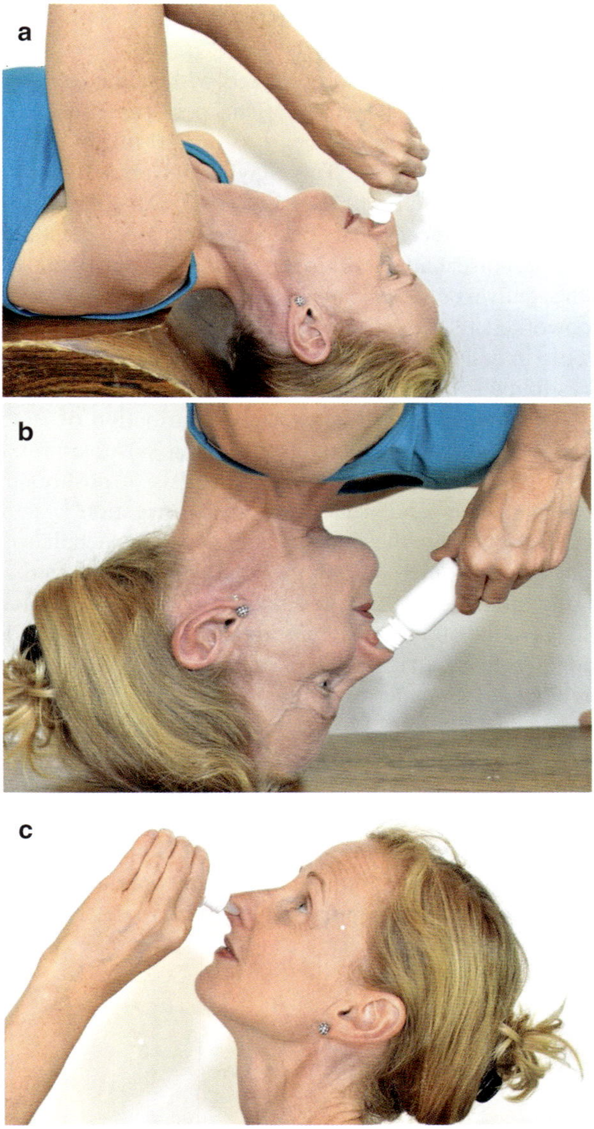

Fig. 16.1 This series of photographs depicts the administration of nasal drops via the Mygind (**a**), head down and forward position (**b**), and head-back (**c**) positions (Photo courtesy of David P. Welch)

Drug delivery via nasal drops appears to be very dependent upon head position, and given the low volume/high concentration of the drug delivered, accurate deposition within the sinuses may provide a viable means for treating some forms of CRS. However, the low volume raises cost issues since otologic and ophthalmic preparations of steroids.

High-Volume/Low-Pressure Bottle Irrigation

Aqueous preparations of steroids can be mixed with saline and used in commercially available bottle irrigation systems. Patients performing medicated irrigations typically add a steroid respule into either 120 or 240 mL of saline solution and irrigate the nasal cavity and sinuses. This may be performed via positive pressure (squeeze bottle) or gravity (neti pot) (See Fig. 16.2). This method of delivery has gained popularity over the recent years because of evidence demonstrating that the irrigant has the widest distribution within the unoperated and operated sinuses when compared to other delivery mechanisms.

Miller and coworkers [21] evaluated the effectiveness of a nebulizer, an atomizer, a spray, and a bulb in delivering dye to the sinuses in seven post-ESS patients. The bulb syringe was found to be the most effective method of delivery to all sinonasal sites. Similarly, Olson et al. [22] evaluated the distribution of isotonic, nonionic contrast material in eight healthy volunteers using positive-pressure irrigation, negative-pressure irrigation, and a nebulizer. Analysis of posttreatment CT scans demonstrated that positive- and negative-pressure irrigation systems resulted in more significant distribution to the sinuses compared to the nebulizer; moreover, the positive-pressure irrigation method provided the best results. Lam and colleagues [23] compared the effectiveness of spray bottles to irrigation bottles in delivering methylene blue dye to the olfactory regions in eight cadaveric heads. Based on blind review of staining patterns, irrigation bottles demonstrated greater penetration of the sphenoethmoidal recess, superior turbinate, and olfactory region.

Finally, Harvey and colleagues [24] evaluated the effects of ESS on sinus distribution of Gastroview in cadaver heads by using a pressurized spray, a neti pot, and a squeeze irrigation bottle. Distribution of Gastroview was significantly higher in the post-ESS cadaver head with the neti pot performing the best. The pressurized spray demonstrated the poorest sinus distribution. It is important to note, however, that even with extensive sinus distribution, the amount of retained irrigant within the sinuses is approximately 2.5 % [25], making it critical to determine the appropriate concentration or dosing of the delivery.

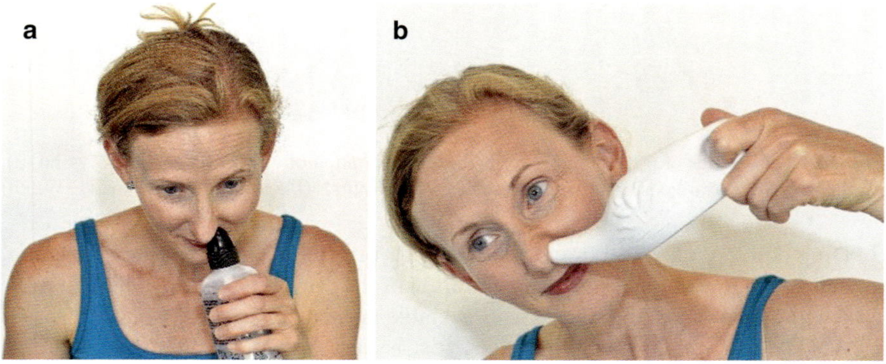

Fig. 16.2 This series of photographs depicts the administration of irrigation via a squeeze bottle (**a**) and neti pot (**b**) (Photo courtesy of David P. Welch)

Based on these studies, the use of a high-volume/low-pressure delivery system such as an irrigation bottle or neti pot allows one to deliver targeted therapy to multiple sinonasal subsites. Since ESS enhances delivery of irrigation bottle content to the sinuses, this represents an important adjunct in the postoperative period.

Biomaterials/Implants

The delivery of topical steroids may also be accomplished through the placement of biomaterials or implants into the sinonasal cavity following surgery. These delivery devices include FDA-approved biomaterials such as mometasone furoate (Propel®, Intersect ENT), which is placed within the ethmoid sinuses during surgery or in the office setting via a delivery catheter, as well as off-label delivery of steroids via temporary, self-absorbing dressings utilized as middle meatus spacers (Gelfoam, XeroGel®, Nasopore®). Biomaterials and implants represent a mechanism for the one-time physician-directed instillation of a topical steroid that is maintenance-free for the patient.

Summary of Methods

There are several options for delivering topical steroids to the nasal cavity and paranasal sinuses, and the choice of delivery method depends on a number of factors. All of these methods are capable of delivering topical steroids to the nasal cavity and sinuses; however, it is clear that some techniques result in more effective delivery. Much of this is dependent upon the device and the operated state of the sinuses. Thomas et al. recently performed an evidence-based review with recommendations on the distribution of topical agents to the sinuses, assessing multiple factors affecting distribution such as delivery device, head position, outcome assessment, anatomy, patient factors, disease states, etc. [26]. The final recommendations based on their pooled assessment include the following:

1. Sinus surgery increases sinus penetration of topical therapies.
2. High-volume delivery devices are recommended.
3. Head position should be down for high-volume delivery devices.
4. High-volume delivery devices overcome "unfavorable" nasal and sinus anatomy.

Topical Steroids for Chronic Rhinosinusitis

Topical Steroids in Chronic Rhinosinusitis Without Polyposis

Several randomized clinical trials (RCT) have evaluated the use of topical steroids in the management of CRSsNP; however, the recommendations remain unclear, given the variability of these multiple studies. Several RCTs have evaluated topical steroid spray against placebo in the management of CRSsNP [27–32]. Sykes and colleagues [27] compared the outcomes in 50 patients with mucopurulent rhinosinusitis treated with combination dexamethasone/tramazoline sprays with or without neomycin against placebo. Patients receiving placebo sprays did worse, and there was no significant difference in groups receiving the antibiotic. Although patients in both dexamethasone/tramazoline groups improved, the addition of the tramazoline component makes it difficult to ascertain the exact effect of the dexamethasone in this study. Parikh et al. [28] followed 22 patients randomly assigned to 200 mcg of fluticasone spray or placebo and, after 16 weeks, noted no difference between the 2 groups in measured parameters (symptoms, endoscopy scores, acoustic rhinometry, and serology studies). Likewise, Dijkstra and colleagues [29] evaluated the effect of fluticasone 400 mcg or 800 mcg vs. placebo on the recurrence rate of CRS and nasal polyps over a 1-year period following ESS and found no significant differences in outcomes.

On the other hand, Lund and coworkers [30] evaluated the efficacy of budesonide aqueous nasal spray against placebo in a multicenter randomized trial and found that in patients with CRSsNP, budesonide significantly decreased combined symptom scores while at the same time improved sense of smell and peak nasal inspiratory flow (PNIF). Jorissen et al. [31] compared mometasone furoate nasal spray and placebo in wound healing following endoscopic sinus surgery for 6 months and found that although total endoscopic scores did not differ, combination scores did improve in the mometasone furoate group, indicating that mometasone furoate may improve healing. Finally, in a 12-week RCT of a bidirectional delivery device (OptiNose) administering fluticasone propionate or placebo, patients with CRSsNP demonstrated improvements in all parameters measured (endoscopy scores, PNIF, symptoms VAS, and RSOM-31scores). Magnetic resonance imaging (MRI) scores did not differ significantly.

In a comprehensive systematic review and meta-analysis, Kalish et al. [33] reviewed the evidence on the use of topical steroids in patients with CRSsNP. Six of the eight trials demonstrated that topical steroids significantly improve symptoms. However, as noted in the review, the studies used different outcome measures, precluding definitive conclusions on the efficacy of topical steroids for CRSsNP other than to say that topical steroids are low-risk interventions that may be beneficial. Snidvongs et al. [34] expanded on this in a more formalized Cochrane Review and evaluated the outcomes in patients without polyps who were treated with topical steroids. Pooled data from ten RCTs in this analysis revealed that patients with CRSsNP treated with topical steroids had significant improvements in overall symptoms as well as objective response to therapy, and this was not influenced in their subgroup analysis by the presence or absence of surgery. A subgroup analysis showed some benefit to using direct sinus application over nasal application of the steroid. This review was unable to determine if topical steroids in patients with CRSsNP resulted in significant radiographic changes, endoscopic scores, or disease-specific quality of life, however. The authors' conclusions were that adverse effects were infrequent and that topical steroids should be utilized as part of a comprehensive management of CRSsNP.

Steinke et al. [35] performed a pilot study in patients with hyperplastic CRS to assess the effects of 0.5 mg budesonide in 100 mL saline. Over 3 months, patients experienced a decrease in symptoms as well as improvement in endoscopy and Lund-MacKay CT scores. Snidvongs and colleagues [36] also evaluated the efficacy of steroid irrigations on CRSsNP. Following surgery, patients received either 1 mg budesonide or 1 mg betamethasone, and significant improvements in baseline compared to posttreatment were noted for SNOT-22 and endoscopic scores.

A recent evidence-based review with recommendations was performed by Rudmik et al. [37] who proposed recommendations after evaluating the data on the use of topical steroids in patients with CRSwNP and CRSsNP. For standard therapies (i.e., nasal steroid spray), the aggregate quality of evidence was given a grade of A. Main benefits were improved symptoms and endoscopic appearance as well as polyp size reduction. Given the lack of significant side effects and adverse events, the use of standard topical steroids was given a "strong recommendation" for routine use with a preponderance of benefit over harm. For nonstandard therapies (irrigations, drops, etc.), the aggregate quality of evidence was given a grade of C. The benefit was reduced ostial stenosis and reduced use of systemic steroids. A recommendation of "option" was given in these cases due to heterogeneity and paucity of studies.

Topical Steroids in Chronic Rhinosinusitis with Polyposis

Topical steroids have long been used to treat nasal polyps [38], and several early RCT studies [39–46] demonstrate consistently that use of topical steroid sprays (when compared to placebo) in patients with CRSwNP results in improved symptoms and quality of life and reduction in polyp size. These studies encompass a wide variety of steroids as demonstrated in Table 16.1; however, none of these studies compare one topical nasal steroid spray to another in the management of CRSwNP. Since the extent of improvement among outcome measures varies from study to study, no conclusion can be drawn as to whether one topical nasal steroid spray is superior to another. Nevertheless, there is some evidence that demonstrates that higher doses of steroid sprays may result in better outcomes [47]. The efficacy of nasal sprays depends in many ways upon compliance and technique; therefore, a cross-hand spray (left hand sprays the right nostril) is frequently advocated, and patients are often reminded to make administration part of a daily ritual.

The utilization of steroid drops has the potential to provide patients with an easily portable delivery system that may work as effectively as nasal sprays in the management of CRSwNP. Unlike nasal sprays which rely on a slightly head-down position, correct placement of nasal drops relies heavily on the Mygind or "head down and forward position" position. A number of studies have evaluated the efficacy of steroid drops. Penttila and coworkers [48] randomized 142 patients with bilateral polyps to receive either fluticasone 400 mcg nasal steroid drops *b.i.d.* or placebo. After a 12-week treatment period, patients receiving fluticasone experienced significant reduction in polyp size and significant improvements in nasal parameters such as PNIF. Similar findings were reported by Chalton et al. [49] with betamethasone drops and by Aukema and colleagues [50] using fluticasone drops.

In contrast, Ehnhage et al. [51] evaluated the effect of ESS on asthma in patients with polyps, and although surgery did benefit asthmatics, an evaluation of fluticasone drops showed no benefit in disease outcomes when compared to placebo. DelGaudio and Wise [52] retrospectively evaluated dexamethasone, prednisolone, and ciprofloxacin/dexamethasone drops in patients undergoing revision ESS at high risk for polyp recurrence and found patients to have decreased ostial stenosis and decreased need for revision surgery. Therefore, while topically placed steroid drops do offer a beneficial alternative therapy for patients with CRSwNP, the likelihood of success may depend upon disease and surgery status and heavily upon head position during administration.

Evidence continues to mount demonstrating positive outcome in administration of steroids via irrigation in CRSwNP patients. Wang and colleagues [53] evaluated the efficacy and safety of budesonide 1 mg/2 mL inhalation suspension via transnasal nebulization compared to budesonide aqueous nasal spray 256 mcg *b.i.d.* in CRSwNP and found that patients experienced significant improvements in all symptoms as well as polyp size. This was also demonstrated by Sachanandani et al. [54] who treated 9 patients with budesonide irrigations; patients experienced significant improvements in SNOT-20 scores after 30 days of treatment. Snidvongs and colleagues [36] also evaluated the effect of betamethasone 1 mg or budesonide 1 mg irrigations on patients with CRSwNP. They recorded significant improvements in SNOT-22 and endoscopy scores after the treatment period of 55.5 ± 33.9 weeks. Jang et al. [55] retrospectively reviewed the efficacy of 0.5 mg/2 mL in 60 patients with CRSwNP, allergic fungal sinusitis (AFS), aspirin-exacerbated respiratory disease (AERD, Samter's triad), and CRSsNP who had previously undergone primary or revision endoscopic sinus surgery. Overall, SNOT-20 scores were significantly improved compared to baseline after use of budesonide irrigations.

Not all groups, however, have been able to demonstrate an effect. Rotenberg et al. [56] performed an RCT evaluating saline irrigation, budesonide nasal spray, and budesonide irrigation following ESS in 60 patients with AERD. Although overall improvement was measured up to 1 year, quality of life and radiographic and endoscopic scores were no different in each of the three groups, suggesting no additional benefit over saline in either the irrigation or spray budesonide groups.

The local delivery of steroids via biomaterials or implants is seen as an attractive alternative to daily steroid administration since it offers the potential to deliver topical steroids to a specific target without having to worry about patient compliance. Côté and Wright [57] evaluated the effectiveness of a triamcinolone-impregnated nasal dressing (Nasopore®) compared to saline-impregnated dressing in patients undergoing ESS for CRSwNP. There was a significant difference in both perioperative endoscopy scores and Kennedy-Lund scores favoring the triamcinolone-impregnated side after both 3 and 6 months. This study involved an off-label use of triamcinolone but did demonstrate the effectiveness of a targeted placement of steroid.

A biodegradable polymer containing 370 μg of mometasone furoate (Propel, Intersect ENT, Palo Alto, CA) is FDA approved for targeted delivery of topical steroids to the ethmoid cavity following ESS. Murr et al. [58] published a multicenter double-blinded RCT trial of 43 patients undergoing ESS, each of whom received mometasone-eluting stent on one side and non-eluting stent on the other. After 60 days, the side containing the steroid-releasing stent demonstrated significantly less inflammation, reduced polyp formation, and significantly fewer adhesions. Forwith and coworkers [59] further reported on a multicenter single-cohort, non-randomized trial assessing safety and efficacy following ESS in 50 patients with CRS. At 1 month, the rate of polypoid edema, adhesions, and middle turbinate lateralization was 10, 1.1, and 4.4 %, respectively. As expected, there were significant improvements in patient-reported outcomes, but whether the improvements in outcomes were due to the surgery, the biomaterial, or both was difficult to assess. Finally, Marple et al. [60] performed another multicenter RCT involving 105 patients with CRS undergoing ESS. Patients were used as their own control, as a drug-eluting stent was placed on one side and non-eluting stent on the other. Sides receiving the drug-eluting stent demonstrated 29 % fewer interventions and a 52 % decrease in adhesion lysis. Sides with the drug-eluting stent also had a 44.9 % reduction in frank polyposis.

Therefore, the targeted delivery of a steroid-eluting stent provides a viable option for the management of polyps following ESS and may spare patients the need for steroid irrigations, steroid sprays, or systemic steroids. Objective parameters improved in these studies; however, quality of life improvements and patient-reported outcomes are more difficult to clarify since the effect of the stent cannot be separated from the effect of surgery. Nevertheless, it remains another option for otolaryngologists for the management of CRSwNP.

Joe et al. [61] performed a systematic review of 13 studies evaluating the effect of topical steroids on CRSsNP and CRSwNP, and 6 concerning CRSwNP were eligible for meta-analysis. They were able to demonstrate a significant reduction in polyp size for the treatment group, indicating at least an objective improvement in patients with polyps who were treated with topical steroids. This analysis did comment on changes in symptoms as would be expected from reduction in polyp size; however, the authors felt the heterogeneity in reporting made it difficult to report this variable as part of this meta-analysis. On the contrary, Rudmik et al. [62] evaluated 12 RCTs to determine the effect of intranasal topical steroids on patient symptoms, and the pooled risk ratio of successful improvement in patient symptoms was 1.72 (95 % CI: 1.41–2.09), indicating significant improvement in symptoms.

Kalish and coworkers [63] performed a Cochrane Collaboration Review of 40 studies, 36 of which compared the effects of topical steroids to placebo in CRSwNP. The authors evaluated a number of primary outcomes, including symptoms, polyp size, and polyp recurrence. Secondary outcomes studied included endoscopic findings, radiologic findings, changes in nasal airflow, change in sense of smell, and quality of life outcomes. For the primary outcomes, the overall results favored the steroid group with respect to symptoms, reduction in polyp size, and less recurrence of polyps. For secondary outcomes, patients receiving steroids had significant improvement in nasal airflow, olfaction (one study), and quality of life (one study). The results of this analysis led the authors to conclude that topical nasal steroids should be utilized in the treatment of CRSwNP.

Side Effects and Safety

The risks and side effects of systemic steroids have been well established. These side effects include sodium/fluid retention, headache, vertigo, nervousness, mood swings, muscle weakness, glucose intolerance, hypokalemia, increases in intraocular pressure, skin changes, and hirsutism. More serious side effects include adrenal insufficiency, immunosuppression, infection, congestive heart failure, diabetes, psychosis, GI ulceration, hypokalemic alkalosis, avascular necrosis of the hip, glaucoma, cataracts, and even anaphylaxis. While these side effects are applicable to all forms of steroids, the typical local side effects of topically applied nasal steroids include pharyngitis, epistaxis, nasal burning, nasal irritation, nausea, cough, and septal perforation [64]. Although commonly cited, mucosal atrophy may be minimal even with long-term use [65–67]. Localized *Candida* infection has been reported as has the increased incidence of upper respiratory illnesses. Many manufactures recommend that topical nasal steroids not be used following nasal surgery since steroids are known to inhibit healing. Patients should be made aware of the significant local and systemic side effects of steroid use since untoward side effects—especially when patients are not made aware of them—may result in legal action. A nice assessment of the legal implications can be understood by reviewing the work of Poetker et al. [68].

No topical steroid is listed as a pregnancy Category A medicine by the FDA; this means that none has been involved in any well-controlled study that has failed to show risk to the fetus. Budesonide is the only Category B drug, which means that animal reproduction studies have failed to show a risk to the fetus. All remaining topical steroids are Category C drugs which means that animal reproduction studies have shown an adverse effect on the fetus; however, these may warrant use if the benefits outweigh the risk to the mother and fetus.

As previously stated, the concept of localized (topical) delivery of steroids is attractive since the direct delivery of steroids to the nasal cavity and sinuses at least in concept should require lower doses of steroid and avoid the systemic side effects of steroids. Hadley and colleagues [69] have detailed the bioavailability of various steroids, and they range from <0.1 % (mometasone furoate) to 20–50 % (flunisolide). The most commonly prescribed topical steroid sprays include fluticasone (<2 % bioavailability), budesonide (11 %), triamcinolone acetonide (22 %), and beclomethasone (17 %). Depending on the lipophilicity, one-third to one-half of nasal steroids may reach the systemic circulation and are not subject to first-pass metabolism since they are directly absorbed by the nasal mucosa. Any steroid cleared by mucociliary clearance will be absorbed by the gastrointestinal system and undergo extensive first-pass metabolism. Stjarne and colleagues [70] looked at the effects of mometasone 200 mcg nasal spray in 298 patients throughout 12 centers in Denmark, Finland, Norway, and Sweden. In addition to the significant improvement in symptoms, side effects were reported as "tolerable" by patients. Fluticasone has been approved for children as young as age 4 while mometasone has been approved for children as young as 2. Neither has been shown to affect the growth of children [71, 72]. Since steroids are known to cause glaucoma and cataracts, the effect of topical steroid sprays on these ocular conditions has been studied as well. Both a controlled trial in 9,000 patients and a retrospective review of nearly 300,000 patients showed no increased incidence of glaucoma or cataracts [73, 74].

The increasing use of *off-label* steroid preparations (e.g., drops and irrigations) have prompted groups to investigate the systemic side effects since these preparations are typically introduced at much more concentrated doses to the nasal cavity and sinuses. DelGaudio and Wise evaluated cortisol levels in patients using dexamethasone, prednisolone, and ciprofloxacin/dexamethasone drops following revision ESS who were at high risk for polyp recurrence; there were no decrease in cortisol levels [52]. Welch et al. [75] performed a prospective study on ten post-ESS patients at risk for polyp recurrence who received *b.i.d.* budesonide 0.5 mg/2 mL irrigations, and over a 6-week period, there were no significant decreases in AM serum cortisol levels or in 24-h urinary cortisol levels. Bhalla and coworkers [76] evaluated the effect of budesonide irrigations on cortisol levels after an 8-week course. Again, there was no significant reduction in cortisol levels, and the ACTH stimulation after 8 weeks of therapy did not detect any HPA suppression. Other studies have evaluated intraocular pressure [77, 78] as well as salivary cortisol levels [78] and found no increased incidence of ocular pathology or reductions in salivary cortisol levels.

Finally, the sustained release of mometasone furoate from an FDA-approved biomaterial stent has been studied over the recent past. These level 1a studies [58–60] looked at cortisol levels [58] and intraocular pressure [59, 60] and found over a short study period no significant changes from baseline.

Conclusion

Topical steroids are a mainstay therapy for patients with CRS. The evidence shows that topical steroids are beneficial in both CRSsNP and CRSwNP. The efficacy and safety of FDA-approved delivery methods (topical nasal steroid spray, steroid-eluting sinus stent (Propel®)) is established with well-performed RCTs. Other methods of delivery such as topical steroid drops and topical steroid irrigations are less well studied, and safety and efficacy remain to be proven. However, at least in the short term, studies involving steroid drops and steroid irrigations do not appear to demonstrate harm to the patient and do seem to provide patients with subjective and objective improvements.

References

1. Kennedy DW. Functional endoscopic sinus surgery. Tech Arch Otolaryngol. 1985;111:643–9.
2. Barnes PJ. Series "signalling and transcriptional regulation in inflammatory and immune cells: importance in lung biology and disease". Eur Respir J. 2006;27:413–26.
3. Dubin MG, Liu C, Lin SY, Senior BA. American Rhinologic Society member survey on "maximal medical therapy" for chronic rhinosinusitis. Am J Rhinol. 2007;21:483–8.

4. Slavin RG, Spector SL, Bernstein IL, et al. The diagnosis and management of sinusitis: a practice parameter update. J Allergy Clin Immunol. 2005;116:S13–47.
5. Fokkens WJ, Lund VJ, Mullol J, et al. European position paper on rhinosinusitis and nasal polyps 2012. Rhinol Suppl 2012;(23) p preceding table of contents, 1–298.
6. Rosenfeld RM, Andes D, Bhattacharyya N, et al. Clinical practice guideline: adult sinusitis. Otolaryngol Head Neck Surg. 2007;137:S1–31.
7. Hardy JG, Lee SW, Wilson CG. Intranasal drug delivery by spray and drops. J Pharm Pharmacol. 1985;37:294–7.
8. Newman SP, Moren F, Clarke SW. Deposition pattern from a nasal pump spray. Rhinology. 1987;25:77–82.
9. Thorsson L, Newman SP, Weisz A, Trofast E, Moren F. Nasal distribution of budesonide inhaled via a powder inhaler. Rhinology. 1993;31:7–10.
10. Keyhani K, Scherer PW, Mozell MM. Numerical simulation of airflow in the human nasal cavity. J Biomech Eng. 1995;117:429–41.
11. Hyo N, Takano H, Hyo Y. Particle deposition efficiency of therapeutic aerosols in the human maxillary sinus. Rhinology. 1989;27:17–26.
12. Saijo R, Majima Y, Hyo N, Takano H. Particle deposition of therapeutic aerosols in the nose and paranasal sinuses after transnasal sinus surgery: a cast model study. Am J Rhinol. 2004;18:1–7.
13. Albu S. Novel drug-delivery systems for patients with chronic rhinosinusitis. Drug Des Devel Ther. 2012;6:125–32.
14. Hwang PH, Woo RJ, Fong KJ. Intranasal deposition of nebulized saline: a radionuclide distribution study. Am J Rhinol. 2006;20:255–61.
15. Negley JE, Krause H, Pawar S, Reeves-Hoche MK. RinoFlow nasal wash and sinus system as a mechanism to deliver medications to the paranasal sinuses: results of a radiolabeled pilot study. Ear Nose Throat J. 1999;78:550–2.
16. Manes RP, Tong L, Batra PS. Prospective evaluation of aerosol delivery by a powered nasal nebulizer in the cadaver model. Int Forum Allergy Rhinol. 2011;1:366–71.
17. Moller W, Schuschnig U, Celik G, et al. Topical drug delivery in chronic rhinosinusitis patients before and after sinus surgery using pulsating aerosols. PLoS One. 2013;8:e74991.
18. Kubba H, Spinou E, Robertson A. The effect of head position on the distribution of drops within the nose. Am J Rhinol. 2000;14:83–6.
19. Homer JJ, Maughan J, Burniston M. A quantitative analysis of the intranasal delivery of topical nasal drugs to the middle meatus: spray versus drop administration. J Laryngol Otol. 2002;116:10–3.
20. Rudman KL, O'Brien EK, Leopold DA. Radiographic distribution of drops and sprays within the sinonasal cavities. Am J Rhinol Allergy. 2011;25:94–7.
21. Miller TR, Muntz HR, Gilbert ME, Orlandi RR. Comparison of topical medication delivery systems after sinus surgery. Laryngoscope. 2004;114:201–4.
22. Olson DE, Rasgon BM, Hilsinger Jr RL. Radiographic comparison of three methods for nasal saline irrigation. Laryngoscope. 2002;112:1394–8.
23. Lam K, Tan BK, Lavin JM, Meen E, Conley DB. Comparison of nasal sprays and irrigations in the delivery of topical agents to the olfactory mucosa. Laryngoscope. 2013;123:2950–7.
24. Harvey RJ, Goddard JC, Wise SK, Schlosser RJ. Effects of endoscopic sinus surgery and delivery device on cadaver sinus irrigation. Otolaryngol Head Neck Surg. 2008;139:137–42.
25. Harvey RJ, Debnath N, Srubiski A, Bleier B, Schlosser RJ. Fluid residuals and drug exposure in nasal irrigation. Otolaryngol Head Neck Surg. 2009;141:757–61.
26. Thomas 3rd WW, Harvey RJ, Rudmik L, Hwang PH, Schlosser RJ. Distribution of topical agents to the paranasal sinuses: an evidence-based review with recommendations. Int Forum Allergy Rhinol. 2013;3:691–703.
27. Sykes DA, Wilson R, Chan KL, Mackay IS, Cole PJ. Relative importance of antibiotic and improved clearance in topical treatment of chronic mucopurulent rhinosinusitis. A controlled study. Lancet. 1986;2:359–60.
28. Parikh A, Scadding GK, Darby Y, Baker RC. Topical corticosteroids in chronic rhinosinusitis: a randomized, double-blind, placebo-controlled trial using fluticasone propionate aqueous nasal spray. Rhinology. 2001;39:75–9.

29. Dijkstra MD, Ebbens FA, Poublon RM, Fokkens WJ. Fluticasone propionate aqueous nasal spray does not influence the recurrence rate of chronic rhinosinusitis and nasal polyps 1 year after functional endoscopic sinus surgery. Clin Exp Allergy. 2004;34:1395–400.
30. Lund VJ, Black JH, Szabo LZ, Schrewelius C, Akerlund A. Efficacy and tolerability of budesonide aqueous nasal spray in chronic rhinosinusitis patients. Rhinology. 2004;42:57–62.
31. Jorissen M, Bachert C. Effect of corticosteroids on wound healing after endoscopic sinus surgery. Rhinology. 2009;47:280–6.
32. Hansen FS, Djupesland PG, Fokkens WJ. Preliminary efficacy of fluticasone delivered by a novel device in recalcitrant chronic rhinosinusitis. Rhinology. 2010;48:292–9.
33. Kalish LH, Arendts G, Sacks R, Craig JC. Topical steroids in chronic rhinosinusitis without polyps: a systematic review and meta-analysis. Otolaryngol Head Neck Surg. 2009;141:674–83.
34. Snidvongs K, Kalish L, Sacks R, Craig JC, Harvey RJ. Topical steroid for chronic rhinosinusitis without polyps. Cochrane Database Syst Rev 2011: (8):CD009274.
35. Steinke JW, Payne SC, Tessier ME, Borish LO, Han JK, Borish LC. Pilot study of budesonide inhalant suspension irrigations for chronic eosinophilic sinusitis. J Allergy Clin Immunol. 2009;124:1352–4.
36. Snidvongs K, Pratt E, Chin D, Sacks R, Earls P, Harvey RJ. Corticosteroid nasal irrigations after endoscopic sinus surgery in the management of chronic rhinosinusitis. Int Forum Allergy Rhinol. 2012;2:415–21.
37. Rudmik L, Hoy M, Schlosser RJ, et al. Topical therapies in the management of chronic rhinosinusitis: an evidence-based review with recommendations. Int Forum Allergy Rhinol. 2013;3:281–98.
38. Badia L, Lund V. Topical corticosteroids in nasal polyposis. Drugs. 2001;61:573–8.
39. Lund VJ, Flood J, Sykes AP, Richards DH. Effect of fluticasone in severe polyposis. Arch Otolaryngol Head Neck Surg. 1998;124:513–8.
40. Tos M, Svendstrup F, Arndal H, et al. Efficacy of an aqueous and a powder formulation of nasal budesonide compared in patients with nasal polyps. Am J Rhinol. 1998;12:183–9.
41. Keith P, Nieminen J, Hollingworth K, Dolovich J. Efficacy and tolerability of fluticasone propionate nasal drops 400 microgram once daily compared with placebo for the treatment of bilateral polyposis in adults. Clin Exp Allergy. 2000;30:1460–8.
42. Day J, Alexander M, Drouin M, et al. Budesonide aqueous nasal spray and pressurized metered dose inhaler in the treatment of adult patients with seasonal allergic rhinitis. Am J Rhinol. 1997;11:77–83.
43. Holmberg K, Juliusson S, Balder B, Smith DL, Richards DH, Karlsson G. Fluticasone propionate aqueous nasal spray in the treatment of nasal polyposis. Ann Allergy Asthma Immunol. 1997;78:270–6.
44. Lildholdt T, Rundcrantz H, Lindqvist N. Efficacy of topical corticosteroid powder for nasal polyps: a double-blind, placebo-controlled study of budesonide. Clin Otolaryngol Allied Sci. 1995;20:26–30.
45. Ruhno J, Andersson B, Denburg J, et al. A double-blind comparison of intranasal budesonide with placebo for nasal polyposis. J Allergy Clin Immunol. 1990;86:946–53.
46. Filiaci F, Passali D, Puxeddu R, Schrewelius C. A randomized controlled trial showing efficacy of once daily intranasal budesonide in nasal polyposis. Rhinology. 2000;38:185–90.
47. Jankowski R, Klossek JM, Attali V, Coste A, Serrano E. Long-term study of fluticasone propionate aqueous nasal spray in acute and maintenance therapy of nasal polyposis. Allergy. 2009;64:944–50.
48. Penttila M, Poulsen P, Hollingworth K, Holmstrom M. Dose-related efficacy and tolerability of fluticasone propionate nasal drops 400 microg once daily and twice daily in the treatment of bilateral nasal polyposis: a placebo-controlled randomized study in adult patients. Clin Exp Allergy. 2000;30:94–102.
49. Chalton R, Mackay I, Wilson R, Cole P. Double blind, placebo controlled trial of betamethasone nasal drops for nasal polyposis. Br Med J (Clin Res Ed). 1985;291:788.

50. Aukema AA, Mulder PG, Fokkens WJ. Treatment of nasal polyposis and chronic rhinosinusitis with fluticasone propionate nasal drops reduces need for sinus surgery. J Allergy Clin Immunol. 2005;115:1017–23.
51. Ehnhage A, Olsson P, Kolbeck KG, et al. Functional endoscopic sinus surgery improved asthma symptoms as well as PEFR and olfaction in patients with nasal polyposis. Allergy. 2009;64:762–9.
52. DelGaudio JM, Wise SK. Topical steroid drops for the treatment of sinus ostia stenosis in the postoperative period. Am J Rhinol. 2006;20:563–7.
53. Wang C, Lou H, Lou W, Zhang L. The efficacy and safety of a short course of budesonide inhalation suspension via transnasal nebulization in chronic rhinosinusitis with nasal polyps. Lin Chung Er Bi Yan Hou Tou Jing Wai Ke Za Zhi. 2012;26:347–50.
54. Sachanandani NS, Piccirillo JF, Kramper MA, Thawley SE, Vlahiotis A. The effect of nasally administered budesonide respules on adrenal cortex function in patients with chronic rhinosinusitis. Arch Otolaryngol Head Neck Surg. 2009;135:303–7.
55. Jang DW, Lachanas VA, Segel J, Kountakis SE. Budesonide nasal irrigations in the postoperative management of chronic rhinosinusitis. Int Forum Allergy Rhinol. 2013;3:708–11.
56. Rotenberg BW, Zhang I, Arra I, Payton KB. Postoperative care for Samter's triad patients undergoing endoscopic sinus surgery: a double-blinded, randomized controlled trial. Laryngoscope. 2011;121:2702–5.
57. Cote DW, Wright ED. Triamcinolone-impregnated nasal dressing following endoscopic sinus surgery: a randomized, double-blind, placebo-controlled study. Laryngoscope. 2010;120:1269–73.
58. Murr AH, Smith TL, Hwang PH, et al. Safety and efficacy of a novel bioabsorbable, steroid-eluting sinus stent. Int Forum Allergy Rhinol. 2011;1:23–32.
59. Forwith KD, Chandra RK, Yun PT, Miller SK, Jampel HD. ADVANCE: a multisite trial of bioabsorbable steroid-eluting sinus implants. Laryngoscope. 2011;121:2473–80.
60. Marple BF, Smith TL, Han JK, et al. Advance II: a prospective, randomized study assessing safety and efficacy of bioabsorbable steroid-releasing sinus implants. Otolaryngol Head Neck Surg. 2012;146:1004–11.
61. Joe SA, Thambi R, Huang J. A systematic review of the use of intranasal steroids in the treatment of chronic rhinosinusitis. Otolaryngol Head Neck Surg. 2008;139:340–7.
62. Rudmik L, Schlosser RJ, Smith TL, Soler ZM. Impact of topical nasal steroid therapy on symptoms of nasal polyposis: a meta-analysis. Laryngoscope. 2012;122:1431–7.
63. Kalish L, Snidvongs K, Sivasubramaniam R, Cope D, Harvey RJ. Topical steroids for nasal polyps. Cochrane Database Syst Rev 2012;(12):CD006549.
64. Cervin A, Andersson M. Intranasal steroids and septum perforation–an overlooked complication? A description of the course of events and a discussion of the causes. Rhinology. 1998;36:128–32.
65. Holm AF, Fokkens WJ, Godthelp T, Mulder PG, Vroom TM, Rijntjes E. A 1-year placebo-controlled study of intranasal fluticasone propionate aqueous nasal spray in patients with perennial allergic rhinitis: a safety and biopsy study. Clin Otolaryngol Allied Sci. 1998;23:69–73.
66. Minshall E, Ghaffar O, Cameron L, et al. Assessment by nasal biopsy of long-term use of mometasone furoate aqueous nasal spray (Nasonex) in the treatment of perennial rhinitis. Otolaryngol Head Neck Surg. 1998;118:648–54.
67. Pipkorn U, Pukander J, Suonpaa J, Makinen J, Lindqvist N. Long-term safety of budesonide nasal aerosol: a 5.5-year follow-up study. Clin Allergy. 1988;18:253–9.
68. Poetker DM, Smith TL. What rhinologists and allergists should know about the medico-legal implications of corticosteroid use: a review of the literature. Int Forum Allergy Rhinol. 2012;2:95–103.
69. Hadley JA, Kavuru MS, Anon JB, Pien LC. Diagnosis and management of rhinitis and rhinosinusitis. New York: Professional Communications Inc; 2005.
70. Stjarne P, Blomgren K, Caye-Thomasen P, Salo S, Soderstrom T. The efficacy and safety of once-daily mometasone furoate nasal spray in nasal polyposis: a randomized, double-blind, placebo-controlled study. Acta Otolaryngol. 2006;126:606–12.

71. Allen DB, Meltzer EO, Lemanske Jr RF, et al. No growth suppression in children treated with the maximum recommended dose of fluticasone propionate aqueous nasal spray for one year. Allergy Asthma Proc. 2002;23:407–13.
72. Schenkel EJ, Skoner DP, Bronsky EA, et al. Absence of growth retardation in children with perennial allergic rhinitis after one year of treatment with mometasone furoate aqueous nasal spray. Pediatrics. 2000;105:E22.
73. Garbe E, LeLorier J, Boivin JF, Suissa S. Inhaled and nasal glucocorticoids and the risks of ocular hypertension or open-angle glaucoma. JAMA. 1997;277:722–7.
74. Derby L, Maier WC. Risk of cataract among users of intranasal corticosteroids. J Allergy Clin Immunol. 2000;105:912–6.
75. Welch KC, Thaler ER, Doghramji LL, Palmer JN, Chiu AG. The effects of serum and urinary cortisol levels of topical intranasal irrigations with budesonide added to saline in patients with recurrent polyposis after endoscopic sinus surgery. Am J Rhinol Allergy. 2010;24:26–8.
76. Bhalla RK, Payton K, Wright ED. Safety of budesonide in saline sinonasal irrigations in the management of chronic rhinosinusitis with polyposis: lack of significant adrenal suppression. J Otolaryngol Head Neck Surg. 2008;37:821–5.
77. Seiberling KA, Chang DF, Nyirady J, Park F, Church CA. Effect of intranasal budesonide irrigations on intraocular pressure. Int Forum Allergy Rhinol. 2013;3:704–7.
78. Man LX, Farhood Z, Luong A, et al. The effect of intranasal fluticasone propionate irrigations on salivary cortisol, intraocular pressure, and posterior subcapsular cataracts in postsurgical chronic rhinosinusitis patients. Int Forum Allergy Rhinol. 2013;3:953–7.

Oral and Topical Antifungals

17

Wytske Fokkens and Vishal Pundir

Key Take-Home Points

- The role of fungi in various forms of CRS remains to be defined.
- The immunocompetence of the patient is of great importance, as invasive fungal rhinosinusitis is usually found in immunosuppressed patients.
- Antifungal drugs and immunotherapy may have a role as adjuvant therapy in allergic fungal rhinosinusitis, but evidence is poor to support recommendations.
- There is no indication for antifungal treatment in CRS with or without nasal polyps.

Introduction

Allergic fungal rhinosinusitis (AFRS) as a distinct clinical entity was first reported in 1976 [1]. In the 1990s it was suggested that fungus could be an important contributor to chronic rhinosinusitis [2]. With new culture techniques, it was possible to culture fungus like *Alternaria* and *Aspergillus* in most patients with CRS. It was hypothesized that fungus might play a causal role in the disease.

For causality, however, we need Koch's postulates. These four criteria are designed to establish a causative relationship between a microbe and a disease:

1. The microorganism must be found in abundance in all organisms suffering from the disease but should not be found in healthy organisms.

W. Fokkens, MD, PhD (✉) • V. Pundir, MS, MRCS
Department of Otorhinolaryngology, Academic Medical Centre,
Meibergdreef 9, Amsterdam NH 1100DD, The Netherlands
e-mail: w.j.fokkens@amc.nl; Vishalpundir@Yahoo.Com

P.S. Batra, J.K. Han (eds.), *Practical Medical and Surgical Management of Chronic Rhinosinusitis*, DOI 10.1007/978-3-319-16724-4_17

2. The microorganism must be isolated from a diseased organism and grown in pure culture.
3. The cultured microorganism should cause disease when introduced into a healthy organism.
4. The microorganism must be reisolated from the inoculated, diseased experimental host and identified as being identical to the original specific causative agent.

The second of Koch's postulates was shown. However, quite soon after the finding of fungus in patients with CRS, the first reports evolved showing that fungus was also found in healthy individuals therewith defying the first Koch's postulate. Also the third postulate about introducing fungus in a healthy individual should create CRS could not be fulfilled and finally also the last postulate could not be fulfilled. This proved that fungus as such cannot cause CRS [3–5].

However, much more interesting than a pure causal relationship might be the option that fungus is a disease modifier within CRS. To prove or disapprove this option has been shown to be much more difficult and the debate is still ongoing [6].

Fungal Colonization

Fungal colonization is usually found in patients with impaired mucociliary transport, particularly on nasal crusts. A fungus ball is a noninvasive, dense conglomeration of fungus hyphae mostly found in the maxillary sinus without tissue invasion but sometimes accompanied by a weak noneosinophilic mucosal inflammatory response [7].

Bent and Kuhn in 1994 published the diagnostic criterion for fungal rhinosinusitis, which is largely regarded as the standard for diagnosis today. Patients must meet all the major criteria for diagnosis, while the minor criteria serve to support the diagnosis and describe individual patients but are not used to make a diagnosis. The major criteria include a history of type I hypersensitivity by history, skin testing, or in vitro testing, nasal polyposis, characteristic computed tomography (CT) scan findings, the presence of eosinophilic mucin without invasion, and a positive fungal stain of sinus contents removed at the time of surgery. The minor criteria include a history of asthma, unilateral predominance of disease, radiographic evidence of bone erosion, fungal cultures, presence of Charcot-Leyden crystals in surgical specimens, and serum eosinophilia [8].

Moreover, special forms of chronic rhinosinusitis exist often referred to as eosinophilic fungal rhinosinusitis (EFRS), including allergic fungal rhinosinusitis.

EFRS is a noninvasive chronic eosinophilic sinus inflammation frequently associated with nasal polyps. A characteristic of eosinophilic fungal rhinosinusitis is the presence of highly viscid sinus secretions with eosinophil decay products, termed eosinophilic mucus by Bent and Kuhn. EFRS may be further divided into allergic fungal rhinosinusitis (AFRS) with a positive diagnostic test for IgE-mediated allergy to the fungal elements detected within the sinus. It is considered an IgE-mediated mucosal hypersensitivity directed against fungal antigens deposited on the sinus mucosa. If type I allergy tests to molds are negative but eosinophilic mucus with fungal elements is found, the term non-allergic EFRS is used [9, 10].

Other Forms of Fungal Sinus Disease

Acute invasive fungal rhinosinusitis almost exclusively occurs in immunocompromised hosts and is characterized by hyphal invasion of surrounding tissues, vascular invasion, and tissue necrosis. Today, mortality ranges between 20 and 50 % and is mainly dependent on the improvement of the immunity of the host [11, 12]. Chronic invasive fungal rhinosinusitis is a non-granulomatous, slowly destructive process with abundant hyphae on histopathologic examination. Chronic invasive fungal rhinosinusitis is commonly seen in patients with less severe immune dysfunction like diabetes mellitus and corticosteroid treatment. A 40 % mortality rate has been reported. In South Asia a granulomatous invasive fungal rhinosinusitis with noncaseating granulomas around sparse hyphae is found. This form also has a significant mortality [11, 12].

Treatment of Fungus in CRS

Potential Indications for Oral and Topical Antifungals

In the rest of this chapter, we will mainly talk about treatment of fungus in patients with a normal immunity. At the end of the chapter, in a short paragraph we will talk about treatment of fungal sinus disease in immunocompromised patients.

As aforementioned, the main forms of fungal disease in patients with normal immunity are the fungus ball [7] and eosinophilic fungal rhinosinusitis [9].

The fungus ball usually appears as a mass within the lumen and is usually unilateral and limited to one paranasal sinus. The maxillary sinus is most frequently affected, followed by the sphenoid sinus. The most common symptoms are purulent nasal discharge, facial pain or fullness, chronic nasal obstruction, fetid smell perception, and postnasal discharge. However, it is not uncommon for these lesions to be recognized as an incidental radiological finding in an asymptomatic patient. Fungus balls typically appear hyperdense on CT scans and frequently show calcifications [7, 13]. Sinus walls may be hypersclerotic or expanded and thinned. On T1-weighted MRI, a fungus ball appears hypointense. Calcifications and paramagnetic metals, such as iron, magnesium, and manganese, generate areas of signal void in T2-weighted images. The treatment of fungus balls is surgical. The goal of the surgery is to remove all fungal material without unnecessary damaging the mucosa. Additional medical treatment is not necessary. The recovery is usually excellent [14, 15].

Eosinophilic Fungal Rhinosinusitis

The concept of AFRS (a subtype of CRS) parallels allergic bronchopulmonary aspergillosis (ABPA), in which hypersensitivity reactions to *Aspergillus* species colonizing the lower respiratory tract result in significant pathology [1]. As clinical evidence for AFRS accumulated, controversy regarding its definition (should fungal allergy be present?), prevalence, and disease mechanisms emerged.

From the immunological point of view, patients with AFRS present (a) type I hypersensitivity to multiple molds and non-fungal aeroallergens demonstrable by immediate skin test reactions and in vitro detection of sIgE, although sensitization rates to fungi do not seem to be higher in patients with AFRS than in patients with other forms of CRS [2] or patients with allergic rhinitis [16]; (b) increased total IgE, which can also be found in the absence of sensitization to fungus at all or sensitization to other fungi than the ones found in the sinus [17]; and (c) increased sIgG to multiple molds [16]. Fungal-specific precipitins and peripheral eosinophilia are presented inconsistently.

Although the exact relevant pathophysiological mechanisms are unclear and widely discussed, we can summarize that it should be questioned whether a type I hypersensitivity to fungi is relevant for the development of CRS, even AFRS. Whether fungal-specific IgG (especially IgG1 and IgG3) is involved in the pathogenesis of CRS requires additional research.

Fungus Anti-host Effects

Besides innate and adaptive antifungal immune responses that may contribute to disease development, fungus anti-host effects may be involved in CRS pathogenesis. Ubiquitous airborne fungi (especially *Alternaria* and *Aspergillus*) are known to produce proteases that bind to protease-activated receptors (PARs) expressed on epithelial cells, airway cells, leukocytes, and blood vessels, thereby activating intracellular signaling pathways that give rise to multiple responses, including the production and release of mediators involved in tissue damage [18, 19].

In addition to an indirect effect, *Alternaria alternata* may activate eosinophils directly. *Alternaria alternata,* but not IL-5, has been shown to induce eosinophil IL-8 synthesis and eosinophil surface expression of CD11b (a β_2-integrin that is used by eosinophils to adhere to β-glucan, a major fungal cell wall component [20]) and CD63 (a component of eosinophil granule membranes) in healthy volunteers, patients with allergic rhinitis, and patients with bronchial asthma.

Upon recognition of *Alternaria alternata*, eosinophil-released eosinophil-derived neurotoxin (EDN) [21] may play a pivotal role in CRS pathogenesis.

Specific Therapy

Oral Antifungals

In contrast to antibacterial antibiotics, the current arsenal of antifungal drugs is limited. Antimycotics have a fungistatic or fungicide mechanism. They can be divided into antimycotic antibiotics (the polyene macrolide amphotericin B and nystatin), imidazoles (ketoconazole, miconazole), triazoles (fluconazole, itraconazole, posaconazole, voriconazole), echinocandin (caspofungin), terbinafine, and flucytosine [22].

In various forms of chronic rhinosinusitis, including AFRS and EFRS, mainly oral itraconazole and ketoconazole have been tried. A recent systematic review on the use of oral antifungals in chronic rhinosinusitis identified 28 studies, majority using azoles [23]. The composite data suggested a beneficial effect of using azoles but the authors admitted that the majority of the studies included were cases series and were confounded by non-validated outcome variables and a need for larger RCTs was identified. Another systematic review of the literature recently published also found no overall benefit of oral antifungals upon endoscopic findings or patient-reported outcome measures in AFRS [24].

Although a significant number of uncontrolled case series have reported a beneficial effect mainly in AFRS, the single double-blind placebo-controlled study of oral antifungals in CRS using terbinafine did not show any effect [25]. As has been suggested by Ponikau et al. [2], fungi reside extramucosally outside the range of the drug circulation. In order to produce an effect, a systemic antifungal must be secreted in sinus mucus, a phenomenon that has not been documented and may not occur.

At this moment, there is no evidence for the use of oral antifungals in CRS. Well-designed RCTs in well-defined patient groups, starting with strict AFRS, are urgently needed.

Topical Antifungals

Topical therapy may be administered by douching, nebulization, atomization, inhalations, irrigation, spray, drops, or powder insufflations. Ideally, treatment should eliminate the fungus without causing harm to the host. Amphotericin B is active against most fungi frequently identified within the nose and paranasal sinuses [26]. Despite its clinical effectiveness, the use of systemic amphotericin B is limited by adverse systemic reactions. Topical treatment may have the advantage in that high concentrations may be achieved locally without causing major systemic side effects. In total 5 RCTs have been performed with amphotericin B nasal lavages [27–31]. However, a meta-analysis combining these five studies concluded that "there is no evidence of any benefit of topical antifungals from the included studies in patients with CRS [32, 33]. Topical antifungal therapy reported beneficial effects in only one of five trials for radiographic and endoscopic scores, but not for symptoms [34]. There was substantial heterogeneity in these two outcomes, possibly because of differences in patient populations and disease factors. The control groups were favored in one of five trials [30] for symptom scores and disease-specific quality-of-life scores. The pooled results showed significant symptom improvement in the placebo group across those studies reporting this outcome [33]."

Also for disease-specific quality-of-life scores, nasal endoscopy scores, and radiograph evaluation, no statistically significant difference was noted between treatment with amphotericin B nasal lavages versus placebo. A meta-analysis of adverse events was performed and found no statistically significant difference between the amphotericin B and placebo groups [33]. Although duration and optimal concentration of amphotericin B nasal lavages have not been established, recent in vitro studies suggest that amphotericin B nasal lavages are ineffective in killing fungi at concentrations of 100 μg/mL when used for 6 consecutive weeks. Irrigation with concentrations of 200 and 300 μg/mL successfully prevents fungal growth at 5 and 6 weeks respectively [35]. Whether prolonged treatment (e.g., 3–6 months) with amphotericin B at a concentration of 100 μg/mL is equal to treatment with topical amphotericin B at a concentration of 200 and 300 μg/mL for shorter periods of time remains unclear.

Immunotherapy

Although there are some studies showing safety [36] and potential efficacy [37, 38] of immunotherapy in AFRS, conclusive evidence of the efficacy of immunotherapy for patients with AFRS in the form of a randomized controlled trial is currently lacking.

Treatment of Fungal Sinus Disease in Immunocompromised Patients

The most important step in treatment of acute invasive fungal sinusitis is the improvement of the immunocompromised state to control the spread of infection. The mainstays of treatment are extensive debridement of the craniofacial lesion and systematic antifungal drugs although the extent of the resection has to be considered carefully in light of their poor survival [39].

A recent prospective randomized unblinded study showed no difference in efficacy of oral amphotericin B and itraconazole in treatment of chronic invasive fungal sinusitis in immunocompetent patients [40]. There are only case series on the treatment of chronic invasive fungal sinusitis in patients with immune dysfunction.

Conclusion

Fungus is likely to be causal in invasive disease (acute invasive fungal rhinosinusitis and chronic invasive fungal rhinosinusitis) and might play a role in noninvasive disease (localized fungal colonization, fungal ball, and allergic fungal rhinosinusitis) but does not seem to play an important role in CRS with or without nasal polyps. Systemic antifungal agents are, together with surgery, a fundamental component in the treatment of invasive forms but are not indicated for the treatment of the noninvasive forms. There is no indication for antifungal treatment in CRS with or without nasal polyps.

References

1. Safirstein BH. Allergic bronchopulmonary aspergillosis with obstruction of the upper respiratory tract. Chest. 1976;70(6):788–90.
2. Ponikau JU, Sherris DA, Kern EB, Homburger HA, Frigas E, Gaffey TA, et al. The diagnosis and incidence of allergic fungal sinusitis. Mayo Clin Proc. 1999;74(9):877–84.

3. Orlandi RR, Marple BF. The role of fungus in chronic rhinosinusitis. Otolaryngol Clin North Am. 2010;43(3):531–7, viii.
4. Ebbens FA, Georgalas C, Luiten S, van Drunen CM, Badia L, Scadding GK, et al. The effect of topical amphotericin B on inflammatory markers in patients with chronic rhinosinusitis: a multicenter randomized controlled study. Laryngoscope. 2009;119(2):401–8.
5. Fokkens WJ, van Drunen C, Georgalas C, Ebbens F. Role of fungi in pathogenesis of chronic rhinosinusitis: the hypothesis rejected. Curr Opin Otolaryngol Head Neck Surg. 2012;20(1):19–23.
6. Fokkens WJ, Ebbens F, van Drunen CM. Fungus: a role in pathophysiology of chronic rhinosinusitis, disease modifier, a treatment target, or no role at all? Immunol Allergy Clin North Am. 2009;29(4):677–88.
7. Broglie MA, Tinguely M, Holzman D. How to diagnose sinus fungus balls in the paranasal sinus? An analysis of an institution's cases from January 1999 to December 2006. Rhinology. 2009;47(4):379–84.
8. Hamilos DL. Allergic fungal rhinitis and rhinosinusitis. Proc Am Thorac Soc. 2010;7(3): 245–52.
9. Chakrabarti A, Denning DW, Ferguson BJ, Ponikau J, Buzina W, Kita H, et al. Fungal rhinosinusitis: a categorization and definitional schema addressing current controversies. Laryngoscope. 2009;119(9):809–18.
10. Ferguson BJ. Eosinophilic mucin rhinosinusitis: a distinct clinicopathological entity. Laryngoscope. 2000;110(5 Pt 1):799–813.
11. Epstein VA, Kern RC. Invasive fungal sinusitis and complications of rhinosinusitis. Otolaryngol Clin North Am. 2008;41(3):497–524, viii.
12. Callejas CA, Douglas RG. Fungal rhinosinusitis: what every allergist should know. Clin Exp Allergy. 2013;43(8):835–49.
13. Kim TH, Na KJ, Seok JH, Heo SJ, Park JH, Kim JS. A retrospective analysis of 29 isolated sphenoid fungus ball cases from a medical centre in Korea (1999–2012). Rhinology. 2013;51(3) :280–6.
14. Eloy P, Grenier J, Pirlet A, Poirrier AL, Stephens JS, Rombaux P. Sphenoid sinus fungall ball: a retrospective study over a 10- year period. Rhinology. 2013;51(2):181–8.
15. Nomura K, Asaka D, Nakayama T, Okushi T, Matsuwaki Y, Yoshimura T, et al. Sinus fungus ball in the Japanese population: clinical and imaging characteristics of 104 cases. Int J Otolaryngol. 2013;2013:731640.
16. Pant H, Kette FE, Smith WB, Wormald PJ, Macardle PJ. Fungal-specific humoral response in eosinophilic mucus chronic rhinosinusitis. Laryngoscope. 2005;115(4):601–6.
17. Collins MM, Nair SB, Wormald PJ. Prevalence of noninvasive fungal sinusitis in South Australia. Am J Rhinol. 2003;17(3):127–32.
18. Vroling AB, Fokkens WJ, van Drunen CM. How epithelial cells detect danger: aiding the immune response. Allergy. 2008;63(9):1110–23.
19. Kauffman HF, Tomee JF, van de Riet MA, Timmerman AJ, Borger P. Protease-dependent activation of epithelial cells by fungal allergens leads to morphologic changes and cytokine production. J Allergy Clin Immunol. 2000;105(6 Pt 1):1185–93.
20. Yoon J, Ponikau JU, Lawrence CB, Kita H. Innate antifungal immunity of human eosinophils mediated by a beta 2 integrin, CD11b. J Immunol. 2008;181(4):2907–15.
21. Inoue Y, Matsuwaki Y, Shin SH, Ponikau JU, Kita H. Nonpathogenic, environmental fungi induce activation and degranulation of human eosinophils. J Immunol. 2005;175(8):5439–47.
22. Francois IE, Aerts AM, Cammue BP, Thevissen K. Currently used antimycotics: spectrum, mode of action and resistance occurrence. Curr Drug Targets. 2005;6(8):895–907.
23. Thanasumpun T, Batra PS. Oral antifungal therapy for chronic rhinosinusitis and its subtypes: a systematic review. Int Forum Allergy Rhinol. 2011;1(5):382–9.
24. Mistry SG, Kumar BN. The value of antifungal therapy in allergic fungal rhinosinusitis. Rhinology. 2014;52(1):9–18.
25. Kennedy DW, Kuhn FA, Hamilos DL, Zinreich SJ, Butler D, Warsi G, et al. Treatment of chronic rhinosinusitis with high-dose oral terbinafine: a double blind, placebo-controlled study. Laryngoscope. 2005;115(10):1793–9.

26. Wildfeuer A, Seidl HP, Paule I, Haberreiter A. In vitro evaluation of voriconazole against clinical isolates of yeasts, moulds and dermatophytes in comparison with itraconazole, ketoconazole, amphotericin B and griseofulvin. Mycoses. 1998;41(7–8):309–19.
27. Ebbens FA, Scadding GK, Badia L, Hellings PW, Jorissen M, Mullol J, et al. Amphotericin B nasal lavages: not a solution for patients with chronic rhinosinusitis. J Allergy Clin Immunol. 2006;118(5):1149–56.
28. Gerlinger I, Fittler A, Fonai F, Patzko A, Mayer A, Botz L. Postoperative application of amphotericin B nasal spray in chronic rhinosinusitis with nasal polyposis, with a review of the antifungal therapy. Eur Arch Otorhinolaryngol. 2009;266(6):847–55.
29. Liang KL, Su MC, Shiao JY, Tseng HC, Hsin CH, Lin JF, et al. Amphotericin B irrigation for the treatment of chronic rhinosinusitis without nasal polyps: a randomized, placebo-controlled, double-blind study. Am J Rhinol. 2008;22(1):52–8.
30. Ponikau JU, Sherris DA, Weaver A, Kita H. Treatment of chronic rhinosinusitis with intranasal amphotericin B: a randomized, placebo-controlled, double-blind pilot trial. J Allergy Clin Immunol. 2005;115(1):125–31.
31. Weschta M, Rimek D, Formanek M, Polzehl D, Podbielski A, Riechelmann H. Topical antifungal treatment of chronic rhinosinusitis with nasal polyps: a randomized, double-blind clinical trial. J Allergy Clin Immunol. 2004;113(6):1122–8.
32. Sacks PL, Harvey RJ, Rimmer J, Gallagher RM, Sacks R. Topical and systemic antifungal therapy for the symptomatic treatment of chronic rhinosinusitis. Cochrane Database Syst Rev. 2011;(8):CD008263.
33. Sacks 4th PL, Harvey RJ, Rimmer J, Gallagher RM, Sacks R. Antifungal therapy in the treatment of chronic rhinosinusitis: a meta-analysis. Am J Rhinol Allergy. 2012;26(2):141–7.
34. Ponikau JU, Sherris DA, Kita H, Kern EB. Intranasal antifungal treatment in 51 patients with chronic rhinosinusitis. J Allergy Clin Immunol. 2002;110(6):862–6.
35. Shirazi MA, Stankiewicz JA, Kammeyer P. Activity of nasal amphotericin B irrigation against fungal organisms in vitro. Am J Rhinol. 2007;21(2):145–8.
36. Greenhaw B, deShazo RD, Arnold J, Wright L. Fungal immunotherapy in patients with allergic fungal sinusitis. Ann Allergy Asthma Immunol. 2011;107(5):432–6.
37. Folker RJ, Marple BF, Mabry RL, Mabry CS. Treatment of allergic fungal sinusitis: a comparison trial of postoperative immunotherapy with specific fungal antigens. Laryngoscope. 1998;108(11 Pt 1):1623–7.
38. Mabry RL, Marple BF, Folker RJ, Mabry CS. Immunotherapy for allergic fungal sinusitis: three years' experience. Otolaryngol Head Neck Surg. 1998;119(6):648–51.
39. Monroe MM, McLean M, Sautter N, Wax MK, Andersen PE, Smith TL, et al. Invasive fungal rhinosinusitis: a 15-year experience with 29 patients. Laryngoscope. 2013;123(7):1583–7.
40. Mehta R, Panda NK, Mohindra S, Chakrabarti A, Singh P. Comparison of efficacy of amphotericin B and itraconazole in chronic invasive fungal sinusitis. Indian J Otolaryngol Head Neck Surg: Off Publ Assoc Otolaryngol India. 2013;65 Suppl 2:288–94.

Leukotriene Modifiers

18

Mark A. Zacharek and Andrew C. Birkeland

Key Take-Home Points

- Leukotriene-modifying agents have been shown to be beneficial in asthma and allergic rhinitis.
- Leukotriene-modifying agent may have benefit in chronic rhinosinusitis with nasal polyposis (aspirin triad) as adjuvant therapy in select patients.
- Further randomized controlled trials are needed to more fully assess benefits of leukotriene-modifying agents.

Introduction

Leukotriene modifiers have been key agents for treatment of asthma and lower airway disease. Under a united airway model, it has been postulated that leukotriene modifiers may be of benefit in reducing inflammation in the upper airway and specifically in the nasal mucosa. In allergic rhinitis, leukotriene modifiers have been shown to be of benefit in symptomatic relief [1, 2]. However, evidence to date in regard to leukotriene-modifying agents in chronic rhinosinusitis (CRS) is limited.

There is considerable overlap between allergic rhinitis and CRS [3]. Chronic allergen exposure in patients leads to increased inflammatory cell recruitment and inflammatory cascades in nasal mucosal tissue. This leads to increased inflammation (both acute and chronic), nasal edema, fibrosis, goblet cell hyperplasia, and mucous production [4–6]. The allergic milieu subsequently leads to nasal polyp

M.A. Zacharek, MD, FACS (✉) • A.C. Birkeland, MD
Department of Otolaryngology – Head and Neck Surgery, University of Michigan Health System, 1904 Taubman Center, 1500 East Medical Center Drive, Ann Arbor, MI 48109, USA
e-mail: zacharek@med.umich.edu; abirkela@med.umich.edu

P.S. Batra, J.K. Han (eds.), *Practical Medical and Surgical Management of Chronic Rhinosinusitis*, DOI 10.1007/978-3-319-16724-4_18

formation and CRS. The exact mechanisms associated with the development of CRS, however, have not yet been elucidated.

Chronic rhinosinusitis is stratified into two groups: chronic rhinosinusitis with nasal polyposis (CRSwNP) and chronic rhinosinusitis without nasal polyposis. The two groups encompass very different inflammatory environments. Chronic rhinosinusitis with nasal polyposis usually exhibits lower regulatory T cell activity, with increased eosinophilia, IgE production, and Th2 activation, with IL-3 and IL-5 production. On the other hand, CRS without polyposis usually entails an environment with increased fibrosis, neutrophilic inflammation, and Th1 activation, with IFN-γ, IL-2, and TNF-β production [7].

Current guidelines for medical management of CRS most frequently recommend treatment with daily intranasal corticosteroids with short courses of oral corticosteroids as needed [8–10]. Additional therapeutic options including antibiotics, nasal rinses, and leukotriene-modifying agents are often used as adjunct therapy. The current guidelines from the European position paper on rhinosinusitis and nasal polyps do not recommend the use of leukotriene-modifying agents, citing a lack of current supportive evidence [8]. The clinical practice guidelines from *Otolaryngology – Head and Neck Surgery* journal acknowledge the role of allergy in CRS, but do not comment on the use of leukotriene modifiers specifically.

Mechanisms of Action

Leukotriene-modifying agents act in one of two ways: decreasing the production of leukotrienes by inhibiting 5-lipooxygenase function or acting as competitive leukotriene receptor antagonists. See Fig. 18.1 for a depiction of the leukotriene pathway. The enzyme phospholipase A_2 is initially activated, which then cleaves arachidonic acid from cell membrane phospholipids via hydrolysis. The enzyme 5-lipoxygenase then converts arachidonic acid to LTA_4. This enzyme is the target of the inhibitor zileuton. Activity of 5-lipoxygenase is enhanced by the protein 5-lipoxygenase-activating protein. LTC_4 synthase adds glutathione to LTA_4 to produce LTC_4. LTA_4 hydrolase converts LTA_4 into LTB_4. Specific transporters target LTB_4 and LTC_4 to export these leukotrienes extracellularly. γ-Glutamyl leukotrienase converts LTC_4 to LTD_4 extracellularly. LTE_4 is created extracellularly as well by a dipeptidase. These cysteinyl leukotrienes (LTC_4, LTD_4, and LTE_4) act as the primary proinflammatory molecules of this pathway [11, 12]. These leukotrienes bind primarily to two G protein-coupled receptors, $CysLT_1$ and $CysLT_2$, in target cells. Montelukast, zafirlukast, and pranlukast act as antagonists of $CysLT_1$ specifically. When leukotriene receptors are activated in target cells, there is an increase in intracellular calcium and decrease in cAMP, with subsequent activation of protein kinases and proinflammatory downstream effects. Notably, the pathway is active in nasal mucosa as well as the lower airway. As is seen in patients with aspirin triad, patients may have effects in the nasal mucosa (polyposis) and the lower respiratory tract (asthma).

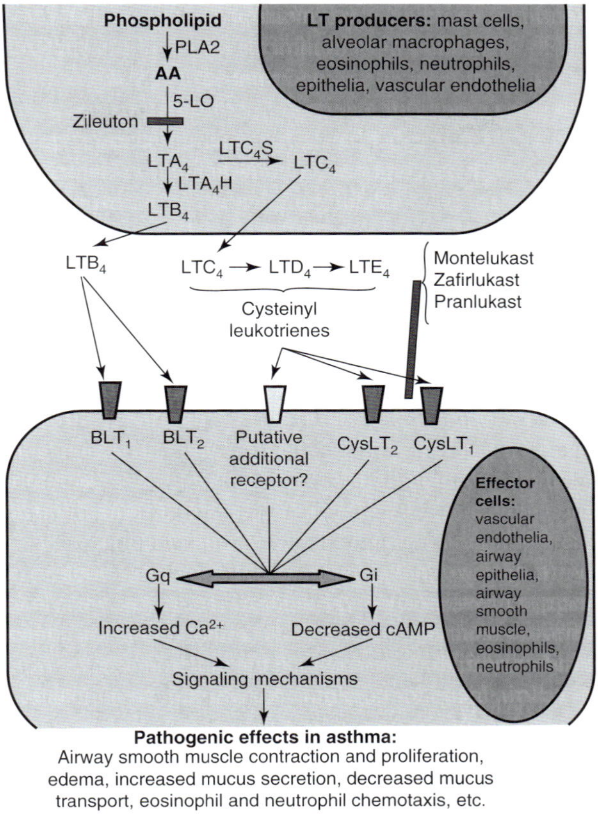

Fig. 18.1 Depiction of the leukotriene pathway

Leukotrienes are produced and secreted by mast cells, eosinophils, and basophils. Normal nasal mucosa has been shown to express leukotriene receptors [13], and nasal polyps, in particular, demonstrate increased upregulation of leukotriene receptors [14]. In the nasal and paranasal sinus mucosa, leukotrienes work by increasing nasal mucosa blood flow, increasing nasal airway edema and resistance, and recruiting and maturing of inflammatory cells. Additionally, they play roles in increasing cytokine and collagen production and increasing vascular permeability with plasma protein exudation [4–6].

Indications

There are no established indications for the use of leukotriene-modifying agents in CRS. These agents are FDA approved for use in patients with allergic rhinitis and asthma and have been shown to be of benefit in these patients [1]. They have been used frequently in the treatment of aspirin triad and CRSwNP. As discussed below, limited studies in regard to use in CRS suggest a benefit of leukotriene-modifying agents in specific cases.

Specific Therapy

The most frequently used leukotriene-modifying agent is montelukast. It is a leukotriene receptor antagonist, specifically against $CysLT_1$. It is usually prescribed as one 10 mg tablet daily. The other commonly used leukotriene receptor antagonist is zafirlukast. Zileuton is the only 5-lipoxygenase inhibitor currently on the market.

In general, these drugs are fairly well tolerated. The most common side effect of zileuton, montelukast, and zafirlukast is headache (25 %, 18 %, and 13 % of patients, respectively). Montelukast and zafirlukast are class B pregnancy category drugs. These agents have been linked to neuropsychiatric changes, with increased agitation, disorientation, irritability, vivid dreams, depression, and suicidal ideation. Additionally, cases have been described of increased eosinophilia and vasculitis in montelukast. Unlike, zafirlukast and zileuton, liver function tests are not necessary for patients taking montelukast. Zafirlukast has been associated with Churg-Strauss syndrome and hepatitis. Careful surveillance should be undertaken when starting patients on this medication, and baseline liver function tests should be performed. It is contraindicated in patients with existing Churg-Strauss syndrome and patients with cirrhosis or liver disease. Zileuton is a class C pregnancy category drug. This drug, as well, can exacerbate underlying liver disease and is contraindicated in patients with a history of liver disease or heavy alcohol use. Zileuton also can cause similar neuropsychiatric effects. It additionally has a higher incidence of gastrointestinal symptoms.

Clinical Efficacy Data (Including Expert Opinion)

A few randomized clinical trials exist studying the effects of antileukotrienes in CRS. There are additionally multiple case series documenting the effects of antileukotrienes on patients with CRS, with the majority of these studying aspirin triad patients.

Leukotriene-modifying agents in comparison to placebo have been studied in CRSwNP. Pauli et al. performed a randomized clinical trial comparing montelukast against placebo in CRSwNP patients [15]. The montelukast group had significant improvements in health-related quality of life symptoms, including headaches, sleep, and emotional problems, as well as objective measurement of polyp burden. Schaper et al. [16] performed a crossover study comparing montelukast to placebo in patients with CRSwNP who also had mild to moderate asthma. Overall, patients demonstrated statistically significant improvement in nasal symptoms (nasal obstruction, rhinorrhea, itching), reduction in nasal edema, increased nasal airflow, and decreased local and systemic eosinophil counts while on montelukast in comparison to placebo. A case series by Kutting et al. [17] provided montelukast to patients who had undergone multiple previous endoscopic surgeries for sinonasal polyposis. Seven out of nine patients noted significant improvement in symptoms up to 1 year out. Notably, when two patients discontinued montelukast, they suffered recurrence of their symptoms. These studies do suggest that antileukotriene medications have an overall beneficial effect when compared to placebos.

Other studies have compared leukotriene modifiers to standard nasal corticosteroids. Mostafa et al. performed a randomized controlled study treating CRS patients with sinonasal polyps postoperatively with either montelukast or beclomethasone [18]. Both groups demonstrated symptomatic improvement postoperatively, with the montelukast group showing greater improvement in postnasal drip, headache, and itching and the beclomethasone group having greater improvement in dysosmia and nasal obstruction. There was no difference in nasal polyp recurrence rates. There was no combination group or negative control group postoperatively in this study, however. Another study by Vuralkan et al. compared treatment with montelukast versus mometasone postoperatively in patients with CRSwNP, with both groups showing improvement on SNOT-22 scores and decreased sinonasal disease on CT imaging [19]. Mometasone performed slightly better than montelukast in preventing polyp recurrence. Overall, studies do not support replacement of standard nasal corticosteroid therapy with leukotriene-modifying agents, but do not symptomatic benefits and objective decrease in nasal polyposis with antileukotriene therapy.

Additional studies have focused on adding leukotriene inhibitors to patients already taking nasal corticosteroid regimens. Parnes and Chuma studied the effect of adding zileuton or zafirlukast to standard therapy in patients with CRS with sinonasal polyposis [20]. Seventy-two percent of patients reported symptomatic improvement with added antileukotriene therapy, although there were no control or comparison groups in this study. Nonaka et al. added montelukast to the treatment regimen of 20 CRSwNP patients who were already taking inhaled corticosteroids for over 1 year [21]. After 1 year of combined treatment, significant reductions in nasal polyp size, sinus disease burden, and peripheral eosinophil counts were noted. Similarly, Kieff and Busaba added montelukast to patients with nasal polyposis who had been taking intranasal corticosteroids for greater than 6 months [22]. After addition of montelukast, 71 % of patients noted symptomatic improvement, and biopsies of nasal polyps demonstrated a significant reduction in eosinophil burden. The greatest effect of montelukast, notably, was found in patients with documented allergic rhinitis, indicating that leukotriene-modifying agents may be ideally suited in CRS patients with an allergic component. Stewart et al. [23] tested for additional benefits of adding montelukast to an oral steroid course and nasal steroids for 8 weeks. They identified statistically significant improvement in headache, facial pain, and sneezing in the montelukast group, although these benefits did not last after discontinuing therapy. Ragab et al. [24] also studied the addition of montelukast to patients with CRSwNP and asthma refractory to treatment with intranasal steroids. The researchers subdivided their subjects into those with aspirin sensitivity and those without. Subjective improvement was noted in patients who were aspirin tolerant. However, other measures such as rhinometry and nasal inspiratory peak flow did not improve. Aspirin sensitivity was not associated with improvement on montelukast in this study. Overall, these studies suggest symptomatic improvement with the addition of leukotriene-modifying therapy to standard steroid therapy, although many of the studies reviewed did not have control groups.

Ulualp et al. [25] surveyed patients with aspirin triad who had functional endoscopic sinus surgery and who underwent trials of postoperative zafirlukast (16) or zileuton (2). Patients reported improvement in CRS symptoms, ranging from slight (seven) to moderate (two) to very good (three).

Notably, in all these studies, leukotriene-modifying agents appeared to be well tolerated. Side effects were minimal in studies that commented on tolerance to medications.

Conclusion

Current evidence does not support the use of leukotriene-modifying drugs in all cases of CRS. The current European Position Paper on Rhinosinusitis and Nasal Polyps 2012 does not recommend the use of leukotriene-modifying agents for the treatment of CRS [8] as there is insufficient data in the literature to support their use. The current clinical practice guideline for adult sinusitis in *Otolaryngology – Head and Neck Surgery* journal does not comment on the role of leukotriene-modifying agents in CRS [10]. A meta-analysis and systematic review by Wentzel et al. in 2013 [26] did find some mild benefit in patients with CRSwNP in symptom management. Overall, the use of leukotriene-modifying agents may be warranted in specific cases of CRS, such as patients with aspirin triad. In patients with a clear component or history of allergic rhinitis or asthma in conjunction with CRSwNP, a trial of leukotriene modifiers may be beneficial. Additionally, patients who do not tolerate, or fail, intranasal corticosteroids therapy may benefit from a trial of leukotriene-modifying agents. The effects of these medications, however, may not last after cessation of treatment. Overall, the use of these medications in carefully chosen patients may provide additional benefit to standard therapy for CRS and in particular CRSwNP. Leukotriene-modifying agents are generally well tolerated, with few side effects, the most notable being headaches, neuropsychiatric changes, and liver injury. Current reports in the literature have small population sizes, with at most a few dozen patients receiving treatments. Given the lack of large, randomized, blinded clinical studies involving leukotriene-modifying agents, further research into the application of these agents in chronic rhinosinusitis is warranted.

References

1. Nayak A, Langdon RB. Montelukast in the treatment of allergic rhinitis: an evidence-based review. Drugs. 2007;67(6):887–901.
2. Cingi C, Gunham K, Gage-White L, Unlu H. Efficacy of leukotriene antagonists as concomitant therapy in allergic rhinitis. Laryngoscope. 2010;120(9):1718–23.

3. Kennedy JL, Borish L. Chronic sinusitis pathophysiology: the role of allergy. Am J Rhinol Allergy. 2013;27(5):367–71.
4. Bisgaard H, Olsson P, Bende M. Effect of leukotriene D4 on nasal mucosal blood flow, nasal airway resistance and nasal secretion in humans. Clin Allergy. 1986;16:289–97.
5. Busse W, Kraft M. Cysteinyl leukotrienes in allergic inflammation: strategic target for therapy. Chest. 2005;127:1312–26.
6. Howarth PH, Salagean M, Dokic D. Allergic rhinitis: not purely a histamine-related disease. Allergy. 2000;55:7–16.
7. Van Zele T, Claeys S, Gevaert P, et al. Differentiation of chronic sinus diseases by measurement of inflammatory mediators. Allergy. 2006;61(11):1280–9.
8. Fokkens WJ, Lund VJ, Mullol J, et al. EPOS 2012: European position paper on rhinosinusitis and nasal polyps 2012. Rhinol Suppl. 2012;23(3):1–298.
9. Cain RB, Lal D. Update on the management of chronic rhinosinusitis. Infect Drug Resist. 2013;6:1–14.
10. Rosenfeld RM, Andes D, Bhattacharyya N, et al. Clinical practice guideline: adult sinusitis. Otolaryngol Head Neck Surg. 2007;137:S1–31.
11. Okunishi K, Peters-Golden M. Leukotrienes and airway inflammation. Biochim Biophys Acta. 2011;1810(11):1096–102.
12. Peters-Golden M, Henderson Jr WR. Leukotrienes. N Engl J Med. 2007;357(18):1841–54.
13. Shirasaki H, Kanaizumi E, Watanabe K, et al. Expression and localization of the cysteinyl leukotriene 1 receptor in human nasal mucosa. Clin Exp Allergy. 2002;32(7):1007–12.
14. Chao SS, Graham SM, Brown CL, et al. Cysteinyl leukotriene 1 receptor expression in nasal polyps. Ann Otol Rhinol Laryngol. 2006;115(5):394–7.
15. Pauli C, Fintelmann R, Klemens C, et al. Polyposis nasi – improvement in quality of life by the influence of leukotriene receptor antagonists. Laryngorhinootologie. 2007;86(4):282–6.
16. Schaper C, Noga O, Koch B, et al. Anti-inflammatory properties of montelukast, a leukotriene receptor antagonist in patients with asthma and nasal polyposis. J Investig Allergol Clin Immunol. 2011;21(1):51–8.
17. Kutting B, Nieschalk M, Brehler R. A new concept for treatment of sinonasal polyposis. Allergy. 2000;55(11):1091–2.
18. Mostafa BE, Abdel Hay H, Mohammed HE, Yamani M. Role of leukotriene inhibitors in the postoperative management of nasal polyps. ORL J Otorhinolaryngol Relat Spec. 2005;67(3): 148–53.
19. Vuralkan E, Saka C, Akin I, Hucumenoglu S, et al. Comparison of montelukast and mometasone furoate in the prevention of recurrent nasal polyps. Ther Adv Respir Dis. 2012;6(1): 5–10.
20. Parnes SM, Chuma AV. Acute effects of antileukotrienes on sinonasal polyposis and sinusitis. Ear Nose Throat J. 2000;79(1):18–20.
21. Nonaka M, Sakanushi A, Kusama K, et al. One-year evaluation of combined treatment with an intranasal corticosteroid and montelukast for chronic rhinosinusitis associated with asthma. J Nippon Med Sch. 2010;77(1):21–8.
22. Kieff DA, Busaba NY. Efficacy of montelukast in the treatment of nasal polyposis. Ann Otol Rhinol Laryngol. 2005;114(12):941–5.
23. Stewart RA, Ram B, Hamilton G, et al. Montelukast as an adjunct to oral and inhaled steroid therapy in chronic nasal polyposis. Otolaryngol Head Neck Surg. 2008;139(5):682–7.
24. Ragab S, Parikh A, Darby YC, Scadding GK. An open audit of montelukast, a leukotriene receptor antagonist, in nasal polyposis associated with asthma. Clin Exp Allergy. 2001;31(9):1385–91.
25. Ulualp SO, Sterman BM, Toohill RJ. Antileukotriene therapy for the relief of sinus symptoms in aspirin triad disease. Ear Nose Throat J. 1999;78(8):604–6.
26. Wentzel JL, Soler ZM, Deyoung K, et al. Leukotriene antagonists in nasal polyposis: a meta-analysis and systematic review. Am J Rhinol Allergy. 2013;27(6):482–9.

Aspirin Desensitization and High-Dose Aspirin Therapy in Aspirin-Exacerbated Respiratory Disease

19

Katherine N. Cahill, Kathleen Buchheit, Carolyn Word, and Larry Borish

Key Take-Home Points

- Seventy to eighty percent of patients with AERD report therapeutic benefit on daily high-dose aspirin therapy.
- The benefits of daily aspirin therapy in patients with AERD include decreased symptoms, corticosteroid use, and rates of revision sinus surgery while improving quality of life.
- Aspirin desensitization followed by daily aspirin therapy is recommended for patients with AERD who are have refractory symptoms despite standard medical and surgical therapy.
- Aspirin desensitization can be safely performed in the outpatient setting for most patients with AERD under the guidance of physicians trained in the management of asthma and allergic reactions.

K.N. Cahill, MD
Department of Medicine/Division of Rheumatology, Immunology, and Allergy, Brigham and Women's Hospital/Harvard Medical School, 1 Jimmy Fund Way, Boston, MA 02115, USA
e-mail: kncahill@partners.org

K. Buchheit, MD
Department of Allergy and Immunology, Brigham and Women's Hospital, 1 Jimmy Fund Way, Boston, MA 02115, USA

C. Word, MD
Department of Allergy and Immunology, University of Virginia Health System, PO Box 801355, Charlottesville, VA 22908, USA
e-mail: cmr6f@hscmail.mcc.virginia.edu

L. Borish, MD (✉)
Department of Medicine (Allergy and Immunology) and Microbiology, University of Virginia Health System, PO Box 801355, Charlottesville, VA 22908, USA
e-mail: lb4m@virginia.edu

P.S. Batra, J.K. Han (eds.), *Practical Medical and Surgical Management of Chronic Rhinosinusitis*, DOI 10.1007/978-3-319-16724-4_19

Introduction

The classic "aspirin triad" consisting of sensitivity to aspirin, bronchial asthma, and nasal polyps was first reported by Widal and colleagues in 1922 [1]. In their original publication, they describe not only the clinical presentation but also the process of aspirin desensitization. In 1968, having followed a large cohort of patients with aspirin sensitivity for over a decade, Samter and Beers published an account of the natural history of the syndrome and further characterized patients with the aspirin triad (subsequently referred to as *Samter's* triad) [2]. This condition is now more commonly termed aspirin-exacerbated respiratory disease (AERD) in recognition that not all of these patients have asthma. The introduction of aspirin desensitization and high-dose aspirin therapy as common medical practice for the treatment of AERD began following the report by Stevenson and colleagues in 1980 on tolerance to aspirin and improvement of asthma and sinusitis symptoms using oral desensitization protocols [3]. Subsequent studies have confirmed aspirin desensitization followed by high-dose aspirin therapy improves asthma and sinus symptoms scores, decreases corticosteroid use, and reduces rates of revision sinus surgery with a low rate of adverse events [4–8]. Thus, as a safe and effective treatment option for patients with AERD, aspirin desensitization is now considered part of the mainstay of the management of patients with AERD.

AERD is defined clinically by the presence of nasal polyps, chronic hypereosinophilic sinusitis, and bronchial asthma, along with the induction of respiratory symptoms upon exposure to aspirin and all other nonsteroidal antiinflammatory drugs (NSAIDs) that nonselectively inhibit cyclooxygenase-1 (COX-1). Upon ingestion of a COX-1 inhibitor, patients with AERD will develop respiratory reactions within 30–120 min and report any combination of upper and/or lower symptoms, including nasal congestion, rhinorrhea, sneezing, ocular injection, and bronchospasm. Many patients with AERD have severe persistent asthma, are steroid dependent prior to desensitization [9], and comprise an asthma phenotype particularly prone to develop irreversible obstruction [10], even with avoidance of all COX-1 inhibitors. Chronic rhinosinusitis (CRS) experienced by aspirin-sensitive patients is particularly severe and includes severe mucosal inflammation with eosinophilia and often complete opacification on sinus computed tomography [11, 12]. The nasal polyposis in this subset is particularly refractory, and recurrence after functional endoscopic sinus surgery (FESS) is common despite aggressive postoperative medical management [13, 14]. These patients are uniquely susceptible to develop complete anosmia and that, along with the nasal obstruction, leads to the profound adverse impact on patients' quality of life (QoL).

Standard Treatment Options for Control of AERD

The underlying pathophysiology of the disease is still not well understood, hindering the development of definitive therapeutics, but includes an extremely robust increase in cysteinyl leukotriene (CysLT) production and responsiveness likely due to CysLT receptor expression [15, 16]. The overexpression of the rate-limiting enzyme for CysLT expression, LTC_4 synthase, may underlie the constitutive overproduction of CysLTs observed at baseline and also drives the further surge seen with ingestion of aspirin or other COX-1 inhibitors [16]. With this central role for CysLTs in AERD, medical management for AERD has typically involved the use of leukotriene-modifying agents including the CysLT receptor antagonists (i.e., montelukast, zafirlukast) [17]. Inhibitors of leukotriene synthesis (5-lipoxygenase (5-LO) inhibitors, i.e., zileuton) may be uniquely beneficial in this disorder [18]. However, leukotriene modifiers alone seldom produce long-term remission of disease. With the severity of the disease, long-term morbidity, adverse impact on QoL, and poor responsiveness to medical and surgical therapies, aspirin desensitization provides one of the most important therapeutic interventions available.

Indications for Aspirin Desensitization

Aspirin desensitization followed by daily high-dose aspirin therapy is a valuable tool for many patients with AERD and is indicated in patients who are refractory to standard medical therapy, require frequent bursts of oral steroids, or have recurrent nasal polyps (Table 19.1) [19]. Nearly all patients with AERD meet one or more of the criteria to recommend aspirin desensitization therapy. Aspirin (or other NSAID) desensitization is also appropriate for patients with an unrelated medical indication for requiring chronic aspirin or NSAID use, such as the primary or secondary prevention of coronary artery disease [20–22], or an ongoing need for an antiinflammatory medication [19, 23]. There is no indication for aspirin desensitization or high-dose aspirin therapy in patients with asthma, chronic rhinosinusitis, or nasal polyposis who are aspirin tolerant.

Table 19.1 Indications and benefits of aspirin desensitization and high-dose aspirin therapy in patients with aspirin-exacerbated respiratory disease (AERD)

Aspirin desensitization and high-dose aspirin therapy	
Indications	Benefits
Any patient with AERD	Slows nasal polyp regrowth and decreases need for repeat FESS
Symptoms refractory to medical therapy	Improves nasal congestion
Frequent use of oral steroids	Decreases sinus infections
Recurrent nasal polyposis requiring repeat FESS	Decreases INS, ICS, and oral steroid use
Need for chronic aspirin or other NSAID use	Decreases asthma-related hospitalizations
	Cross-desensitization with all other NSAIDs
	Improves quality of life
	Cost-effective

FESS functional endoscopic sinus surgery, *NSAIDs* nonsteroidal antiinflammatory drugs, *INS* intranasal steroids, *ICS* inhaled corticosteroids

Benefits of Aspirin Desensitization

Patients with AERD often develop progressive upper and lower airway disease despite treatment with maximum medical and surgical management, such as CysLT receptor antagonists, 5-LO inhibitors, topical or systemic corticosteroids, and repeat FESS. Aspirin desensitization and subsequent high-dose aspirin therapy are known to alter the trajectory of nasal polyp regrowth, to improve upper and lower respiratory symptoms, and to improve QoL (Table 19.1). Aspirin desensitization improves nasal congestion, increases the interval of time between surgeries, decreases the frequency of sinus infections, and lessens the need for topical or oral corticosteroids in patients with AERD [7, 24–27]. In the month following aspirin desensitization, many patients can experience near-immediate improvement in sense of smell, decreased need for prednisone, and improvement in nasal congestion [25]. In the long-term, patients continue to experience increased sense of smell, fewer purulent sinus infections, and a reduction in steroid treatment [24].

Patients with rapid regrowth of nasal polyps benefit from aspirin desensitization as it slows the regrowth of nasal polyps and decreases the need for repeated surgeries. One retrospective analysis assessed AERD patients with nasal polyps over a 2-year period. None of the aspirin desensitization patients required repeat surgery, whereas 80 % of the non-desensitized patient underwent repeat procedures [7]. Another study demonstrated that even AERD patients on low maintenance doses of aspirin (100 mg) required fewer nasal polypectomies than patients who were not taking aspirin at all [26]. In long-term follow-up of aspirin-desensitized patients, the need for sinus surgery decreased from once every 3 years to once every 10 years [27].

Although symptom improvement is typically more profound in the upper airway than the lower airway, asthma control often improves following aspirin desensitization as well. During a mean follow-up of 3.1 years, an uncontrolled study of 65 patients showed a significant decrease in asthma-related hospitalizations following aspirin desensitization [27]. A decrease in inhaled corticosteroid (ICS) dose following aspirin desensitization has been reported, although the number of patients requiring an ICS did not change [24].

A side benefit of aspirin desensitization is cross-desensitization to all other COX-1 inhibitors. This allows the desensitized patients to use NSAIDs for pain and antiinflammatory treatment. Cross tolerance only lasts as long as the desensitized state is maintained. Therefore, if a patient were to stop taking aspirin, they would also lose tolerance to all other COX-1 inhibitors.

Desensitization also serves as a diagnostic procedure to confirm the diagnosis of AERD. In this setting, the procedure is referred to as an aspirin challenge, and the protocol remains the same as described below. Aspirin challenges are often necessary to confirm the diagnosis of AERD in the setting of an appropriate clinical history and to rule out the diagnosis when a patient has no prior history of NSAID exposure. Clinical history of respiratory reaction to NSAIDs is not sufficient alone to make a diagnosis of AERD. In 15 % of subjects with a clinical history consistent with AERD, aspirin challenge is negative [25]. Additionally, patients with nasal polyposis and asthma who are on daily low-dose aspirin therapy may deny history of clinical reaction to NSAIDs but when formally challenged after having stopped their daily aspirin exhibit a reaction. Confirming the diagnosis of AERD with aspirin challenge is important for patient safety and optimization of treatment.

Aspirin desensitization is a cost-effective intervention for patients with moderate-to-severe AERD. In an economic analysis that accounted for the up-front cost of aspirin desensitization in a hospital or ambulatory setting, patients who underwent successful aspirin desensitization required fewer costly subsequent medical interventions and surgeries [22]. The same analysis also revealed it is more cost-effective to desensitize patients who require aspirin for secondary cardiovascular prophylaxis than to prescribe them other antiplatelet agents.

Despite the ability to successfully desensitize nearly all patients with AERD to aspirin, there remains a subset of patients with AERD who do not experience improvement in symptoms on high-dose aspirin therapy. A retrospective study of 172 AERD patients showed that 78 % of patients improved following aspirin desensitization [24]. The other 22 % of patients either did not improve on aspirin or discontinued it due to side effects. Currently, there are no available biomarkers or clinical parameters to help preselect for aspirin responders. Patients must first undergo aspirin desensitization and initiate aspirin therapy to determine if they will benefit from the treatment. Prior to aspirin desensitization, physicians should inform patients of the possibility that high-dose aspirin may not alleviate symptoms of AERD.

Safety of Aspirin Desensitization

Aspirin desensitization is not without risk but generally can be performed in the ambulatory setting. In this controlled environment of aspirin desensitization, where the provocative dose of aspirin averages around 100 mg and patients are on montelukast, prior history of reaction severity to NSAID ingestion does not predict the severity of the clinical reaction [28]. In a study of 210 patients with AERD undergoing aspirin challenges, the majority of reactions involved naso-ocular symptoms or mild decreases in FEV_1. Only 9 % of patients in the study had a greater than 30 % decrease in FEV_1 [28]. History of emergency department visits for asthma independent of aspirin use, baseline FEV_1 of 60–80 %, and lack of leukotriene receptor antagonist use at time of challenge are predictors of a fall in FEV_1 of 21 % or greater during aspirin challenge [29]. In one retrospective series of over 670 aspirin desensitizations, no emergency room visits or hospitalizations and only one administration of intramuscular epinephrine were required during aspirin desensitization [30]. In our experience, a small subset of patients report persistent asthma symptoms that do not improve despite having been desensitized to 650 mg of aspirin. Additionally, the occurrence of rash, urticaria, or angioedema on high-dose aspirin therapy occasionally necessitates discontinuing aspirin therapy. High-dose aspirin therapy for AERD provides the same amount of antiplatelet effect as 81 mg of aspirin and therefore the same bleeding risk with doses of 650 mg twice daily showing the same or less gastrointestinal side effects, such as dyspepsia, than 325 mg twice daily [31].

Performance of Aspirin Desensitization

Aspirin desensitization can be carried out safely in the outpatient clinic by physicians trained in the treatment of asthma and allergic diseases with experience performing aspirin desensitization and the capability to treat anaphylaxis. Typically this procedure is performed over 1–2 days. Protocols outlined in the literature involve either oral aspirin or a combination of intranasal ketorolac [32] and oral aspirin starting at doses between 20 and 40 mg of aspirin (1.26 mg of ketorolac) and doubling the dose every 90–180 min until a dose of 325 mg oral aspirin has been reached [29]. These starting doses and rate of dose escalation are in stark contrast to aspirin desensitization protocols employed in the setting of aspirin-induced urticaria or anaphylaxis which are beyond the scope of this review and are discussed elsewhere [33]. It is to be expected that patients with AERD undergoing aspirin desensitization will experience a clinical reaction, most often involving upper and lower respiratory symptoms, such that a baseline FEV_1 <50 % predicted or <1 L is the primary contraindication to performing an aspirin desensitization [34]. Premedication with montelukast and zileuton is associated with increased patient safety, decreasing airway bronchospasm and the severity of naso-ocular symptoms [30]. Use of montelukast is associated with the small (10 %) risk of completely blocking all reaction symptoms in patients with AERD [35], and a clinician may elect to withhold this premedication during a challenge procedure in order to ensure the correct diagnosis is made. Patient history of abdominal symptoms during aspirin exposure may be overcome in our experience by premedication with oral cromolyn sodium, H_2-receptor antagonists, or proton pump inhibitors (PPIs). Once a patient reaches the dose of aspirin that induces a clinical reaction (provocative dose), the reaction is treated symptomatically, and the patient is observed for the resolution of symptoms. Once aspirin-induced symptoms have resolved, repeat administration of the provocative aspirin dose and then subsequent doses of aspirin are typically well tolerated without further respiratory reaction. Patients are discharged home on 650 mg aspirin twice daily with a potential to decrease the dose to 325 mg twice daily in a subset of patients and still maintain the therapeutic benefit [31]. The best available data support the use of aspirin 650 mg twice daily as the dose that offers the most benefit in preventing nasal polyp regrowth and improving asthma control [31]. In some patients, high-dose aspirin therapy is associated with gastrointestinal side effects such as gastritis, acid reflux, and ulcer formation, and the use of PPIs (and often additional therapies such as sucralfate) to treat such side effects is warranted.

Proposed Mechanisms of Aspirin Desensitization

The mechanism of how aspirin ameliorates the severity of AERD remains an enigma. The process of aspirin desensitization allows patients to clinically tolerate the surge in CysLTs [36] and mast cell mediators, such as histamine, tryptase, and prostaglandin D_2 [36–38], seen following the ingestion of the provocative dose during the desensitization procedure. However, what allows the patient to go on to tolerate subsequently higher doses of aspirin without further clinical reaction is unknown. What is known is that the continued administration of aspirin after desensitization mitigates many of the features characteristic of the AERD phenotype. Desensitized subjects no longer have the characteristic surge in LT production after taking each dose of aspirin yet continue to produce CysLTs at levels unchanged from baseline levels on high-dose aspirin therapy [8]. They display diminished responsiveness to the CysLTs, reflecting, in part, decreased expression of CysLT1R in their airways following aspirin desensitization [39]. What happens to the other mediators involved in the clinical reaction to aspirin following long-term high-dose aspirin therapy has not been systematically studied.

There are several plausible mechanisms that could underlie the benefits of high-dose aspirin therapy. The baseline and reaction-induced overproduction of CysLTs reflects, in part, the striking adherence of platelets to neutrophils and eosinophils in these patients and subsequent transcellular arachidonate metabolism [40]. A clinical trial is underway exploring whether the antiplatelet effects of aspirin diminish the adherence of platelets to granulocytes (http://clinicaltrials.gov/ct2/show/NCT01597375). In addition to supporting CysLT production, platelet-derived TxA_2 is likely pathogenic in this disorder by its direct ability to induce bronchospasm, effects that are diminished with continuous aspirin administration. Other "on-target" (cyclooxygenase-targeting) effects of aspirin include inhibited synthesis of proinflammatory and bronchospastic prostaglandins such as $PGF_2\alpha$ and PGD_2. Diminished PGD_2 is a particularly inviting target for investigation given its recently reported ability to induce recruitment and secretion of cytokines associated with a Th2 "signature" from type 2 innate lymphoid cells [41].

There are numerous facets of aspirin desensitization that cannot be directly explained by "on-target" influences on the cyclooxygenases, for example, the influences noted above on downregulation of CysLT1R expression. Aspirin has an impressive array of these "off-target" effects that invite consideration as a basis for these observations. However, among the most intriguing observations is its ability to modulate gene transcription through influences on the nuclear pores responsible for transcription factor trafficking in and out of the nucleus such as its ability to downregulate NF-κB entry into the nucleus [42, 43]. Of direct relevance to AERD, aspirin-mediated modulation of both CysLT1R and LTC_4S expressions has been ascribed to aspirin's influences on nuclear expression of the IL-4-/IL-13-dependent transcription factor STAT6 [44]. Thus, at the higher doses used after desensitization, aspirin blocks STAT6 trafficking into the nucleus, providing a molecular basis for the downregulation of these transcripts. It is, again, reasonable to speculate that similar influences may underlie modulation of the dysregulation of other genes associated with the AERD phenotype such as COX-1, prostaglandin E_2 (EP2) receptor, perhaps the LTE_4 receptor, and others. However, an understanding of the mechanism of high-dose aspirin therapy in AERD remains largely speculative, and, although an inviting area for future research, at present what exists is just the tantalizing observation that aspirin desensitization does somehow work.

Conclusion

Although the mechanism of action of desensitization and high-dose aspirin therapy remains unknown and further research is needed, the clinical benefit of high-dose aspirin therapy for 70–80 % of subjects with AERD is well established. Referral to a physician trained in the treatment of asthma and allergic diseases with experience with aspirin desensitization protocols should be strongly considered for any patient with AERD who fails standard medical management of their upper or lower airway disease. Aspirin desensitization followed by high-dose aspirin therapy is a safe, clinically effective, and cost-effective option for almost all patients with AERD.

References

1. Widal F, Abraimi P, Lermoyez J. Anaphylaxie et idiosyncrasie. Presse Med. 1922;30:189–92.
2. Samter M, Beers Jr RF. Intolerance to aspirin: clinical studies and considerations of its pathogenesis. Ann Intern Med. 1968;68:975–83.
3. Stevenson DD, Simon RA, Mathison DA. Aspirin-sensitive asthma: tolerance to aspirin after positive oral aspirin challenges. J Allergy Clin Immunol. 1980;66:82–8.
4. Xu JJ, Sowerby L, Rotenberg BW. Aspirin desensitization for aspirin-exacerbated respiratory disease (Samter's Triad): a systematic review of the literature. Int Forum Allergy Rhinol. 2013;3:915–20.
5. Williams AN, Woessner KM. The clinical effectiveness of aspirin desensitization in chronic rhinosinusitis. Curr Allergy Asthma Rep. 2008;8:245–52.
6. Stevenson DD. Aspiring desensitization in patients with AERD. Clin Rev Allergy Immunol. 2003;24:159–68.
7. McMains KC, Kountakis SE. Medical and surgical considerations in patients with Samter's triad. Am J Rhinol. 2006;20:573–6.
8. Swierczynska-Krepa M, Sanak M, Bochenek G, Strek P, Cmiel A, Gielicz A, et al. Aspirin desensitization in patients with aspirin-induced and aspirin-tolerant asthma: a double-blind study. J Allergy Clin Immunol. 2014;134(4):883–90.
9. Szczeklik A, Nizankowska E, Duplaga M. Natural history of aspirin-induced asthma. AIANE Investigators. European Network on Aspiring-Induced Asthma. Eur Respir J. 2000;16:432–6.
10. Mascia K, Haselkorn T, Deniz Y, Miller DP, Bleecker ER, Borish L. Aspirin sensitivity and severity of asthma: evidence for irreversible airway obstruction in patients with severe or difficult-to-treat asthma. J Allergy Clin Immunol. 2005;116:970–5.
11. Kowalski ML. Rhinosinusitis and nasal polyposis in aspirin sensitive and aspirin tolerant patients: are they different? Thorax. 2000;55:S84–6.
12. Mascia K, Borish L, Patrie J, Hunt J, Phillips CD, Steinke J. Chronic hyperplastic eosinophilic sinusitis as a predictor of aspirin-exacerbated respiratory disease. Ann Allergy Asthma Immunol. 2005;94:652–7.
13. Havel M, Ertl L, Braunschweig F, Markmann S, Leunig A, Gamarra F, Kramer MF. Sinonasal outcomes under aspirin desensitization following functional endoscopic sinus surgery in patients with aspirin triad. Eur Arch Otorhinolaryngol. 2013;270:571–8.
14. Kennedy DW. Prognostic factors, outcomes and staging in ethmoid sinus surgery. Laryngoscope. 1992;102:1–18.
15. Palikhe NS, Kim JH, Parks HS. Update on recent advances in the management of aspirin exacerbated respiratory disease. Yonsei Med J. 2009;50:744–50.
16. Laidlaw TM, Boyce JA. Pathogenesis of aspirin-exacerbated respiratory disease and reactions. Immunol Allergy Clin North Am. 2013;33:195–210.
17. Dahlen SE, Malstrom K, Nizankowska E, Dahlen B, Kuna P, Kowalski M, et al. Improvement of aspirin-intolerant asthma by montelukast, a leukotriene antagonist: a randomized, double-blind, placebo-controlled trial. Am J Respir Crit Care Med. 2002;165:9–14.

18. Dahlen B, Nizankowska E, Szczeklik A, Zetterstrom O, Bochenek G, Kumlin M, et al. Benefits from adding the 5-lipoxygenase inhibitor zileuton to conventional therapy in aspirin-intolerant asthmatics. Am J Respir Crit Care Med. 1998;157:1187–94.
19. Macy E, Bernstein JA, Castells MC, Gawchik SM, Lee TH, Settipane RA, et al. Aspirin challenge and desensitization for aspirin-exacerbated respiratory disease: a practice paper. Ann Allergy Asthma Immunol. 2007;98:172–4.
20. Gollapudi RR, Teirstein PS, Stevenson DD, Simon RA. Aspirin sensitivity: implications for patients with coronary artery disease. JAMA. 2004;292:3017–23.
21. Woessner KM, Simon RA. Cardiovascular prophylaxis and aspirin "allergy". Immunol Allergy Clin North Am. 2013;33:263–74.
22. Shaker M, Lobb A, Jenkins P, O'Rourke D, Takemoto SK, Sheth S, et al. An economic analysis of aspirin desensitization in aspirin-exacerbated respiratory disease. J Allergy Clin Immunol. 2008;121:81–7.
23. Stevenson DD, Simon RA. Selection of patients for aspirin desensitization treatment. J Allergy Clin Immunol. 2006;118:801–4.
24. Berges-Gimeno MP, Simon RA, Stevenson DD. Long-term treatment with aspirin desensitization in asthmatic patients with aspirin-exacerbated respiratory disease. J Allergy Clin Immunol. 2003;111:180–6.
25. Berges-Gimeno MP, Simon RA, Stevenson DD. Early effects of aspirin desensitization treatment in asthmatic patients with aspirin-exacerbated respiratory disease. Ann Allergy Asthma Immunol. 2003;90:338–41.
26. Fruth K, Pogorzelski B, Schmidtmann I, Springer J, Fennan N, Fraessdorf N, et al. Low-dose aspirin desensitization in individuals with aspirin-exacerbated respiratory disease. Allergy. 2013;68:659–65.
27. Stevenson DD, Hankammer MA, Matthison DA, Christiansen SC, Simon RA. Aspirin desensitization treatment of aspirin-sensitive patients with rhinosinusitis-asthma: long-term outcomes. J Allergy Clin Immunol. 1996;98:751–8.
28. Williams AN, Simon RA, Woessner KM, Stevenson DD. The relationship between historical aspirin induced asthma and severity of asthma induced during oral aspirin challenges. J Allergy Clin Immunol. 2007;120:273–7.
29. Hope AP, Woessner KM, Simon RA, Stevenson DD. Rational approach to aspirin dosing during oral challenges and desensitization of patients with aspirin-exacerbated respiratory disease. J Allergy Clin Immunol. 2009;123:406–10.
30. White A, Ludington E, Mehra P, Stevenson DD, Simon RA. Effect of leukotriene modifier drugs on the safety of oral aspirin challenges. Ann Allergy Asthma Immunol. 2006;97:688–93.
31. Lee JY, Simon RA, Stevenson DD. Selection of aspirin dosages for aspirin desensitization treatment in patients with aspirin-exacerbated respiratory disease. J Allergy Clin Immunol. 2007;119:157–64.
32. Lee RU, White AA, Ding D, Dursun AB, Woessner KM, Simon RA, Stevenson DD. Use of intranasal ketorolac and modified oral aspirin challenge for desensitization of aspirin-exacerbated respiratory disease. Ann Allergy Asthma Immunol. 2010;105:130–5.
33. Wong JT, Nagy CS, Krinzman SJ, Maclean JA, Bloch KJ. Rapid oral challenge-desensitization for patients with aspirin-related urticarial-angioedema. J Allergy Clin Immunol. 2000;105:997–1001.
34. Crapo RO, Casaburi R, Coates AL, Enright PL, Hankinson JL, Irvin CG, et al. Guidelines for methacholine and exercise challenge testing – 1999. Am J Respir Crit Care Med. 2000;161:309–29.
35. Stevenson DD, Simon RA, Mathison DA, Christiansen SC. Montelukast is only partially effective in inhibiting aspirin responses in aspirin-sensitive asthmatics. Ann Allergy Asthma Immunol. 2000;85:477–82.
36. Kumlin M, Dahlén B, Björck T, Zetterström O, Granström E, Dahlén SE. Urinary excretion of leukotriene E4 and 11-dehydro-thromboxane B2 in response to bronchial provocations with allergen, aspirin, leukotriene D4, and histamine in asthmatics. Am Rev Respir Dis. 1992;146:96–103.

37. Bochenek G, Nagraba K, Nizankowska E, Szczeklik A. A controlled study of 9α,11β-PGF2 (a prostaglandin D2 metabolite) in plasma and urine of patients with bronchial asthma and healthy controls after aspirin challenge. J Allergy Clin Immunol. 2003;111:743–9.
38. Fischer AR, Rosenberg MA, Lilly CM, Callery JC, Rubin P, Cohn J, et al. Direct evidence for a role of the mast cell in the nasal response to aspirin in aspirin-sensitive asthma. J Allergy Clin Immunol. 1994;94:1046–56.
39. Sousa AR, Parikh A, Scadding G, Corrigan CJ, Lee TH. Leukotriene-receptor expression on nasal mucosal inflammatory cells in aspirin-sensitive rhinosinusitis. N Engl J Med. 2002;347:1493–9.
40. Laidlaw TM, Kidder MS, Bhattacharyya N, Xing W, Shen S, Milne GL, et al. Cysteinyl leukotriene overproduction in aspirin-exacerbated respiratory disease is driven by platelet-adherent leukocytes. Blood. 2012;119:3790–8.
41. Barnig C, Cernada M, Dutile S, Liu Z, Perrella MA, Kazani S, et al. Lipoxin A_4 regulates natural killer cell and type 2 innate lymphoid cell activation in asthma. Sci Transl Med. 2013;174:174ra26.
42. Kopp E, Ghosh S. Inhibition of NF-kappa B by sodium salicylate and aspirin. Science. 1994;265:956–9.
43. Tegeder I, Pfeilschifter J, Geisslinger G. Cyclooxygenase-independent actions of cyclooxygenase inhibitors. FASEB J. 2001;15:2057–72.
44. Steinke JW, Culp JA, Kropf E, Borish L. Modulation by aspirin of nuclear phospho-signal transducer and activator of transcription 6 expression: possible role in therapeutic benefit associated with aspirin desensitization. J Allergy Clin Immunol. 2009;124:724–30.

Saline Irrigations

20

Niall Jefferson and Richard Harvey

Key Take-Home Points

- Nasal irrigation has a limited role in the unoperated patient.
- High-volume, positive-pressure devices offer the most reliable delivery to the paranasal sinuses after sinus surgery.
- Saline nasal irrigation alone has been shown to modify the disease process through a likely mechanical effect.

Introduction

Chronic rhinosinusitis (CRS) is one of the commonest conditions to present to primary care providers and a range of subspecialists. It is currently thought to affect up to 9 % of the population and comparable to rates of asthma. While symptom relief is always the goal, contemporary management of CRS is primarily focused on reducing bacterial colonization or infection, suppressing inflammation and restoring mucociliary function.

N. Jefferson, MBBCh, BAO, FRACS (OHNS) (✉)
Department of Otolaryngology Head and Neck Surgery,
St Vincent's Hospital, Victoria Street, Darlinghurst, Sydney, NSW Australia
e-mail: niallj99@yahoo.com

R. Harvey, MD, PhD
Department of Otolaryngology Head and Neck Surgery,
St Vincent's Hospital, Victoria Street, Darlinghurst, Sydney, NSW Australia

Department of Otolaryngology and Skull Base Surgery,
Rhinology and Skull Base, Applied Medical Research Centre,
University of New South Wales, Sydney, NSW 2010, Australia

Australian School of Advanced Medicine, Macquarie University,
Darlinghurst, Sydney, NSW Australia
e-mail: Richard@sydneyentclinic.com

P.S. Batra, J.K. Han (eds.), *Practical Medical and Surgical Management of Chronic Rhinosinusitis*, DOI 10.1007/978-3-319-16724-4_20

Nasal saline irrigation is a common adjunct treatment in the management of CRS. Its favorable safety profile, minimal systemic risks, and good patient acceptance make it a successful therapy in the long-term management of CRS. Evidence exists that saline is not simply a symptom reliever but a potential disease-modifying intervention. Nasal irrigation can be used as a sole modality of treatment, as a treatment adjunct, or as a vehicle to deliver local therapies to the paranasal sinuses. Its simplicity allows it to be integrated into a disease process that spans a spectrum of disease severity.

Pathophysiology of CRS

The pathophysiology of CRS is discussed elsewhere in this book, but the different theories relating to the mechanisms contributing to chronic mucosal inflammation in this disease state have evolved over time. Current theories surrounding the nature of CRS broadly fall into debate over the influence of local microenvironment versus a "disease-differentiated" mucosal barrier that inherently activates an inappropriate proinflammatory immune response.

Local microenvironment has focused on the role of superantigens and their modification of eicosanoid metabolism as well as enhancing Th2-mediated immunity [1, 2]. It has also examined the effect of Staphylococcus aureus biofilms influencing the local immune response in the direction of a Th2-modulated pathway [3, 4], and the effect of fungal proteases [5, 6]. The immune barrier hypothesis describes epithelial barrier dysfunction, innate immune dysregulation, and an inappropriate activation of the acquired immune system resulting in the pathogenetic changes seen in CRS [7]. The shift away from environmental and microbial agents as the cause of CRS toward determining the hosts' epithelial susceptibility has been established in other chronic inflammatory disease states such as atopic dermatitis and asthma. Evidence now exists demonstrating barrier disruption as a result of diminished tight junctions and increased ion permeability [8, 9]; in addition, a complex interplay between proteases and antiproteases, activated toll-like receptors (TLR) [10], and the subsequent activation of an adaptive-immunity response lead to the development of CRS. This chapter will discuss the factors that influence saline irrigation therapy, including distribution, effects on the microenvironment, and clinical recommendations from a blend of evidence base and expert opinion.

Effective Topical Distribution to the Paranasal Sinuses

The paranasal sinuses are a complex network of interconnected cavities lined by respiratory epithelium. The ability of saline or any other topical therapy to reach the paranasal sinuses has been the focus of recent research. Surgical state, delivery device, volume, pressure, and position all impact the distribution of irrigant into the sinonasal cavity [11].

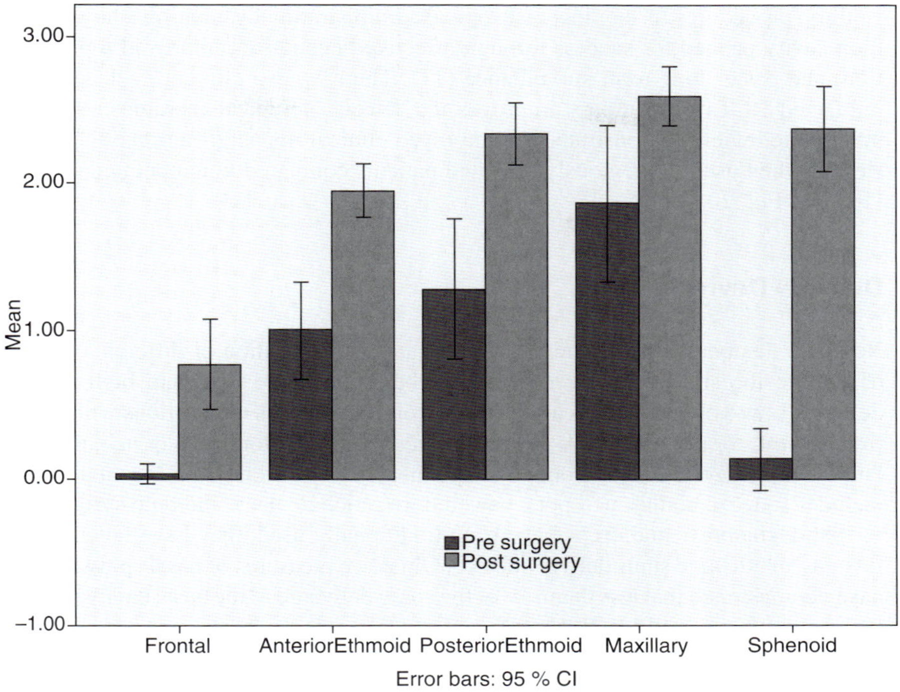

Fig. 20.1 Sprays have almost no sinus distribution to the paranasal sinuses prior to surgery. Mean sinus dispersion of radiographic contrast is extremely limited without surgical exposure of the sinus mucosa. This is particularly true of the frontal and sphenoid sinuses (Reprinted by permission of SAGE Publications, Harvey et al. [15])

Surgical State

It is widely recognized that unoperated patients have both inconsistent and limited sinus distribution of topical therapies regardless of the delivery device, head position, or volume [12, 13], and in the CRS patient with mucosal edema, this penetration is further reduced [14]. It has long been thought that sinus surgery results in improved delivery of topical preparations to the sinuses, but only recently has evidence become available to support this assertion [15, 16]. See Fig. 20.1.

Heterogeneity within published series in relation to the extent of surgery performed has made comparison of outcomes in interventions utilizing topical therapies difficult to assess, as some institutions will create widely connected cavities whereas others favor balloon dilatation or more conservative sinusotomies. Current evidence supports larger ostial remodeling, thereby permitting more effective delivery of topical therapies. A minimal size for effective penetration to the maxillary sinus is described as at least 4–5 mm [16–18]. For frontal and sphenoid sinuses, their more remote locations result in sinus surgery greatly influencing delivery of irrigation. More extensive surgeries such as medial maxillectomy and endoscopic

Lothrop procedures further increase topical administration by creating a large, common cavity primed for success through effective penetration, improved topicalization, and easier long-term surveillance [11]. There is also clinical evidence from published RCTs that surgery improves the effects of topical therapies. A recent systematic review demonstrated the improved clinical impact of intranasal corticosteroid when used in previously operated patients compared to unoperated patients [19] (see Fig. 20.2).

Delivery Device

Research demonstrates significant variation in the distribution of different delivery devices to the sinuses. These devices can be divided into low- and high-volume delivery. Low-volume devices are typically common rhinitis medications which vary from 0.1 mL for a "spray" to 1–5 mL delivered by drops, atomizers, or nebulizers. A large volume device ranges from 60 mL to the more common 240 mL container and includes squeeze bottles, neti pots, powered irrigation devices, and bulb syringes.

Although sprays and drops have been traditionally used, they have fallen out of favor as an effective sinus delivery device. Objective measures of nasal spray devices have demonstrated that less than 1 % of the spray delivered to the nasal cavity reaches the paranasal sinuses [20]. Even with an optimal angle of delivery, nasal sprays are limited to the inferior and middle turbinate [21]. In the operated patient, nasal sprays fail to reliably reach the middle meatus least the paranasal sinuses, thus limiting their useful application in the pre- or postoperative state of the CRS patient [22]. While drops have been demonstrated to reach the olfactory cleft in a dependent position, overall, they are equivalent to nasal sprays in their limited distribution.

Nebulizers demonstrate limited delivery to the paranasal sinuses even in the postoperative state. There remains a lack of agreement in the literature in relation to the optimal particle size varying from small particles (<5 um) to larger particles [23]. Overall, nebulizers are good at moisturizing the nasal cavity but, like the other low-volume devices, fail to effectively penetrate the paranasal sinuses, even in the operated patient. Studies comparing the various low-volume devices have failed to demonstrate clear superiority of one over the others [12, 24]. The low volume of specialized pulsing nebulizers that might provide improved sinus penetration only works by delivering the fluid, and the mechanical action of clearing mucus is lost.

There are a range of high-volume devices; however when the volume delivered is >100 mL, the effective delivery to the paranasal sinuses is far more reliable. The sinuses represent a significant "dead space" beyond the nasal cavity, and a 100 mL + volume has been shown to most effectively penetrate these cavities [25].

Squeeze bottles, passive-flow devices such as neti pots, and pulsed irrigators all result in improved sinonasal distribution compared to low-volume devices. Clinical studies have also demonstrated improved patient symptoms and endoscopic appearance in postoperative patients with mild CRS [26], though in the same study, there

a

Study or Subgroup	steroid Mean	SD	Total	placebo Mean	SD	Total	Weight	Std, Mean Difference IV,Fixed, 95% CI
1 Patients with sinus surgery (all or majority)								
Holopainen 1982	-3.43	4.74	10	-1 .71	2.11	8	2.6%	-0.43 [-1 .37, 0.51]
Jorissen 2009	-14.3	9.1	46	-13.8	8.63	45	13.7%	-0.06 [-0.47, 0.36]
Lavigne 2002	-5	2.05	11	-1 .82	2.56	11	2.6%	-1.32 [-2.26, -0 .38]
Lund 1998	2	4.44	10	4	4.44	9	2.8%	-0.43 [-1 .34, 0.48]
Mygind 1975	-1.72	1.07	19	-0.76	1.09	16	4.7%	-0.87 [-1 .57, -0 .17]
Vlckova 2009	-1.11	1.91	54	0.31	1.93	52	14.9%	-0.73 [-1 .13, -0 .34]
Subtotal (95% CI)			150			**141**	**41.2%**	**-0.52 [-0.76, -0.29]**
Heterogeneity: Chi²= 9.84, df= 5 (P = 0.08); I²= 49%								
Test for overall effect: z = 4.33 (P < 0.0001)								
2 Patients wtthout sinus surgeJY (all, majority or undefined)								
Filiaci 2000	-1.15	0.91	36	-0.15	0.95	31	8.7%	-1 .06 [-1 .58, -0 .55]
Furukido 2005	-6.18	4.44	15	-5.71	5.21	10	3.6%	-0.10 [-0.90, 0.71]
Johansson 2002	-11.41	4.32	50	0.84	42.07	48	14.4%	-0.41 [-0.81, -0 .01]
Lund 2004	-1.85	1.93	81	-1.02	2.88	86	24.7%	-0.34 [-0.64, -0 .03]
Mastalerz 1997	-1.62	2.86	15	0.59	4.53	15	4.3%	-0.57 [-1.30, 0.16]
Parikh 2001	-21.3	32.9	9	3.6	73	13	3.1%	-0.40 [-1.26, 0.46]
Subtotal (95% CI)			206			**203**	**58.8%**	**-0.47 [-0.67, -0.27]**
Heterogeneity: Chi²= 6.89, df= 5 (P = 0.23); I²= 27%								
Testfor overall effect: Z = 4.62 (P < 0.00001)								
Total (95% CI)			**356**			**344**	**100.0%**	**-0.49 [-0.64, -0.34]**
Heterogeneity: Chi²= 16.85, df= 11 (P = 0.11); I²= 35%								
Test for overall effect: z = 6.32 (P < 0.00001)								
Test for subgroup differences: Chi²= 0.12. df= 1 (P = 0.73).1²= 0%								

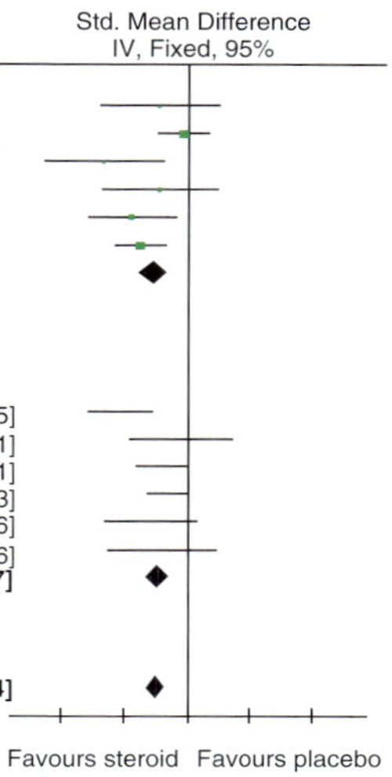

b

Study or Subgroup	placebo Events	Total	steroid Events	Total	Weight	Risk Ratio M-H,Fixed,95% CI
1 Patients with sinus surgery (all or majority)						
Holopainen 1982	2	8	8	10	4.4%	0.31 [0.09, 1.08]
Keith 2000	8	52	14	52	8.7%	0.57 [0.26, 1.25]
Penttila 2000	7	47	19	47	11.8%	0.37 [0.17, 0.79]
Vickova 2009	5	55	31	54	19.4%	0.16 [0.07, 0.38]
Subtotal(95% CI)		**162**		**163**	**44.2%**	**0.31[0.20, 0.48]**
Total events	22		72			
Heterogeneity: Chi²= 4.86, df= 3 (P = 0.18); I²= 38%						
Test for overall effect: z = 5.38 (P < 0.00001)						
2 Patients without sinus surgery (all or majority)						
Chalton 1985	2	15	9	15	5.6%	0.22 [0.06, 0.86]
Holmstrom 1999	8	51	15	49	9.5%	0.51 [0.24, 1.10]
Lang 1983	6	18	4	14	2.8%	1.17 [0.41, 3.35]
Stjarne 2006b	39	145	63	153	38.0%	0.65 [0.47, 0.91]
Subtotal(95% CI)		**229**		**231**	**55.8%**	**0.61[046,0.81]**
Total events	55		91			
Heterogeneity: Chi²= 3.94, df= 3 (P = 0.27); I²= 24%						
Test for overall effect: z = 3.42 (P = 0.00006)						
Total (95% CI)		**391**		**394**	**100.0%**	**0.48[0.38, 0.60]**
Total events	77		163			
Heterogeneity: Chi²= 14.85, df= 7 (P = 0.04); I²= 53%						
Test for overall effect: z = 6.18 (P < 0.00001)						
Test for subgroup differences: Chi²= 6.78, df= 1 (P = 0.099).1²= 85.3%						

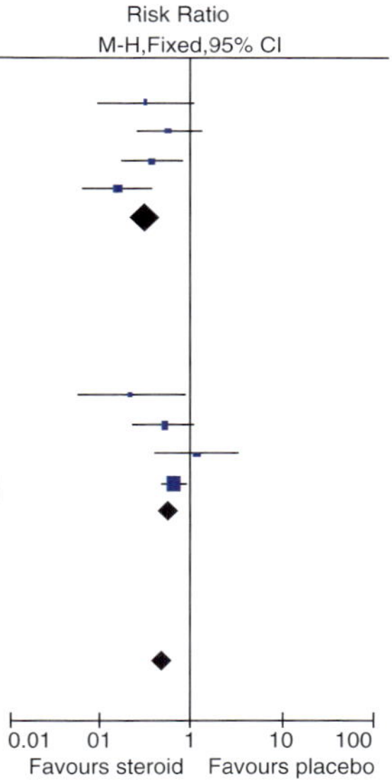

Fig. 20.2 Forest plot from meta-analysis of RCTs demonstrating benefit of nasal steroids versus placebo in patients undergoing sinus surgery from CRS. A meta-analysis demonstrating that the effects of INCS in the treatment of CRS are greater when looking at a group of randomized controlled trials if the studies are sub-analyzed by prior sinus surgery. (**a**) The standardized mean difference for symptom scores is greater in the studies that used groups of patients that have had prior sinus surgery, and the difference for overall "responders" to INCS therapy (**b**) is "significant" (Reprinted with permission from Snidvongs et al. [19])

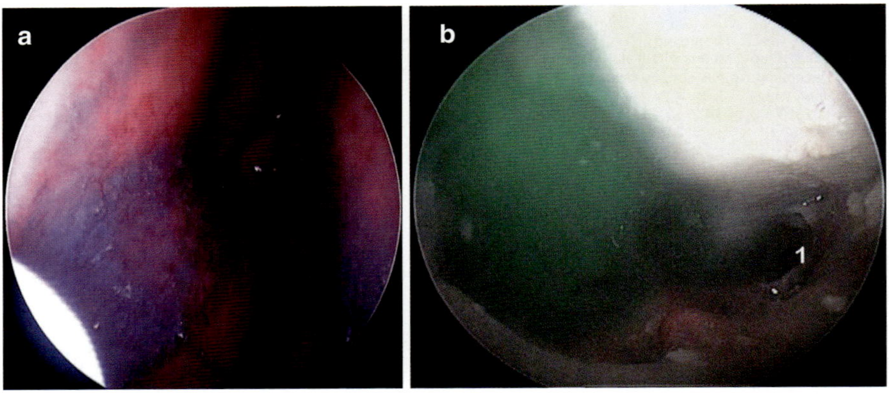

Fig. 20.3 Image (**a**) demonstrating the limited penetration of intranasal sprays with the nozzle of the nasal spray (*a*) seen in the nasal vestibule and the limited amount of methylene blue within the anterior nasal cavity. Even after endoscopic sinus surgery (ESS), the frontal recess (*1*) is not well penetrated with simple delivery. Only with head-down positioning and high-volume, positive-pressure irrigation does frontal sinus recess delivery occur (Image **b**)

was no improvement in the same outcomes versus sinus debridement alone for those patients with moderate to severe CRS. Pynnonen et al. [27] compared high-volume (240 mL) low-pressure isotonic irrigation to low-volume nasal spray and evaluated QOL and symptom scores in the postoperative period. They demonstrated improved QOL in both groups at 8 weeks but a significant improvement in both QOL and symptoms in the high-volume irrigation group.

Fluid dynamics between the different high-volume devices is likely to be very different. The high-pressure devices generate greater shearing forces on the mucous blanket; however, this is something that is very difficult to quantify at the research level (see Fig. 20.3).

Radiographic studies as well as endoscopic grading systems do not tend to distinguish between high-volume high-pressure devices, such as a squeeze bottle, and high-volume low-pressure devices, such as neti pots. It is not currently known whether high-pressure delivery offers an advantage over a high-volume low-pressure device. It has been demonstrated, however, that increasing the volume delivered results in improved sinonasal distribution [28, 29].

Position

A number of positions are available; these include the Mygind position (lying head back), the Ragan position (lying head lateral and low), and the kneeling position (head down and forward) (see Fig. 20.4).

Regardless of head position, sinus delivery is not reliably seen in the unoperated patient. For the operated patient, delivery to the paranasal sinuses is best seen in the kneeling position, though this is also found to be the most uncomfortable for many patients [11]. Well-designed studies seem to suggest that head position can affect sinus distribution when using positive-pressure devices such as a neti pot or bulb

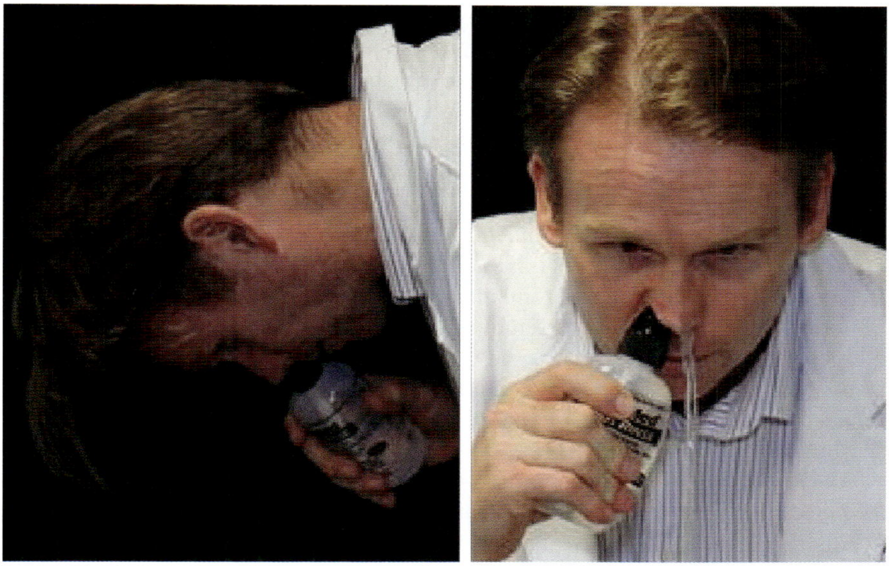

Fig. 20.4 The ideal position for maximal sinus penetration with an irrigation bottle is the "vertex down" position using sinus irrigation bottle (Model: A/professor Richard Harvey, Rhinology and skull base surgeon, Department of Otorhinolaryngology, St. Vincent's hospital, Sydney)

syringes. The lateral position appears more favorable for the neti pot [15], whereas the kneeling position results in improved sinus delivery (particularly to the frontal sinus) when using a "squeeze bottle" [25]. Most of the studies in position have used low-volume sprays and drops, and it is highly likely that a large volume mostly overcomes an advantage of positioning.

An important consideration is that in the elderly or the physically impaired, achieving these positions becomes increasingly challenging. In such a circumstance, a "head-over-sink" position may be preferable.

Based on the best available research, high-volume, positive-pressure irrigation devices appear to be the most effective delivery modality for penetrating the paranasal sinuses and overcome head position. In addition, both patients and prescribers require appropriate education on optimal volume and positioning based on the device used and the underlying mobility and dexterity of the patient.

Factors Influencing the Microenvironment

Mucous Blanket and Rheology

Nasal mucus is an important part of the body's innate protection and represents the first line of defense to inspired particles. Up to 25 million particles are managed by the airway epithelium every hour with more than 500 l of air filtered in the same time period [30, 31]. The mucous blanket is a non-Newtonian shearing blanket that is composed of a watery periciliary layer and a viscoelastic gel outer layer. The thickness of these layers can be challenging to measure accurately; the inner layer in which the cilia reside is estimated to be about 5–10 um and the outer layer approximately 7–30 um in healthy mucosa [32, 33]. This can increase by as much as ten times in the diseased state thereby affecting mucociliary function as well as limiting diffusion of medications [34, 35].

This gel blanket that covers the respiratory epithelium is highly inducible and can increase in thickness by as much as 10 um per second when stimulated [36]. Hypersecretion of nasal mucus is a feature of CRS [37] as well as rhinitis [38] and is a recognized element in other inflammatory airway conditions. The implied role of sprays and irrigations is to remove particulate matter and reduce the load of antigenic or inflammatory debris; however, there is only limited evidence to substantiate this claim. There does exist indirect evidence in allergic rhinitis of reduced antigen-specific IgE in allergy sufferers who use saline during the allergy season [39].

Mucociliary clearance is comprised of a number of factors including ciliary beat frequency (CBF), ciliary structure, ciliary orientation, gel and sol composition, and mucus rheology. Studies have failed to demonstrate direct evidence of improved CBF with the topical delivery of saline; in fact, there is evidence of ciliostasis with hypertonic solutions at 7 and 14 % and reduced CBF with isotonic saline by as much as 46 % [40].

The effect of differing tonicities on mucociliary clearance and its effect on mucus rheology have also been explored. A blinded controlled study [41] (albeit in normal healthy adult patients) comparing buffered isotonic against buffered hypertonic saline demonstrated improved saccharine clearance time (SCT) for both. This reduction has been purported to be secondary to rehydration of the sol layer and better viscoelastic properties as a result of the increased ionic load, thus leading to more efficient movement of the cilia within the mucous blanket [42].

Effect on the Nasal Mucosa

Traditionally, it has been posited that saline irrigations are protective to the sinonasal mucosa by reducing mucosal dryness and by facilitating the clearance of thickened secretions and crusts. It has been further proposed that this could lead to improved IgA-mediated innate mucosal defense [43]. In vitro studies however have demonstrated morphologic changes in previously healthy mucosa with both hypo- (0.3 %) and hypertonic (3 %) saline solutions [44]. In the 0.3 % saline treatment group, normal human nasal epithelial (NHNE) cells were moderately damaged, and the total number of cilia-containing cells was also significantly decreased. In the 0.9 % saline treatment group, the epithelium appeared normal and was covered with healthy cilia. Cell-to-cell integrity also appeared to be maintained. When cells were treated with 3 % saline, holes appeared in places where secretory cells exfoliated, but cell-to-cell integrity was maintained. No studies to date have demonstrated beneficial changes histologically from isotonic solutions.

Tonicity

While there is a wide variation in individual thresholds and tolerance, the potential exists for increasing pain, secretions, and vasodilation with increasing tonicity. A number of randomized controlled trials have been performed evaluating outcomes in relation to symptoms and quality of life (QOL) comparing isotonic and hypertonic preparations [45], hypertonic versus no treatment [46], and isotonic irrigation versus reflexology [1]. Hypertonic saline has certainly been shown to stimulate the nasal mucosa. Hyperosmolar challenges have led to an increase in nasal secretions in concert with increasing osmolarity. A significant increase in secretions is seen first at 3.6 % in healthy patients [47], but even with 2.7 % solutions, burning and discomfort are experienced. In the viral rhinosinusitis sufferer, hypertonic saline solutions have demonstrated greater burning and discomfort when compared with an isotonic preparation, 32 % versus 13 % ($p<0.05$) [48].

Proposed Decongestant Effect of Hypertonic Solutions

While there has been much speculation relating to the potential decongestant effect of hypertonic saline, this has not been supported in the scientific literature. This potential decongestant effect has been proposed through the effect of an osmotic process leading to reduced edema thereby improving nasal patency [48]. No statistically significant difference has been demonstrated at commonly used concentrations (0.3 % versus 3 % saline preparations) on rhinometric studies [49], and decreased airspace measurements have been seen on rhinometry following hypertonic saline exposure [50].

Adverse Effects

Overall, the use of nasal saline irrigation is regarded as low risk as demonstrated in the Cochrane review [51]. Often overlooked side effects however include cost, preparation time, and delivery effort. Some patients will find the practice of irrigation uncomfortable due to burning sensation, Eustachian tube dysfunction, and nausea. Our current protocols recommend twice-daily or less frequency schedules; more frequent protocols are simply not practical nor is there adequate evidence to support it.

The first description of contamination was by Heatley et al. in 2001 [52]. While not the main focus of the paper, it was recognized by the authors that colonization with bacteria happened in up to 30 % of neti pots or bulb syringes within 2 weeks. This is reflective of subsequent research evaluating colonization varying from 20 to 100 % of devices. While an in vitro study by Williams et al. demonstrated bacterial colonization of bulb syringes in the absence of human contact [53], it is widely accepted that device contamination is a result of colonized or infected sinonasal cavities [54].

Overall, *Staphylococcus aureus* and *Pseudomonas aeruginosa* are the most commonly isolated bacteria from irrigation devices. Geographical differences have been noted, with *Pseudomonas* more commonly isolated in the North American studies and *S. aureus* found to predominate in Australia.

Only one study to date has compared contamination between devices. Heatley et al. [52] found no statistically significant difference in contamination rate between open neti pots and the closed bulb syringe systems, although there was a trend toward fewer infections in the neti pot group [53]. Williams et al. also assessed the effect of tonicity and buffering and their effect on bacterial load. Unbuffered isotonic saline resulted in the highest contamination rates, with increasing tonicity producing an almost protective effect likely as a result of the optimal pH conditions for the proliferation of microorganisms (particularly *S. aureus* and *Pseudomonas*), seen at neutral/slightly acidic conditions.

Keen et al. [55] in an attempt to document the most effective cleaning method examined the success rates of the five most commonly recommended cleaning methods: rinsing with cold water, boiling water, detergents, Milton's antibacterial solution, and microwaving. Although contamination still occurred with all cleaning practices, rinsing with boiling water or Milton's solution or microwaving for 1.5 min on high appeared to reduce the degree of contamination.

While most manufacturers recommend changing the irrigation device every 3 months, a recently published small survey reported that most patients continue to use them for much longer, with the median duration of bottle use as high as 12 months [56]. A number of studies have assessed the effect of duration of use on colonization. While it was not found to be a linear effect, in most cases contamination increased with the duration of use. Despite the clear evidence of device contamination, the clinical effect is unclear. At the present time, it is recommended that devices be changed every 3 months and be washed between uses with clear education for the user on the optimal methods for sterilization and storage to reduce the burden of contamination.

Clinical Applications

Rhinitis

There are several well-performed clinical studies with patient-reported outcomes to support saline therapy in rhinitis management. In 2012, ten studies were identified that assessed the intervention of saline in patients with allergic rhinitis defined by a positive patient history or skin tests (skin prick) or blood test [57–65]. All ten studies were prospective and controlled with randomization not performed in only one [58] of the ten studies. The saline intervention was compared to no treatment in six studies [58–62], to INCS in one [63], to cetirizine in one [64], and to oil drops in one [57] and directly comparing isotonic versus hypertonic in one [65]. Combined analysis of eight of these studies demonstrated that the nasal symptom score improvement ranged from 3.150 to 67.159 % [66]. Saline irrigation failed to result in symptom improvement in pregnant patients and in fact caused mild worsening [62]. However, when compared to the control group that did not use nasal irrigation, the symptom score and consumption of anti-histamines were significantly reduced. Only two studies [63, 67] used high-volume nasal irrigation and four used a spray [57–59, 64] with the remainder using either drops or syringes. Sprays resulted in improvements ranging from 22.7 to 45 % compared with irrigation (200–400 mL) which generated improvements between 3.2 and 45 %. The question as to the optimal volume required and the best delivery method for nasal saline in the management of AR remains unanswered. Significantly, little differentiation exists to distinguish mild, moderate, and severe AR. Future research may clarify whether SNI alone is sufficient in mild cases or an adjunct to pharmacotherapy in moderate to severe cases.

Clinical Studies in CRS

Saline as an intervention for CRS has been well studied. A review by an American Rhinologic Society (ARS) consensus group in 2013 identified eight RCTs and one meta-analysis evaluating the impact of saline irrigation on clinical outcomes on adult CRS. The studies identified included five presurgical and three post-ESS and were restricted to the adult population with a diagnosis of CRS based on current diagnostic criteria.

All five presurgical studies demonstrated improvement in symptoms and health-related quality-of-life (HRQoL) outcomes from sinonasal irrigation in CRS. Two studies evaluated the effect of isotonic versus hypertonic irrigation [45, 68]; while not demonstrating a significant difference between both groups, the two studies found improvement in subjective sinonasal symptoms defined as "nasal stuffiness" and "nasal obstruction."

Of the eight studies identified, three involved high-volume (>100 mL) irrigation for comparison [26, 27, 68]. While one study [68] assessed a preoperative population and found benefit in primary clinical end points as discussed previously, the two assessing high-volume saline irrigation in the postoperative setting [26, 27] warrant discussion.

The first compared high-volume (240 mL) low-pressure irrigation to an isotonic saline spray with twice-daily treatment for 8 weeks [27]. Though both groups demonstrated improvement in HRQoL at 8 weeks, high-volume irrigation was superior, with a significant improvement in both HRQoL and symptoms when directly comparing the two treatments.

The second study [26] evaluated the effect of once-daily saline irrigation (240 mL) as an adjunct to postoperative debridement. The authors found an improvement in symptoms and endoscopic appearance in the mild CRS population when combining irrigation and debridement compared to debridement alone but failed to demonstrate any significant improvement in the moderate-to-severe CRS group.

The Cochrane review published in 2007 included a mixed group of pediatric and adult patients with both persistent rhinitis and CRS patients [51] as at the time of its review, many studies did not clearly define their patient populations. Standardized mean differences (SMD) were obtained from the reported results in order to compare the trials. The SMD of 1.42 between saline versus no treatment represented a very significant shift favoring saline in the treatment of CRS. The review also concluded that saline irrigation was a useful adjunct in the treatment of CRS but was inferior when compared directly with INS.

Likewise, European guidelines support the use of saline therapy for CRS [69]. In the position paper released in 2012 by aggregate evidence appraised by leaders in the field, saline irrigation was recommended in both the pre- and postoperative setting for patients with CRS without nasal polyposis. The same paper cited insufficient quality evidence to make the same recommendation in CRS with nasal polyposis; however, insufficient evidence does not imply a lack of effect and denotes an area requiring more robust evidence.

Further evidence for the efficacy of saline irrigation exists indirectly through clinical trials. The SINUNASE trial compared an antifungal lavage (amphotericin B 0.01 %) with a placebo arm which consisted of saline irrigation only. An unexpected therapeutic benefit was seen in objective markers, with the saline irrigation arm demonstrating a reduction in the levels of nasal mucus testing of eosinophilic major basic protein (eMBP); it was proposed that saline irrigation reduced the fungal load within the sinuses and consequently resulted in reduced sinonasal inflammation.

Conclusion

There is substantial body of evidence supporting the use of saline irrigation in the management of CRS. Its excellent safety profile and good patient acceptance make it an appealing adjunct to a long-term management strategy. Without effective delivery to the paranasal sinuses however, its application is limited even for the high-volume devices. There is now strong evidence supporting the role of sinus surgery in improving effective delivery of sinus irrigation. Once surgery has resulted in an appropriate corridor, a high-volume device can deliver the irrigation to the paranasal sinuses, regardless of the head position. However, the optimal frequency remains a subject of ongoing debate and research.

References

1. Rudmik L, Hoy M, Schlosser R, Harvey H, Welch K, Lund V, Smith T. Topical therapies in the management of chronic rhinosinusitis: an evidence-based review with recommendations. Int Forum Allergy Rhinol. 2013;3(4):281–98.
2. Okano M, Fujiwara T, Haruna T, Kariya S, Makihara S, Higaki T, et al. Prostaglandin E(2) suppresses staphylococcal enterotoxin-induced eosinophilia-associated cellular responses dominantly through an E-prostanoid 2-mediated pathway in nasal polyps. J Allergy Clin Immunol. 2009;123(4):868–74. 4.
3. Krysko O, Holtappels G, Zhang N, Kubica M, Deswarte K, Derycke L, et al. Alternatively activated macrophages and impaired phagocytosis of S. aureus in chronic rhinosinusitis. Allergy. 2011;66(3):396–403.
4. Poposki JA, Uzzaman A, Nagarkar DR, Chustz RT, Peters AT, Suh LA, et al. Increased expression of the chemokine CCL23 in eosinophilic chronic rhinosinusitis with nasal polyps. J Allergy Clin Immunol. 2011;128(1):73–81. 1.

5. Tieu DD, Kern RC, Schleimer RP. Alterations in epithelial barrier function and host defense responses in chronic rhinosinusitis. J Allergy Clin Immunol. 2009;124(1):37–42.
6. Kern RC, Conley DB, Walsh W, Chandra R, Kato A, Tripathi-Peters A, et al. Perspectives on the etiology of chronic rhinosinusitis: an immune barrier hypothesis. Am J Rhinol. 2008;22(6):549–59.
7. Tan BK, Schleimer RP, Kern RC. Perspectives on the etiology of chronic rhinosinusitis. Curr Opin Otolaryngol Head Neck Surg. 2010;18(1):21–6.
8. Zuckerman JD, Lee WY, DelGaudio JM, Moore CE, Nava P, Nusrat A, et al. Pathophysiology of nasal polyposis: the role of desmosomal junctions. Am J Rhinol. 2008;22(6):589–97.
9. Dejima K, Randell SH, Stutts MJ, Senior BA, Boucher RC. Potential role of abnormal ion transport in the pathogenesis of chronic sinusitis. Arch Otolaryngol Head Neck Surg. 2006;132(12):1352–62.
10. Vroling AB, Fokkens WJ, van Drunen CM. How epithelial cells detect danger: aiding the immune response. Allergy. 2008;63(9):1110–23.
11. Thomas 3rd WW, Harvey RJ, Rudmik L, Hwang PH, Schlosser RJ. Distribution of topical agents to the paranasal sinuses: an evidence-based review with recommendations. Int Forum Allergy Rhinol. 2013;3(9):691–703.
12. Harvey RJ, Debnath N, Srubiski A, Bleier B, Schlosser RJ. Fluid residuals and drug exposure in nasal irrigation. Otolaryngol Head Neck Surg: Off J Am Acad Otolaryngol Head Neck Surg. 2009;141(6):757–61.
13. Manes RP, Tong L, Batra PS. Prospective evaluation of aerosol delivery by a powered nasal nebulizer in the cadaver model. Int Forum Allergy Rhinol. 2011;1(5):366–71.
14. Snidvongs K, Chaowanapanja P, Aeumjaturapat S, Chusakul S, Praweswararat P. Does nasal irrigation enter paranasal sinuses in chronic rhinosinusitis? Am J Rhinol. 2008;22(5):483–6.
15. Harvey RJ, Goddard JC, Wise SK, Schlosser RJ. Effects of endoscopic sinus surgery and delivery device on cadaver sinus irrigation. Otolaryngol Head Neck Surg: Off J Am Acad Otolaryngol Head Neck Surg. 2008;139(1):137–42.
16. Grobler A, Weitzel EK, Buele A, Jardeleza C, Cheong YC, Field J, et al. Pre- and postoperative sinus penetration of nasal irrigation. Laryngoscope. 2008;118(11):2078–81.
17. Saijo R, Majima Y, Hyo N, Takano H. Particle deposition of therapeutic aerosols in the nose and paranasal sinuses after transnasal sinus surgery: a cast model study. Am J Rhinol. 2004;18(1):1–7.
18. Singhal D, Weitzel EK, Lin E, Feldt B, Kriete B, McMains KC, et al. Effect of head position and surgical dissection on sinus irrigant penetration in cadavers. Laryngoscope. 2010;120(12):2528–31.
19. Snidvongs K, Kalish L, Sacks R, Sivasubramaniam R, Cope D, Harvey RJ. Sinus surgery and delivery method influence the effectiveness of topical corticosteroids for chronic rhinosinusitis: systematic review and meta-analysis. Am J Rhinol Allergy. 2013;27(3):221–33.
20. Moller W, Schuschnig U, Khadem Saba G, Meyer G, Junge-Hulsing B, Keller M, et al. Pulsating aerosols for drug delivery to the sinuses in healthy volunteers. Otolaryngol Head Neck Surg: Off J Am Acad Otolaryngol Head Neck Surg. 2010;142(3):382–8.
21. Charlton S, Jones NS, Davis SS, Illum L. Distribution and clearance of bioadhesive formulations from the olfactory region in man: effect of polymer type and nasal delivery device. Eur J Pharm Sci: Off J Eur Fed Pharm Sci. 2007;30(3–4):295–302.
22. Wormald PJ, Cain T, Oates L, Hawke L, Wong I. A comparative study of three methods of nasal irrigation. Laryngoscope. 2004;114(12):2224–7.
23. Hilton C, Wiedmann T, St Martin M, Humphrey B, Schleiffarth R, Rimell F. Differential deposition of aerosols in the maxillary sinus of human cadavers by particle size. Am J Rhinol. 2008;22(4):395–8.
24. Brenner PS, Abadie WM, Weitzel EK, Thomas RF, McMains KC. Unexpected consequences of transnasal balloon dilation of the maxillary ostium. Int Forum Allergy Rhinol. 2011;1(6):466–70.
25. Beule A, Athanasiadis T, Athanasiadis E, Field J, Wormald PJ. Efficacy of different techniques of sinonasal irrigation after modified Lothrop procedure. Am J Rhinol Allergy. 2009;23(1):85–90.

26. Liang KL, Su MC, Tseng HC, Jiang RS. Impact of pulsatile nasal irrigation on the prognosis of functional endoscopic sinus surgery. J Otolaryngol Head Neck Surg. 2008;37(2):148–53.
27. Pynnonen MA, Mukerji SS, Kim HM, Adams ME, Terrell JE. Nasal saline for chronic sinonasal symptoms: a randomized controlled trial. Arch Otolaryngol Head Neck Surg. 2007;133(11):1115–20.
28. Bleier BS, Debnath I, Harvey RJ, Schlosser RJ. Temporospatial quantification of fluorescein-labeled sinonasal irrigation delivery. Int Forum Allergy Rhinol. 2011;1(5):361–5.
29. Miller TR, Muntz HR, Gilbert ME, Orlandi RR. Comparison of topical medication delivery systems after sinus surgery. Laryngoscope. 2004;114(2):201–4.
30. Seaton A, MacNee W, Donaldson K, Godden D. Particulate air pollution and acute health effects. Lancet. 1995;345(8943):176–8.
31. Rogers DF. Mucoactive agents for airway mucus hypersecretory diseases. Respir Care. 2007;52(9):1176–93; discussion 93–7.
32. Matsui H, Grubb BR, Tarran R, Randell SH, Gatzy JT, Davis CW, et al. Evidence for periciliary liquid layer depletion, not abnormal ion composition, in the pathogenesis of cystic fibrosis airways disease. Cell. 1998;95(7):1005–15.
33. Tarran R, Grubb BR, Gatzy JT, Davis CW, Boucher RC. The relative roles of passive surface forces and active ion transport in the modulation of airway surface liquid volume and composition. J Gen Physiol. 2001;118(2):223–36.
34. Widdicombe J. Airway and alveolar permeability and surface liquid thickness: theory. J Appl Physiol. 1997;82(1):3–12.
35. Widdicombe JG. Airway liquid: a barrier to drug diffusion? Eur Respir J. 1997;10(10): 2194–7.
36. Rogers DF, Lethem M. Airway mucus: basic mechanisms and clinical perspectives. 1st ed. Basel: Birkhauser; 1997. 388 p.
37. Kim DH, Chu HS, Lee JY, Hwang SJ, Lee SH, Lee HM. Up-regulation of MUC5AC and MUC5B mucin genes in chronic rhinosinusitis. Arch Otolaryngol Head Neck Surg. 2004; 130(6):747–52.
38. Martinez-Anton A, Roca-Ferrer J, Mullol J. Mucin gene expression in rhinitis syndromes. Curr Allergy Asthma Rep. 2006;6(3):189–97.
39. Subiza JL, Subiza J, Barjau MC, Rodriguez R, Gavilan MJ. Inhibition of the seasonal IgE increase to Dactylis glomerata by daily sodium chloride nasal-sinus irrigation during the grass pollen season. J Allergy Clin Immunol. 1999;104(3 Pt 1):711–2.
40. Boek WM, Keles N, Graamans K, Huizing EH. Physiologic and hypertonic saline solutions impair ciliary activity in vitro. Laryngoscope. 1999;109(3):396–9.
41. Keojampa BK, Nguyen MH, Ryan MW. Effects of buffered saline solution on nasal mucociliary clearance and nasal airway patency. Otolaryngology Head Neck Surg: Off J Am Acad Otolaryngol Head Neck Surg. 2004;131(5):679–82.
42. Wabnitz DA, Wormald PJ. A blinded, randomized, controlled study on the effect of buffered 0.9% and 3% sodium chloride intranasal sprays on ciliary beat frequency. Laryngoscope. 2005;115(5):803–5.
43. Passali D, Damiani V, Passali FM, Passali GC, Bellussi L. Atomized nasal douche vs nasal lavage in acute viral rhinitis. Up-regulation of MUC5AC and MUC5B mucin genes in chronic rhinosinusitis. Archiv Otolaryngol Neck Surg. 2005;131(9):788–90.
44. Kim CH, Hyun Song M, Eun Ahn Y, Lee JG, Yoon JH. Effect of hypo-, iso- and hypertonic saline irrigation on secretory mucins and morphology of cultured human nasal epithelial cells. Acta Otolaryngol. 2005;125(12):1296–300.
45. Hauptman G, Ryan MW. The effect of saline solutions on nasal patency and mucociliary clearance in rhinosinusitis patients. Otolaryngol Head Neck Surg: Off J Am Acad Otolaryngol Head Neck Surg. 2007;137(5):815–21.
46. Rabago D, Zgierska A, Mundt M, Barrett B, Bobula J, Maberry R. Efficacy of daily hypertonic saline nasal irrigation among patients with sinusitis: a randomized controlled trial. J Fam Pract. 2002;51(12):1049–55.

47. Cassano P, Latorre F. Nasal provocation test with hyperosmolar solutions: normal values. Boll Soc Ital Biol Sper. 1991;67(3):311–8.
48. Adam P, Stiffman M, Blake Jr RL. A clinical trial of hypertonic saline nasal spray in subjects with the common cold or rhinosinusitis. Arch Fam Med. 1998;7(1):39–43.
49. Haavisto L, Sipila J, Suonpaa J. Nonspecific nasal mucosal reactivity, expressed as changes in nasal airway resistance after bilateral saline provocation. Am J Rhinol. 1998;12(4):275–8.
50. Baraniuk JN, Ali M, Naranch K. Hypertonic saline nasal provocation and acoustic rhinometry. Clin Exp Allergy: J Br Soc Allergy Clin Immunol. 2002;32(4):543–50.
51. Harvey R, Hannan SA, Badia L, Scadding G. Nasal saline irrigations for the symptoms of chronic rhinosinusitis. Cochrane Database Syst Rev. 2007;(3):CD006394.
52. Heatley DG, McConnell KE, Kille TL, Leverson GE. Nasal irrigation for the alleviation of sinonasal symptoms. Otolaryngol Head Neck Surg: Off J Am Acad Otolaryngol Head Neck Surg. 2001;125(1):44–8.
53. Williams GB, Ross LL, Chandra RK. Are bulb syringe irrigators a potential source of bacterial contamination in chronic rhinosinusitis? Am J Rhinol. 2008;22(4):399–401.
54. Psaltis AJ, Foreman A, Wormald PJ, Schlosser RJ. Contamination of sinus irrigation devices: a review of the evidence and clinical relevance. Am J Rhinol Allergy. 2012;26(3):201–3.
55. Keen M, Foreman A, Wormald PJ. The clinical significance of nasal irrigation bottle contamination. Laryngoscope. 2010;120(10):2110–4.
56. Foreman A, Wormald PJ. Can bottle design prevent bacterial contamination of nasal irrigation devices? Int Forum Allergy Rhinol. 2011;1(4):303–7.
57. Barbieri M, Salami A, Mora F, Casazza A, Sovatzis A, Teglia R, et al. [Behavior of serum IgE and IgA in patients with allergic rhinitis treated with iodine bromide thermal water]. Acta Otorhinolaryngol Ital. 2002;22(4):215–9.
58. Cingi C, Unlu HH, Songu M, Yalcin S, Topcu I, Cakli H, et al. Seawater gel in allergic rhinitis: entrapment effect and mucociliary clearance compared with saline. Ther Adv Respir Dis. 2010;4(1):13–8.
59. Cordray S, Harjo JB, Miner L. Comparison of intranasal hypertonic dead sea saline spray and intranasal aqueous triamcinolone spray in seasonal allergic rhinitis. Ear Nose Throat J. 2005;84(7):426–30.
60. Garavello W, Romagnoli M, Sordo L, Gaini RM, Di Berardino C, Angrisano A. Hypersaline nasal irrigation in children with symptomatic seasonal allergic rhinitis: a randomized study. Pediatr Allergy Immunol: Off Publ Eur Soc Pediatr Allergy Immunol. 2003;14(2):140–3.
61. Garavello W, Di Berardino F, Romagnoli M, Sambataro G, Gaini RM. Nasal rinsing with hypertonic solution: an adjunctive treatment for pediatric seasonal allergic rhinoconjunctivitis. Int Arch Allergy Immunol. 2005;137(4):310–4.
62. Garavello W, Somigliana E, Acaia B, Gaini L, Pignataro L, Gaini RM. Nasal lavage in pregnant women with seasonal allergic rhinitis: a randomized study. Int Arch Allergy Immunol. 2010;151(2):137–41.
63. Li H, Sha Q, Zuo K, Jiang H, Cheng L, Shi J, et al. Nasal saline irrigation facilitates control of allergic rhinitis by topical steroid in children. ORL J Otorhinolaryngol Relat Spec. 2009;71(1):50–5.
64. Rogkakou A, Guerra L, Massacane P, Baiardini I, Baena-Cagnani R, Zanella C, et al. Effects on symptoms and quality of life of hypertonic saline nasal spray added to antihistamine in persistent allergic rhinitis – a randomized controlled study. Eur Ann Allergy Clin Immunol. 2005;37(9):353–6.
65. Ural A, Oktemer TK, Kizil Y, Ileri F, Uslu S. Impact of isotonic and hypertonic saline solutions on mucociliary activity in various nasal pathologies: clinical study. J Laryngol Otol. 2009;123(5):517–21.
66. Hermelingmeier KE, Weber RK, Hellmich M, Heubach CP, Mosges R. Nasal irrigation as an adjunctive treatment in allergic rhinitis: a systematic review and meta-analysis. Am J Rhinol Allergy. 2012;26(5):e119–25.

67. Klimek LJVHF, Hommmel G, Hormann K. Lässt sich der Medikamentenverbrauch bei Patienten mit saisonaler Rhinitis allergica durch Nasenspülbehandlungen mit isoosmotischer Emser Salzlösung reduzieren. Allergologie. 2001;24:309–15.
68. Bachmann G, Hommel G, Michel O. Effect of irrigation of the nose with isotonic salt solution on adult patients with chronic paranasal sinus disease. Eur Arch Otorhinolaryngol: Off J Eur Fed Otorhinolaryngol Soc. 2000;257(10):537–41.
69. Fokkens WJ, Lund VJ, Mullol J, Bachert C, Alobid I, Baroody F, et al. European Position Paper on Rhinosinusitis and Nasal Polyps 2012. Rhinol Suppl. 2012;(23):3 p preceding table of contents, 1-298.

Emerging Innovative Topical Therapies 21

Josh Meier and Eric H. Holbrook

Key Take-Home Points

- Recalcitrant chronic rhinosinusitis (CRS) refractory to traditional medical and maximal therapies represents a significant clinical challenge.
- Manuka honey has shown promise in treating recalcitrant CRS in vitro and in animal models; however, clinical efficacy data are lacking, and a recommendation for use cannot be given.
- Xylitol has been shown to be safe for use in humans and appears to have some effectiveness in treating CRS. Xylitol could be considered for topical use in patients that have failed conventional treatments.
- Surfactants have deleterious effects on sinonasal ciliary and olfactory function and should be used with caution in patients with CRS.

Conflicts: No authors have conflicts of interest to disclose

J. Meier, MD
Nevada ENT and Hearing Associates,
9770 S. McCarran Boulevard, Reno, NV 89523, USA
e-mail: meier_josh@yahoo.com

E.H. Holbrook, MD (✉)
Department of Otolaryngology,
Harvard Medical School, Boston, MA USA

Division of Rhinology, Massachusetts Eye and Ear Infirmary,
243 Charles Street, Boston, MA 02114, USA
e-mail: eric_holbrook@meei.harvard.edu

P.S. Batra, J.K. Han (eds.), *Practical Medical and Surgical Management of Chronic Rhinosinusitis*, DOI 10.1007/978-3-319-16724-4_21

Introduction

Chronic rhinosinusitis (CRS) represents a spectrum of disease with a common end result of sinonasal mucosal inflammation. The cause of the inflammation can be multifactorial, including infections and allergies. Although defined recommendations for optimal treatment are lacking, typical therapeutics include antibiotics and steroids in systemic and topical forms. Endoscopic sinus surgery is recommended when medical management fails. The benefits of sinus surgery in creating enlarged sinus ostia are twofold: optimization of drainage and deposition of topical therapies. Once exposed surgically, the air-filled sinus cavities are ideal for topical therapies, providing a larger surface area for distribution. Topical therapies are ideal for providing increased local drug concentration while decreasing systemic side effects. However, local mucosal irritation, physically challenging delivery methods, higher costs, and unclear pharmacokinetics provide limitation to their use [1]. Besides saline irrigation, common topical therapies include steroids and antibiotics, but alternative topical therapies have been investigated as an adjunct to these more standard therapies. Manuka honey, xylitol, and surfactants are three frequently used topical therapies that reportedly exert an anti-inflammatory or antimicrobial effect. This chapter will focus on these three alternative topical therapies and provide current data supporting or refuting their benefit in the treatment of CRS.

Manuka Honey

Mechanism of Action

The honeybee (*Apis mellifera*) produces honey by collecting and modifying nectar from local flowers [2]. It is inexpensive and simple to obtain, but various types are available, depending on the plant source (i.e., Manuka, Kanuka, Sidr, clover). The full therapeutic effect of medicinal honeys has not been fully elucidated; however, many properties have been identified that are potentially antibacterial in effect. Honey is a supersaturated sugar solution, with a high osmolarity and a low pH, and can create hydrogen peroxide via endogenous glucose oxidase activity [3]. Manuka honey is produced in New Zealand and is derived from the Manuka plant (*Leptospermum scoparium*). The phenol compound methylglyoxal (MGO) has been implicated as a major bactericidal compound in Manuka honey. MGO is cytotoxic and is produced chiefly in glycolysis. These qualities provide an adverse environment for bacterial growth [3]. Manuka honey has been shown to prevent and disrupt preexistent biofilms and is effective against planktonic bacteria and yeast. Honey has also been shown to stimulate the immune system as well as promote wound healing [3]. Lu et al. evaluated the effect of Manuka, Kanuka, and clover honeys against four strains of bacteria, including *S. aureus* and *P. aeruginosa*. Manuka honey, with the highest concentration of endogenous MGO, was the most effective strain in slowing bacterial growth. When catalase was added to the honeys, rendering the hydrogen peroxide inactive, Manuka honey (with its high concentration of MGO) still resulted in the greatest inhibition of bacterial growth. Even if hydrogen peroxide and MGO were neutralized, the honeys still maintained their growth inhibitory effect, suggesting the presence of other antibacterial compounds besides hydrogen peroxide and MGO [3].

Jervis-Bardy et al. evaluated the effect of the MGO present in Manuka honey in an in vitro system. They found that honey with endogenous MGO was bactericidal to four strains of *S. aureus* biofilms and honey without endogenous MGO was not. Exogenous MGO alone or in combination with a non-MGO honey reinstituted bactericidal activity [4]. This suggests that naturally occurring MGO in the Manuka honey is the cause of the bactericidal effect on biofilm-forming *S. aureus*. Some Manuka/Kanuka blends of honey have endogenous MGO; however, Kanuka honey has very low levels [2]. The presence of endogenous MGO in Manuka suggests why this honey has been found to have superior antibacterial properties to others [5].

Indications

Manuka honey can be considered for use in patients with CRS that continue to have symptoms despite maximal traditional antibacterial and surgical therapy, especially when attributed to biofilm-producing bacteria.

Specific Therapy

The inflammation from CRS may be directly or indirectly caused by the body's host response to bacterial infection. Biofilms have been implicated as a causative and complicating factor of CRS management. Typically biofilms are difficult to treat with traditional medical and surgical methods. Alandejani et al. evaluated the effect of various honeys, including gamma-irradiated Manuka, in the treatment of biofilm-producing *Pseudomonas aeruginosa* and *Staphylococcus aureus* in vitro. Gamma-irradiation was performed to ensure sterility. Manuka honey was found to be bactericidal to 82 % of MSSA biofilms, 63 % of MRSA biofilms, and 91 % of *Pseudomonas* [5]. Manuka honey was found to be superior in this study to traditional antibiotic therapy in the treatment of biofilm-producing MSSA, MRSA, and *Pseudomonas*. Rifampin was the only antibiotic of those tested that had bactericidal activity against the biofilms (only to 18 % of the strains however) [5].

Side Effects

Kilty et al. treated nasal mucosa with Manuka honey once daily in one of the nasal cavities of rabbits and used the other nasal cavity as a control. Light and transmission electron microscopy revealed no epithelial damage. Mouse trachea was used to evaluate Manuka honey's effect on ciliary beat frequency and was found to not alter motility of cilia. When the olfactory mucosa was examined, there was a higher rate of cell proliferation in the epithelium (as measured by Ki-67 staining) when samples treated with Manuka honey were compared to control, suggesting olfactory injury [6]. Paramasivan et al. used a sheep model to evaluate the efficacy of Manuka honey with varying concentrations of MGO. They found that increasing MGO levels resulted in a dose-related decrease in *S. aureus* biofilm levels. At MGO concentrations of 3.6 mg/ml, there was loss of cilia seen on scanning electron microscopy (SEM). At 7.2 mg/ml of MGO, the sinus mucosa appeared grossly inflamed and demonstrated squamous metaplasia on light microscopy. Furthermore, ciliary denudation and cellular detachment were seen on electron microscopy [7].

Clinical Efficacy Data

A Cochrane review of the use of honey in wound care and burns found that honey may shorten healing times for moderate burns when compared with conventional dressings. Honey was not found to improve healing of chronic venous ulcers and may delay healing in deep burns [2]. Thamboo et al. have performed the only clinical study of Manuka honey for treating CRS. They conducted a single-blind randomized prospective study in patients with allergic fungal sinusitis. Thirty-four patients sprayed their postsurgical sinus cavities with 2 ml of 50:50 saline to Manuka honey solution daily for 30 days. The primary outcome (endoscopic score of the sinonasal cavity) showed no difference between the honey group and control. There was no effect on culture results from the ethmoid cavities. However, SNOT-22 symptom scores were significantly improved in patients that used the Manuka honey sprays [8].

The EPOS 2012 guidelines [9] and a systemic review of topical therapies [1] concluded that there was insufficient evidence to recommend for or against the use of Manuka honey to treat CRS. Given the lack of significant evidence for efficacy and possible adverse effect on olfactory epithelium, we would suggest caution in utilizing this therapy for routine treatment of refractory CRS.

Xylitol

Mechanism of Action

Xylitol is a natural, nonionic, five-carbon sugar alcohol found in low concentrations in the fibers of fruits and vegetables. Xylitol was first used as a diabetic sweetener in Europe, as it has a similar sweetness, and results in less blood glucose rise and insulin rise than with the ingestion of glucose. Xylitol is safe for human use and was used for parenteral nutrition in the 1970s. Xylitol is non-fermentable, and bacteria cannot use it as an energy source thereby inhibiting growth. Making use of this property, xylitol has been utilized in prevention of infection. It has been shown to decrease dental caries when used in chewing gums and decreased the rate of acute otitis media in children [10].

Many different molecules such as lysozyme, lactoferrin, and human beta defensins have been implicated in the process of innate host defense in the human respiratory system [11]. These molecules exist in a thin layer along the entire lining of the human respiratory tract, termed the airway surface liquid (ASL). Changes in the composition of the ASL, such as by changing the salt concentration of the fluid, can have profound effects on innate defense. An example of this is in cystic fibrosis, where the salt concentration of the ASL is increased by altered chloride transport. This increase in salt concentration in the ASL is thought to decrease the activity of innate host molecules, increasing bacteria's ability to cause infection. Given that the airway epithelium is water permeable, the addition of a nonionic osmolyte such as xylitol, with low transmembrane permeability, would result in increased water transport to the ASL, reducing the effective salt concentration and possibly enhancing innate host defense [11].

Indications

Xylitol can be considered for use in patients with recalcitrant CRS attributed to a bacterial source who have failed traditional medical and surgical therapy.

Specific Therapy

Zabner et al. evaluated the effect of xylitol on innate defense. They demonstrated that xylitol is nonpermeable and that it decreased ASL chloride concentration in explanted cystic fibrosis epithelia in vitro. They further demonstrated that xylitol cannot be fermented by bacteria. Xylitol itself did not result in bacterial killing; however, when placed in ASL, increased bacterial killing was seen, suggesting that xylitol enhances endogenous innate defense mechanisms [11].

Brown et al. demonstrated that the addition of xylitol resulted in increased killing of *Pseudomonas aeruginosa* in a rabbit maxillary sinus model of sinusitis. They attributed this effect to xylitol lowering the ASL ionic strength and enhancing endogenous antimicrobials [12].

Side Effects

No specific toxicity has been attributed to xylitol. It has a long history of use as a sweetener in gums and lozenges. It was used previously for IV nutrition as well [11]. Other hypertonic solutions have been used safely in CF patients, such as mannitol and hypertonic saline [11]. Zabner et al. performed a randomized trial of xylitol, in which there were no reported adverse events. Patients received 4 days of four times a day xylitol or saline sprays in their nostrils, then switched. Xylitol, compared to saline, resulted in a statistically significant decrease in colony-forming units of coagulase-negative *Staphylococcus* [11].

Clinical Efficacy Data

Weissman et al. performed a randomized clinical trial comparing 5 % xylitol to saline irrigations. Subjects irrigated with xylitol or saline for 10 days and switched after a 3-day washout period to the other irrigant. Blinding was difficult given the sweet taste of xylitol. Sinonasal Outcomes Test-20 (SNOT-20) scores and visual analog scores were obtained after each irrigant course was finished. On average, SNOT-20 scores increased from 15 to 18.93 with saline irrigations and improved from 17.93 to 15.5 with xylitol irrigations. The difference in the average change between xylitol and saline was statistically significant ($p = 0.044$). In this study, xylitol irrigations were well tolerated, with one patient reported nasal stinging [13].

In a systematic review of topical therapies for CRS, the authors were unable to make a recommendation on the use of xylitol irrigations because of the lack of studies evaluating xylitol [1]. The EPOS 2012 guidelines regarding CRS without nasal polyps stated that current data do support the use of xylitol irrigations (recommendation A) [9]. Although convincing evidence for broad use in treatment of CRS is lacking, xylitol appears to be safe and warrants further investigation for efficacy in treatment of CRS.

Surfactants

Mechanism of Action

Surfactants are molecules that possess both hydrophilic and hydrophobic properties. These characteristics result in the ability to form micelles, decrease surface tension, and disrupt cell membranes [14]. Bacterial biofilms are thought to play a role in patients with CRS that are recalcitrant to conventional surgical and medical therapies. Through their amphipathic properties, surfactants can potentially dislodge biofilms from the underlying nasal mucosa [14]. Surfactants also work by reducing the adherence of mucus from the underlying epithelium, and this may represent a novel therapy for patients with thick, recalcitrant mucus [15]. For this reason, products such as baby shampoo (containing three surfactants – PEG-80 sorbitan laurate, cocamidopropyl betaine, and sodium trideceth sulfate) [14] or a combination of hypertonic citric acid and a zwitterionic surfactant (caprylyl sulfobetaine) have been evaluated in the treatment of recalcitrant CRS.

Indications

As with Manuka honey and xylitol, surfactants would be used in patients with continuing symptoms despite maximal medical therapy after endoscopic sinus surgery, especially in patients where biofilm formation is a concern.

Side Effects

Chiu et al. demonstrated that a surfactant developed by their group resulted in a brief increase, then a return to baseline in ciliary beat frequency in a murine explanted mucosa model. No toxic effects were seen on the cilia [15]. Valentine et al. used a sheep frontal sinus model to evaluate the effects of a citric acid/zwitterionic surfactant (CAZS) on biofilms and cilia morphology. They demonstrated a negative impact on cilia. There was a reduction in biofilm levels in sheep treated with CAZS; however, this was not statistically significant. When CAZS treatment was stopped, this group showed a trend toward increased biofilm growth, which was not seen in the saline control group. The authors suggested that CAZS leads to ciliary morphologic changes, which in turn results in an opportunity for increased biofilm growth [16]. Tamashiro et al. used a rabbit maxillary sinus model to investigate the effects of CAZS on healthy mucosa. They found marked loss of cilia at days 1 and 3 after CAZS irrigation; however, at day 6, regeneration was near complete. CAZS caused a decrease in ciliary beat frequency at days 1 and 3, but this also recovered at day 6 [17]. This implies that CAZS produces a nonpermanent deleterious effect on sinonasal mucosa that is reversible, at least over short-term use. In a prospective study, Isaacs et al. evaluated the effect on saccharine mucociliary clearance times (MCT) with irrigation containing 1 % baby shampoo in saline. They found that this irrigation significantly increased the MCT, suggesting that baby shampoo has a negative effect on mucociliary function [14].

The effect of surfactant irrigations on olfactory function became of interest with consumer reports of smell loss after use of a previous commercially available product. In a randomized controlled trial by Farag et al., 40 patients that had recently undergone ESS received either surfactant (1 % baby shampoo with isotonic saline) or hypertonic saline. Phenyl ethyl alcohol smell tests were administered to patients. There was no significant difference between groups; however, patients in the surfactant group were three times more likely to have a decrease in olfaction. Side effects were experienced in 52 % of the surfactant group compared to 6 % in the hypertonic saline group ($p=0.002$). Common complaints were nasal burning and headache. Five subjects from the surfactant group withdrew from the study compared to zero withdrawals in the hypertonic saline patients [18].

Clinical Efficacy Data

Chiu et al. performed a prospective study in patients that were symptomatic despite intensive medical and surgical management using baby shampoo concentrations that were determined in vitro. In vitro testing revealed that baby shampoo was unable to eradicate existing *Pseudomonas* biofilms but was effective in killing planktonic *Pseudomonas*. Fifteen patients completed the study, 7 patients showed improvement in SNOT-22 scores, and 7 of 11 patients studied had improvement in UPSIT smell testing [19].

In the randomized trial by Farag et al., both the surfactant and saline groups had significant improvement in RSOM-31 and SNOT-22 quality of life scores after sinus surgery and irrigations; however, there was not a statistically significant difference between the groups [18].

Rudmik et al. were unable to make a recommendation on the use of baby shampoo irrigations because of the lack of studies evaluating the harm and benefits of these compounds [1]. The EPOS 2012 guidelines regarding CRS without nasal polyps recommended against the addition of baby shampoo to nasal irrigations (recommendation D) [9]. Given the lack of convincing data to support the use of currently available surfactants in the treatment of CRS along with reports of potential harm, we would suggest caution in the use of this therapy.

Conclusion

Patients with recalcitrant symptoms after exhausting the medical and surgical armamentarium of modern rhinology represent a significant challenge. Alternative topical treatments such as Manuka honey, xylitol, and surfactants provide options for additional therapy in the management of challenging patients failing conventional treatment. The ease of use and avoidance of direct systemic effects make them attractive supplements. Unfortunately, available guidelines are limited in their recommendations due to insufficient proper studies on efficacy and safety. There is soft support for the use of xylitol irrigations with minimal side effects. However, the benefits of Manuka honey or surfactant irrigations are weak, and there is considerable concern that surfactants may have deleterious effects upon nasal mucosa and negative impact on olfaction. Until larger studies are performed, caution and close observation are advised when offering these therapies in clinical practice.

References

1. Rudmik L, Hoy M, Schlosser RJ, et al. Topical therapies in the management of chronic rhinosinusitis: an evidence-based review with recommendations. Int Forum Allergy Rhinol. 2013;3:281–98.
2. Jull AB, Walker N, Deshpande S. Honey as a topical treatment for wounds. Cochrane Database Syst Rev. 2013;(2):CD005083.
3. Lu J, Carter DA, Turnbull L, et al. The effect of New Zealand Kanuka, Manuka and clover honeys on bacterial growth dynamics and cellular morphology varies according to the species. PLoS One. 2013;8:e55898.
4. Jervis-Berdy J, Foreman A, Bray S, et al. Methylglyoxal-infused honey mimics the anti-staphylococcus aureus biofilm activity of manuka honey: potential implication in chronic rhinosinusitis. Laryngoscope. 2011;121:1104–7.
5. Alandejani T, Marsan J, Ferris W, et al. Effectiveness of honey on *Staphylococcus aureus* and *Pseudomonas aeruginosa* biofilms. Otolaryngol Head Neck Surg. 2009;141:114–8.
6. Kilty SJ, Almutari D, Duval M. Manuka honey: histological effect on respiratory mucosa. Am J Rhinol Allergy. 2010;24:e63–6.
7. Paramasivan S, Drilling AJ, Jardeleza C. Methylglyoxal-augmented manuka honey as a topical anti-Staphylococcus aureus biofilm agent: safety and efficacy in an in vivo model. Int Forum Allergy Rhinol. 2014;4:187–95.

8. Thamboo A, Thamboo A, Philpott C, et al. Single-blind study of manuka honey in allergic fungal rhinosinusitis. J Otolaryngol Head Neck Surg. 2011;40:238–43.
9. Fokkens WJ, Lund VJ, Mullol J. EPOS 2012: European position paper on rhinosinusitis and nasal polyps. Rhinol Suppl. 2012;23:1–298.
10. Azarpazhooh A, Limeback H, Lawrence HP, Shah PS. Xylitol for preventing acute otitis media in children up to 12 years of age. Cochrane Database Syst Rev. 2011;(11):CD007095.
11. Zabner J, Seiler MP, Launspach JL, et al. The osmolyte xylitol reduces the salt concentration of airway surface liquid and may enhance bacterial killing. Proc Natl Acad Sci U S A. 2000;97:11614–9.
12. Brown CL, Graham SM, Cable BB. Xylitol enhances bacterial killing in the rabbit maxillary sinus. Laryngoscope. 2004;11:2021–4.
13. Weissman JD, Fernandez D, Hwang PH. Xylitol nasal irrigation in the management of chronic rhinosinusitis: a pilot study. Laryngoscope. 2011;121:2468–72.
14. Isaacs S, FAkhri S, Luong A, et al. The effect of dilute baby shampoo on nasal mucociliary clearance in healthy subjects. Am J Rhinol Allergy. 2011;25:e27–9.
15. Chiu AG, Chen B, Palmer JN, et al. Safety evaluation of sins surfactant solution on respiratory cilia function. Int Forum Allergy Rhinol. 2011;1:280–3.
16. Valentine R, Jervis-Bardy J, Psaltis A. Efficacy of using a hydrodebrider and of a citric acid/zwitterionic surfactant on a *Staphylococcus aureus* bacterial biofilm in the sheep model of rhinosinusitis. Am J Rhinol Allergy. 2011;25:323–6.
17. Tamashiro E, Banks CA, Chen B. *In vivo* effects of citric acid/zwitterionic surfactant cleansing solution on rabbit sinus mucosa. Am J Rhinol Allergy. 2009;23:597–601.
18. Farag AA, Deal AM, McKinney KA, et al. Single-blind randomized controlled trial of surfactant vs hypertonic saline irrigation following endoscopic endonasal surgery. Int Forum Allergy Rhinol. 2013;3:276–80.
19. Chiu AG, Palmer JN, Woodworth BA, et al. Baby shampoo nasal irrigations for the symptomatic post-functional endoscopic sinus surgery patient. Am J Rhinol. 2008;22:34–7.

Part III

Surgical Therapy of Chronic Rhinosinusitis

Endoscopic Sinus Surgery: Rationale, Indications, and Techniques

22

Marie Bussières and Erin D. Wright

Key Take-Home Points

- Endoscopic sinus surgery (ESS) is a procedure that is now performed worldwide, mainly in patients suffering from chronic rhinosinusitis (CRS) who have failed medical therapy.
- The goal of ESS has evolved, initially described as a way of relieving sites of anatomical obstruction in the paranasal sinuses to now providing symptomatic relief while also optimizing access to the sinus cavities for long-term topical nasal therapies.
- The indications for surgery are multiple, primarily being CRS with or without nasal polyps, but also to treat recurrent acute sinusitis or the complications of acute sinusitis, fungal disease, and mucoceles, among others.
- The key to safe and effective surgery is refined anatomical knowledge that can be applied to a surgical 3-D setting in order to prevent potentially serious complications such as orbital or neurological injuries.

M. Bussières, MD, FRCSC (✉)
Division of Otolaryngology – Head and Neck Surgery,
Université de Sherbrooke, 580 rue Bowen sud, Sherbrooke, QC J1G 2E8, Canada
e-mail: marie.bussieres@usherbrooke.ca

E.D. Wright, MDCM, MED
Division of Otolaryngology – Head and Neck Surgery, University of Alberta,
Room 1E4 WMC 8440 – 112 Street, Edmonton, AB T6M 2K8, Canada
e-mail: erin.wright@ualberta.ca

P.S. Batra, J.K. Han (eds.), *Practical Medical and Surgical Management of Chronic Rhinosinusitis*, DOI 10.1007/978-3-319-16724-4_22

Historical Background

Sinus surgery has evolved and advanced considerably since Molinetti first accessed the maxillary sinus in 1675. It was not until 1890 before Caldwell and Luc described their classic approach to the maxillary sinus, adding an inferior antrostomy to the maxillary sinus anterior wall fenestration. In 1901, Hirschmann was the first to visualize the nasal cavities using a cystoscope, which would eventually revolutionize sinus surgery in the 1950s with the development of the rod optic telescopes by Harold H. Hopkins. It gave surgeons better illumination and field of vision compared to preexisting endoscopes. Advancements in rhinology accelerated with Walter Messerklinger, who used this improved technology to gain further understanding of the lateral nasal wall anatomy as well as the mucociliary clearance patterns of the paranasal sinuses. He also described the importance of the ostiomeatal complex (OMC) in the pathophysiology of chronic rhinosinusitis (CRS). The integration of these concepts led him to pioneer the development of endoscopic sinus surgery (ESS). Heinz Stammberger, who trained with Messerklinger, subsequently popularized their work outside Germany and Austria in the late 1970s and early 1980s. The introduction of this revolutionary surgical approach in North America is attributed to David Kennedy in 1985. He observed the techniques of Messerklinger and Stammberger and also visited Wigand and Draf in Germany. It gave him the opportunity to integrate all these different practices into his own. More recent technological developments such as powered instrumentation and image-guided surgery have allowed ESS to be done in a more safe, efficient, and complete manner. Endoscopic sinus surgery is now performed worldwide and is considered the standard of care for patients suffering from CRS having failed medical therapy.

Rationale

ESS as described by Stammberger and Kennedy has as its main goal the physiologic restoration of ventilation and mucociliary clearance to the diseased sinuses [1, 2]. A lot of emphasis is placed on the importance of the ostiomeatal complex in the pathophysiology of CRS. The middle meatus and ethmoid infundibulum are composed of many narrow channels. Chronic inflammation in these constricted spaces can easily lead to mucosal contact points, disruption of the normal mucociliary clearance, and retention of secretions leading to chronic sinonasal inflammation or infection. As the OMC represents the final drainage pathway of the maxillary, frontal, and anterior ethmoid sinuses, obstruction of this area has the potential to cause chronic disease in these three major sinuses. Therefore, relieving the blockage in a limited way should then be sufficient to treat the affected sinuses without the need to address the sinuses themselves.

Knowledge acquired from the study of normal mucociliary flow in the sinuses by Proctor and Messerklinger [3] was critical to the development of such focused sinus surgery. In the maxillary sinus, the mucus typically flows toward the natural ostium. If a posterior fontanel breaks down to form an accessory ostium separate from the natural ostium, secretions will continue to flow toward the natural ostium, and this dual ostium configuration will result in a recirculation phenomenon and chronic inflammation and potential infection. Mucociliary flow in the frontal sinus has also been described: going upward medially over the intersinus septum and then flowing laterally over the roof and the walls of the sinus. It finally runs medially on the floor to the lateral wall of the frontal recess. Approximately 60 % of the mucus recirculates, and only 40 % actually drains toward the infundibulum or the middle meatus. The upgoing flow of secretions on the medial wall of the frontal recess can explain why infection in the anterior ethmoid cells could be the culprit to frontal sinus disease. This once again may explain the preponderant role of the OMC in the historic explanation of chronic disease of some of the major sinuses.

The last few decades have given us a further refined understanding of the pathophysiology of CRS beyond the fact that chronic sinus disease is more complex than simply obstruction of the OMC and mucociliary disruption. Chronic sinonasal inflammation is now seen as a multifactorial process rather than a disease attributed only to anatomical factors. The role of many systemic and local host factors as well as environmental factors has been put forward, and the chronic mucosal reaction that is seen in CRS may be a maladaptive host immune response to environmental elements or a shift in the local microbiome as well as other factors. Thus, there has been a shift from primary surgical treatment toward more medically oriented therapy, keeping the surgical options only for those patients failing medical therapies.

The previously described physiological approach to performing sinus surgery still applies today but with the shift in treatment orientations came the change in surgical goals. Nowadays, improving access for the nasal topical treatments to the sinus cavities is one of the main reasons to perform ESS. A review published in 2013 by Thomas derived at the conclusion that standard ESS does improve nasal irrigation's delivery to the sinuses. More aggressive surgeries may further increase distribution [4]. Consequently, wide marsupialization of the sinonasal cavities and in particular of the ethmoid labyrinth should be done in order to try to optimize patients' outcomes. This also decreases the inflammatory load present in the sinuses and removes most of the bony partitions that would otherwise tend to become osteitic and contribute to persistent inflammation.

Even after over 30 years of practicing endoscopic sinus surgery, the exact extent to which ESS should be performed is still not clearly delineated. There are still proponents of very limited approaches. The best example is resources placed into the development of balloon catheter technology (BCT). The first large-scale clinical studies done by Bolger demonstrated the safety of the procedure and the durability of ostial patency [5]. In 2011 Batra reviewed this literature and stated that even though this technique seems to be safe, there is a lack of comparative data to create clear clinical indications and guidelines, thus limiting its applicability in day-to-day patient care [6]. More recently, the first randomized controlled trial comparing BCT to standard ESS showed equivalence of both techniques in terms of symptom improvement but a lesser need for postoperative debridement in the BCT group. The downfall of that study was the limited clinical applicability, having included only patients suffering from sole maxillary disease without polyposis [7]. Slightly more invasive than BCT, a minimally invasive sinus technique (MIST) has been described by Setliff in 1996 and further advocated by Catalano and Roffman [8]. They described a surgery during which the drainage pathways of the sinuses and not the sinuses themselves are addressed with utmost importance on the preservation of mucosa. This is very similar to the first descriptions of ESS by Messerklinger and Kennedy. At the other hand of the surgical spectrum, more aggressive approaches have been adopted to treat this benign but often recalcitrant disease. In Australia, Wormald has used the endoscopic modified Lothrop procedure for revision cases of nasal polyposis involving the frontal sinuses [9]. He reports good long-term outcomes with a 5 % revision rate over a mean follow-up period of 45 months. Jankowski, from France, is renowned for the nasalization procedure, which he described in 1997 [10]. This consists of complete exenteration of the ethmoid labyrinth, including complete removal of the middle turbinate and mucosal stripping over the lamina papyracea and the skull base. His retrospective study showed an improvement in nasal function and sense of smell compared to a more conventional limited ethmoidectomy.

Current Indications

Chronic Rhinosinusitis With or Without Nasal Polyposis

This is the primary reason for patients to undergo endoscopic sinus surgery, though it is also a relative, subjective indication. While most experts agree that patients with CRS failing maximal medical management can be offered surgery, the definition of what is considered "maximal" treatment varies considerably among practitioners. Nasal saline irrigations, topical steroids, oral steroids, and oral antibiotics are the most frequently prescribed therapies, either alone or in combination, according to a survey conducted of rhinologists in 2007 [11]. Similar conclusions were reached more recently in a study done in the United Kingdom where otolaryngologists were mainly using nasal irrigations, topical steroids, and oral antibiotics as their maximal treatment before considering a patient candidate for surgery [12]. Thus, this surgical indication is not an absolute but rather a matter of quality of life; the extent of surgery should be tailored to the severity of the disease affecting the sinuses.

A subset of CRS patients that also have the potential to benefit from surgery are the ones suffering from both upper and lower respiratory diseases. The concept of unified airway disease (UAD) has been codified in the last two decades from the observation of "both epidemiologic and pathophysiologic links among diseases such as allergic rhinitis, CRS and asthma" [13]. As such, multiple studies have investigated the possible effects of treatment of the upper airway over asthma control, and there seems to be objective measurements confirming the improvement in asthma management when CRS is treated either medically or surgically [14–16].

Individuals plagued with CRS as the result of a systemic disease process represent another subgroup of patients that can be helped with judicious use of ESS. Some degree of CRS has been found in approximately 90 % of patients suffering from cystic fibrosis. These patients can have quite severe polypoid disease, and the process affecting their mucosa leads to even further impaired mucociliary function, sometimes making more conventional and functional surgery unsuccessful. Revision rates are higher, and wide marsupialization of the sinuses, especially of the maxillary sinus in which the mucus flows against gravity, is sometimes recommended in refractory cases [17]. Granulomatosis with polyangiitis (GPA), formerly known as Wegener's granulomatosis, can affect the sinonasal mucosa significantly. The role of surgery is to address specific problems (e.g., scarring, mucoceles) when the disease is inactive; otherwise, one risks additional unnecessary scarring and worsened iatrogenic disease [18]. Two other granulomatous diseases that are worth mentioning are Churg-Strauss disease and sarcoidosis. The former can present with polyposis with a strong tendency for early recurrence postoperatively, and the introduction of appropriate medical therapy may lessen the need for surgery [19]. The latter seldom presents with sinonasal findings, but when it does, the role of surgery is first to help establish the diagnosis through mucosal biopsies and second to improve quality of life when the disease is under good medical control.

Fungal Rhinosinusitis

Endoscopic sinus surgery can be an important component of the treatment regimen for most forms of fungal disease. In cases of fungus ball, it represents the sole treatment modality. A wide opening of the affected sinus(es) with complete removal of the fungal concretions suffices. This is associated with excellent outcomes with high patient satisfaction and low recurrence rate [20, 21]. Allergic fungal sinusitis is another noninvasive form of fungal disease. Although surgery is not intended to be curative, removal of the polyps and allergic mucin should be performed to stop the benign but potentially expansive nature of this process. Concomitant treatment with corticosteroids, both oral and topical, is also required for long-term disease control [22]. Chronic invasive fungal rhinosinusitis, granulomatous or non-granulomatous variants, is a rare disease entity. Surgical removal of the disease process, while respecting natural boundaries such as periorbita or dura, is part of the overall treatment plan. On the other hand, when faced with acute invasive fungal sinusitis, endoscopic sinus surgery with debridement of the devitalized tissue is required until healthy, bleeding tissues are encountered. Serial debridements might be needed during the course of the disease. Surgery should be performed concurrently with the administration of antifungals and the reversal of the underlying core process [23].

Infectious Complications of Sinusitis

In the advent of an acute sinusitis with intraorbital or intracranial complications, drainage of the affected sinus(es) should be performed to facilitate resolution of the acute infection. Extra care should be taken in such cases given that tissues are extremely inflamed and bleeding may limit visualization. Select complications can also be addressed with the use of ESS. Most often this will be the case of an orbital subperiosteal abscess. After complete ethmoidectomy, the lamina papyracea can be removed allowing the abscess to drain intranasally, obviating the need for an external Lynch incision.

Recurrent Acute Bacterial Rhinosinusitis (R-ABRS)

The 2007 American clinical practice guidelines on sinusitis have suggested a cutoff of 4 ABRS per year for diagnosis of this entity. As most adults will suffer of 1.4–2.3 upper respiratory tract infections (viral and otherwise) a year, placing the cutoff too low would result in diagnostic overlap and unnecessary surgery. Endoscopic diagnostic confirmation of at least 1 episode is required to ensure the true bacterial nature of the infection. CT imaging should be performed to assess anatomical factors that can predispose to sinus obstruction [24]. In 2008, Poetker et al. reported that ESS seems to improve patients' quality of life similarly to patients with CRS [25]. A recent productivity-based analysis suggested establishing a new threshold for surgery in R-ABRS at 6 episodes per year. As this study does not take quality of life into account, a discussion about the risks versus benefits of the surgery should take place between each patient and the surgeon [26].

Mucoceles

Historically, the management of mucoceles has been through external approaches and obliterative procedures, completely removing the lining of the mucocele. Though potentially effective, these are associated with higher rate of morbidity than endoscopic approaches [27]. Since Kennedy's description in 1989, endoscopic marsupialization of the mucoceles has become the preferred surgical technique. The goal is to perform a "wide opening into the cyst so that its lining practically becomes part of the roof of the nose" [28]. Even with extensive disease, such as in the setting of erosion of the posterior table of the frontal sinus or the roof of the orbit, ESS offers a minimally invasive surgical procedure with low recurrence rates and morbidity.

Other Indications

Although this chapter focuses on inflammatory disease, a brief overview of the other possible indications for endoscopic surgery is worthwhile. Most benign and some malignant tumors can be removed endoscopically. It is also utilized for endoscopic resection of pituitary tumors; further, with accrued experience, neoplasms located in the clivus, middle cranial fossa, or posterior cranial fossa can be addressed [29]. Orbital pathology can also be addressed, ranging from dacryocystorhinostomy and orbital or optic nerve decompression to resection of medially located intraorbital masses. Posterior epistaxis not responding to conventional packing treatments may be brought to the operating room for endoscopic ligation or cautery of the sphenopalatine artery. Finally, in the pediatric population, choanal atresia repair can also be managed endoscopically.

Surgical Technique

Two main philosophies exist for performing a complete sphenoethmoidectomy. Stammberger's original description in 1986 slightly differs from the more commonly employed current approach [2]. He started with an infundibulotomy followed by an anterior ethmoidectomy. Identification of the skull base at that level allowed for exploration of the frontal recess and removal of any intervening bony partitions. Following the lamina papyracea and skull base closely through the posterior ethmoids, identification of the sphenoid ostium and subsequent sphenoidotomy was performed, if clinically indicated. The maxillary ostium was visualized last. In contrast, in 1981 Wigand described a posterior to anterior approach [30]. After the anterior ethmoidectomy is performed, the approach traverses the basal lamella and identifies the skull base in the posterior ethmoids, then skeletonizing the ethmoid partitions from posterior to anterior. The surgery ends with the frontal sinusotomy, if clinically warranted. This technique is purported to be safer as the dissection of the skull base proceeds by working away from it rather than toward it.

Preoperative Evaluation

A complete history and physical exam are requisite in the evaluation of a patient suffering from CRS. Diagnostic nasal endoscopy, in particular, can afford important information in the surgical planning. Another essential component of the preoperative workup is thorough assessment of the preoperative CT imaging. A standardized fashion to review the images is critical to first clarify the extent of surgery required and also identify potential pitfalls that may increase the risk of complications. A formal checklist is imperative to proceed with a comprehensive evaluation in a systematic manner.

The skull base is first assessed for its integrity, clearly delineating any preexisting zones of thinning or erosion. Its slope in the posterior ethmoid is also evaluated through the use of the sagittal views. The depth of the skull base at the level of the olfactory fossa is an important indicator of the risk of inadvertent CSF leak given that the medial wall, the lateral lamella of the cribriform plate, is the thinnest portion of the skull base and thus can be injured easily. It has been classified by Keros into four types: type A from 1 to 3 mm, type B from 4 to 7 mm, type C from 8 to 16 mm, and type D being oblique or asymmetrical. The medial orbital wall is the second structure to be evaluated. Its integrity should be ascertained as unrecognized protrusion of orbital content in the ethmoid sinus can lead to unintended injury to the extraocular muscles or optic nerve. Knowing the position of the uncinate process relative to the lamina papyracea is critical to avoid orbital injury at the time of uncinectomy. This unfortunate complication could occur if the uncinate is severely lateralized as seen in patients with chronic maxillary atelectasis. Next, the ethmoid vessels are identified, and their relationship to the skull base, more particularly the anterior ethmoid artery, should be evaluated. The arteries more frequently lie within the skull base itself but can be encased in bony mesentery below the skull base. If not previously identified, while skeletonizing the skull base from the ethmoid cavity to the frontal recess, one could curette the mesentery and injure the artery, leading to an orbital hematoma.

The major sinuses are subsequently checked for additional specific features. The position of the medial maxillary sinus wall is evaluated relative to the medial orbital wall. This serves as the lateral limit of dissection in the posterior ethmoid region. The presence of any infraorbital cell is noted so that it can be addressed during the performance of the maxillary antrostomy. The vertical height of the posterior ethmoid and the existence of a sphenoethmoid cell are assessed since the latter can place the optic nerve at risk of injury. Then, the sphenoid sinuses are inspected for the site of attachment of the intersinus septum and the relationship of the internal carotid artery to the optic nerve. It has been demonstrated that 22 % of the internal carotid artery canals show some level of clinical bony dehiscence in the lateral wall of the sphenoid sinus [31]. Finally, the frontal sinus is reviewed. The degree of development of the sinus itself, and the different cells that pneumatize the frontal recess are carefully assessed. Three-dimensional knowledge of the drainage pathway can be acquired by studying the axial and sagittal cuts and will prove invaluable during surgery.

Computer-Aided Surgery

Another significant development that has been introduced in the ESS paradigm is computer-aided surgery (CAS). This technology utilizes the preoperative sinus CT images to offer real-time tracking of calibrated instruments in the surgical field to a precision of 1–2 mm. The use of CAS should theoretically decrease the risk of orbital or skull base complications given the ability to dynamically ascertain these relationships during surgery. A recent meta-analysis published in 2013 demonstrated that the number of both major and total complications was significantly lower in the group of patients where CAS was used [32]. Though no official indications are available for the use of image-guided surgery, American Academy of Otolaryngology and Head and Neck Surgery (AAO-HNS) has provided recommendations for its utilization including, but not limited to revision ESS, cases where the anatomy has been distorted by a developmental or traumatic process, extensive sinonasal polyposis, disease involving the frontal and posterior ethmoid or sphenoid sinuses, pathologies abutting the skull base, optic nerve or carotid artery, CSF rhinorrhea or skull base defects, and benign or malignant neoplasms.

Anesthesia

In the early years of sinus surgery, topical and local anesthesia were the most commonly employed anesthetic techniques. There were some benefits reported, such as identifying the skull base more easily as this structure is more sensitive to pain than the ethmoid partitions. Also, in the setting of an orbital complication, the vision could be monitored more easily with the patient being awake. With the increased safety of anesthetic techniques in conjunction with increased experience with the surgical techniques, the procedure is now most frequently conducted under general anesthesia. Because of the more extensive nature of the surgery performed nowadays, it is also more comfortable for the patients to have a general anesthetic. In addition, it is easier for the anesthesiologist to adjust the hemodynamic parameters if needed. Keeping the mean arterial pressure between 60–70 and the heart rate below 60 bpm is ideal to decrease blood loss and hence improve visualization [33]. The controversy regarding the possible benefit of total intravenous anesthesia (TIVA) over inhalational anesthesia on surgical field visualization is still a matter of debate. A systematic review and meta-analysis published in 2013 reported a trend toward improved visualization when using TIVA, but the studies were of heterogeneous quality, hence no definitive conclusion could be drawn [34].

Patient Preparation

The following steps are performed with the goal of optimizing the surgical field through decreased bleeding. The patient is placed in a mild reverse Trendelenburg position, and the nose is decongested with 0.1 % xylometazoline. 1:1,000 adrenaline wringed cotton pledgets can then be introduced into the nasal cavities. A recent systematic review published in 2011 evaluated the safety of various vasoconstrictor agents in order to provide a protocol for surgeons performing ESS. In adults, topical epinephrine 1:1,000 or 1:2,000 is deemed safe, but caution must be exercised in patients with a history of cardiovascular disease. They recommended against topical phenylephrine in children and extreme caution with the use of cocaine [35]. Many surgeons utilize a throat pack inserted transorally to keep the blood from pooling around the endotracheal tube or being swallowed during the surgery, as this could otherwise place the patient at risk of aspiration or postoperative nausea and vomiting.

In order to optimize the surgical field further, a greater palatine or sphenopalatine block can also be performed. We prefer the second option to reduce the possible risks of blindness or infraorbital nerve injury described with the greater palatine foramen block. Infiltration of vasoconstrictive agents has been shown to reduce the bleeding and to aid with visualization during sinus surgery [36, 37]. Under endoscopic guidance, a mildly bent spinal needle (alternatively a tonsil needle) is inserted in the region of the sphenopalatine foramen close to the posterior attachment of the middle turbinate. Infiltration of 1 % lidocaine with 1:100,000 adrenaline is then performed until the mucosa blanches around the needle insertion point. The greater palatine block is performed transorally. The greater palatine foramen is located with manual palpation close to the second maxillary molar. The needle should be bent at 25 mm from the tip and at an angle of 45° to prevent insertion of the needle further into the pterygopalatine fossa [38].

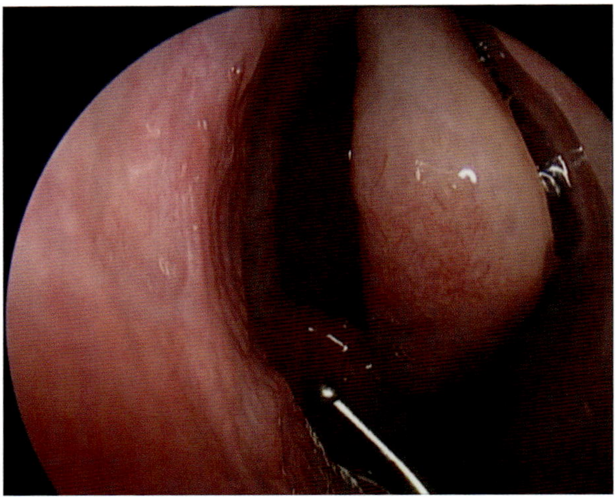

Fig. 22.1 Superior uncinectomy

Maxillary Antrostomy

A 0° endoscope is next inserted in the nasal cavity. If the axilla of the middle turbinate cannot be easily seen at this point because of the presence of a septal deviation, a septoplasty is performed to facilitate intraoperative surgical access and postoperative care. When the middle turbinate is easily visualized, it is gently medialized along its lower edge, being cautious not to fracture its attachment to the skull base superiorly. The most important step is then the performance of a complete uncinectomy using a retrograde approach. First, its posterior free edge is identified with an ostium seeker. A backbiting forceps is positioned as low as possible on the uncinate, and the cut is brought forward toward the anterior fontanel/membranous attachment of the uncinate to the lacrimal bone. Next its superior portion is medially rotated and resected with a forceps or the microdebrider (Fig. 22.1). Although an anterograde approach with the use of a sickle knife has been well described, it places the patient at an unnecessary increased risk of orbital penetration. This is especially true if the uncinate process is retracted laterally close to the lamina papyracea. A 30° endoscope is sometimes useful to confirm complete resection of the uncinate process, especially its most inferior portion (remnant often present after the initial resection) that often overlies the infundibulum.

Once this step is completed, visualization of the natural maxillary ostium should be possible with the use of an angled scope (Fig. 22.2). Proper identification and inclusion of the natural ostium in the surgically created antrostomy is of critical importance [39]. Creation of posterior antrostomy will result in a dual ostial configuration resulting in mucus recirculation and predispose to recurrent infections. If an accessory ostium is already present, it is joined to the natural ostium using through-cutting instruments. If an infraorbital or Haller cell is present, it should be addressed. Its presence narrows the infundibulum and may be a contributing factor in the pathophysiology of recurrent acute sinusitis.

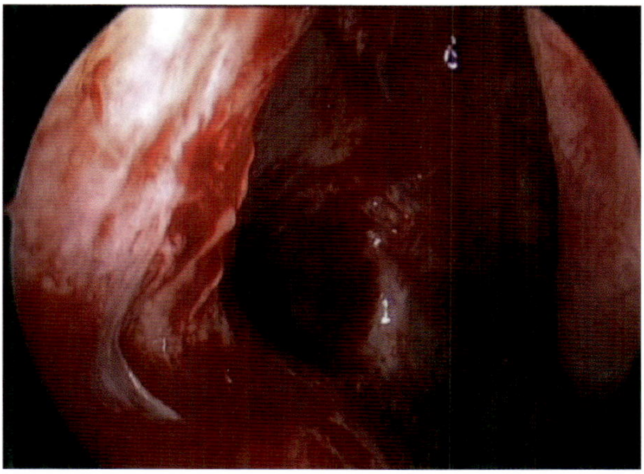

Fig. 22.2 Maxillary antrostomy

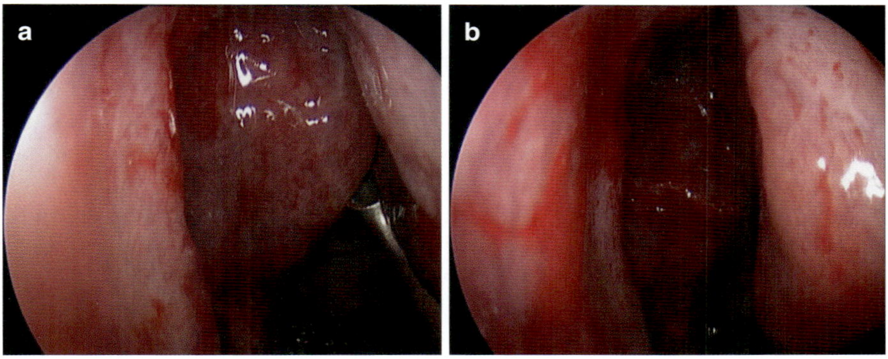

Fig. 22.3 (**a**) Before anterior ethmoidectomy. (**b**) After anterior ethmoidectomy

The optimal size of the antrostomy itself is still a matter of debate. Proponents of a small opening state that a larger ostium may have a drying effect of the sinus mucosa and that there may be a decrease in nitric oxide (NO) concentration after surgery. The clinical importance of such a reduction in NO level is still not well defined as evidenced by a recent meta-analysis [40]. On the other hand, a large antrostomy may lessen the risk of restenosis and improve access to topical therapies and cultures in the postoperative period.

Sphenoethmoidectomy

The next step is the performance of an anterior ethmoidectomy. The ethmoid bulla is the largest of the ethmoidal cells and the most prominent structure visualized when the uncinate is removed. With the use of a 0° scope, the middle turbinate is once again gently medialized in order to visualize the cleft between the bulla and the middle turbinate, the superior hiatus semilunaris. A curette is slid in that space and then more posterolaterally if a retrobullar recess exists. The bulla as a whole can be brought forward with the curette making this approach very safe for the orbit (Fig. 22.3a, b).

The remaining mucosa and bony lamellae are cleared to expose the basal lamella of the middle turbinate and to begin skeletonizing the lamina papyracea. The basal lamella often is not smooth but rather has indentations from ethmoid cells. Entry into the posterior ethmoid cells is through this lamella in an inferior and medial position immediately superior to the horizontal portion of the middle turbinate. This avoids injury to the middle turbinate branch of the sphenopalatine artery. The same low and medial approach is also used in the posterior ethmoid region to avoid injury to the lamina papyracea and the skull base until they can be definitively identified later in the procedure. The basal lamella of the superior turbinate is then traversed to bring the dissection into the sphenoethmoidal recess. At this point, the superior turbinate can be identified, and its inferior third is resected using through-cutting instruments in order to preserve the olfactory mucosa. Next, the natural sphenoid ostium is identified and opened to a diameter of at least 5–6 mm while preventing circumferential damage to the mucosa, which could lead to future ostium stenosis. A circular mushroom punch is useful for this maneuver.

An alternative way of entering the sphenoid has been described by Bolger using the parallelogram-shaped box [41]. The borders are the medial orbital wall laterally, the skull base superiorly, the superior turbinate medially, and the basal lamella of the superior turbinate inferiorly. The sphenoidotomy should be safe if performed low and medial in that box. However, this could be problematic if the superior turbinate attaches very laterally on the sphenoid face because this could potentially put the posterior orbit, optic nerve, or internal carotid injury at risk [42].

Following the sphenoidotomy, the skull base can be identified in the sphenoid sinus. Completing the ethmoidectomy entails removal of all the bony partitions comprising the posterior ethmoids, allowing for skeletonization of the skull base and lamina papyracea. Cells are often left undissected posteriorly close to the orbital wall since the orbit is cone shaped and the ethmoid cavity is larger posteriorly than anteriorly. Probing behind these lamellae and then curetting them or removing them with through-cutting instruments will ensure complete marsupialization of the ethmoid cavity (Fig. 22.4).

The complete removal of the bony lamellae is imperative, as residual partition may thicken causing ongoing inflammation and chronic osteitis. The same process may also happen if mucosal stripping occurs. Exposure of the bony surfaces can lead to mucosal metaplasia and non-physiological healing.

Frontal Recess Surgery

The extent of frontal sinus surgery should be individualized based on the extent of disease, frontal recess anatomy, and associated patient symptomatology.

The surgical anatomy of the frontal recess represents the most complex region of the sinonasal anatomy. It is an inverted funnel-shaped space from the frontal ostium to the ethmoid infundibulum or middle meatus, depending on the superior attachment of the uncinate process. It is bordered by the anterior attachment of the middle turbinate medially and by the medial orbital wall laterally. A sagittal view of the

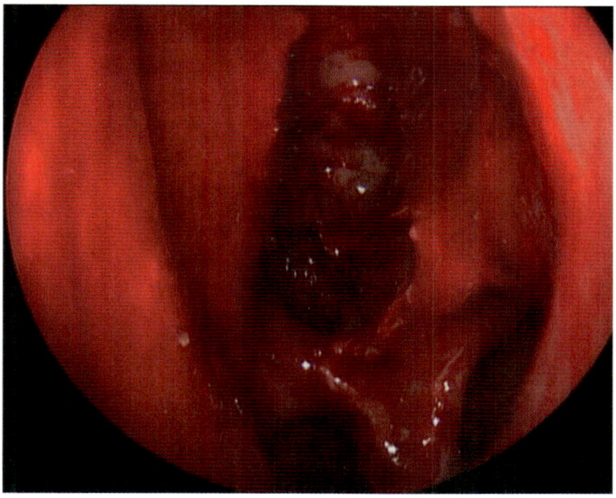

Fig. 22.4 Complete left sphenoethmoidectomy cavity

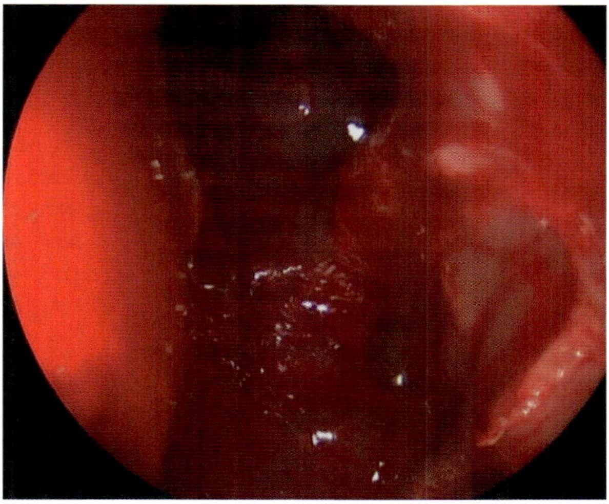

Fig. 22.5 Left frontal recess dissection

frontal recess is key to understanding its relationship with the skull base and the ethmoid bulla posteriorly and the agger nasi cell and frontal beak anteriorly. The goal of frontal recess surgery is to remove all the bony partitions that are present within these previously described limits in order to create wide access to the frontal sinus (Fig. 22.5).

CT imaging is also essential to understanding the various cells that occupy the frontal recess. Agger nasi cell, the most constant anterior cell, is present over 95 % of the time [43]. Kuhn described four different types of frontal cells that can pneumatize over the agger nasi cell potentially narrowing the recess anteriorly. His classification system has been further revised by Wormald and Chan [44]. Type 1 cell describes 1 cell above the agger nasi cell, while type 2 denotes 2 or more cells above the agger nasi cell. Type 3 and 4 cells signify pneumatization above the frontal beak under 50 % of the sinus height or 50 % above the sinus height, respectively. These frontal cells have the potential to be large enough to be mistaken for the frontal sinus itself during surgery. Supraorbital cells are also a common finding. Visualization of a vertical septation in the frontal sinus on the preoperative CT scan is often correlated with the presence of these cells [45]. The supraorbital cell opening is posterior and lateral to the frontal sinus proper. Ideally, both these openings should be connected by removal of the intervening septation to prevent future stenosis.

Endoscopic frontal sinus surgery ensues with the use of angled scopes (30°, 45°, and 70°) and appropriately curved instruments. Navigating instruments are also helpful since the dissection will proceed in the vicinity of the skull base and orbit. Surgical navigation is also helpful for corroborating the surgeons' impression of location of the recess and the intervening cells. Removing the most superior portion of the uncinate process and reshaping/widening the axilla of the middle turbinate are helpful steps at the beginning of the frontal sinusotomy, as these structures have the potential to obstruct optimal view.

The skull base is identified just posterior to the recess, and the bony partitions found anteriorly are brought forward with a 90° curved curette. A small tip navigating frontal seeker is then used to probe the frontal recess. Often this can be done between the medial wall of the agger nasi cell and the middle turbinate. The importance of completely "uncapping the egg" cannot be overstated as advocated by Stammberger. If these partitions are left undissected, the sinus will not drain adequately and potentially lead to scarring in the frontal recess. Preservation of the mucosa is also critical to prevent stenosis in these narrow confines. The role of stenting in the postoperative period is controversial, but it is generally reserved for revision and complex cases rather than primary surgeries.

Management of the Middle Turbinate

Ideal management of the middle turbinate signifies another important area of controversy. Two areas of thought have emerged since the beginning of ESS. Proponents of middle turbinate preservation argue that this leads to protection of the sinuses from inhaled irritants and maintenance of surgical landmarks for future surgeries and leaves intact the structures that are not affected by the disease process. Others have proposed routine turbinectomy while performing ESS especially in cases of nasal polyposis. Bulky middle turbinates because of either polypoid degeneration or pneumatization can contribute to OMC obstruction. Also, a "floppy" middle turbinate may have a tendency to scar to the lateral wall, compromising the delivery of topical therapies in the postoperative period. Despite the retrospective and prospective data demonstrating potentially better outcomes with partial turbinectomy, none of these studies was randomized thus introducing a major bias in the interpretation of the results [46, 47]. Consequently, there is still no definitive answer to the question of whether or not to resect all or a portion of the middle turbinate.

If the decision is to preserve the middle turbinate, then, measures to prevent lateralization are important. Multiple techniques and devices have been used with variable success. "Bolgerization" has been described which consists of creating a controlled synechiae between the medial aspect of the middle turbinate and the corresponding nasal septum, which would serve to maintain the turbinate in a medialized position [48]. Transseptal sutures holding both middle turbinates against the septum have also been described but are technically more difficult to perform. The use of middle meatal stents is often used, though options abound, ranging from resorbable to non-resorbable materials. A randomized controlled trial by Côté and Wright in 2010 established the efficacy of an absorbable dressing for the prevention of middle turbinate synechiae against the lateral nasal wall. The possibility of impregnating this dressing with a steroid solution had the added benefit of improved healing of the sinonasal cavities up to 6 months after surgery [49].

Conclusion

Over the past 30 years, there has been considerable evolution of the surgical paradigm in endoscopic sinus surgery. The main goal of surgery has changed from a strictly anatomically oriented approach to a wider marsupialization of the sinus cavities in order to optimize the delivery of topical nasal therapies in the postoperative period. Multiple technologies are also available to the otolaryngologist to enhance the safety and completeness of surgery, though intimate understanding of the anatomy and mucosal preservation technique remain key prerequisites to sinus surgery.

References

1. Kennedy DW, Zinreich SJ, Rosenbaum AE, Johns ME. Functional endoscopic sinus surgery. Theory and diagnostic evaluation. Arch Otolaryngol (Chicago: 1960). 1985;111(9):576–82.
2. Stammberger H. Endoscopic endonasal surgery–concepts in treatment of recurring rhinosinusitis. Part II. Surgical technique. Otolaryngol Head Neck Surg. 1986;94(2):147–56.
3. Messerklinger W. On the drainage of the normal frontal sinus of man. Acta Otolaryngol. 1967;63(2):176–81.
4. Thomas 3rd WW, Harvey RJ, Rudmik L, Hwang PH, Schlosser RJ. Distribution of topical agents to the paranasal sinuses: an evidence-based review with recommendations. Int Forum Allergy Rhinol. 2013;3(9):691–703.
5. Bolger WE, Brown CL, Church CA, Goldberg AN, Karanfilov B, Kuhn FA, et al. Safety and outcomes of balloon catheter sinusotomy: a multicenter 24-week analysis in 115 patients. Otolaryngol Head Neck Surg. 2007;137(1):10–20.
6. Batra PS, Ryan MW, Sindwani R, Marple BF. Balloon catheter technology in rhinology: reviewing the evidence. Laryngoscope. 2011;121(1):226–32.
7. Cutler J, Bikhazi N, Light J, Truitt T, Schwartz M. Standalone balloon dilation versus sinus surgery for chronic rhinosinusitis: a prospective, multicenter, randomized, controlled trial. Am J Rhinol Allergy. 2013;27(5):416–22.
8. Catalano P, Roffman E. Outcome in patients with chronic sinusitis after the minimally invasive sinus technique. Am J Rhinol. 2003;17(1):17–22.

9. Naidoo Y, Bassiouni A, Keen M, Wormald PJ. Long-term outcomes for the endoscopic modified Lothrop/Draf III procedure: a 10-year review. Laryngoscope. 2014;124(1):43–9.
10. Jankowski R, Pigret D, Decroocq F. Comparison of functional results after ethmoidectomy and nasalization for diffuse and severe nasal polyposis. Acta Otolaryngol. 1997;117(4):601–8.
11. Dubin MG, Liu C, Lin SY, Senior BA. American Rhinologic Society member survey on "maximal medical therapy" for chronic rhinosinusitis. Am J Rhinol. 2007;21(4):483–8.
12. Sylvester DC, Carr S, Nix P. Maximal medical therapy for chronic rhinosinusitis: a survey of otolaryngology consultants in the United Kingdom. Int Forum Allergy Rhinol. 2013;3(2):129–32.
13. Krouse JH, Veling MC, Ryan MW, Pillsbury 3rd HC, Krouse HJ, Joe S, et al. Executive summary: asthma and the unified airway. Otolaryngol Head Neck Surg. 2007;136(5):699–706.
14. Ragab S, Scadding GK, Lund VJ, Saleh H. Treatment of chronic rhinosinusitis and its effects on asthma. Eur Respir J. 2006;28(1):68–74.
15. Meena RS, Meena D, Aseri Y, Singh BK, Verma PC. Chronic rhino-sinusitis and asthma: concept of unified airway disease (UAD) and its impact in otolaryngology. Indian J Otolaryngol Head Neck Surg. 2013;65 Suppl 2:338–42.
16. Batra PS, Kern RC, Tripathi A, Conley DB, Ditto AM, Haines 3rd GK, et al. Outcome analysis of endoscopic sinus surgery in patients with nasal polyps and asthma. Laryngoscope. 2003;113(10):1703–6.
17. Crosby DL, Adappa ND. What is the optimal management of chronic rhinosinusitis in cystic fibrosis? Curr Opin Otolaryngol Head Neck Surg. 2014;22(1):42–6.
18. Cannady SB, Batra PS, Koening C, Lorenz RR, Citardi MJ, Langford C, et al. Sinonasal Wegener granulomatosis: a single-institution experience with 120 cases. Laryngoscope. 2009;119(4):757–61.
19. Bacciu A, Buzio C, Giordano D, Pasanisi E, Vincenti V, Mercante G, et al. Nasal polyposis in Churg-Strauss syndrome. Laryngoscope. 2008;118(2):325–9.
20. Lai JC, Lee HS, Chen MK, Tsai YL. Patient satisfaction and treatment outcome of fungus ball rhinosinusitis treated by functional endoscopic sinus surgery. Eur Arch Otorhinolaryngol. 2011;268(2):227–30.
21. Ledderose GJ, Braun T, Betz CS, Stelter K, Leunig A. Functional endoscopic surgery of paranasal fungus ball: clinical outcome, patient benefit and health-related quality of life. Eur Arch Otorhinolaryngol. 2012;269(10):2203–8.
22. Laury AM, Wise SK. Chapter 7: Allergic fungal rhinosinusitis. Am J Rhinol Allergy. 2013;27 Suppl 1:S26–7.
23. Duggal P, Wise SK. Chapter 8: Invasive fungal rhinosinusitis. Am J Rhinol Allergy. 2013;27 Suppl 1:S28–30.
24. Rosenfeld RM. Clinical practice guideline on adult sinusitis. Otolaryngol Head Neck Surg. 2007;137(3):365–77.
25. Poetker DM, Litvack JR, Mace JC, Smith TL. Recurrent acute rhinosinusitis: presentation and outcomes of sinus surgery. Am J Rhinol. 2008;22(3):329–33.
26. Leung R, Almassian S, Kern R, Conley D, Tan B, Chandra R. Patient level decision making in recurrent acute rhinosinusitis: a cost-benefit threshold for surgery. Laryngoscope. 2013; 123(1):11–6.
27. Courson AM, Stankiewicz JA, Lal D. Contemporary management of frontal sinus mucoceles: a meta-analysis. Laryngoscope. 2014;124(2):378–86.
28. Kennedy DW, Josephson JS, Zinreich SJ, Mattox DE, Goldsmith MM. Endoscopic sinus surgery for mucoceles: a viable alternative. Laryngoscope. 1989;99(9):885–95.
29. Prevedello DM, Ditzel Filho LF, Solari D, Carrau RL, Kassam AB. Expanded endonasal approaches to middle cranial fossa and posterior fossa tumors. Neurosurg Clin N Am. 2010;21(4):621–35. 4.

30. Wigand ME. [Transnasal, endoscopical surgery for chronic sinusitis. III. Endonasal ethmoidectomy (author's transl)]. Hno. 1981;29(9):287–93.
31. Kennedy DW, Zinreich SJ, Hassab MH. The internal carotid artery as it relates to endonasal sphenoethmoidectomy. Am J Rhinol. 1990;4(1):7–12.
32. Dalgorf DM, Sacks R, Wormald PJ, Naidoo Y, Panizza B, Uren B, et al. Image-guided surgery influences perioperative morbidity from endoscopic sinus surgery: a systematic review and meta-analysis. Otolaryngol Head Neck Surg. 2013;149(1):17–29.
33. Wormald PJ, van Renen G, Perks J, Jones JA, Langton-Hewer CD. The effect of the total intravenous anesthesia compared with inhalational anesthesia on the surgical field during endoscopic sinus surgery. Am J Rhinol. 2005;19(5):514–20.
34. DeConde AS, Thompson CF, Wu EC, Suh JD. Systematic review and meta-analysis of total intravenous anesthesia and endoscopic sinus surgery. Int Forum Allergy Rhinol. 2013;3(10):848–54.
35. Higgins TS, Hwang PH, Kingdom TT, Orlandi RR, Stammberger H, Han JK. Systematic review of topical vasoconstrictors in endoscopic sinus surgery. Laryngoscope. 2011;121(2):422–32.
36. Wormald PJ, Athanasiadis T, Rees G, Robinson S. An evaluation of effect of pterygopalatine fossa injection with local anesthetic and adrenalin in the control of nasal bleeding during endoscopic sinus surgery. Am J Rhinol. 2005;19(3):288–92.
37. Eloy JA, Kovalerchik O, Bublik M, Ruiz JW, Casiano RR. Effect of greater palatine canal injection on estimated blood loss during endoscopic sinus surgery. Am J Otolaryngol. 2014;35(1):1–4.
38. Douglas R, Wormald PJ. Pterygopalatine fossa infiltration through the greater palatine foramen: where to bend the needle. Laryngoscope. 2006;116(7):1255–7.
39. Kennedy DW, Adappa ND. Endoscopic maxillary antrostomy: not just a simple procedure. Laryngoscope. 2011;121(10):2142–5.
40. Phillips PS, Sacks R, Marcells GN, Cohen NA, Harvey RJ. Nasal nitric oxide and sinonasal disease: a systematic review of published evidence. Otolaryngol Head Neck Surg. 2011;144(2):159–69.
41. Bolger WE, Keyes AS, Lanza DC. Use of the superior meatus and superior turbinate in the endoscopic approach to the sphenoid sinus. Otolaryngol Head Neck Surg. 1999;120(3):308–13.
42. Gheriani H, Flamer D, Orton T, Mechor B, Javer AR. A comparison of two sphenoidotomy approaches using a novel computerized tomography grading system. Am J Rhinol Allergy. 2009;23(2):212–7.
43. Bolger WE, Butzin CA, Parsons DS. Paranasal sinus bony anatomic variations and mucosal abnormalities: CT analysis for endoscopic sinus surgery. Laryngoscope. 1991;101(1 Pt 1):56–64.
44. Wormald PJ, Chan SZ. Surgical techniques for the removal of frontal recess cells obstructing the frontal ostium. Am J Rhinol. 2003;17(4):221–6.
45. Comer BT, Kincaid NW, Smith NJ, Wallace JH, Kountakis SE. Frontal sinus septations predict the presence of supraorbital ethmoid cells. Laryngoscope. 2013;123(9):2090–3.
46. Soler ZM, Hwang PH, Mace J, Smith TL. Outcomes after middle turbinate resection: revisiting a controversial topic. Laryngoscope. 2010;120(4):832–7.
47. Wu AW, Ting JY, Platt MP, Tierney HT, Metson R. Factors affecting time to revision sinus surgery for nasal polyps: a 25-year experience. Laryngoscope. 2014;124(1):29–33.
48. Bolger WE, Kuhn FA, Kennedy DW. Middle turbinate stabilization after functional endoscopic sinus surgery: the controlled synechiae technique. Laryngoscope. 1999;109(11):1852–3.
49. Cote DW, Wright ED. Triamcinolone-impregnated nasal dressing following endoscopic sinus surgery: a randomized, double-blind, placebo-controlled study. Laryngoscope. 2010;120(6):1269–73.

Medical Therapy in the Preoperative and Postoperative Period

23

Opeyemi O. Daramola and Rakesh K. Chandra

Key Take-Home Points

- Oral antibiotics are an option in perioperative care of patients with chronic rhinosinusitis.
- Short course of perioperative oral steroids may improve surgical field and limit postoperative morbidity.
- There is no proven role for topical or oral antifungal medications.
- Aspirin desensitization and postoperative immunotherapy have been associated with better outcomes when indicated.

Introduction

Chronic rhinosinusitis (CRS) is a complex disease process that manifests in diverse phenotypes that may have different responses to treatment. There are multiple potential etiologies including allergic, infectious, anatomic, and immunologic in nature. The first line of treatment for CRS typically consists of medical therapies that are based on physiologic principles of restoring natural mucociliary function, ventilation of paranasal sinuses, and eradication of any underlying infection.

O.O. Daramola, MD
Department of Otolaryngology – Head and Neck Surgery, Northwestern University
Feinberg School of Medicine, 676 N St. Clair Street, Suite 15-200, Chicago, IL 60611, USA
e-mail: ODaramola@beckerentcenter.com

R.K. Chandra, MD (✉)
Department of Otolaryngology – Head and Neck Surgery, Vanderbilt University
School of Medicine, 1215 21st Ave. South Suite 7209 Medical Center East,
South Tower, Nashville, TN 37232, USA
e-mail: rakesh.chandra@vanderbilt.edu

P.S. Batra, J.K. Han (eds.), *Practical Medical and Surgical Management of Chronic Rhinosinusitis*, DOI 10.1007/978-3-319-16724-4_23

Surgical intervention, in the form of endoscopic sinus surgery, is indicated for complicated cases, patients with abnormal anatomic features precluding adequate delivery of topical therapies, and cases refractory to medical therapy. Notably, CRS is primarily an inflammatory disease; endoscopic sinus surgery (ESS) is not curative but can be instrumental in improving access for optimal topical treatment, alleviating complicated situations, and limiting the severity and frequency of exacerbations. There is little doubt that properly vetted and performed ESS plays a vital role in the comprehensive management of CRS. ESS is associated with significantly higher quality of life compared to medical therapy alone [1, 2]. Thus, it is intuitive to infer that optimization of preoperative and postoperative care of CRS patients undergoing ESS will further enhance clinical outcomes and, in turn, patient's quality of life.

Given the potential myriad of precipitating events and patient factors that contribute to the development and persistence of inflammation in CRS, the preoperative, perioperative, and postoperative regimen should be tailored to the clinical profile and prevailing comorbidities. This chapter presents existing medical practices and available evidence regarding medical therapies in the perioperative management of CRS patients with emphasis on preoperative and immediate postoperative period of patients undergoing ESS. The main decisions regarding perioperative care in ESS revolve around antibiotics, anti-inflammatory regimen, treatment of allergic disease, and office debridement.

Antibacterial Therapy

Preoperative Oral Antibiotics

For the purposes of a concise discussion, the preoperative phase of the ESS patient will be regarded as the time period between provision of consent for surgery and initiation of anesthetic on the day of surgery. Preoperative treatment of patients should include measures that can provide immediate improvement in symptoms and/or reduce risk of complications. These measures should also optimize intraoperative milieu by limiting inflammatory load and addressing infectious agents. The utility of oral antibiotics should be examined in the context of challenges involved in determining the etiologic role of bacteria in CRS.

The role of microbes in CRS is unclear, but the use of therapies targeting potential microorganisms is a mainstay feature in the medical treatment of CRS [3]. These organisms may be viral, bacterial, or fungal. The rationale behind antibacterial therapy is based on the inference that these organisms act as pathogens or incite inflammatory response in CRS. Debate on the use of preoperative antibiotics is valid as the pathogenicity of bacteria is frequently challenged. The microbiology of isolates from the nasal cavity, middle meatus, or postsurgical cavities of patients with CRS is often polymicrobial with a preponderance of aerobic bacteria such as *Staphylococcus aureus* and *Pseudomonas aeruginosa* [4–7]. Anaerobes and fungi are also present in clinically significant frequencies. While there may be discovery of rare organisms in CRS patients, the nasal cavity and paranasal sinuses in 18–50 % of healthy patients are colonized with similar bacteria found in CRS [4–6]. Multiple studies have demonstrated that bacteria can be recovered from purulent and non-purulent fluid from CRS patients regardless of the collection technique. These findings confound the ability to differentiate between pathogens and colonizers, and bacteria may also exist as complex biofilms.

On an individual level, physicians may offer anecdotal reports of improvement in patient symptoms and healing time; however, there is little evidence specifically addressing preoperative antibiotic use. In a systematic review and meta-analysis of perioperative antibiotic use in ESS, there was no significant reduction in the incidence of infection, symptoms scores, and endoscopic scores [8]. However, there is evidence supporting the recommendation of oral antibiotics as an option in the overall management of CRS exacerbations for as long as 3 weeks [3]. Macrolide and non-macrolide agents used in this context have been found to alleviate symptoms and reduce polyposis. There is recommendation against treatment longer than 3 weeks because of the lack of studies demonstrating clear benefit. Longer courses of antibiotics may place the patient at risk for resistant organisms, medication side effects, and unnecessary financial investment. Regardless of the level of available evidence, in practicality, preoperative antibiotic therapy is widely practiced and regarded by sinus surgeons as an important modality to decrease inflammation, improve wound healing, and reduce patient morbidity [8, 9].

The choice of preoperative antibiotic agent should be ideally culture directed. If culture result and sensitivity are not available, empiric treatment should note that bacteria in chronically inflamed sinuses tend to be resistant to penicillin due to beta-lactamase production [7, 10, 11]. Useful oral agents in CRS patients must have good activity against aerobic and anaerobic beta-lactamase-producing bacteria. These include penicillin combined with a beta-lactamase inhibitor, macrolides, quinolones, and clindamycin. Surgeons seeking to reduce disease burden from *Pseudomonas aeruginosa* and other gram-negative bacteria have limited options with oral fluoroquinolones, with intravenous aminoglycosides, fourth-generation cephalosporins, and fluoroquinolones being options in exceptional cases. As a matter of routine practice, intravenous preoperative antibiotics are not generally recommended given lack of demonstrated benefit, potential for catheter-related complications, and significant expense. Agent-specific risks of short-term oral courses should be discussed with patients. Rosenfeld et al. noted a relative risk of 83 % of adverse events such as gastrointestinal events, including *Clostridium difficile colitis*, skin rash, vaginal discharge, headache, dizziness, and fatigue in patients treated with similar agents in an acute setting [12].

There is some objective evidence that supports the use of macrolides for their anti-inflammatory potential [13–16]. Specifically, in vitro studies have demonstrated macrolide reduction of proinflammatory cytokines such as IL-5, IL-6, and IL-8. Macrolides have also been found to inhibit oxidative burst and stimulate phagocytosis. Although anti-inflammatory mechanism in vivo is not clear, macrolide treatment has been associated with reduction in IL-6 and IL-8. Long-term use of low-dose roxithromycin (daily 150 mg orally for three months) in a placebo-controlled single-center study was associated with statistically significant improvement in nasal endoscopy, saccharin transit time, reduction in nasal lavage IL-8 and SNOT-20 scores [15]. This study also illustrated that individuals with lower baseline immunoglobulin E levels (<200 μg/L) are better responders across outcome measures, thus suggesting a potential selective criterion if this therapy is considered in clinical practice. There is a plethora of level 4 studies that have investigated or reported the role of clarithromycin, azithromycin, and roxithromycin with trend toward objective improvement of inflammatory findings [7]. Notably, the anti-inflammatory properties of macrolides were evident at low concentrations than normally prescribed, thus likely limiting side effects. Notably, a majority of these studies were not intended for outcome evaluation in the perioperative period, but it is not unreasonable to favor macrolides preoperatively given the prevailing evidence.

Other non-macrolide antibiotics have been investigated as well. Doxycycline is an option with anti-inflammatory properties that has been studied in patients diagnosed with chronic rhinosinusitis with nasal polyposis (CRSwNP) [17]. Van Zele et al. conducted a level 1b study demonstrating endoscopic reduction in polyp load in patients treated with 20 days of oral doxycycline (200 mg once, then 100 mg daily for 20 days) compared to placebo. There was no difference in subjective outcomes. In an observational study of patients with chronic rhinosinusitis without polyposis (CRSsNP), treatment with 6 weeks of clindamycin (150 mg orally three times daily) was associated with improvement in computed tomography (CT) scores [18]. No subjective outcome measures were evaluated. Overall, it is difficult to draw relevant conclusions regarding the choice and duration of non-macrolide therapy based on existing literature because of lack of controls and randomization or comparisons of multiple antibiotics in a single study.

Perioperative Intravenous Antibiotics

The infusion of intravenous antibiotics perioperatively is practiced as a measure to reduce surgical site infection. The role of the antibiotic varies based on the wound classification. The classification of operative wounds stems from the classic study from the National Academy of Sciences–National Research Council published in 1964 [19]. The risk for postoperative surgical site infection has been further modified by additional studies such as the National Nosocomial Infection Surveillance study which highlighted major risk factors including wound classification, American Society of Anesthesiologists (ASA) class III, IV, or V, and length of surgery [20, 21]. Surgeries of the aerodigestive tract, including ESS, are classified as clean-contaminated. Clean-contaminated cases are associated with operative wound infection rate of up to 10 % or less [22]. Generally, antibiotic prophylaxis not exceeding 24 h postoperatively is recommended for clean-contaminated head and neck cases, but studies involved in this recommendation are dominated by soft tissue oncologic procedures [23]. Consideration of intravenous antibiotic prophylaxis on the day of surgery should proceed in the context of three important considerations: indication, timing, and selection of appropriate agent. In practice, perioperative antibiotics should be provided within 30 min of incision time. However, with regard to indication, there is a lack of evidence to support the use of perioperative antibiotics in ESS [8, 24]. This lack of solid empiric evidence is acknowledged by otolaryngologists, but the practice to infuse intravenous perioperative antibiotic prophylaxis is adopted by reasonable portion of the specialty [25].

The perpetuation of intravenous antibiotic prophylaxis use in ESS is complex and may be related to the strong ties between perioperative antibiotic prophylaxis in surgical fields to pay for performance measures. The use and timing of antibiotic prophylaxis for all surgeries is a nationally tracked and publicly reported quality metric sponsored by the Centers for Medicare and Medicaid Services Surgical Care Improvement Project. Thus, surgeons may feel pressure to be included in such reporting even if their operative wounds and nature of surgery do not call for perioperative antibiotics. When perioperative antibiotics are used by a surgeon, the preferred regimens for "clean-contaminated head and neck procedures" are cefazolin, or cefuroxime plus metronidazole, and ampicillin–sulbactam [24]. Clindamycin may be used in patients with documented beta-lactam allergy.

There are certain categories of patients in which intravenous perioperative antibiotics are recommended despite the weak evidence. Immunocompromised patients should be given prophylactic antibiotics. Another group consists of patients with cardiovascular or valvular disease. Studies of the incidence of endocarditis associated with dental procedures and endoscopy-related surgeries are lacking, but transient bacteremia consistent with operative-site bacteriology has been documented in as many as 7 % of patients undergoing ESS [26]. Antibiotic prophylaxis should be performed with guidance provided by cardiologists, infectious disease specialists, and primary care physicians involved in the perioperative care of the patient. Nevertheless, the consensus is that patients with specific cardiac and vascular conditions are at risk for endocarditis or vascular prosthetic infection when undergoing certain procedures, and these patients should receive prophylactic antibiotics [27].

It is not uncommon to recommend nasal surgeries such as turbinate reduction and septoplasty to CRS patients in addition to ESS. The use of perioperative antibiotics for these procedures is also based on surgeon preference. This is a low-risk practice, but patients receiving systemic antibiotics for septal surgery and/or turbinate reduction do not have reduced morbidity or infection rates, and prophylaxis does not provide protection against *S. aureus* colonization [28, 29].

Postoperative Oral Antibiotics

Similar to pre- and perioperative antibiotics, there is also a lack of consensus regarding the use of antibiotics in the postoperative period. However, up to 86 % of otolaryngologists self-reported providing postoperative antibiotics after ESS [9]. Most responders in the referenced survey study by Portelo et al. prescribed postoperative antibiotics to cover routinely discovered organisms in the paranasal sinuses but tailored their regimen based on culture results. Outcomes based on postoperative antibiotics have demonstrated mixes results. Postoperative amoxicillin–clavulanate has been shown to significantly decrease crusting, nasal obstruction, and drainage [30]. In contrast, a level 2b randomized study without placebo by Jiang et al. (using amoxicillin-clavulanate) found no differences in the symptom and endoscopic scores, rates of bacterial culture, and drug sensitivity [31]. In addition, other studies have found no significant difference in patients receiving postoperative amoxicillin versus homeopathic treatment or placebo [32]. Notably, there is a variation in the doses and randomization techniques used in referenced studies, but a review of available studies at different levels appears to suggest an overall benefit in the early postoperative period within 2 weeks [33]. A macrolide or penicillin agent is recommended for nonallergic patients. Treatment should be tailored according to final culture results as culture-inappropriate therapy may actually decrease quality of life, while culture-directed therapy may improve short-term ESS outcome [34].

Topical Antibiotics

The use of off-label intranasal topical antibiotics is relatively unproven practice but attractive idea because of the potential to avoid side effects from systemic treatment while attempting to improve the local health of the paranasal sinuses. In addition, the possibility of addressing biofilms may confer another potential benefit. There is an abundance of literature, ranging from case series to randomized controlled trials, evaluating antimicrobials in nebulized, metered-dose spray or lavage administrations [3, 35, 36]. Randomized controlled trials investigating the role of neomycin, bacitracin/colimycin, and tobramycin in CRS have failed to consistently demonstrate clear, clinically significant benefit. However, postoperative topical tobramycin has been retrospectively shown to decrease frequency of subsequent sinus surgeries in the pediatric cystic fibrosis population [37]. Mupirocin irrigation has also been shown in uncontrolled studies effective in eradicating *Staphylococcus aureus* in colonized subjects, providing subjective and objective improvement [3, 35]. While the risk of an adverse event associated with topical antibiotics is low, the benefits derived from the antimicrobial potential (which should not be confounded with the mechanical debridement afforded by lavage) in the perioperative period are questionable. Furthermore, the decision to use topical antimicrobials is expensive and time consuming even with the compliant patient. However, it is reasonable option in diseased postoperative sinuses refractory to oral antimicrobials, especially if compelling culture results are obtained.

Antifungal Therapy

Oral and Topical Antifungals

Historically, Ponikau et al. suggested fungi as a major potential cause of CRS [38]. Hence, topical and systemic antifungals were suggested as treatment options. However, the use of topical and systemic antifungals is controversial, especially when viewed through the lens of potential side effects. Furthermore, the idea of eradicating fungal colonization appears impractical given the known ubiquity of the fungal biomass. The majority of original publications dedicated to outcomes of oral antifungals in CRS are level 4 and expert opinions with the exception of a level 1 study by Kennedy et al. [39]. These subjects in the experimental arm in this study used 625 mg of terbinafine for 6 weeks without any benefit in subjective and objective outcome measures. There are other studies reporting the use of itraconazole and ketoconazole in uncontrolled prospective studies, retrospective series, and case reports [40–42]. These series investigated the use of antifungals in CRS treatment and as a postoperative adjunct. There is considerable heterogeneity in these studies, but the lack of consistent, reproducible objective and subjective benefit remains a common denominator. There is a collective higher level of evidence with topical amphotericin B irrigations with aggregate evidence from randomized control trials demonstrating no consistent, clear, clinical benefit [3, 40]. Oral antifungals have been associated with hepatoxicity, cardiotoxicity, and nephrotoxicity, while topical antifungals can cause nasal irritation. While they may be considered on individual basis, the preponderance of harm over benefit has resulted into multiple reviewers recommending against the routine use of systemic and topical antifungals. Thus, antifungals do not currently have a role in perioperative care of patients undergoing ESS for CRS.

Anti-inflammatory Therapies

The diagnosis of CRS requires confirmation of sinonasal inflammation via nasal endoscopy or imaging. Subsequently, topical and systemic medical treatments that primarily address sinonasal inflammation are widely used, with corticosteroids acting as the cornerstone of nonsurgical CRS management. Dosing regimen and delivery methods for corticosteroids vary in the preoperative and postoperative phases depending on the patient context.

Oral Steroids

The role of oral corticosteroids in treating symptomatic CRS patient is well documented and is summarized in a systematic review by Poetker et al. [43]. There is strong evidence supporting the recommendation of oral steroids in the short-term management of patients with CRSwNP. There is limited data available regarding the role of oral steroids in CRSsNP secondary to the paucity of high-quality studies investigating oral steroids as sole medical treatment in these patients. There is a lower number of high level evidence specifically on perioperative use of oral steroids in CRS. Nevertheless, it is not imprudent to contemplate their use in the perioperative period to improve the intraoperative course.

Three studies are worth mentioning regarding perioperative oral steroids in ESS. Wright and Aggarwal conducted a randomized, double-blind, placebo-controlled study (level 1b) on objective and subjective outcome measures in 26 patients with CRSwNP undergoing ESS [44]. Patients randomized to the treatment group received 30 mg of prednisone daily for 5 days preoperatively and 9 days postoperatively without tapering. The selection of dose was based on investigator experience as a sufficient dose to achieve clinical effect while limiting short-term side effects. There was no difference in postoperative subjective symptoms except improved olfaction in the treatment group at 2 weeks with a significant trend of persistent improvement toward the fourth week. Improved endoscopic appearance up to six months was reported in the treatment group as well. There was a statistically insignificant higher level of difficulty in ESS in the placebo subjects without difference in duration or blood loss. Similarly, Giordano et al. reported no difference in blood loss, but a significant reduction in duration after preoperative prednisone dosed at 1 mg/kg for 7 days [45]. Sieskiewicz et al. reported reduced difficulty, better visibility, and shorter operative time in subjects treated with preoperative 30 mg of prednisone for 5 days preoperatively [46].

Two studies have reported benefit with postoperative oral steroids greater than 2 weeks in patients with allergic fungal rhinosinusitis (AFRS). In a case control study, Ikram et al. reported a recurrence rate of 15.2 % in experimental subjects who received a month of oral prednisone (0.5 mg/kg) postoperatively followed by 5 months of beclomethasone spray. This recurrence rate was lower in comparison to historical controls who underwent surgery alone and had a recurrence rate of 50 % within a 2-year follow-up [47]. Duration of treatment was even longer in a study by Rupa et al. where experimental subjects with AFRS were treated with 50 mg daily for 6 weeks with additional tapering over the next 6 weeks with adjunctive oral ranitidine, oral itraconazole, and fluticasone nasal spray [48]. These experimental patients had no endoscopic evidence of disease after treatment. However, dermatologic, diabetic, and cushingoid complications were reported.

Most experienced otolaryngologists would agree that a short course of oral steroids perioperatively has the potential to improve the surgical field and to alleviate postoperative morbidity in moderate to severe CRSwNP. Ideally, surgeons who routinely treat with steroids perioperatively should adopt a weight-based protocol with a ceiling dose for consistency. If a decision to treat with steroids is made, there is no strong evidence available to suggest doses higher than 30 mg 5–7 days preoperatively. Postoperative duration and tapering is surgeon specific, but overall treatment is not recommended to exceed 14–21 days in patients without AFRS [43, 44]. An open dialogue centered on side effects of steroids should be held during the informed consent process as there is potential for major adverse reactions with serious medicolegal ramifications (Table 23.1) [49, 50].

Topical Intranasal Corticosteroids

Topical steroids are commonly prescribed as a component of first-line treatment in CRS. They are recommended as monotherapy or adjunctive to oral antibiotics in acute rhinosinusitis [51]. It is rare to see a CRS patient scheduled for ESS who is naïve to topical nasal corticosteroids. There is no contraindication to continuation of nasal spray preoperatively in the context of positive objective and/or subjective results. Table 23.2 lists some commonly prescribed nasal steroids in the adult population [52–59].

Table 23.1 Side effects of oral steroid use [49, 50]

Common side effects	Infrequent side effects	Rare side effects
Insomnia Increased appetite Anxiety Acid reflux Hyperglycemia	Peptic ulcer Osteoporosis Diabetes Dry skin Cushing's syndrome	Avascular necrosis of the hip Congestive heart failure Depression (suicidal ideation) Hypertension Heart block Hallucination Hepatomegaly Increased intraocular pressure of the eye Mood lability Pseudotumor cerebri Paranoia Pulmonary edema Psychosis Esophageal ulcers Seizures Tendon rupture

Table 23.2 Commonly used topical corticosteroids [52–59]

Generic name	Dose (ug/ inhalation)	Active metabolite	Systemic absorption%	Serum half-life (h)	Common dosage
Nasal sprays					
Beclomethasone dipropionate	80/actuation	Beclomethasone-17-monopropionate	44	2.8	1-2 sprays/ nostril daily
Ciclesonide (aqueous)	50	Des-ciclesonide	<1	6–7	2 sprays/ nostril daily
Budesonide	32	None	34	2–3	
Flunisolide	25-29	6-beta-hydroxylated metabolite	<7	1–2	2 sprays/ nostril twice daily
Fluticasone furoate	27.5	None	1.2 6(oral)	15.1[a]	2 sprays/ nostril daily
Fluticasone propionate	50	None	2	7.8[a]	2 sprays/ nostril daily
Mometasone	50	None	<1	5.8	2 sprays/ nostril daily
Triamcinolone	55	None	Minimal	18–36	
Off-label drops					
Ciprofloxacin/ dexamethasone	0.1–0.3 % otic drops				
Dexamethasone	0.1 % ophthalmic drops				
Prednisolone	1 % ophthalmic drops				
Other off-label drops					
Budesonide saline irrigation					

[a]After intravenous administration

In chronic rhinosinusitis with nasal polyposis, topical corticosteroids have been shown in multiple studies to be beneficial in improving patient symptoms, reducing polyp size, and preventing polyp recurrence after surgery. Results are more pronounced in patients with previous ESS [60, 61]. Although there are few studies regarding the use of topical corticosteroids in patients with CRSsNP, there is ample information showing symptomatic improvement in this population as well [62, 63]. The response may be greater with direct application of the corticosteroid via cannulation of the sinuses or nasal irrigation compared to drops or sprays. Off-label drops (prednisolone, dexamethasone, ciprofloxacin/dexamethasone) may be useful in limiting the need for postoperative oral steroids and reducing risk of ostial stenosis in patients undergoing revision endoscopic sinus surgery at high risk for ostial obstruction [64]. Challenging patients with eosinophilic chronic rhinosinusitis (tissue eosinophil >10 eosinophils/HPF) may specifically benefit from budesonide and betamethasone irrigations postoperatively [65].

The timing of postoperative topical steroids depends on multiple factors such as endoscopic appearance of the dissected sinuses, debridement status, and patient compliance. Ideally, topical steroids may be more effective when initiated after the first debridement 1–2 weeks postoperatively when there is more mucosal surface area for distribution. Common local adverse effects such as ulceration and epistaxis can be prevented by teaching patients proper technique of spraying and irrigating away from the nasal septum.

Perioperative Management of Allergy/Immunology Comorbidities

A detailed discussion of the management of allergic disease in the CRS patient is outlined in Chap. 10. Nonetheless, treatment of allergic and immunologic aspects of CRS is key in overall management preoperatively and postoperatively. Dedicated treatment of chronic allergic rhinitis should include accurate diagnosis with skin or in vitro testing, address environmental contributors, and trial of appropriate pharmacotherapy. There are multiple options for pharmacotherapy regardless of the surgical phase of the patient. Topical options include nasal corticosteroids, antihistamines, and anticholinergics. Decongestants can serve as temporary adjuncts especially during acute exacerbations. Oral antihistamines and leukotriene receptor antagonist also provide benefit in select patients. Intranasal corticosteroids may be more effective than topical antihistamines, but combination therapy of both produces significantly greater benefit than monotherapy with either class or oral antihistamines [66–68]. Patients with a history of positive response to topical and oral treatment of their allergic disease should continue their treatment in the context of planned ESS continuing in the postoperative period. If a patient has aspirin-exacerbated airway disease (AERD), postoperative aspirin desensitization should be considered as this is associated with improved symptoms, better olfaction, and lower recurrence rates relative to AERD patients that do not undergo aspirin desensitization [69, 70]. Postoperative immunotherapy in patients with allergic rhinitis has also been associated with decreased need for revision surgery and reduced usage of intranasal and oral steroids [71].

Patients with nasal polyposis and asthma tend to exhibit marked local production of immunoglobulin E (IgE). Human monoclonal anti-IgE antibody, omalizumab, utilizes this feature as a novel target. This antibody binds circulating IgE and prevents binding of available IgE to the IgE receptor. Omalizumab is approved for moderate-to-severe asthma in the United States; further, results in clinical study of patients with CRSwNP and comorbid asthma are encouraging. Gevaert et al. reported a decrease in total nasal endoscopic scores and radiologic improvement in disease load in subjects who received 4–8 subcutaneous injections of omalizumab [72]. Though this study was not conducted in the perioperative phase, given the challenging sinonasal disease exhibited by this phenotype, omalizumab may be a promising adjunct for future perioperative medical care in this cohort of CRSwNP with comorbid asthma.

Nasal Saline Irrigation

The use of nasal saline irrigation alone or as an adjunct to other medical therapies is an important postoperative practice. Nasal saline irrigation can be instrumental in mobilizing crusts and blood clots, moisturizing biodegradable dressing, and removing antigens which may contribute to postoperative edema. The body of literature regarding postoperative nasal irrigation consists of heterogenous studies but favors an overall benefit. A Cochrane review by Harvey et al. reported eight randomized trials with different experimental regimens which compared isotonic nasal saline to placebo, no treatment, and hypertonic saline [73]. Large volume saline irrigation (>240 ml daily) is recommended over saline mist alone or low volume irrigation [74]. Lactated Ringer's may play a role in postoperative sinonasal toilet, and it has been shown to result to better symptom improvement relative to normal or hypertonic saline [75]. Patients are typically instructed to start irrigation 24–48 h after surgery.

Postoperative Debridement

Unlike skin wounds that are immediately accessible for necessary dressing changes and suture removal, the paranasal sinuses require endoscopic-guided care to promote postoperative healing and limit complications. Clinical experience and available evidence suggest that debridement in 1 week is useful in removing crusts and clot and any residual biomaterials and nasal dressing that may promote synechiae and ostial stenosis [33]. Additional debridements are performed dependent on patient outcome and surgeon preference.

Conclusion

Perioperative care in CRS patient can be a complex undertaking due to the different subtypes and plurality of contributing etiologies. Preoperative antibiotics are an option but not a universal practice given the lack of clear benefit. Available evidence favors nasal saline irrigation commencing within 1–2 days postoperatively, use of perioperative intranasal corticosteroids, and debridement within a week of surgery. A short postoperative course of macrolide or penicillin antibiotic may alleviate patient symptoms and improve objective outcomes as well. Potent corticosteroid irrigation such as budesonide suspension in saline is an off-label option in patients with moderate to severe CRS, especially in the setting of polyposis. Aspirin desensitization should be considered in postoperative AERD patients. Patients with comorbid asthma and refractory CRSwNP should be considered for omalizumab treatment. Ongoing investigations are underway to identify novel therapeutic approaches, including other monoclonal antibodies and immune modulators that may modify various components of both innate and adaptive immunity in the CRS patient.

References

1. Smith TL, Kern R, Palmer JN, Schlosser R, Chandra RK, Chiu AG, Conley D, Mace JC, Fu RF, Stankiewicz J. Medical therapy vs surgery for chronic rhinosinusitis: a prospective, multi-institutional study. Int Forum Allergy Rhinol. 2011;1:235–41.
2. Smith TL, Kern R, Palmer JN, Schlosser R, Chandra RK, Chiu AG, Conley D, Mace JC, Fu RF, Stankiewicz J. Medical therapy vs surgery for chronic rhinosinusitis: a prospective, multi institutional study with 1-year follow-up. Int Forum Allergy Rhinol. 2013;3(1):4–9.
3. Soler ZM, Over SL, Kern SC, Senior BA, Kountakis SE, Marple BF, Smith TL. Antimicrobials and chronic rhinosinusitis with or without polyposis in adults: an evidence-based review with recommendations. Int Forum Allergy Rhinol. 2013;3(1):31–4.
4. Gluck U, Gebbers JO. The nose as bacterial reservoir: important differences between the vestibule and cavity. Laryngoscope. 2000;110(3 Pt 1):426–8.
5. Bhattacharyya N. Antimicrobial therapy in chronic rhinosinusitis. Curr Allergy Asthma Rep. 2009;9(3):221–6.
6. Bhattacharyya N. Bacterial infection in chronic rhinosinusitis: a controlled paired analysis. Am J Rhinol. 2005;19(6):544–8.
7. Araujo E, Palombini BC, Cantarelli V, Pereira A, Mariante A. Microbiology of middle meatus in chronic rhinosinusitis. Am J Rhinol. 2003;17(1):9–15.
8. Saleh AM, Torres KM, Murad MH, Erwin PJ, Driscoll CL. Prophylactic perioperative antibiotic use in endoscopic sinus surgery: a systematic review and meta-analysis. Otolaryngol Head Neck Surg. 2012;146(4):533–8.
9. Portela RA, Hootnick J, McGinn J. Perioperative care in functional endoscopic sinus surgery: a survey study. Int Forum Allergy Rhinol. 2012;2(1):27–33.
10. Brook I, Yocum P, Frazier EH. Bacteriology and beta-lactamase activity in acute and chronic maxillary sinusitis. Arch Otolaryngol Head Neck Surg. 1996;122:418–23.
11. Brook I. Treatment modalities for bacterial rhinosinusitis. Expert Opin Pharmacother. 2010;11(5):55–69.
12. Rosenfeld RM, Singer M, Jones S. Systematic review of antimicrobial therapy in patients with acute rhinosinusitis. Otolaryngol Head Neck Surg. 2007;137(3 Suppl):S32–45.
13. Wallwork B, Coman W, Feron F, Mackay-Sim A, Cervin A. Clarithromycin and prednisolone inhibit cytokine production in chronic rhinosinusitis. Laryngoscope. 2002;112(10):1827–30.
14. Wallwork B, Coman W, Mackay-Sim A, Cervin A. Effect of clarithromycin on nuclear factor-kappa B and transforming growth factor-beta in chronic rhinosinusitis. Laryngoscope. 2004;114(2):286–90.
15. Wallwork B, Coman W, Mackay-Sim A, Greiff L, Cervin A. A double-blind, randomized, placebo-controlled trial of macrolide in the treatment of chronic rhinosinusitis. Laryngoscope. 2006;116(2):189–93.
16. Cervin A, Wallwork B. Efficacy and safety of long-term antibiotics (macrolides) for the treatment of chronic rhinosinusitis. Curr Allergy Asthma Rep. 2014;14(3):416.

17. Van Zele T, Gevaert P, Holtappels G, Beule A, Wormald PJ, Mayr S, Hens G, Hellings P, Ebbens FA, Fokkens W, Van Cauwenberge P, Bachert C. Oral steroids and doxycycline: two different approach to treat nasal polyps. J Allergy Clin Immunol. 2010;125:1069–76.
18. Dubin MG, Kuhn FA, Melroy CT. Radiographic resolution of chronic rhinosinusitis without polyposis after 6 weeks vs 3 weeks of oral antibiotics. Ann Allergy Asthma Immunol. 2007;98:32–5.
19. Berard F, Gandon J. Postoperative wound infections: the influence of ultraviolet irradiation of the operating room and of various other factors. Ann Surg. 1964;160(Suppl 2):1–192.
20. Mangram AJ, Horan TC, Pearson ML, Silver LC, Jarvis WR. The Hospital Infection Control Practices Advisory Committee: guideline for prevention of surgical site infection, 1999. Infect Control Hosp Epidemiol. 1999;20:247.
21. Culver DH, Horan TC, Gaynes RP, Martone WJ, Jarvis WR, Emori TG, Banerjee SN, Edwards JR, Tolson JS, Henderson TS, et al. Surgical wound infection rates by wound class, operative procedure and patient risk index. Am J Med. 1991;91(Suppl 3B):153S.
22. Cruse PJ, Foord R. The epidemiology of wound infection. A 10-year prospective study of 62,939 wounds. Surg Clin North Am. 1980;60:27–40.
23. Russell MD, Goldberg AN. What is the evidence for use of antibiotic prophylaxis in clean-contaminated head and neck surgery? Laryngoscope. 2012;122(5):945–6.
24. Bratzler DW, Dellinger EP, Olsen KM, et al. Clinical practice guidelines for antimicrobial prophylaxis in surgery. Am J Health Syst Pharm. 2013;70:195–283.
25. Chandra RK, Conley DB, Kern RC. Prophylactic i.v. antibiotics in functional endoscopic sinus surgery: trends and attitudes of the American Rhinologic Society membership. Am J Rhinol Allergy. 2009;23(4):448–50.
26. Rontal M, Bernstein JM, Rontal E, Anon J. Bacteriologic findings from the nose, ethmoid, and bloodstream during endoscopic surgery for chronic rhinosinusitis: implications for antibiotic therapy. Am J Rhinol. 1999;13(2):91–6.
27. American Heart Association. Prevention of infective (bacterial) endocarditis. http://www.heart.org/idc/groups/heart-public/@wcm/@hcm/documents/downloadable/ucm_307684.pdf. Accesed 11 May 2014.
28. Caniello M, Passerotti GH, Goto EY, Voegels RL, Butugan O. Antibiotics in septoplasty: is it necessary? Rev Bras Otorrinolaringol. 2005;71(6):734–8.
29. Karaman E, Alimoglu Y, Aygun G, Kilic E, Yagiz C. Effect of septoplasty and per-operative antibiotic prophylaxis on nasal flora. B-ENT. 2012;8(1):13–9.
30. Albu S, Lucaciu R. Prophylactic antibiotics in endoscopic sinus surgery: a short follow-up study. Am J Rhinol Allergy. 2010;24(4):306–9.
31. Jiang RS, Liang KL, Yang KY, Shiao JY, Su MC, Hsin CH, Lin JF. Postoperative antibiotic care after functional endoscopic sinus surgery. Am J Rhinol. 2008;22(6):608–12.
32. Liang KL, Su YC, Tsai CC, Lin JS, Jiang RS, Su MC. Postoperative care with Chinese herbal medicine or amoxicillin after functional endoscopic sinus surgery: a randomized, double-blind, placebo-controlled study. Am J Rhinol Allergy. 2011;25(3):170–5.
33. Rudmik L, Smith TL. Evidence-based practice: postoperative care in endoscopic sinus surgery. Otolaryngol Clin North Am. 2012;45(5):1019–32.
34. Zhang Z, Palmer JN, Morales KH, Howland TJ, Doghramji LJ, Adappa ND, Chiu AG, Cohen NA, Lautenbach E. Culture-inappropriate antibiotic therapy decreases quality of life improvement after sinus surgery. Int Forum Allergy Rhinol. 2014;4(5):403–10.
35. Wei CC, Adappa ND, Cohen NA. Use of topical nasal therapies in the management of chronic rhinosinusitis. Laryngoscope. 2013;123(10):234–59.
36. Lim M, Citardi MJ, Leong JL. Topical antimicrobials in the management of chronic rhinosinusitis: a systematic review. Am J Rhinol. 2008;22(4):381–9.
37. Moss RB, King VV. Management of sinusitis in cystic fibrosis by endoscopic surgery and serial antimicrobial lavage. Reduction in recurrence requiring surgery. Arch Otolaryngol Head Neck Surg. 1995;121(5):566–72.
38. Ponikau JU, Sherris DA, Kern EB, Homburger HA, Frigas E, Gaffey TA, Roberts GD. The diagnosis and incidence of allergic fungal sinusitis. Mayo Clin Proc. 1999;74(9):877–84.

39. Kennedy DW, Kuhn FA, Hamilos DL, Zinreich SJ, Butler D, Warsi G, Pfister PJ, Tavakkol A. Treatment of chronic rhinosinusitis with high-dose oral terbinafine: a double blind, placebo-controlled study. Laryngoscope. 2005;115:1793–9.
40. Sacks PL, Harvey RJ, Rimmer J, Gallagher RM, Sacks R. Topical and systemic antifungal therapy for the symptomatic treatment of chronic rhinosinusitis. Cochrane Database Syst Rev. 2011;(8):CD008263.
41. Sacks 4th PL, Harvey RJ, Rimmer J, Gallagher RM, Sacks R. Antifungal therapy in the treatment of chronic rhinosinusitis: a meta-analysis. Am J Rhinol Allergy. 2012;26(2):141–7.
42. Thanasumpun T, Batra PS. Oral antifungal therapy for chronic rhinosinusitis and its subtypes: a systematic review. Int Forum Allergy Rhinol. 2011;1(5):382–9.
43. Poetker DM, Jakubowski LA, Lal D, Hwang PH, Wright ED, Smith TL. Oral corticosteroids in the management of adult chronic rhinosinusitis with and without nasal polyps: an evidence-based review with recommendations. Int Forum Allergy Rhinol. 2013;3:104–20.
44. Wright ED, Agrawal S. Impact of perioperative systemic steroids on surgical outcomes in patients with chronic rhinosinusitis with polyposis: evaluation with the novel perioperative sinus endoscopy (POSE) scoring system. Laryngoscope. 2007;117(11 Pt 2 Suppl 115):1–28.
45. Giordano J, Darras J, Chevalier D, Mortuaire G. Preoperative corticosteroid treatment and nasal polyposis. Ann Otolaryngol Chir Cervicofac. 2009;126:120–4.
46. Sieskiewicz A, Olszewska E, Rogowski M, Grycz E. Preoperative corticosteroid oral therapy and intraoperative bleeding during functional endoscopic sinus surgery in patients with severe nasal polyposis: a preliminary investigation. Ann Otol Rhinol Laryngol. 2006;115:490–4.
47. Ikram M, Abbas A, Suhail A, Onali MA, Akhtar S, Iqbal M. Management of allergic fungal sinusitis with postoperative oral and nasal steroids: a controlled study. Ear Nose Throat J. 2009;88:E8–11.
48. Rupa V, Jacob M, Mathews MS, Seshadri MS. A prospective, randomised, placebo-controlled trial of postoperative oral steroid in allergic fungal sinusitis. Eur Arch Otorhinolaryngol. 2010;267:233–8.
49. Poetker DM, Smith TL. What rhinologists and allergists should know about the medico-legal implications of corticosteroid use: a review of the literature. Int Forum Allergy Rhinol. 2012;2(2):95–103.
50. Poetker DM, Reh DD. A comprehensive review of the adverse effects of systemic corticosteroids. Otolaryngol Clin North Am. 2010;43(4):753–68.
51. Zalmanovici A, Yaphe J. Intranasal steroids for acute sinusitis. Cochrane Database Syst Rev. 2009;(7):CD005149.
52. QNASL® [package insert]. Horsham: Teva Respiratory, LLC. Prescribing information. http://qnasl.com/Content/pdf/pi.pdf. Accessed 11 May 2014.
53. Rhinocort AQ® AstraZeneca LP Wilmington (DE). Product information. http://www1.astrazeneca-us.com/pi/Rhinocort_Aqua.pdf Accessed 11 May 2014.
54. Omnaris® Sunovion Pharmaceuticals. Marlborough: Prescribing information. http://www.omnaris.com/OMNARIS-Prescribing-Information.pdf. Accessed 11 May 2014.
55. Flunisolide [package insert]. Tampa: Bausch & Lomb Inc.; 2008.
56. Fluticasone propionate. GlaxoSmithKline. Research Triangle Park (NC). https://www.gsksource.com/gskprm/htdocs/documents/FLONASE-PI-PIL-COMBINED.PDF. Accessed 11 May 2014.
57. Fluticasone furoate. GlaxoSmithKline. Research Triangle Park (NC). https://www.gsksource.com/gskprm/htdocs/documents/VERAMYST-PI-PIL-COMBINED.PDF. Accessed 11 May 2014.
58. Nasonex ®Product information. Whitehouse Station: Merch & CO.,INC. http://www.merck.com/product/usa/pi_circulars/n/nasonex/nasonex_pi.pdf.
59. Nasacort AQ® [package insert]. Bridgewater: Sanofi-Aventis U.S. LLC; 2010.
60. Kalish L, Snidvongs K, Sivasubramaniam R, Cope D, Harvey RJ. Topical steroids for nasal polyps. Cochrane Database Syst Rev. 2012;(12):CD006549.
61. Joe SA, Thambi R, Huang J. A systematic review of the use of intranasal steroids in the treatment of chronic rhinosinusitis. Otolaryngol Head Neck Surg. 2008;139:340–7.

62. Kalish LH, Arendts G, Sacks R, et al. Topical steroids in chronic rhinosinusitis without polyps: a systematic review and meta-analysis. Otolaryngol Head Neck Surg. 2009;141:674–83.
63. Snidvongs K, Kalish L, Sacks R, Craig JC, Harvey RJ. Topical steroid for chronic rhinosinusitis without polyps. Cochrane Database Syst Rev. 2011;(8):CD009274.
64. DelGaudio JM, Wise SK. Topical steroid drops for treatment of sinus ostia stenosis in the postoperative period. Am J Rhinol. 2006;20(6):565–7.
65. Snidvongs K, Pratt E, Chin D, Sacks R, Earls P, Harvey RJ. Corticosteroid nasal irrigations after endoscopic sinus surgery in the management of chronic rhinosinusitis. Int Forum Allergy Rhinol. 2012;2(5):415–21.
66. Corren J, Storms W, Bernstein J, Berger W, Nayak A, Sacks H. Effectiveness of azelastine nasal spray compared with oral cetirizine in patients with seasonal allergic rhinitis. Azelastine Cetirizine Trial No. 1 (ACT 1) Study Group. Clin Ther. 2005;27(5):543–53.
67. Ratner PH, Hampel F, Van Bavel J, Amar NJ, Daftary P, Wheeler W, Sacks H. Combination therapy with azelastine hydrochloride nasal spray and fluticasone propionate nasal spray in the treatment of patients with seasonal allergic rhinitis. Ann Allergy Asthma Immunol. 2008;100(1):74–81.
68. Hampel FC, Ratner PH, Van Bavel J, Amar NJ, Daftary P, Wheeler W, Sacks H. Double-blind, placebo-controlled study of azelastine and fluticasone in a single nasal spray delivery device. Ann Allergy Asthma Immunol. 2010;105(2):168–73.
69. Klimek L, Dollner R, Pfaar O, Mullol J. Aspirin desensitization: useful treatment for chronic rhinosinusitis with nasal polyps (CRSwNP) in aspirin-exacerbated respiratory disease (AERD)? Curr Allergy Asthma Rep. 2014;14(6):441.
70. Havel M, Ertl L, Braunschweig F, Markmann S, Leunig A, Gamarra F, Kramer MF. Sinonasal outcome under aspirin desensitization following functional endoscopic sinus surgery in patients with aspirin triad. Eur Arch Otorhinolaryngol. 2013;270(2):571–8.
71. Deyoung K, Wentzel JL, Schlosser RJ, Nguyen SA, Soler ZM. Systematic review of immunotherapy for chronic rhinosinusitis. Am J Rhinol Allergy. 2014;28(2):145–50.
72. Gevaert P, Calus L, Van Zele T, Blomme K, De Ruyck N, Bauters W, Hellings P, Brusselle G, De Bacquer D, van Cauwenberge P, Bachert C. Omalizumab is effective in allergic and nonallergic patients with nasal polyps and asthma. J Allergy Clin Immunol. 2013;131(1):110–6.
73. Harvey R, Hannan SA, Badia L, Scadding G. Nasal saline irrigations for the symptoms of chronic rhinosinusitis. Am J Rhinol Allergy Cochrane Database Syst Rev. 2007;(3):CD006394.
74. Liang KL, Su MC, Tseng HC, et al. Impact of pulsatile nasal irrigation on the prognosis of functional endoscopic sinus surgery. J Otolaryngol Head Neck Surg. 2008;37:148–53.
75. Low TH, Woods CM, Ullah S, Carney AS. A double-blind randomized controlled trial of normal saline, lactated Ringer's, and hypertonic saline nasal irrigation solution after endoscopic sinus surgery. Am J Rhinol Allergy. 2014;28(3):225–31.

Surgery of the Maxillary Sinus

24

Jeremiah A. Alt and Richard R. Orlandi

Key Take-Home Points

- Understanding paranasal sinus development and recognizing preoperative surgical anatomy helps guide the endoscopic surgeon intraoperatively.
- When maxillary sinus surgery is indicated, performing a complete uncinectomy is critical.
- Identifying the infundibulum that leads to the natural maxillary ostium enables the surgeon to incorporate the natural ostium into the surgical antrostomy to prevent the recirculation phenomenon.

Introduction

As the understanding of the pathophysiology of maxillary sinusitis has evolved, so has the approach and treatment of the disease. Patients that fail medical management, which includes, but is not limited to, culture-directed or empiric antibiotics, saline irrigations, topical and/or oral steroids, decongestants, and, in select cases, dental consultation for suspected odontogenic source, may be candidates for surgical management. The technological advancements in rhinology have enabled us to treat maxillary disease in a minimally invasive manner.

J.A. Alt, MD, PhD (✉) • R.R. Orlandi, MD
Division of Otolaryngology – Rhinology, Sinus and Skull Base Surgery Program, Otolaryngology, University of Utah, 50 N. Medical Drive, SOM 3C120, Salt Lake City, UT 84132, USA
e-mail: jeremiah.alt@hsc.utah.edu; richard.orlandi@hsc.utah.edu

P.S. Batra, J.K. Han (eds.), *Practical Medical and Surgical Management of Chronic Rhinosinusitis*, DOI 10.1007/978-3-319-16724-4_24

Surgical Anatomy

Embryology and Postnatal Development

The sinonasal cavity begins to develop early in fetal life. At the 8th week of gestation, the septum and small ridges begin to appear on the lateral nasal sidewall. By the 9th week, cartilaginous tissue encapsulates the forming sinonasal cavity that provides outgrowths into these small ridges. These ridges correspond to the developing turbinates and are termed the ethmoturbinals. Between the primordial turbinates, spaces are created termed primary furrows that serve as the precursors to meatus that separate the turbinates. The first primary furrow that separates the inferior and middle turbinate becomes the middle meatus, maxillary infundibulum, and the hiatus semilunaris. Shortly after the 9th week and extending into the 10th week, the primordial uncinate can be seen extending upward into the first primary furrow. This early bud of cartilaginous tissue further divides the first primary furrow into forming the primordial ethmoid infundibulum.

Maxillary Sinus

The maxilla begins ossification at 11–12 weeks of gestation [1]. This is in conjunction with the formation of the ethmoid air cells, which are the first air cells to develop. The ethmoid air cells can expand beyond the limits of the ethmoid bone and extend into the maxillary bone resulting in infraorbital ethmoid (Haller) cells. The primordial ethmoid infundibulum develops around the 14–16th weeks as an invagination just lateral to the uncinate process. By the 15–16th weeks of gestation, the inferior, middle, and superior turbinates are fully formed, and there are hints of a forming maxillary sinus. By 17–18 weeks gestation, there is an air space within the maxillary bone that continues to expand into the maxilla through the second and third trimester. When the fetus is greater than 30 weeks to birth, the maxillary sinus is approximately 7 mm anteroposterior and 3 mm in vertical height [2]. By 4 years of age, the maxillary sinus has expanded laterally to the infraorbital nerve and inferior to the level of the inferior turbinate. The maxillary sinus continues to expand and reaches the zygomatic recess laterally, the floor of the nose inferiorly, and the nasolacrimal duct medially by age 12. The adult maxillary sinus continues to expand toward the maxillary alveolar ridge and further into the zygomatic recess [3]. The maxillary tooth roots commonly reach to the floor of the maxillary sinus (Fig. 24.1).

The maxillary sinus communicates with the nasal cavity through its ostium. The size of the ostium varies but is generally 1–3 mm in size [4]. The maxillary sinuses have a reliably defined drainage pattern that is based on mucociliary clearance. The maxillary sinus is lined by pseudostratified ciliated columnar epithelium (Fig. 24.2). The cilia beat in a coordinated fashion to transport mucus from the point of its secretion in the sinus toward its natural ostium. The maxillary sinus ostium drains into

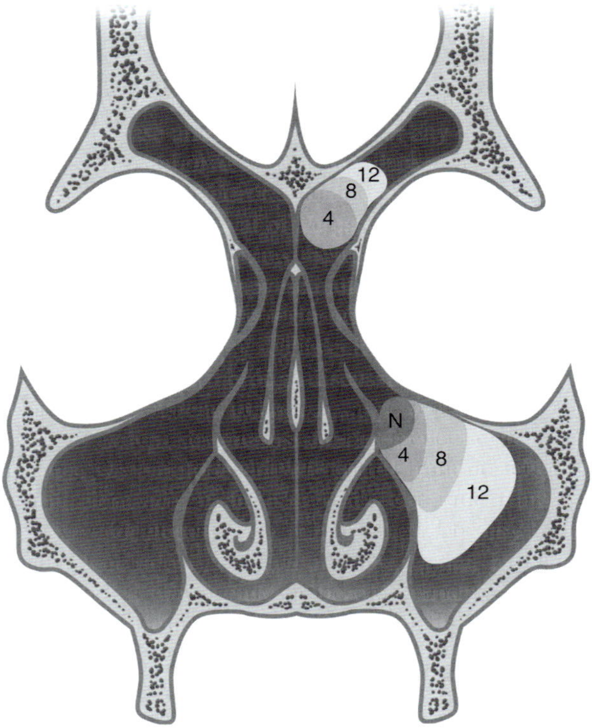

Fig. 24.1 Coronal representation of the development of the frontal and maxillary sinus. The frontal sinus begins to develop at age of 4 and does not reach adulthood until after 12 years old. The newborn (*N*) has a small maxillary sinus that continues to expand in a lateral inferior direction reaching adult pneumatization after 12 years of age. Note the potential association of the maxillary tooth roots as the maxillary sinus pneumatizes completely. *4, 8 and 12* are represent years of age

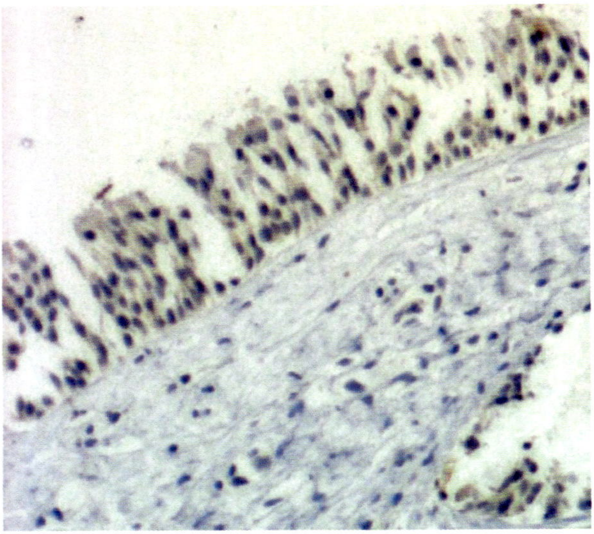

Fig. 24.2 Immunohistochemistry slide demonstrating pseudostratified epithelium from the anterior ethmoid tissue (40× magnification) with human calgranulin (S100A12) staining (innate bacterial peptide)

the ethmoid infundibulum, eventually draining into the middle meatus. Once the secretions have reached the nasal cavity, they are carried into the nasopharynx and then pass into the digestive tract, where the secretions and whatever debris they carry are destroyed.

Lateral Nasal Wall

Understanding the anatomy of the lateral nasal sidewall with its associated anatomical structures, spaces, and sinus ostia is critical for the endoscopic surgeon before surgically approaching the maxillary sinus. Projecting from the lateral nasal sidewall are three conchae or turbinate bones. They are named in ascending sequential order according to their position on the lateral nasal wall. The turbinates in ascending order from inferior to superior are as follows: the inferior turbinate, middle turbinate, superior turbinate, and, if present, there is a fourth turbinate termed the supreme turbinate. Below each turbinate is a meatus or space, whereby its name is derived from the turbinate above. Each meatus receives unique drainage from corresponding paranasal sinuses.

The nasolacrimal duct empties into the inferior meatus, which sits below the inferior turbinate. A small mucosal flap called Hasner's valve covers the distal opening of the nasolacrimal duct. The nasolacrimal duct is best identified on axial CT cuts and becomes the most anterior limit of dissection when opening the maxillary sinus. The middle meatus is located lateral to the middle turbinate and is the most complex and utmost important to the endoscopic sinus surgeon. The middle meatus receives drainage from the frontal, maxillary, and the anterior ethmoid sinuses. Posteriorly, the superior meatus is below the superior turbinate, which collects drainage from the posterior ethmoid air cells. The drainage continues medially into the sphenoethmoidal recess, which also receives drainage from the sphenoid sinus.

Ostiomeatal Unit

The ostiomeatal unit (OMU) is a complex anatomic area within the middle meatus, which can be defined as the functional designation of the anterior ethmoid complex, thereby acting as the common drainage pathway of the frontal, anterior ethmoid, and maxillary sinuses [5]. The OMU includes the following structures:

- Anterior ethmoid cells
- Uncinate process
- Ethmoid bulla
- Ethmoid infundibulum
- Hiatus semilunaris

Obstruction of the OMU is commonly the cornerstone seen in the pathophysiology of chronic maxillary sinus disease. Obstruction may be secondary to inflammation or anatomic variations of the OMU such as a paradoxical middle turbinate, concha bullosa, Haller cell, agger nasi cell, or nasal septal deviation. Endoscopic sinus surgery (ESS) specifically addresses the OMU as a functional unit by targeting diseased cells while preserving sinonasal mucosa. This enables the return of normal mucociliary drainage within the OMU. The endoscopic surgeon should carefully evaluate the anatomic variations within the OMU on preoperative imaging to adequately address the underlying disease process. However, there is still a lack of consensus in regard to the role those anatomical variations of the OMU play in the pathogenesis of CRS.

Uncinate Process

The uncinate process is a sickle-shaped bone that appears as a fold on the lateral nasal sidewall that extends from the inferior turbinate to its anterior-superior attachments at the skull base and lamina papyracea. The inferior-posterior most portion of the uncinate has no bony attachment and inserts into the ethmoid complex of the inferior turbinate bone. The middle portion of the uncinate has a bony attachment to the maxillary and lacrimal bones as it extends superiorly. The superior attachment of the uncinate process has a tremendous amount of variation. The location of its attachments has direct consequence on drainage patterns of the frontal sinus and dictates the surgical approach. The uncinate process can also present with pneumatization occluding the infundibulum of the maxillary sinus.

Understanding the variations of the superior insertion of the uncinate process will enable the endoscopic surgeon to protect the frontal sinus drainage pathway when performing an uncinectomy in conjunction with a maxillary antrostomy. Its superior attachment is highly variable and was originally classified with three distinct attachment sites including the lamina papyracea, skull base, and middle turbinate. A more detailed classification has been described classifying the insertion into six different categories [6]. When the uncinate process inserts into the lamina papyracea, the ethmoid infundibulum ends as a blind pouch named the recess terminalis [7]. In this instance, the frontal sinus will drain medially into the middle meatus or the suprabullar recess. However, when the uncinate attaches to either the skull base or the middle turbinate, the frontal recess drains into the middle meatus through the ethmoid infundibulum.

The uncinate process can be atelectatic and intimately opposed to the lamina papyracea seen in conditions such as silent sinus syndrome or chronic maxillary atelectasis, or it can be pushed medially as a result of nasal polyposis (Fig. 24.3). If the laterally rotated uncinate is not recognized, the surgeon may inadvertently enter the orbital cavity as the distance between the uncinate process and the lamina papyracea can be as narrow as 0.1 mm [8]. Likewise, natural congenital dehiscence of the lamina is reported to be as high as 10 % and should be avoided at the time of surgery. Temporally remote trauma can also cause lamina dehiscence, which can alter lateral nasal wall anatomy, causing increased potential for intraoperative injury to orbital contents while performing the uncinectomy. Therefore, careful dissection

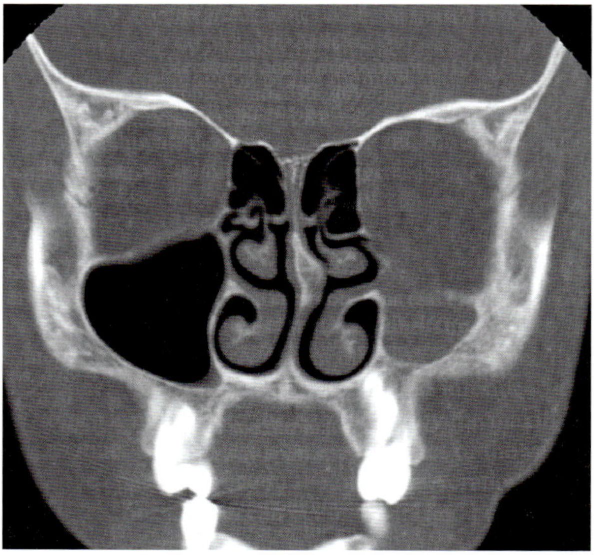

Fig. 24.3 Coronal bone window CT shows an atelectatic left uncinate process that is intimately opposed to the lamina

is required in these instances to prevent lamina penetration and can be assessed intraoperatively with gentle external orbital pressure while visualizing the lamina endoscopically.

Infundibulum and Hiatus Semilunaris

The infundibulum is a three-dimensional space that is bounded by the lamina papyracea laterally, the uncinate process medially, and the ethmoid bulla posteriorly. The infundibulum can be likened to a hallway, which collects drainage from the frontal, ethmoid, and the maxillary sinus and subsequently directs the secretions medially to the hiatus semilunaris. The hiatus semilunaris or "exit" is a two-dimensional space that is defined by the free edge of the uncinate and the anterior face of the ethmoid bulla. The hiatus semilunaris can be seen with nasal endoscopy at the most posterior-inferior portion of the uncinate, is difficult to identify on coronal images, and is best seen on sagittal cuts. In contrast, the infundibular space cannot be visualized endoscopically unless the uncinate is removed, which is the first step to surgically access the natural maxillary ostium.

Anatomic Variations

Anatomic variations of sinus anatomy may predispose patients to developing sinus infections. Although the cumulative evidence is unclear in regard to the extent structural changes play in sinonasal pathophysiology, it is apparent that understanding

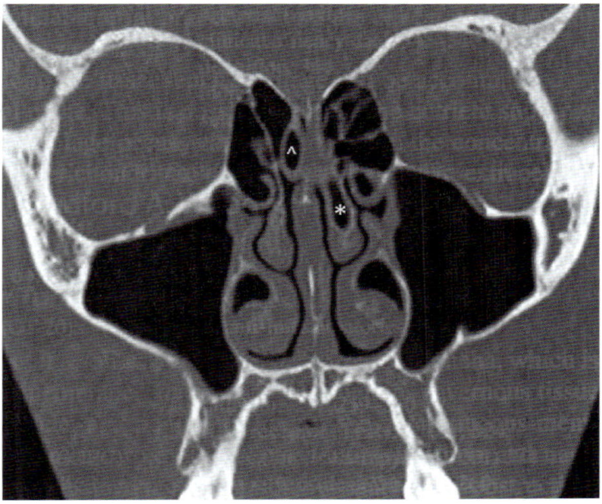

Fig. 24.4 Coronal bone window CT demonstrates pneumatization into the head of the left middle turbinate (*) also called a concha bullosa. There is also a right-sided superior turbinate concha (^)

the anatomy and its variations is critical to performing safe endoscopic surgery and improving surgical outcomes. Several key anatomical variations that should be assessed prior to surgery are discussed.

- Concha bullosa
- Infraorbital recess cells (Haller Cells)
- Septal deviation

Concha Bullosa

Zuckerkandl coined the term concha bullosa when pneumatization of the middle turbinate was present. Pneumatization of the middle turbinate can narrow the OMC and can be involved in the pathophysiology of maxillary sinus disease. Large concha bullosa function as large "balloons" in the middle meatus obstructing normal mucociliary drainage. The amount and location of the pneumatization vary, with the most common location being the head of the middle turbinate (Fig. 24.4). This anatomic variation can easily be seen on CT in both coronal and axial views.

Infraorbital Ethmoid Cells (Haller Cells)

Infraorbital ethmoid air cells (Haller cells) are seen as pneumatized air cells that grow out of the inferior orbital floor at the roof of the maxillary sinus (Fig. 24.5). Infraorbital ethmoid cells are seen as distinctive air cells separate from the anterior ethmoid bulla. These cells are important to identify as they have the potential to narrow the maxillary sinus drainage, which may predispose the patient to sinusitis [9]. The coronal CT is the best view for identifying these air cells.

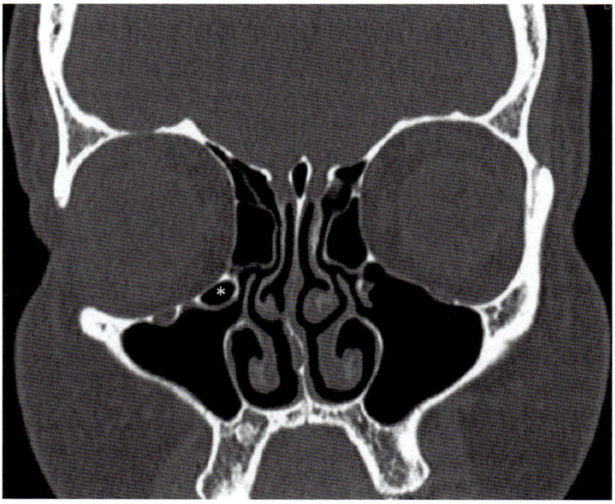

Fig. 24.5 Coronal bone window CT illustrates a right infraorbital ethmoid air cell (Haller cell). Can be visualized as pneumatized air cells of the inferior orbital floor (*)

Nasal Septal Deviation

Significant nasal septal deviation and septal spurs can prevent access to the sinuses during ESS. Surgical planning can be improved by using CT coronal and axial views of the nasal septum in conjunction with nasal endoscopy. In certain circumstances, the septum may need to be addressed with functional rhinoplasty due to severe septal deviation, very anterior caudal deflection, or dynamic valve collapse that can be addressed with concurrent ESS.

Indications

Prior to discussion about surgery, an appropriate workup is required to diagnose sinusitis of the maxillary sinus. This workup is based upon findings in the patient's medical history, physical examination, nasal endoscopy, and CT imaging.

Clinicians should distinguish between the different subclassifications of rhinosinusitis including (1) acute bacterial rhinosinusitis (ABRS), (2) acute viral rhinosinusitis, (3) chronic rhinosinusitis, and (4) recurrent acute rhinosinusitis.

Acute Rhinosinusitis

It is important to delineate presumed acute bacterial rhinosinusitis (ABRS) from acute rhinosinusitis caused by viral upper respiratory infections and noninfectious conditions. ABRS is more likely the diagnosis when (a) symptoms or signs of acute rhinosinusitis are present 10 days or more beyond the onset of upper respiratory symptoms, or (b) symptoms or signs of acute rhinosinusitis worsen within 10 days after an initial improvement (double worsening). *Acute rhinosinusitis* is diagnosed as up to 4 weeks of purulent (not clear) nasal drainage accompanied by nasal obstruction, facial pain/pressure/fullness, or both. Surgery is not recommended for those patients with uncomplicated ABRS.

Chronic Rhinosinusitis

Patients commonly present with nasal obstruction, facial congestion, facial pressure or fullness, discolored nasal drainage, and hyposomia. The American Academy of Otolaryngology-Head and Neck Surgery has utilized these cardinal symptoms as a part of diagnostic criteria for CRS. The presence of two or more of these symptoms beyond 12 weeks is needed to diagnose CRS. In addition, the diagnosis of CRS requires that inflammation is present and documented with either nasal endoscopy or imaging. Surgery for chronic maxillary sinusitis is indicated for those patients who meet diagnostic criteria and have failed medical treatment, typically consisting of oral, broad spectrum, or culture-directed antibiotics ($\geq$2 weeks duration) and either topical nasal corticosteroid sprays ($\geq$3 week duration) or a trial of systemic steroid therapy [10].

Recurrent Acute Rhinosinusitis

Recurrent acute rhinosinusitis (RARS) is diagnosed when the patient develops four or more episodes of ABRS per year, with complete resolution between episodes [10, 11]. Each episode of ABRS should meet the criteria as stated above. Although surgery does not have a role in uncomplicated ABRS, limited ESS may play a role in RARS [12].

Possible Causes of Maxillary Sinusitis

There are many possible etiologies that can potentially contribute to maxillary sinus disease including allergies, structural abnormalities (septal deviation, concha bullosa, Haller cells), nasal polyps, cystic fibrosis, immune deficiency, ciliary dysmotility, smoking and second-hand smoke, silent sinus syndrome caused by chronic maxillary atelectasis [13], maxillofacial trauma that narrows or obstructs the drainage of the maxillary sinus, and dental origin (odontogenic sinusitis).

Surgical Technique

History

Drs. George Walter Caldwell and Henri Luc first described the open surgical approach to the maxillary sinus, termed the Caldwell-Luc, in 1893 and 1895, respectively. This surgery involved an incision in the upper gum, creating an opening in the anterior wall of the maxillary sinus, followed by the removal of the entire diseased maxillary sinus mucosa. Drainage was directed toward the inferior meatus by creating a large window in the lateral nasal wall. This approach persisted for nearly 70 years until advances in the physiologic drainage of the sinuses were appreciated in the late 1960s. This knowledge led to newer intranasal endoscopic techniques that preserved sinonasal mucosa while enlarging the maxillary ostia through the middle meatus. This technique is still useful today as an adjunct to endoscopic techniques, especially in those cases when anatomy limits complete dissection. This primarily occurs when dealing with tumors or complicated cases with inferiorly or anteriorly based disease.

Functional endoscopic sinus surgery (FESS) was first described by Walter Messerklinger via the OMC that is now the standard surgical technique for addressing maxillary sinus disease. The following points should be noted when performing an endonasal infundibulotomy and maxillary antrostomy. Although we acknowledge there are technically many different techniques, the following general take-away points should be considered.

Preoperative

- Epinephrine soaked neuropledgets 1:1,000 are placed in the middle meatus and left in place for 8–10 min. Pledgets are normally placed immediately after intubation to allow preoperative vasoconstriction to occur while patient is being prepped and draped.
- The head of the table is elevated 15–20° to reduce intraoperative bleeding while improving visualization. The table is air planed approximately 5 % to the patient's right for a right-handed surgeon. This maneuver facilitates access to the patient's right maxillary sinus. The converse is true for the left maxillary sinus for surgeons positioned at the patient's left side.
- After the patient is draped for endoscopic sinus surgery, endonasal injections are performed with 1 % lidocaine with 1:100,000 epinephrine. Injections are performed, with a 25- or 27-gauge needle, along the inferior border of the middle turbinate, the lateral nasal wall at the insertion of the uncinate near the maxillary line, and at the axilla or insertion of the middle turbinate. Sphenopalatine artery (SPA) injections are not normally performed, as the SPA vasculature does not significantly contribute to the infundibulum. These injections are reserved for cases where dissection will take place posterior to the basal lamella of the middle turbinate.

Infundibulotomy

- Care should be taken when palpating the uncinate to prevent destabilization and mucosal damage to the middle turbinate.
- We prefer a retrograde approach to the ethmoid infundibulum, where a backward biting forceps is used to transect the uncinate process. We feel this approach

reduces the risk of inadvertent injury to the lamina or orbital contents. Displacing (infracturing) the uncinate medially away from the lamina papyracea, prior to using backbiting forceps, delineates the free posterior margin and demonstrates the uncinate process attachment to the lateral wall. This maneuver defines the anterior limits of the uncinectomy. In cases of silent sinus syndrome, the uncinate process must be distracted medially from the lamina papyracea in order to avoid orbital injury [13]. This can be done gently with a blunt-tipped probe or sharply angled curette.

- Small pediatric backbiting forceps are used to incise the uncinate near its inferior attachment, allowing visualization of the ethmoid infundibulum that leads to the maxillary ostium. This transection of the uncinate process takes place in the same axial plane as the bottom of the ethmoid bulla. The superior and inferior portions of the uncinate process can then be removed with forceps or a microdebrider. The microdebrider can be used with the opening oriented superiorly or inferiorly but not laterally in order to avoid injury to the lamina papyracea. Care must be taken to avoid unnecessary mucosal removal anterior to the uncinate insertion on the maxillary crest.
- Caution should also be used while dissecting anteriorly to prevent damage to the nasolacrimal duct. If the duct is entered with the backbiting forceps, bone fragments should be removed. If the duct is otherwise not obstructed, no further measures are needed.
- An alternative approach to the ethmoid infundibulum is anterograde. In this approach, the surgeon incises the uncinate with a sickle knife at its insertion to the lateral nasal sidewall, usually from superior to inferior. The detached uncinate process is then removed.
- Once the majority of the uncinate process is removed, either retrograde or anterograde, remaining pieces near the lamina can be removed with 45° Blakesley forceps.
- Care should be taken to make sure the anterior dissection is complete, as this will expose the natural maxillary ostium. Failure to expose this can lead to the creation of a second ostium posterior to the natural ostium. Furthermore, an incomplete uncinectomy can lead to scarring off of the maxillary or frontal sinus.

Maxillary Antrostomy

- In more mild cases of maxillary sinusitis, opening of the ethmoid infundibulum may be enough to promote drainage and ventilation of the maxillary sinus. Relieving obstruction within the ethmoid infundibulum may relieve secondary obstruction of the maxillary ostium. In more severe cases, especially those involving polyposis, the surgeon may wish to create a larger maxillary antrostomy.
- A common error when performing a maxillary antrostomy is not identifying and incorporating the natural maxillary sinus ostium. This results in performing a separate antral opening in the posterior fontanelle. The presence of a second antral window interferes with the normal mucociliary clearance of the maxillary sinus, leading to recirculation phenomenon (Fig. 24.6). For this reason, we also

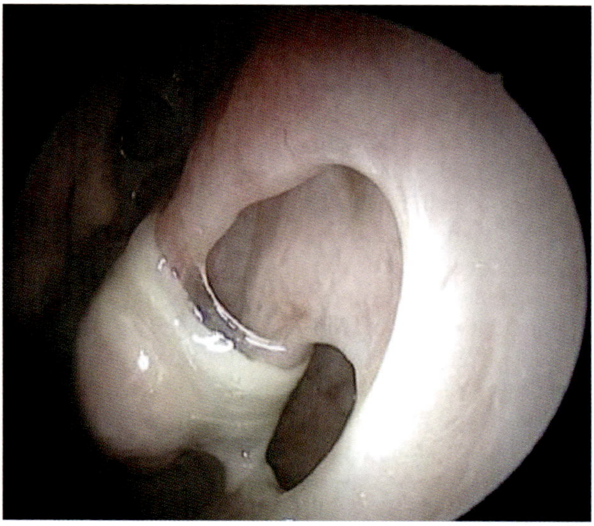

Fig. 24.6 Nasal endoscopy demonstrating recirculation seen in the left maxillary sinus that resulted in tenacious secretions and recurrent sinus infections

recommend considering incorporating a naturally occurring accessory ostium with the natural maxillary ostium.

- Using a 30–45° scope is generally recommended to make sure the natural maxillary ostium is identified after the uncinectomy.
- The natural maxillary ostium is enlarged in a posterior and inferior direction into the posterior fontanelle through cutting instruments and microdebrider.
- Dissecting anterior from the maxillary ostia should be done carefully or not at all, as the nasolacrimal duct is approximately 4 mm anterior and should not be entered inadvertently. Disrupting the natural ostial mucosal lining anteriorly as well as posteriorly and inferiorly predisposes to circumferential ostial scarring and stenosis postoperatively.

Balloon Sinus Dilation

Sinus balloon dilation is a technique that can be used in select cases of maxillary sinusitis. It is used to dilate the natural ostium of the maxillary sinus to restore normal drainage and ventilation, with less overall mucosal damage. It has been used in the operating room and in clinics under local anesthesia, alone or conjunction with traditional techniques.

- The transnasal approach is the most commonly used technique to address the maxillary sinus. Although different manufacturers have their unique systems, the basic premise is the same. Different angled introducers guide the device through the hiatus semilunaris into the natural ostium. An inflation device is attached to the balloon catheter to inflate the balloon. A manometer is used to measure the pressure applied, and a sinus lavage catheter can be used to irrigate the sinus following treatment.

- The transantral approach to the maxillary sinus involves a sublabial incision or puncture to allow placement of a trocar into the maxillary sinus. The balloon catheter can be introduced through the trocar and into the maxillary ostium under direct visualization. The balloon is then inflated to dilate the ostium. The trocar is removed, and the small sublabial incision is allowed to close on its own.

The benefits of balloon sinus dilation show promise in properly selected patients. It is particularly useful in those patients with medical comorbidities that preclude anesthesia for standard ESS and patients with limited sinus disease. Several studies have demonstrated that balloon dilation may be a safe and feasible option for select patients with chronic sinus disease. One of the drawbacks of balloon sinus dilation techniques is the inability to remove polyps or diseased bone from the sinuses. Moreover, the transnasal route does not allow for visualization of the maxillary ostium making the creation of a posterior accessory ostium a distinct risk.

Complications

Endoscopic sinus surgery is an effective treatment for maxillary sinus disease, and maxillary antrostomy is one of the most commonly performed endoscopic procedures. Failed maxillary antrostomy are not uncommon however. Causes of failure are well described (Table 24.1), and need for subsequent revision surgery can be avoided by following a stepwise surgical approach and using angled endoscopes as outlined above. For those that need revision surgery of the maxillary sinus due to chronically diseased maxillary sinuses, poor mucociliary clearance from long-standing inflammation, or scarring from previous surgery, they can be rehabilitated with an endoscopic maxillary mega-antrostomy (Fig. 24.7), a mucosal sparing technique that facilitates recovery in a dysfunctional maxillary sinuses with a 75 % success rate [14]. Furthermore, surrounding structures including the nasolacrimal duct, orbit and its contents (inferior orbital floor and lamina papyracea), the sphenopalatine artery, and structures behind the posterior maxillary wall (trigeminal nerve V2 and internal maxillary artery) can be damaged during endoscopic maxillary antrostomy. Removing polyps or other lesions from the roof of the maxillary sinus may lead to injury of the infraorbital nerve. Extensive opening of the antrostomy beyond the limits of the posterior fontanelle can lead to injury of the greater palatine nerve and the descending palatine artery.

Table 24.1 Revision surgery of the maxillary sinus

Iatrogenic causes	Local causes	Systemic causes
Retained uncinate process Retained Haller cell Recirculation Scarring Previous mucosal stripping such as in Caldwell-Luc Prior inferior meatal window	Polyp recurrence Stenosis of middle meatal antrostomy	Impaired mucociliary clearance Ciliary dysfunction (e.g., Kartagener's syndrome) Cystic fibrosis Autoimmune (e.g., granulomatosis with polyangiitis) Immunodeficiency (e.g., IgG deficiency)

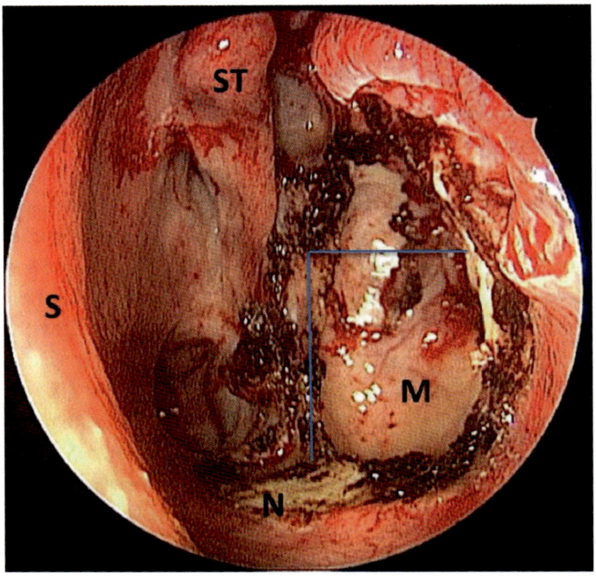

Fig. 24.7 Example of a surgical mega-antrostomy of the left maxillary sinus. The vertical line represents the posterior limit of the maxillary sinus, while the horizontal line represents the superior limit (inferior orbital floor), nasal septum (*S*), maxillary sinus (*M*), nasal floor (*N*), and superior turbinate (*ST*)

References

1. Wang RG, Jiang SC, Gu R. The cartilaginous nasal capsule and embryonic development of human paranasal sinuses. J Otolaryngol. 1994;23:239–43.
2. Farah G, Ahmad FN. Morphometric analysis of developing maxillary sinuses in human foetuses. Int J Morphol. 2006;24:303–8.
3. Lawson W, Patel ZM, Lin FY. The development and pathologic processes that influence maxillary sinus pneumatization. Anat Rec. 2008;291:1554–63.
4. Aust R, Drettner B. The functional size of the human maxillary ostium in vivo. Acta Otolaryngol. 1974;78:432–5.
5. Stammberger HR, Kennedy DW. Paranasal sinuses: anatomic terminology and nomenclature. Ann Otol Rhinol Laryngol Suppl. 1995;167:7–16.
6. Landsberg R, Friedman M. A computer-assisted anatomical study of the nasofrontal region. Laryngoscope. 2001;111:2125–30.
7. Kennedy DW, Senior BA. Endoscopic sinus surgery. A review. Otolaryngol Clin North Am. 1997;30:313–30.
8. Awad Z, Bhattacharyya M, Jayaraj SM. Anatomical margins of uncinectomy in endoscopic sinus surgery. Int J Surg. 2013;11:188–90.
9. Alkire BC, Bhattacharyya N. An assessment of sinonasal anatomic variants potentially associated with recurrent acute rhinosinusitis. Laryngoscope. 2010;120:631–4.
10. Rosenfeld RM, Andes D, Bhattacharyya N, et al. Clinical practice guideline: adult sinusitis. Otolaryngol Head Neck Surg. 2007;137:S1–31.
11. Bhattacharyya N, Lee KH. Chronic recurrent rhinosinusitis: disease severity and clinical characterization. Laryngoscope. 2005;115:306–10.
12. Bhattacharyya N. Surgical treatment of chronic recurrent rhinosinusitis: a preliminary report. Laryngoscope. 2006;116:1805–8.
13. Suh JD, Ramakrishnan V, Lee JY, Chiu AG. Bilateral silent sinus syndrome. Ear Nose Throat J. 2012;91:E19–21.
14. Cho DY, Hwang PH. Results of endoscopic maxillary mega-antrostomy in recalcitrant maxillary sinusitis. Am J Rhinol. 2008;22:658–62.

Ethmoid Sinus Surgery

25

Andrew N. Goldberg and Chase M. Heaton

Key Take-Home Points

- Preoperative nasal endoscopy for identification of bony and soft tissue landmarks
- Systematic assessment of ethmoid anatomy on CT scan with special attention to the slope of the ethmoid roof in the coronal and sagittal planes
- Preoperative control of inflammation to reduce intraoperative bleeding and maintain orientation
- Mucosal preservation whenever possible
- Complete uncinectomy
- Maxillary antrostomy sufficient to identify landmarks in the maxillary sinus
- Removal of the ethmoid bulla with identification of and cleaning of the medial orbital wall
- Preservation of a horizontal strut of the basal lamella
- Penetration of the medial and inferior basal lamella and removal of posterior ethmoid septations in the medial-lateral direction to the medial orbital wall
- Identification of the skull base in the posterior ethmoid
- Use of angled telescopes and instruments to visualize the skull base and removal of septations in a posterior to anterior direction

A.N. Goldberg, MD, MSCE, FACS (✉)
Division of Rhinology and Sinus Surgery, Department of Otolaryngology – Head and Neck Surgery and Neurological Surgery, University of California, San Francisco, 2233 Post Street, Room 309, San Francisco, CA 94115-1225, USA
e-mail: andrew.goldberg@ucsf.edu, agoldberg@ohns.ucsf.edu

C.M. Heaton, MD
Department of Otolaryngology – Head and Neck Surgery, University of California, San Francisco, 2233 Post Street, Room 323, San Francisco, CA 94115-1225, USA
e-mail: chase.heaton@ucsf.edu, cheaton@ohns.ucsf.edu

P.S. Batra, J.K. Han (eds.), *Practical Medical and Surgical Management of Chronic Rhinosinusitis*, DOI 10.1007/978-3-319-16724-4_25

> If the ethmoid labyrinth was placed in any other part of the body, it would be an insignificant and harmless collection of bony cells. Placed where nature has put it, it has a number of major relationships, so that disease and surgery of this labyrinth can often lead to tragedy. Theoretically, an ethmoidal operation is easy; in practice, however, it has proved to be one of the easiest operations with which to kill a patient. [1]
>
> Mosher, 1929

Introduction

Surgery can be defined as the systematic movement from landmark to landmark, whether in soft tissue or bony anatomy. Critical to the ethmoidectomy is the proper identification of each landmark and execution of a systematic surgical plan. The complex, unique, and variable anatomy of the ethmoid sinuses makes ethmoidectomy a challenging surgery even for the well-experienced sinus surgeon. For this reason, developing a systematic approach to management of patients with ethmoid sinus disease is paramount. This chapter will review the complex anatomy of the ethmoid sinuses, discuss clinical indications for ethmoid surgery, and describe how to perform a safe and successful surgical ethmoidectomy.

Surgical Anatomy

The ethmoid sinus is a three-dimensional, air-filled bony labyrinth situated in the superior nasal cavity. With one ethmoid on each side of the nasal cavity, they compromise one pair of the commonly described four pairs of paranasal sinuses. Along with the maxillary sinuses, they are normally present at birth and continue to grow and pneumatize to adult size during puberty. The frontal, palatine, lacrimal, maxillary, and sphenoid bones all contribute to the ethmoid sinus walls. Bony septations create multiple air-filled, mucosal-lined cells. The orientation, number, and size of these cells vary not only from person to person but may also be markedly different in opposing sides of the same patient.

The anatomic boundaries of the ethmoid sinus and the relationship to vital surrounding structures make the understanding of ethmoid anatomy very important for the surgeon. On endoscopic visualization, the first ethmoid air cell generally encountered is the ethmoid bulla within the middle meatus (Fig. 25.1). However, anterior and superior to this is the most anterior of the ethmoid air cells, commonly referred to as an agger nasi cell. Laterally, the medial orbital wall, and aptly named paper-thin lamina papyracea, separates the ethmoid air cells from the orbital contents. The floor of the ethmoid air cells makes up the roof of the nasal cavity. Medially, the complex anatomy of the skull base and fovea ethmoidalis contributes

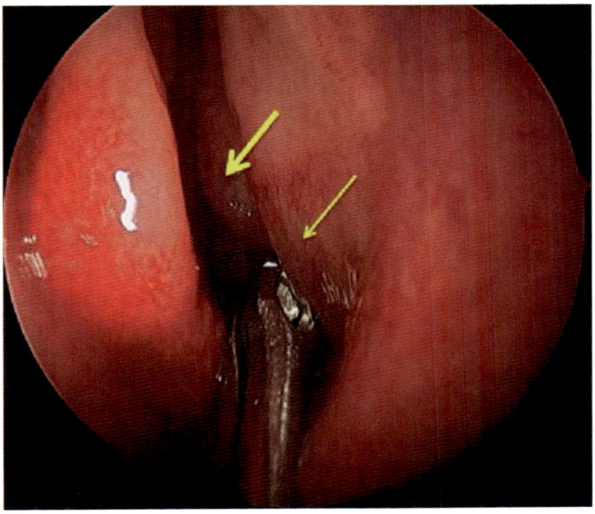

Fig. 25.1 Endoscopic view of left middle meatus. *Thin arrow* pointing to the uncinate process; *thick arrow* pointing to the bulla ethmoidalis (With permission Andrew N. Goldberg, MD, MSCE, FACS)

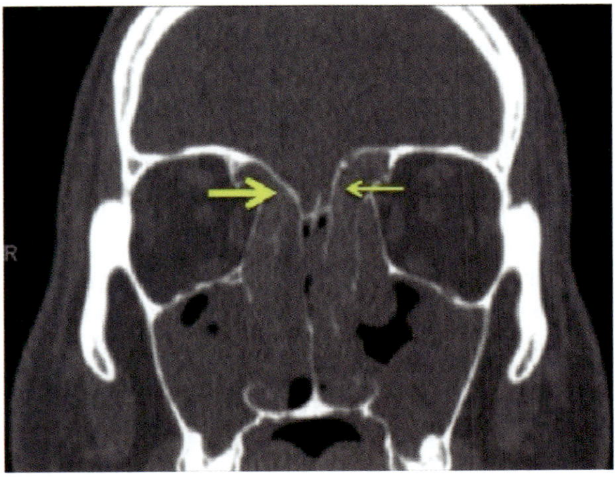

Fig. 25.2 Coronal CT demonstrating slope variation of the fovea ethmoidalis. Note the more steeply oriented left fovea (*thin arrow*) as compared to the right fovea (*thick arrow*) (With permission Andrew N. Goldberg, MD, MSCE, FACS)

to variable ethmoid sinus anatomy. Generally, more anteriorly, a sloping fovea ethmoidalis and adjacent cribriform plate bring the skull base in closer proximity to the superomedial ethmoid air cells (Fig. 25.2). The inferomedial boundary of the ethmoids abuts the middle and superior turbinate, separating the sinus from the nasal cavity. The anterior face of the sphenoid makes up the posterior boundary of the ethmoids. Finally, the skull base, separating the anterior cranial fossa from the sinuses, defines the superior limit of the ethmoid sinuses.

In part due to differing drainage pathways, the ethmoid sinus is subdivided into anterior and posterior groups. The separation of the anterior and posterior ethmoids is the middle turbinate attachment to the lateral nasal wall, also known as the basal lamella. Anteriorly, cells drain into the middle meatus; posteriorly, drainage occurs into the superior meatus.

Variations of air cell anatomy exist throughout the paranasal sinuses. One variant unique to the ethmoid sinus is the Haller cell, described as an infraorbital cell that may cause narrowing of the infundibulum and maxillary sinus ostium. This cell can originate from either the anterior or posterior ethmoid group. A sphenoethmoidal air cell, or Onodi cell, is a posterior ethmoid air cell that aerates the optic nerve and typically extends superior or superior/lateral to the sphenoid sinus. Ethmoid air cells may also be found in a supraorbital location extending into the frontal bone.

Arterial supply to the ethmoid mucosa is primarily from the anterior and posterior ethmoid arteries. These are located in a septation of bone traversing lateral to medial from the orbit across the roof of the ethmoid sinus. Anterior and posterior ethmoidal nerves, arising from the nasociliary nerve, and parasympathetic branches of the pterygopalatine ganglion provide sensory innervation to the ethmoid sinus mucosa. On a coronal CT scan, the anterior and posterior ethmoid arteries can be identified medially and superiorly in the orbit, exiting the orbit medially from a pinch in the bone (Fig. 25.3). The anterior ethmoid artery can also be identified approximately 24 mm posterior to the anterior lacrimal crest roughly corresponding with the posterior end of the globe and is usually associated with the basal lamella. The posterior ethmoid artery is located an additional 12 mm posterior to the exit of the anterior ethmoid artery and is associated with the anterior face of the sphenoid sinus. Both arteries are typically located in the bone of the skull base, but with pneumatization of a supraorbital ethmoid cell, the vessels can also traverse the ethmoid inferior to the skull base in what is characterized as a "low-hanging ethmoid artery" (Fig. 25.4). The optic canal is located an additional 6 mm posterior to the posterior ethmoid artery.

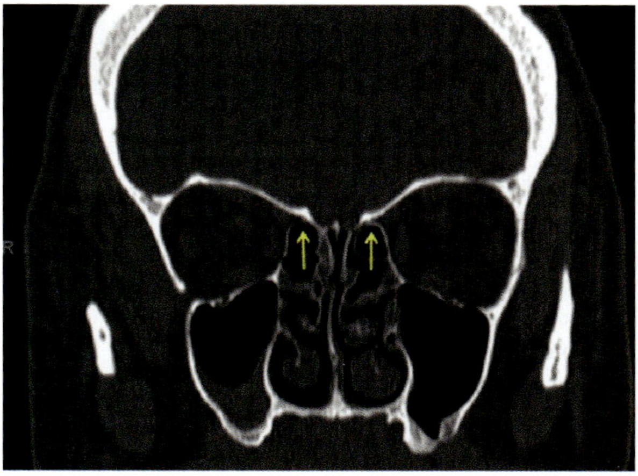

Fig. 25.3 Coronal CT, *arrows* pointing to anterior ethmoid arteries (With permission Andrew N. Goldberg, MD, MSCE, FACS)

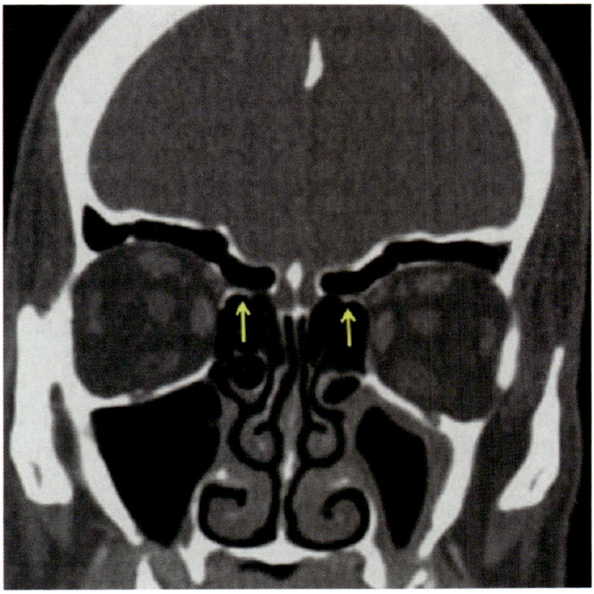

Fig. 25.4 *Arrows* pointing to "low-hanging" anterior ethmoid arteries (With permission Andrew N. Goldberg, MD, MSCE, FACS)

CT Scan Review

A systematic review of the CT scan is performed in the operating room prior to surgery. The review is conducted from anterior to posterior on the coronal CT one image at a time for the medial orbital wall and then for the skull base. This is followed by inspection of the height of the posterior ethmoid and sphenoid sinus configuration. Then the axial and sagittal images are then reviewed. The sagittal view is specifically inspected for the slope of the skull base from anterior to posterior.

Coronal CT

Medial orbital wall (integrity/dehiscence, relationship to uncinate, anterior ethmoid artery, Haller cell).

Skull base (integrity/dehiscence, lateral to medial slope, depth of cribriform).

Height of posterior ethmoid (measure from roof of maxillary sinus to fovea).

Sphenoid sinus configuration (integrity/dehiscence, course of sphenoid septum, Onodi cell).

Diseased areas and synthesis of the above features for formulation of a surgical plan. Special attention is paid to the frontal recess if it is to be addressed surgically.

Axial and Sagittal CT

Slope of the skull base
Ethmoid boundaries

Indications

Typically, the principal indication for surgical ethmoidectomy is for adult patients with chronic sinusitis or recurrent acute sinusitis that fail to respond to appropriate, maximal medical therapy. Generally, it is thought that enhanced drainage and ventilation of the sinuses may restore mucociliary clearance, encourage drainage through natural ostia, and facilitate the delivery of patient-administered nasal irrigations and topical medications. In the case of surgical ethmoidectomy, rarely is it performed alone. Most often, ethmoidectomy is performed in concert with a maxillary antrostomy to facilitate middle meatus drainage. In patients with diffuse pansinus disease, total ethmoidectomy is part of the surgical procedure to open all the involved paranasal sinuses.

Rarely is ethmoidectomy required urgently. However, in the case of rapidly progressive sinusitis with orbital and/or intracranial extension, formation of abscesses, or threat to patient survival, surgery may be more acutely indicated.

There are few absolute contraindications to ethmoidectomy. As with any surgery, patients not healthy enough to undergo anesthesia are considered poor surgical candidates. Caution should be used in any patient with a bleeding disorder, and appropriate preoperative counseling and referrals should be made. With the advent of image guidance and high-resolution video imaging, dehiscent orbital wall and skull base with exposed contents do not preclude the patient from undergoing surgery.

Surgical Technique

The ethmoid operation begins with ensuring appropriate exposure, proper lighting and visualization, and orientation to the ethmoid labyrinth and its associated anatomy and possible tissue planes. Deficiency in any of these three key areas can lead to incomplete surgery, violation of the surrounding structures, and unintended complications. Bleeding and loss of orientation are typically the key culprits in incomplete surgery or surgical misadventure. Control of bleeding begins preoperatively with appropriate treatment of inflammation and may include a combination of corticosteroid administration, antibiotic use, and nasal irrigation. Operating in a clean and quiet field reduces bleeding, improves visualization, decreases operating time, and likely lessens the incidence of complications in this complex region of bony anatomy [2, 3].

Proper orientation on intranasal examination begins with a preoperative endoscopic examination carefully noting the position and presence or absence of surgical landmarks. Specifically, the orientation of and position of the head and body of the middle turbinate, uncinate process, bulla ethmoidalis, and basal lamella should be assessed. A systematic review of imaging, typically triplanar CT scanning and endoscopic visualization of the ethmoid sinuses, is critical to anticipating the configuration of the ethmoid labyrinth and identifying key relationships that will aid in maintaining orientation in surgery.

Intraoperative anatomical orientation includes identification of the middle turbinate as well as the uncinate process, sinus lateralis, basal lamella, skull base, and bulla ethmoidalis. The middle turbinate can be medialized, and the inferior turbinate can be lateralized to improve exposure and access to the region of the middle meatus.

Anterior Ethmoidectomy

Anterior ethmoidectomy begins with complete removal of the uncinate process, which aids in the exposure of the most lateral limits of the ethmoid labyrinth at the lamina papyracea. Identification of the natural ostium of the maxillary sinus in conjunction with performing a maxillary antrostomy can greatly assist in orientation to the ethmoid labyrinth. A maxillary antrostomy of sufficient size to allow for exposure of (1) the floor of the orbit, (2) the posterior wall of the maxillary sinus, and (3) the medial and then superior curve of the orbit toward the lamina papyracea can greatly aid in orientation during ethmoidectomy. Identification of these structures provides information on the position of the ethmoid labyrinth in the superior-inferior direction, anterior-posterior direction, and medial-lateral direction, respectively, and can be an important reason for enlarging the maxillary antrostomy. Accuracy of image-guidance probes, and they are used, can be assessed with relation to these known bony anatomic landmarks.

After a complete uncinectomy and maxillary antrostomy, the ethmoid bulla is fully exposed and can be identified anterior to the basal lamella. Numerous methods for anterior ethmoidectomy have been described including a purely anterior approach through the face of the bulla and use of a curette at the basal lamella and between the middle turbinate and ethmoid bulla to remove the bulla from a posterior to anterior direction. A "J" curette inserted at the medial and inferior attachment of the basal lamella can be gently inserted posterior to the bulla ethmoidalis. The curette should slide smoothly lateral to the middle turbinate into position posterior to the bulla, pointing superiorly and laterally. With the J curette inserted, force is applied anteriorly, laterally, and inferiorly to release the ethmoid bulla from its attachments (Fig. 25.5). The bulla can then be removed with a Blakesley forceps. Remnants of the bulla can be removed using cut instruments such as the straight and upbiting Matsui, straight and upbiting Blakesley, and Kerrison forceps. Identification of and cleaning of the medial orbital wall is a critical step in the performance of a complete ethmoidectomy and helps the surgeon maintain orientation and aids in the completeness of dissection. The philosophy that structures that are to be preserved should be exposed and visualized applies here. The lateral skull base is typically thicker than the medial component and is therefore a safer area to dissect. Removal

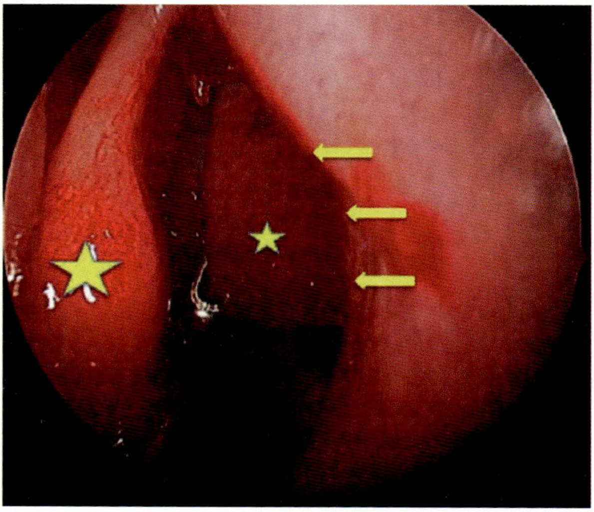

Fig. 25.5 Left anterior ethmoidectomy using a J curette to detach the bulla ethmoidalis. *Large star* – middle turbinate; *small star* – bulla; *arrows* – cut edge of excised uncinate process (With permission Andrew N. Goldberg, MD, MSCE, FACS)

of septations from the medial orbital wall assures complete surgery and aids in orientation. If the middle turbinate is insufficiently medialized, then the medial lamina of the bulla ethmoidalis may inadvertently be left behind and become a source for chronic inflammation. At this point, the medial wall of the orbit in the anterior ethmoid should be completely exposed and clean, the basal lamella should likewise be exposed, and the patient is ready for posterior ethmoidectomy if it is to be performed.

Posterior Ethmoidectomy

As with anterior ethmoidectomy, identification of the superior turbinate, skull base, and medial orbital wall guides posterior ethmoidectomy. Identification of the middle turbinate medially, the lamina papyracea laterally, and the horizontal strut of the basal lamella inferiorly oriented the surgeon to the face of the posterior ethmoid labyrinth or commonly the basal lamella. Use of landmarks in the maxillary sinus also aids in orientation in all three planes. A J curette pointing posteriorly and inferiorly can be used to perforate the face of the posterior ethmoid labyrinth in the medial inferior quadrant of the face of the posterior ethmoid. This orientation of the J curette is roughly parallel to the fovea ethmoidalis and skull base and provides proper orientation for the direction of force applied to the instrument. The horizontal strut of the basal lamella at its inferior border should be preserved to maintain stability of the middle turbinate. Attention to preservation of this horizontal strut is necessary if this stability is to be maintained. After the curette penetrates the basal lamella, fragments of bone of the basal lamella can be displaced anteriorly and removed to expose the superior turbinate medially. Careful use of

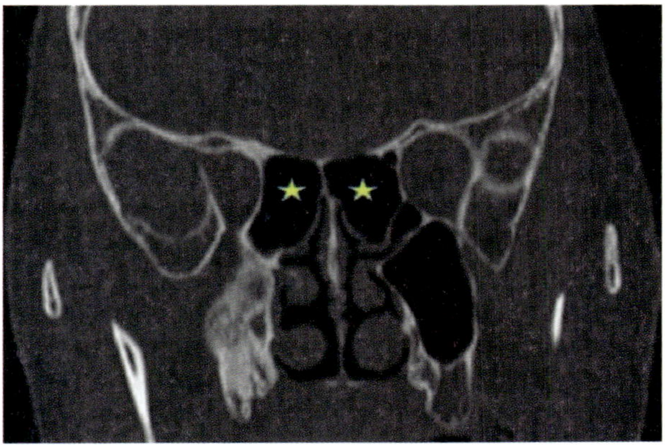

Fig. 25.6 The *star* marks a "Queen" cell bilaterally (With permission Andrew N. Goldberg, MD, MSCE, FACS)

through-biting instrumentation should then be used lateral to the superior turbinate to remove septations of the posterior ethmoid labyrinth with the overarching goal of exposure of the medial orbital wall and cleaning septations that are attached to it. The straight 3 mm Kerrison forceps is particularly useful in removing the septations in a medial-to-lateral direction toward the medial orbital wall. The footplate, or shoe, of the Kerrison forceps is useful in feeling behind each septation before a bite is taken and the septation is removed. The roof of the maxillary sinus can be used to orient the surgeon to the position of the fovea ethmoidalis as the next important landmark is the skull base in the posterior ethmoid. The preoperative CT scan can be used to both assess the likely point for visualization of the skull base in the posterior ethmoid labyrinth and to reveal to the surgeon the expected distance from the orbital floor to the fovea ethmoidalis. In many patients, the posterior-most ethmoid cell may fully pneumatize to expose the medial orbital wall, the skull base, the face of the sphenoid, and the medial limit of the ethmoid to the superior turbinate. If this configuration is present, this posterior ethmoid cell is termed the "Queen cell." In patients with this pneumatization pattern, entry into the Queen cell can greatly facilitate the identification of key landmarks for orientation (Fig. 25.6). The skull base is then identified through careful removal of posterior ethmoid septations, maintaining orientation to the medial orbital wall for medial-lateral orientation and roof of the maxillary sinus for superior-inferior orientation. If a sphenoidotomy is to be performed, it can be performed at this time, but the opening of the sphenoid sinus ostium is medial to the superior turbinate in the sphenoid ethmoidal recess.

After the skull base is identified, surrounding septations should be removed extending from the vertical lamella of the middle turbinate to the medial orbital wall and superiorly to the skull base. A 30° endoscope can then be used to better visualize the skull base. Angled instrumentation including the 45° forward/backward and side-to-side punch, the curved articulated Kerrison, and a gently curved Kerrison are used to completely remove septations attached to the skull base and medial orbital wall.

Complications

Due to the complex variability and close proximity of the ethmoid sinus to vital surrounding structures, many described complications of endoscopic sinus surgery often occur during or following ethmoidectomy. Synechia and lateralization of the middle turbinate are among the most common, and fortunately most minor, of unwanted consequences of ethmoidectomy. A lateralized middle turbinate is best avoided, as it can lead to impaired sinus drainage and return of the sinuses to an obstructed, inflammatory state. Suture medialization of the middle turbinate to the septum and conscientious removal of free mucosa and bone will prevent these complications [4].

As previously described, the ethmoid sinus and the orbit have a close relationship, separated by a thin layer of bone. For this reason, the potential for orbital complications during ethmoidectomy is real. Orbital hematoma can occur after injury to the anterior ethmoid artery. When injured adjacent to the lamina papyracea, the artery may retract into the orbit and cause a hematoma. Accumulation of blood in the intraorbital space can lead to increased orbital pressures with resulting blindness. All surgeons should be familiar with both medical and surgical treatment for this acute complication, starting with an immediate lateral canthotomy and cantholysis as well as a medial decompression. Visual disturbance including blindness can occur in other ways as well during ethmoidectomy. Especially in cases of medial orbital wall dehiscence from sinus or polyp disease where orientation is difficult, aggressive use of the microdebrider may result in direct injury to the medial rectus muscle, globe, or optic nerve. As with all orbital complications, prevention is key. Early identification of the medial orbital wall with continued checks of anatomic landmarks to maintain orientation will lessen the risk of these complications.

Skull base injury with resultant CSF leak or brain parenchyma injury is also possible during ethmoidectomy. This most often occurs medially, especially in patients with a low skull base, sharply sloping fovea ethmoidalis, or steep skull base in the sagittal plane [5]. Identification of the skull base posteriorly with removal of septations from a posterior to anterior direction using angled instruments and telescopes is useful for prevention. In the event that this complication does occur, immediate closure with free or pedicled mucosal grafting and neurosurgical consultation can be considered.

Image guidance systems have emerged as a new tool in the arsenal of sinus surgeons. It allows for real-time assessment of imaging and instrument localization during surgery. It has been shown to improve completeness of ethmoidectomy and, within selected populations, is associated with a lower risk of complications compared to non-image guidance surgeries [6]. However, it is important to understand that though this tool may be used to corroborate intraoperative findings, it should not replace the necessity of understanding anatomy nor replace clinical judgment during ethmoidectomy.

Finally, the key to prevention is done preoperatively with a thorough review of the patient's imaging. An understanding of the unique anatomic variation prior to surgery will help maintain orientation during the operation.

Conclusion

Ethmoidectomy is an integral part of complete endoscopic sinus surgery performed for appropriate clinical indications. Surgeons should be aware of the complex, unique, and variable anatomy that may exist in this confined area. This surgery can be performed safely and effectively using the methods and precautions outlined in this chapter. In order to perform complete surgery and avoid complications, surgeons should develop a systematic way to review preoperative CT imaging to detect anatomic variations that may predispose the surgeon to surgical misadventures. The surgeon must proceed systematically from landmark to landmark intraoperatively and not proceed if anatomic uncertainty exists.

References

1. Mosher HP. The surgical anatomy of the ethmoid labyrinth. Ann Otol Rhinol Laryngol. 1929;38:869–901.
2. Albu S, Gocea A, Mitre I. Preoperative treatment with topical corticoids and bleeding during primary endoscopic sinus surgery. Otolaryngol Head Neck Surg. 2013;149(1):17–29.
3. Tewfik MA, Wormald PJ. Ten pearls for safe endoscopic sinus surgery. Otolaryngol Clin North Am. 2010;43(4):933–44.
4. Hewitt KM, Orlandi RR. Suture medialization of the middle turbinates during endoscopic sinus surgery. Ear Nose Throat J. 2008;87(12):E11.
5. Heaton CM, Goldberg AN, Pletcher SD, Glastonbury CM. Sinus anatomy associated with inadvertent cerebrospinal fluid leak during functional endoscopic sinus surgery. Laryngoscope. 2012;122(7):1446–9.
6. Dalgorf DM, Sacks R, Wormald PJ, Naidoo Y, et al. Image-guided surgery influences perioperative morbidity from endoscopic sinus surgery: a systematic review and meta-analysis. Otolaryngol Head Neck Surg. 2013;149(1):17–29.

Surgery for Frontal Sinus Disease

26

Caitlin McLean, Nathan A. Deckard, and Pete S. Batra

Key Take-Home Points

- The management algorithm for surgical intervention of chronic frontal sinusitis commences when disease is refractory to maximal medical therapy.
- The aim of frontal sinus surgery is to relieve diseased sinuses in a minimally invasive fashion with mucosal preservation, which can be achieved with endoscopic frontal sinusotomy in the majority of patients.
- Endoscopic modified Lothrop provides broad access to the frontal sinus for inflammatory and neoplastic pathology.
- Frontal sinus obliteration should be used as a last resort.

Financial Disclosures:
McLean: None
Deckard: None
Batra: consultant (Medtronic), SAB (Merck)

C. McLean, MD
Department of Otolaryngology-Head and Neck Surgery, Temple University School of Medicine, 3401 North Broad Street, Philadelphia, PA, USA
e-mail: caitlin.mclean@tuhs.temple.edu

N.A. Deckard, MD
Division of Otolaryngology – Head and Neck Surgery, Department of Surgery, Cooper University Hospital, 3 Cooper Plaza, Suite 404, Camden, NJ, USA
e-mail: Deckard-nathan@cooperhealth.edu

P.S. Batra, MD, FACS, FARS (✉)
Department of Otorhinolaryngology – Head and Neck Surgery, Rush Center for Skull Base and Pituitary Surgery, Rush University Medical Center, 1611 W. Harrison St, Suite 550, Chicago, IL, USA
e-mail: pete_batra@rush.edu

P.S. Batra, J.K. Han (eds.), *Practical Medical and Surgical Management of Chronic Rhinosinusitis*, DOI 10.1007/978-3-319-16724-4_26

Introduction/History of Frontal Sinus Surgery

Frontal sinus surgery remains a considerable surgical challenge, given narrow confines of the frontal recess, need for angled scopes and instruments, and proximity to critical structures. Since the late nineteenth century, surgical management of frontal sinus disease has engendered significant controversy, with the pendulum swinging between open and endoscopic approaches. Perhaps its challenge is best summarized by Ellis in 1954 who noted that surgery for frontal sinusitis "…has always been difficult, often unsatisfactory, and sometimes disastrous. The frequency with which we discuss the problem of treating it, and the diverse methods which have been proposed, are clear expression of the uncertainty, and perhaps of our failure" [1].

Sir Ogston published the first account of external frontal surgery for infection when he performed an anterior wall trephination and placed a "drainage tube" [2]. In 1898 Riedel described radical obliterative surgery with ablation of the anterior wall of the frontal sinus, while Hajek introduced the concept of osteoplastic flap operation in 1903 [3]. This was followed by external frontoethmoidectomy approaches via the medial orbital wall to establish the frontonasal connection. In 1914 Lothrop proposed a wide nasofrontal opening with resection of the frontal sinus floor, intersinus septum, and upper nasal septum, while in 1921 Lynch advocated a medial periorbital incision to address the frontoethmoid complex [4, 5]. However, both approaches were associated with a high failure rate due to formation of scar tissue and medial prolapse of orbital contents.

In 1958 Goodale and Montgomery performed the first osteoplastic flap (OPF) with frontal sinus obliteration which served as the workhorse for frontal sinus disease from the 1960s to 1980s [6]. The introduction of the paradigm of functional endoscopic sinus surgery (FESS) by Kennedy and Stammberger facilitated the consideration of endoscopic frontal sinus surgery [7, 8]. Improved understanding of frontal recess anatomy, advances in paranasal sinus computed tomography (CT) imaging, and refinement of frontal instrumentation have all contributed to the technical capability of purely endoscopic approaches.

Frontal Sinus Anatomy/Physiology

The frontal sinuses are typically paired, asymmetric cells that are variably pneumatized and separated by a central intersinus septum. Traditionally, it was thought that the frontal sinus was connected to the anterior ethmoid region by a tubular duct-like structure termed the "nasofrontal duct." However, the nasofrontal duct is an anatomic misnomer and does not exist. In a sagittal section, the transition from the frontal sinus to the frontal recess can be conceptualized as an hourglass configuration. The frontal sinus infundibulum, frontal sinus ostium, and frontal recess comprise a functional unit for drainage referred to as the frontal sinus outflow tract. The superior portion represents the frontal infundibulum, which is the cleft at floor of the frontal sinus that narrows toward the ostium. The middle third, or isthmus, is the point of narrowest diameter and corresponds to the frontal ostium which is

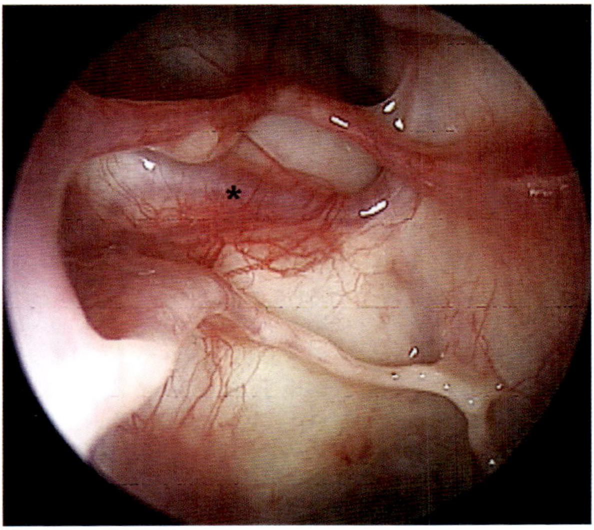

Fig. 26.1 Endoscopic view of anterior ethmoid artery (*asterisk*) at the left ethmoid roof. Patent frontal sinus ostium noted just anterior to the artery

generally positioned in a medial location. The inferior extent is formed by the frontal recess, the inverted portion of the funnel that widens in the posteroinferior direction and blends into the anterior ethmoid region.

The anatomic configuration (e.g., shape and width) and limits of the frontal recess are determined by adjacent structures. The medial and lateral limits are formed by the anterior superior middle turbinate and lamina papyracea, respectively. The anterior boundary is the agger nasi, Latin for "mound" or "eminence," which is formed by the frontal process of the maxilla. The ethmoid bulla provides a good landmark for the posterior margin of the frontal recess, particularly when the bulla lamella extends to the skull base. The skull base delineates the superior boundary of the frontal recess. Anterior ethmoid artery can form the posterior boundary of the frontal recess along the skull base but may vary based on the pneumatization of the suprabullar recess (Fig. 26.1). The anterior ethmoid artery exits the orbit as a terminal branch of the ophthalmic artery and mostly travels in an anteromedial direction to enter the lateral lamella of the cribriform plate. The path of the anterior ethmoid artery is important to recognize when performing frontal sinus surgery; the skull base at the site of entry of the artery, or the ethmoid sulcus, has been measured to be only 0.05 mm thick, placing the skull base at risk for iatrogenic injury [9].

The frontal recess opens into the ethmoid infundibulum inferiorly. The uncinate process can represent the medial or lateral boundary of the frontal recess depending on its development and position. Most often, the anterior superior portion of the uncinate is fused to the lamina papyracea and the ethmoid infundibulum is closed superiorly, forming a blind pouch called the recess terminalis. As a result, the frontal recess communicates with the middle meatus or suprabullar recess. Alternately, the uncinate can extend directly superior to the skull base or fuse with the middle turbinate. In these latter two configurations, the uncinate process forms the medial wall of the frontal recess as it drains directly into the ethmoid infundibulum.

The exact configuration of the frontal recess can be quite variable and is dependent on the three-dimensional pneumatization pattern of the ethmoidal cells in the frontal recess. Various cells can potentially populate the frontal recess, including the agger nasi, supraorbital, frontal, frontal bullar, suprabullar, and intersinus septal cells. The rate of pneumatization of the agger nasi region has been reported as high as 98.5 % [10]. The agger nasi cell (ANC) represents the most anterior and constant frontal recess cell, located at the anterior boundary of the frontal recess. Supraorbital ethmoid cell (SOEC) may determine the frontal recess caliber from a lateral aspect. Traditional teaching holds the cell is present 6–15 % of the time, though recent work has demonstrated its presence in 62 % of cases [11]. SOECs pneumatize the orbital plate of the frontal bone posterior to the frontal recess and lateral to the frontal sinus. Thus, the SOEC ostium is located posterolateral to the frontal recess, whereas the frontal sinus ostium is usually in an anteromedial position. The supraorbital ethmoid cell has been incorrectly recognized as a septated frontal sinus; missed SOECs represent a frequent source of iatrogenic frontal sinus disease (Fig. 26.2).

Frontal cells are ethmoid air cells that pneumatize the frontal recess anteriorly and are found superior to the ANC. Bent and Kuhn grouped these cells into four different types based on their location: type I describes a single cell above the agger nasi, type II refers to a tier of two or more cells superior to the agger nasi, type III is a single cell that pneumatizes into the frontal sinus, and type IV is contained entirely within the frontal sinus [12]. Suprabullar and frontal bullar cells pneumatize along the skull base, residing above the ethmoid bulla, and encroach the frontal recess from posteriorly. The frontal bullar cell extends into the frontal sinus proper, while the suprabullar cell has the same configuration but does not extend into the frontal sinus. The intersinus septal cell is a midline cell that pneumatizes the frontal intersinus septum and may narrow the recess medially.

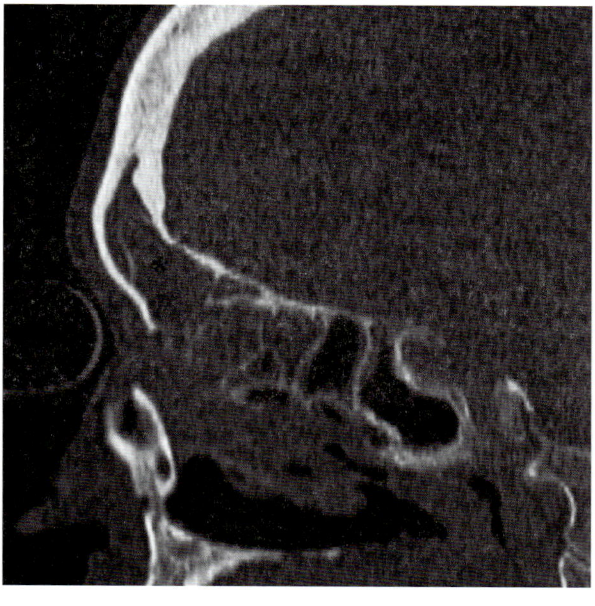

Fig. 26.2 Sagittal CT image depicts a type III frontal cell (*asterisk*) extending into the frontal sinus proper. The cell was dissected with standard endoscopic frontal instrumentation

The physiology of the frontal sinus relies on normal mucociliary transport for drainage and ventilation. The frontal sinus is the only sinus in which an inherent recirculation phenomenon occurs wherein mucus is actively transported into the sinus superiorly along the intersinus septum and then travels across the frontal sinus roof to the lateral frontal sinus and finally medially along the frontal sinus floor. Approximately 60 % of the mucus recirculates to the intersinus septum, while 40 % is swept down into the middle meatus [13].

Decision Making in Frontal Sinus Surgery

The management algorithm for chronic frontal sinusitis commences when the disease is deemed refractory to maximal medical therapy. With widespread adoption of FESS techniques, the central concept of frontal sinus surgery has shifted from ablative to preservative approaches. The primary goals are preservation of mucosa of the frontal outflow tract and establishment of frontal ventilation and drainage. The following surgical options are currently available for treatment of frontal sinus disease:

- Balloon catheter dilation (BCD)
- Endoscopic frontal sinusotomy
- Endoscopic frontal trephination
- Endoscopic modified Lothrop
- Osteoplastic flap (OPF) without obliteration
- Osteoplastic flap with frontal sinus obliteration (FSO)
- Riedel's procedure

Some central tenets must be considered when formulating the surgical approach:

- Majority of frontal sinus disease is amenable to endoscopic frontal sinusotomy.
- Balloon catheter technology may serve as an adjunct in select cases.
- Endoscopic frontal trephination may provide an additional porthole for difficult-to-reach frontal sinus pathology.
- Frontal drillout procedures may be required for refractory disease with new-bone and/or scar formation in the setting of previous failed surgery.
- OPF can be performed without obliteration.
- Riedel's procedure should be considered a last resort.

Frontal Instrumentation

The refinement of rigid endoscopes and advances in frontal instrumentation has been crucial for implementation of the endoscopic frontal surgery paradigm. The following instruments are critical for facilitating frontal sinus surgery:

- Angled scopes (30°, 45°, and 70°)
- Angled frontal recess suctions

- Giraffe (grasping and thru-cutting) 60° and 90° forceps
- Frontal 45° and 90° curettes
- Frontal sinus seekers
- Angled microdebrider attachments
- Drills

Image Guidance

The advent of image-guided surgery (IGS) has been an important advance for management of frontal sinus disease. Preoperatively, image guidance enables triplanar review of the complex frontal recess anatomy, thus facilitating the ability to devise a detailed plan to the frontal sinus. Intraoperatively, IGS allows for sound execution of the surgical strategy and correlation of the preoperative imaging with the endoscopic anatomy. This, in turn, translates into a better safety profile with reduction in complications and more comprehensive frontal recess dissection. Despite its utility, surgical navigation platforms have inherent limitations and do not represent a substitute for intimate knowledge of the frontal sinus anatomy and sound surgical technique [14]. Further, mucosal preservation remains a paramount goal.

Postoperative Care

An important factor in the success of frontal sinus surgery rests on commitment to meticulous postoperative care and close long-term endoscopic surveillance. Saline irrigations are instituted on the first postoperative day. Antibiotics, preferably culture directed, and systemic steroids, if clinically indicated, are utilized until complete mucosal healing is achieved. The patients are typically seen weekly or biweekly with careful removal of fibrin clots and debris to ensure proper mucosal healing. Any early synechiae are lysed with thru-cutting frontal instrumentation to ensure frontal patency and to facilitate unobstructed endoscopic view of the internal ostium (Fig. 26.3) [15].

Endoscopic Frontal Balloon Dilation

Indications

BCD of the sinus ostia is a relatively new tool in the management of chronic rhinosinusitis (CRS). Data has suggested potential utility of this device for treatment of adult and pediatric medically refractory CRS, limited CRS, recurrent acute rhinosinusitis, and frontal sinusitis. Additionally, studies have also shown efficacy in the office and ICU setting [16, 17].

Surgical Technique

Balloon dilation devices may be used as the sole tool in select patients with isolated, unilateral frontal disease. Alternately, concurrent FESS may be performed to

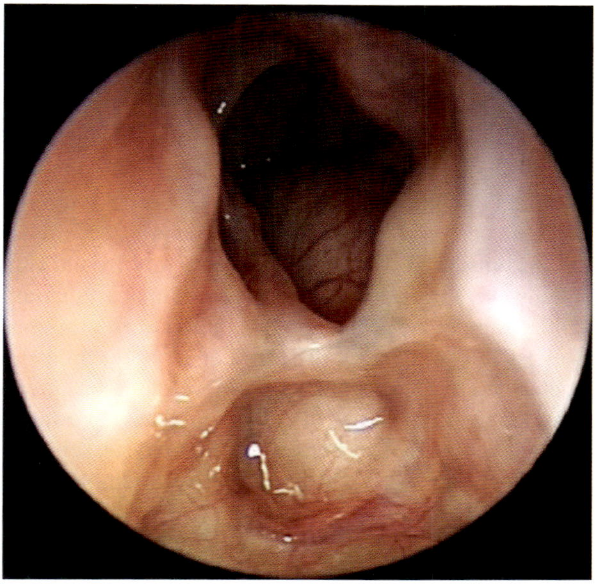

Fig. 26.3 Endoscopic view of healed right frontal internal ostium

address disease in the adjacent sinuses or to achieve optimal exposure of the frontal recess to facilitate successful frontal dilation [18].

Topical and injected local anesthetic can be used for office-based BCD, while general anesthesia is often employed for cases in the operative suite. Balloon Sinuplasty™ (Acclarent, Inc., Menlo Park, CA) employs the Seldinger technique under endoscopic visualization with 30°, 45°, and/or 70° telescopes. A guide catheter is introduced and positioned in the middle meatus posterior to the uncinate process, directed toward the frontal recess. A flexible guide wire is inserted through the guide catheter to cannulate the frontal sinus. Fluoroscopic guidance or a lighted guide wire can be used to confirm frontal sinus position. After successful cannulation, an uninflated balloon catheter is advanced over the wire into position at the frontal sinus ostium. The balloon is inflated and deflated sequentially along the frontal sinus drainage pathway. Alternatively, a newer balloon catheter is available with a malleable tip which can also serve as a frontal seeker and can be directed into the frontal recess under endoscopic visualization during sinus surgery (XprESS™, Entellus Medical, Plymouth, MN). Once dilated by BCD, the sinus ostial region is inspected with angled telescopes to visually confirm successful dilation and patency [17, 19].

Outcomes

Catalano and Payne reported on the utility of BCD to achieve patency for frontal BCD performed on 29 frontal sinuses in 20 patients with medically refractory chronic frontal sinusitis. Success rate by disease subtype for aspirin triad, CRS with nasal polyps, and CRS without nasal polyps was approximately 36, 40, and 62 %, respectively. Viewed differently, this signifies a failure rate approaching 60–64 % in patients with hyperplastic disease and suggests that BCD may not be an appropriate intervention for frontal disease in patients with significant polyp burden [20].

Heimgartner et al. retrospectively evaluated BCD for medically refractory frontal sinus disease to determine the intraoperative technical failure rate and to analyze reasons for failed access. They noted failures in 12 % of cases, most commonly due to complex frontal recess pneumatization pattern or significant neo-osteogenesis [21].

There is a single randomized trial to prospectively evaluate BCD vs. endoscopic frontal sinusotomy for medically refractory frontal sinus disease in 32 patients. All patients were treated with hybrid procedures using multiple subjective and objective validated outcome measures. Resolution of frontal sinus disease was more common after BCD compared with Draf I or Draf IIa procedures (80.8 % vs. 75 %), and frontal patency was statistically more common after BCD (73.1 % vs. 62.5 %), although neither was statistically significant. The study suffers from several limitations, including lack of pretrial power analysis, selective reporting bias given failure to conduct a between-group analysis for multiple parameters, and omitting statistical data, such as p-values and confidence intervals. Nonetheless, this is an important step in the right direction with need for additional more robust studies comparing efficacy of BCD directly to FESS techniques [18].

Endoscopic Frontal Sinusotomy

Indications

Endoscopic frontal sinusotomy is considered the standard for surgical treatment of frontal sinus disease. This is used to address complicated acute sinusitis, chronic or recurrent frontal sinus disease with associated symptoms and radiographic findings, iatrogenic disease of the frontal sinus outflow tract, frontal sinus mucoceles, and limited frontal recess inverted papilloma.

Surgical Technique

Endoscopic frontal sinusotomy can be functionally defined as endoscopic removal of frontal recess cells to restore frontal sinus ventilation and drainage. This approach may include removal of frontal recess cells and/or the common wall between the frontal sinus and SOE cell.

Draf has defined a classification scheme from type I to III of progressively more extended frontal sinus surgery that can be adapted to the specific underlying pathology. Type I drainage is established by ethmoidectomy and serves to remove obstructing disease inferior to the frontal ostium. The frontal infundibulum and its mucosa are preserved, and the frontal sinus heals by improved drainage of the ethmoid cavity. Types IIa and IIb consist of enlargement of the frontal sinus outflow tract. Type IIa involves removal of ethmoid cells protruding into the frontal sinus to create a larger opening of the frontal sinus floor between the lamina papyracea and the middle turbinate. Draf type IIb involves extending the frontal sinus floor removal medially to the nasal septum to provide a maximal ipsilateral frontal opening. Draf type

III, or endoscopic modified Lothrop (EML) procedure, creates a maximal bilateral frontal opening from orbit to orbit [22]. This is described in greater detail later in the chapter.

Key tenets in frontal recess dissection should be observed to optimize results.

1. Careful review of the frontal recess anatomy is essential. Ideally, this should be a composite of the preoperative endoscopic examination and triplanar CT anatomy.
2. The entire frontal recess dissection is performed with 30°, 45°, and 70° endoscopes.
3. Limited or total ethmoidectomy should be first performed to create access for frontal recess dissection. In select cases, a complete anterior ethmoidectomy alone may resolve frontal sinus disease.
4. Frontal recess dissection should proceed carefully from a posterior to anterior and medial to lateral direction to avoid inadvertent skull base penetration.
5. All obstructive frontal recess cells should be gently fractured from posterior to anterior with curettes. Residual bony fragments should be carefully removed with angled giraffe forceps. Angled microdebrider blades should be used very judiciously given risk of inadvertent mucosal trauma.
6. Frontal sinus seekers can also be used to gently probe clefts and recesses to determine depth or visualize/ensure patency, to retrieve obstructing bone fragments, or to redrape mucosa for bony coverage [23].

Once frontal recess surgery is completed, there should be a smooth transition between the anterior ethmoid roof and the posterior wall of the frontal sinus to prevent scar tissue formation and stenosis. Stents can be placed through the enlarged frontal ostium at the conclusion of surgery if there is concern for stenosis or scarring. There are no standardized indications for stent use.

In general terms, endoscopic frontal sinus surgery can be executed safely in most patients. The narrow confines, proximity to orbit and skull base, and need for angled scopes can result in disorientation and place the patient at higher risk of complications than standard FESS procedures. Complications from endoscopic frontal sinus surgery include hemorrhage, scarring resulting postoperative frontal stenosis and mucocele formation, anterior ethmoid artery injury with resultant retro-orbital hematoma, orbital entry from breach of the lamina papyracea, and skull base injury with ensuing CSF leakage. Powered instrumentation, especially microdebriders, can increase the magnitude of injury if the orbital or skull base interface is violated.

Outcomes

The efficacy of endoscopic frontal sinus surgery suffers from lack of randomized blinded placebo controlled trials. Further, the data is confounded by use of differing parameters in various studies, including symptom scores, CT imaging, and/or endoscopic patency. A patent frontal sinus outflow tract does not necessarily mean the patient is asymptomatic [24].

A retrospective evaluation of 200 patients undergoing endoscopy frontal sinusotomy by the Messerklinger technique found a 19 % recurrence rate for frontal sinus disease, with 8 % requiring revision surgery. The Lund-Mackay scores showed no statistical correlation between disease severity and incidence of recurrence; further, no difference was noted between polyp and non-polyp forms of CRS. Incidentally, recurrence and revision rate improved considerably over the 4-year period, suggesting a positive learning curve [25].

Chan et al. evaluated long-term frontal sinus patency after endoscopic frontal sinusotomy in 294 frontal sinuses in 161 CRS patients at an average follow-up of 45.9 months. Durable patency was achieved in 87 % after initial surgery and in 94 % with revision surgery. The non-eosinophilic and eosinophilic CRS patients had a documented endoscopic frontal sinus patency of 90 and 85 %, respectively [26].

Endoscopic Frontal Trephination

Indications

Frontal sinus trephination is a useful adjunct to standard endoscopic frontal sinus surgery when an additional porthole for access is required for visualization and/or instrumentation for difficult-to-reach frontal sinus pathology. This includes complex frontal recess pneumatization patterns beyond the reach of standard frontal recess instrumentation and significant alteration of frontal anatomy due to extensive inflammatory disease, previous surgery, or neoplasm.

Surgical Technique

The procedure starts with the standard endoscopic frontal sinusotomy, with consideration of frontal trephination if the endoscopic approach is unable to achieve the surgical objective. A small curvilinear incision is placed approximately 5–15 mm from midline at the supraorbital rim, at the inferomedial margin of the brow or within the brow. The location of underlying frontal sinus pathology and proximity of supratrochlear and supraorbital neurovascular bundles should also be taken into account in incision placement.

The trephine should be designed at the greatest depth of the frontal sinus to minimize risk of posterior table penetration. Lee et al. showed no statistically significant difference in measurement of frontal sinus depth at 0.5, 1.0, and 1.5 cm from the midline. However, they did note an increased risk of cross trephination in 21.2 % of patients when performed only 5 mm from midline due to the variable location of the frontal intersinus septum [27]. Image-guided surgery can be helpful to identify the safest area for the trephine, to localize the target lesion, to minimize size of the skin incision, and to lower the risk of intracranial entry.

Traditionally, trephination was performed close to the frontal sinus floor to allow gravity dependent drainage in acute frontal sinusitis to avoid inadvertent seeding of the frontal bone with bacteria. However, the trephine placement may be varied based on the clinical scenario at hand. Trephination of the anterior table, typically 4 to

5 mm in size, provides a panoramic view into the frontal sinus and guides removal of frontal cells, drilling of osteoma, or aspiration of pus. Conversely, trephination in the medial frontal sinus floor can be $\leq$10 mm in size; this allows for simultaneous introduction of scope and frontal instruments, soft tissue shaver, or drill and facilitates removal of frontal cells or soft tissue neoplasms, such as inverted papilloma [28].

Outcomes

Batra et al. reported on 22 patients managed with a combined endoscopic trephination and endoscopic frontal sinusotomy. Postoperatively, headaches resolved in 47 %, improved in 35 %, and remained unchanged in 18 % of the patients. Orbital symptoms resolved in 63 %, improved in 25 %, and remained unchanged in 12 % of the patients. They noted patency of the frontal sinusotomy in 86 % of cases at a mean follow-up of 16.2 months [28].

Endoscopic Modified Lothrop Procedure

Indications

EML procedure, or Draf III frontal sinusotomy, is frequently utilized for refractory frontal disease with new-bone and/or scar formation, especially in the setting of previously failed frontal sinus procedures. It affords a wide frontal opening to address severe frontal hyperplastic or fungal disease or to enhance topical medication delivery in the postoperative period. The technique is ideal in those patients with large frontal sinuses, wide intranasal anatomy, a shallow nasion, a frontal sinus floor >1.5 cm in anteroposterior (AP) diameter, and a nasofrontal beak that is not excessively thick, but these are not limiting factors to performing this procedure. This approach provides the largest anatomical opening possible to drain the frontal sinuses into the nasal cavity [29].

Surgical Technique

The adjacent paranasal sinus disease, which is often present due to previous surgeries, should be addressed first. The drillout is started by first identifying the frontal sinus floor by either image guidance or using surgical landmarks to help gauge the relative position of the sinus. The first olfactory fiber can also be used as the posterior limit of dissection, which helps to minimize potential intracranial injury. A superiorly based 2 cm iatrogenic septal perforation is first created just across from the leading edge of the middle turbinate/agger nasi region. This greatly enhances exposure for the procedure and facilitates postoperative endoscopic inspection and debridement.

The anterosuperior portion of the middle turbinate is next removed sharply to further improve exposure to the frontal sinus floor. If possible, at least one frontal internal ostium is first identified, typically on the least involved side utilizing a frontal curette, thru-cutting forceps, or drill. The frontal sinus floor is now removed from orbit to orbit utilizing diamond bur drills and thru-cutting frontal punches. Note that the frontal recess is located posteriorly relative to the midline

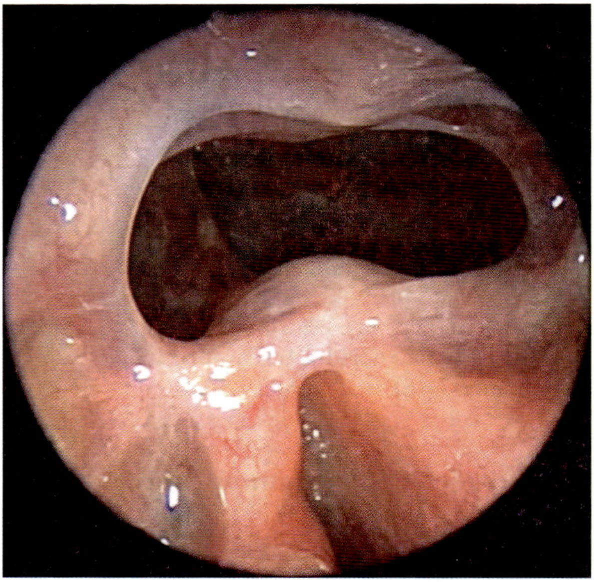

Fig. 26.4 Endoscopic view of healed frontal neo-ostium after Draf III procedure

frontal sinus floor and, thus, drilling directly across from one frontal recess to the other should be avoided. This straight path of drilling will traverse the olfactory fossa and place the patient at risk for iatrogenic CSF leak or even intracranial injury. The final opening will be crescent shaped at the completion of the drillout (Fig. 26.4). Mucosal preservation at the posterior margin of the neo-ostium is crucial. This decreases the risk of circumferential mucosal denudation intraoperatively and lessens the risk of scarring postoperatively. Further, this forces the surgeon to avoid the relatively thin posterior skull base and the risk of inadvertent CSF leak [30].

Outcomes

A meta-analysis of 18 studies published between 1990 and 2008 illustrated that EML is both safe and effective. Postoperative qualitative analysis of 394 patients demonstrated symptom improvement in 82.2 %, with frontal sinus patency in 95.9 % of patients at the last follow-up. Revision surgery was required in 13.9 % of patients; 80 % underwent revision EML and 20 % elected for frontal sinus obliteration [31].

A more recent retrospective study of 229 patients undergoing EML reported a longer follow-up period with mean of 45 months. The success rate of EML was reported at 95 %, defined by no further need for surgery. Frontal ostium patency was reported at 97 %, and all patients reported improvement in postoperative symptoms. Only 12 patients required revision EML, and none required more invasive procedures, such as an osteoplastic flap [32].

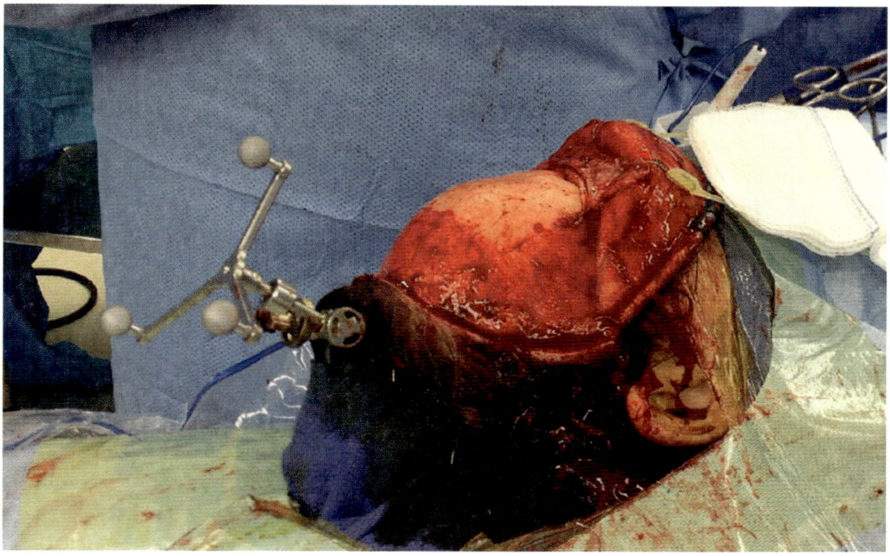

Fig. 26.5 Intraoperative view of bicoronal incision for extensive frontal sinus osteoma removal. Note the image guidance reference frame in place to help outline the frontal bony cuts

Osteoplastic Flap with Obliteration

Indications

OPF with FSO once served as the gold standard for surgical management of frontal sinus disease. The core principle of the procedure rests on complete removal of all frontal mucosal remnants to obliterate the frontal sinus, so it no longer functions as a potentially aerated space. However, given the success of endoscopic techniques, it serves as the last resort for management of recalcitrant frontal sinus disease in the current paradigm of frontal sinus surgery. Current indications for FSO include chronic frontal sinusitis refractory to previous procedures, especially in the setting of extensive scarring and/or neo-osteogenesis, frontal bone osteomyelitis, and frontal sinus fractures with posterior table or frontal recess involvement (Fig. 26.5) [33]. It is also important to note that FSO is contraindicated in cases of allergic fungal sinusitis, mucoceles with orbital and skull base erosion, and frontal sinus neoplasms as this precludes the ability to monitor disease progression.

Surgical Technique

The anterior table of the frontal sinus is typically accessed through a bicoronal incision, although direct brow (gull-wing), mid-forehead, and pretrichial incisions have been previously utilized for the same purpose. The confines of the frontal sinus were traditionally demarcated with a 6-ft Caldwell. However, intraoperative surgical navigation is now employed to more accurately identify the margins (Fig. 26.5). The incision over the periosteum is made with at least a 5 mm cuff beyond the planned osteotomy site. This ensures the blood supply for the flap, which is derived inferiorly from the periosteum.

Beveled bone cuts are performed using a saw or drill 1–2 mm inside the peripheral border of the frontal sinus to prevent inadvertent entry into the anterior cranial fossa. Meticulous removal of all bony septations and diseases mucosa is performed with drills and curettes. The frontal sinus is most commonly obliterated with a fat autograft, although other autologous materials, such as bone, muscle, and hydroxyapatite, may be used. The OPF is then replaced and secured with microplates.

Outcomes

Hardy and Montgomery retrospectively reviewed FSO in 250 patients with symptomatic and/or complicated frontal sinus disease, including primary chronic sinusitis, osteoma, or trauma. Success rate as defined by symptom-free period postoperatively was 93 %. The overall complication rate was 19 % including abdominal wound complications in 5 %, acute postoperative infection in 3 %, and chronic sinusitis in 3 %. Rates of intraoperative CSF leak and postoperative neuralgia were 2.8 and 1 %, respectively [6].

In a more recent review, OPF has been described to have a significant failure rate between 6 and 25 % and significant associated morbidity, including incorrect placement of the OPF (17 %), dural injury (9.8 %), frontal bossing/depression (10.2 %), unfavorable aesthetic result (5 %), and mucocele formation (9.8 %). In addition, less than 20 % of the sinus was filled with adipose tissue on the most recent scan in the majority of cases (53 %) and decreased significantly with time [34].

Frontal Osteoplastic Flap Without Obliteration

The role of OPF continues to diminish with the advances in endoscopic frontal techniques. However, in select cases, OPF may still be required to provide wide exposure to the frontal sinus. Osteoplastic frontal sinusotomy combines OPF with either an endoscopic frontal sinusotomy or endoscopic modified Lothrop procedure to typically address scenarios with complex disease such as frontal sinus neoplasms, trauma with posterior table or frontal recess involvement, and mucoceles with intracranial or orbital extension. It may also be utilized to unobliterate a previously obliterated frontal sinus. Importantly, OPF without obliteration restores physiologic drainage of the frontal sinus and affords the ability of perform endoscopic surveillance in the postoperative period.

Conclusion

Despite the technical advances in the past quarter century, frontal sinus surgery remains a significant surgical challenge. Intimate knowledge of the frontal recess anatomy and physiology is a prerequisite to the successful execution of frontal techniques. The advent of angled endoscopes, sophisticated frontal instrumentation, and surgical navigation has resulted in paradigm shift from open to endoscopic approaches for majority of frontal sinus disease. Indeed, majority of chronic frontal sinusitis can be managed by endoscopic frontal sinusotomy, even in tertiary care referral practices. Open approaches may still be required for select indications, though they should be employed as the last resort in the treatment paradigm. Irrespective of the surgical philosophy, commitment to postoperative care and long-term follow-up remain absolute requisites to the success of frontal sinus surgery.

References

1. Ellis M. The treatment of frontal sinusitis. J Laryngol Otol. 1954;68:478–90.
2. Ogston A. Trephining the frontal sinus for catarrhal diseases. Men Chron Manchester. 1884;3:235–8.
3. Riedel-Schenke H. Cited by Gosdale RH. The radical obliterative frontal sinus operation: A consideration of technical factors in difficult cases. Ann Otol Rhinol Laryngol. 1955;64:470–85.
4. Lothrop HA. Frontal sinus suppuration. Ann Surg. 1914;59:937–57.
5. Lynch RC. The technique of a radical frontal sinus operation which has given me the best results. Laryngoscope. 1921;31:1–5.
6. Hardy JM, Montgomery WW. Osteoplastic frontal sinusotomy: an analysis of 250 operations. Ann Otol Rhinol Laryngol. 1976;85:523–32.
7. Kennedy D. Functional endoscopic sinus surgery technique. Arch Otolaryngol. 1985;111:643–9.
8. Stammberger H. Endoscopic endonasal surgery—concepts in treatment of recurring rhinosinusitis. Part II. Surgical technique. Otolaryngol Head Neck Surg. 1986;94:14–56.
9. McLaughlin RB, Rehl RM, Lanza DC. Clinically relevant frontal sinus anatomy and physiology. Otolaryngol Clin North Am. 2001;34:1–22.
10. Bolger W, Butzin C, Parsons D. Paranasal sinus bony anatomic variations and mucosal abnormalities: CT analysis for endoscopic sinus surgery. Laryngoscope. 1991;101:56–64.
11. Lee W, Kuhn F, Citardi M. 3D computed tomographic analysis of frontal recess anatomy in patients without frontal sinusitis. Otolaryngol Head Neck Surg. 2004;131:164–73.
12. Bent JP, Cuilty-Siller C, Kuhn FA. The frontal cell as a cause of frontal sinus obstruction. Am J Rhinol. 1994;8:185–91.
13. Messerklinger W. On the drainage of the normal frontal sinus of man. Acta Otolaryngol. 1967;63:176–81.
14. Citardi MJ, Batra PS. Intraoperative surgical navigation for endoscopic sinus surgery: rationale and indications. Curr Opin Otolaryngol Head Neck Surg. 2007;15:23–7.
15. Kuhn FA, Citardi MJ. Advances in postoperative care following functional endoscopic sinus surgery. Otolaryngol Clin North Am. 1997;30:479–90.
16. Batra PS. Evidence-based practice: balloon catheter dilation in rhinology. Otolaryngol Clin North Am. 2012;45:993–1004.
17. Bolger WE, Brown CL, Church CA, et al. Safety and outcomes of balloon catheter sinusotomy: a multicenter 24-week analysis in 115 patients. Otolaryngol Head Neck Surg. 2007;137:10–20.
18. Plaza G, Eisenberg G, Montojo J, et al. Balloon dilation of the frontal recess: a randomized clinical trial. Ann Otol Rhinol Laryngol. 2011;120:511–8.
19. Brown CL, Bolger WE. Safety and feasibility of balloon catheter dilation of paranasal sinus ostia: a preliminary investigation. Ann Otol Rhinol Laryngol. 2006;115:293–9.
20. Catalano PJ, Payne SC. Balloon dilation of the frontal recess in patients with chronic frontal sinusitis and advanced sinus disease: an initial report. Ann Otol Rhinol Laryngol. 2009;118:107–12.
21. Heimgartner S, Eckardt J, Simmen D, et al. Limitations of balloon sinuplasty in frontal sinus surgery. Eur Arch Otorhinolaryngol. 2011;268:1463–7.

22. Weber R, Draf W, Kratzsch B, et al. Modern concepts of frontal sinus surgery. Laryngoscope. 2001;111:137–46.
23. Kuhn FA. Chronic frontal sinusitis: the endoscopic frontal recess approach. Op Tech Otolaryngol Head Neck Surg. 1996;7:222–9.
24. Silverman JB, Prasittivatechakool K, Busaba NY. An evidence-based review of endoscopic frontal sinus surgery. Am J Rhinol Allergy. 2009;23:e59–62.
25. Philpott CM, Thamboo A, Lai L, et al. Endoscopic frontal sinusotomy-preventing recurrence or a route to revision? Laryngoscope. 2010;120:1682–6.
26. Chan Y, Melroy CT, Kuhn CA, et al. Long-term frontal sinus patency after endoscopic frontal sinusotomy. Laryngoscope. 2009;119:1229–32.
27. Lee AS, Schaitkin BM, Gillman GS. Evaluating the safety of frontal sinus trephination. Laryngoscope. 2010;120:639–42.
28. Batra PS, Citardi MJ, Lanza DC. Combined endoscopic trephination and endoscopic frontal sinusotomy for management of complex frontal sinus pathology. Am J Rhinol. 2005;19:435–41.
29. Gross CW, Schlosser RJ. The modified Lothrop procedure: lessons learned. Laryngoscope. 2001;111:1302–5.
30. Batra PS, Cannady SB, Lanza DC. Surgical outcomes of drillout procedures for management of complex frontal sinus pathology. Laryngoscope. 2007;117:927–31.
31. Anderson P, Sindwani R. Safety and efficacy of the endoscopic modified Lothrop procedure: a systematic review and meta-analysis. Laryngoscope. 2009;119:1828–33.
32. Naidoo Y. Long-term outcomes for the endoscopic modified Lothrop/Draf III procedure: a 10-year review. Laryngoscope. 2014;124:43–9.
33. Hahn S, Palmer JN, Purkey MT, et al. Indications for external frontal sinus procedures for inflammatory sinus disease. Am J Rhinol Allergy. 2009;23:342–7.
34. Weber R, Draf W, Keerl R, et al. Osteoplastic frontal sinus surgery with fat obliteration: technique and long-term results using magnetic resonance imaging in 82 operations. Laryngoscope. 2000;110:1037–44.

Surgery for Sphenoid Sinus Disease

27

Stanley W. McClurg, Brian D. Thorp, and Brent A. Senior

Key Take-Home Points

- The sphenoid sinus is a variably pneumatized portion of the sphenoid bone, making it a unique structure within the sinonasal cavity.
- The location of the sphenoid sinus at the junction of the posterior aspect of the sinonasal cavity and the central skull base requires intimate knowledge of the anatomic relationships and their surrounding variations.
- It is of utmost importance to recall that the natural sphenoid sinus ostium is always medial to the superior turbinate (Fig. 27.1).
- An array of surgical approaches have been described for optimal management of inflammatory and neoplastic processes involving the sphenoid sinus.

S.W. McClurg, MD • B.D. Thorp, MD
Department of Otolaryngology/Head and Neck Surgery,
University of North Carolina – Chapel Hill, 170 Manning Drive,
CB 7070, Chapel Hill, NC 27599, USA
e-mail: stan_mcclurg@med.unc.edu; brian_thorp@med.unc.edu

B.A. Senior, MD, FACS, FARS (✉)
Division of Rhinology, Allergy and Endoscopic Skull Base Surgery,
Department of Otolaryngology/Head and Neck Surgery,
University of North Carolina – Chapel Hill,
170 Manning Drive, CB 7070, Chapel Hill, NC 27599, USA
e-mail: brent_senior@med.unc.edu

P.S. Batra, J.K. Han (eds.), *Practical Medical and Surgical Management of Chronic Rhinosinusitis*, DOI 10.1007/978-3-319-16724-4_27

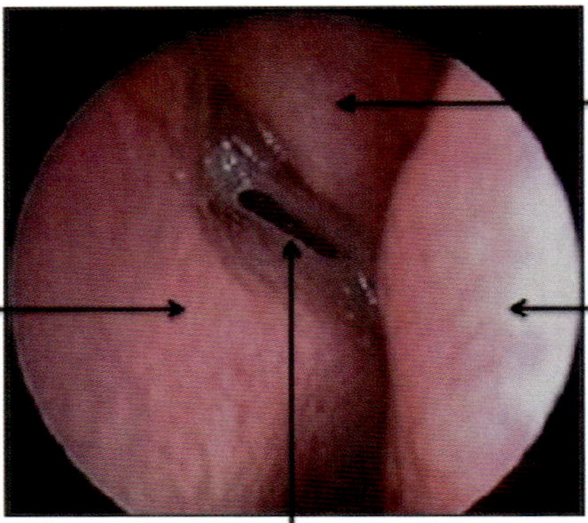

Fig. 27.1 Transnasal view of the left sphenoid ostium showing its position medial to the superior turbinate

Introduction

Sphenoid sinus surgery is an important component of the management of inflammatory sinus disease, as well as integral to the approaches to the sellar and parasellar regions for skull base lesions. Given this dual perspective, the surgeon must carefully appraise the surgical goals in the setting of the patient's anatomy and pathology. Successful surgery requires these considerations, in addition to knowledge of the variable anatomy and anatomic relationships in the region. While complications can occur in any surgical procedure, complications in this delicate region can be devastating and, as with all complications, are best managed with prevention. If encountered, rapid identification and initiation of further diagnostic and/or therapeutic measures is critical.

The embryologic development of the sphenoid sinus typically begins in the third to fourth month of fetal life. It develops from an invagination of the nasal cavity mucosa into the cartilaginous nasal capsule, termed the "cartilaginous cupolar recess of the nasal cavity" [1]. This invagination originates from the posterior ethmoid and does not actually come in contact with the sphenoid bone as it is separated by a cartilaginous plate [2]. This cartilage is resorbed over the first few years of life, allowing the sphenoid sinus to progress into the sphenoid bone. Pneumatization of the sphenoid sinus typically begins at age 1, with the most rapid growth present between 3 months and 5 years of age. Adult size is reached by approximately 12 years of age [3].

The degree of pneumatization of the sphenoid sinus can vary widely and is most often described with respect to orientation in the sagittal plane, termed conchal, presellar, sellar, and postsellar. These terms are defined by pneumatization extending posterior to a vertical line drawn through the tuberculum sellae [1, 2]. Historically, a plain radiograph was used to evaluate this degree of pneumatization leading to the Hamberger classification system of conchal, presellar, and sellar [4]. In a more recent computed tomographic (CT) study assessing the bony configuration in 296 patients, Hamid et al. noted that 2 % had conchal, 21 % had presellar, 54.7 % had sellar, and 22.3 % had postsellar pneumatization [5]. While sphenoid pneumatization in the sagittal plane is of critical importance and drives the nomenclature, aeration into the surrounding bony processes including the greater and lesser sphenoid wings, anterior clinoid processes, pterygoid processes, and palatine bones must also be critically appraised as increasing aeration results in further definition of the surrounding neurovascular structures in the sphenoid walls [2].

The sphenoid bone consists of the following components, each with important neurovascular anatomic relationships: body, lesser wings, greater wings, and pterygoid processes with the medial and lateral pterygoid plates. The body of the sphenoid bone contains the sphenoid sinus and contacts the pituitary fossa, cavernous sinuses with cavernous segments of the internal carotid artery, brainstem with vertebrobasilar arterial system, and nasopharynx on the superior, lateral, posterior, and inferior surfaces, respectively. The greater and lesser wings contribute to the superior orbital fissure, transmitting the oculomotor, trochlear, ophthalmic, and maxillary divisions of the trigeminal nerve and abducens nerves. Of note, the greater wing forms a large portion of the middle cranial fossa and lateral orbital wall, while the lesser wing forms the posterior portion of the orbital roof. The optic nerves are transmitted through the optic canals, which are located superior to the superior orbital fissure and separated from this space by the optic strut, which in the sphenoid sinus is consistent with the lateral opticocarotid recess. At the junction of the greater wing and body, the foramen rotundum transmits the maxillary division of the trigeminal nerve, the foramen ovale transmits the mandibular division of the trigeminal nerve, and the foramen spinosum transmits the middle meningeal artery [6].

Surgical Anatomy of the Sphenoid Sinus

The sphenoid sinus drains into the sphenoethmoidal recess through its natural ostium which is located on the face of the sphenoid. This natural ostium is typically located approximately 1–1.5 cm above the posterior choana and sphenoid sinus floor, situated between the posterior septum and the medial surface of the superior turbinate [2]. This relationship of the natural sphenoid ostium being located medial to the superior turbinate is a guiding principle in safely approaching the sinus. However, in addition to this landmark, other helpful relationships include the face of the sphenoid located at approximately the same depth as the posterior wall of the maxillary sinus (~7 cm from the nasal spine), with the natural ostium at the approximate height of the roof of the maxillary sinus. These relationships emphasize the importance of visualizing the maxillary sinus during sinus surgery to assist with the localization of the suspected position of the natural sphenoid sinus ostium.

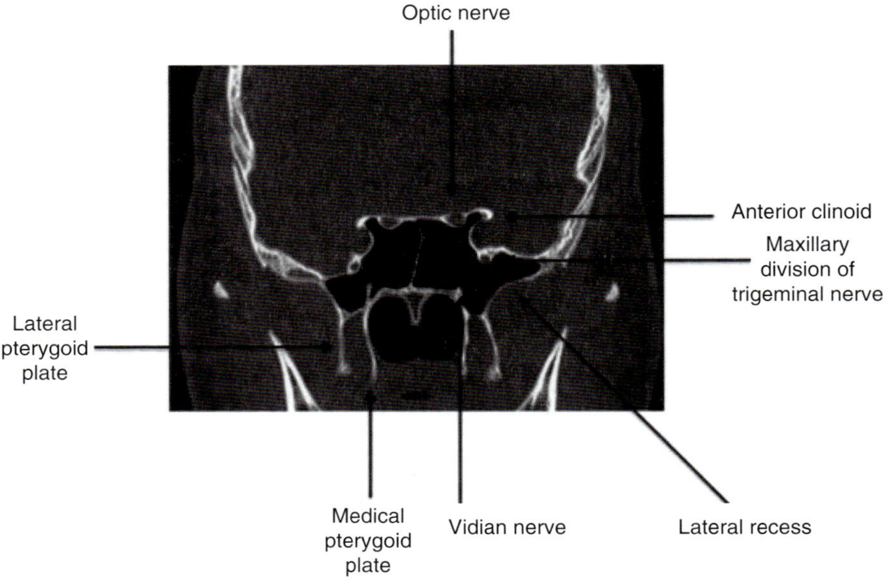

Fig. 27.2 Coronal computed tomography view of a well-pneumatized sphenoid sinus

Within the sphenoid sinus, there are multiple bony landmarks and walls present with their appearance highly dependent upon the degree of sphenoid bone/sinus pneumatization. The roof of the sphenoid sinus antrum is termed the *planum sphenoidale*. In well-aerated sinuses, the posterior aspect of the sphenoid sinus will reveal the *sella turcica*, or the bony covering over the pituitary gland. Just inferior to the sella turcica is the *clival recess*, which is a portion of the middle third of the clivus. The *sphenoid rostrum*, or keel, articulates anteriorly with the vomer to form the face and the floor of the sphenoid sinus [2]. If the pterygoid processes (fused portion of the pterygoid plates) have been pneumatized, these extensions of the sphenoid are deemed *lateral recesses* (Figs. 27.2 and 27.3). Typically, there is a bony indentation at the intersection of the optic nerve and carotid artery located at the posterior-superior aspect of the sphenoid sinus antrum deemed the *opticocarotid recess*. It should be noted that the optic nerve may be dehiscent in 12.5 % of cases, while the carotid arteries have been found to be dehiscent in as many as 19.5–23 % of cases [7, 8]. Given the highly variable anatomy and very close proximity to vital intracranial and neurovascular structures, careful preoperative planning is of the utmost importance.

The presence and location of the intersphenoid sinus septum are also highly variable. In an evaluation of CT axial cuts of 296 patients, Hamid et al. found that no septum was present in 10.8 % of the patients and a single intersphenoid septum was present in 71.6 % of the cohort. The insertion of the septum was at the lowest point in the sellar floor, in a central point, in 66.9 %, and the intersphenoid septum pointed toward the carotid canal in 4.7 %. An accessory septum was also seen in 10.8 % of

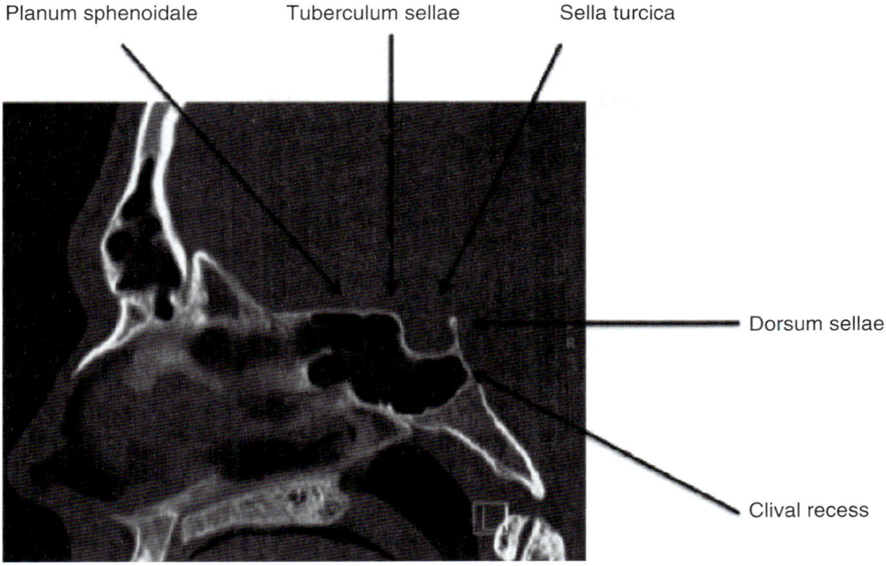

Fig. 27.3 Sagittal computed tomography view of the sphenoid sinus

patients. These visualized accessory septa were attached to the sellar floor in 37.5 % of the cohort and extended into the carotid canal in 62.5 % of patients. Multiple intersphenoid septa were found in 6.8 % of patients. In this study, the intercarotid distance ranged from 12 to 30 mm with a mean of 23 mm [5].

Importantly, the degree of pneumatization within the sphenoid sinus can be significantly affected by chronic sinonasal disease. Frequent examples of this can be seen in patients with cystic fibrosis (CF) or primary ciliary dyskinesia (PCD) as these patient cohorts tend to have under-pneumatization with resultant hypoplastic sphenoid sinuses. While the definitive reason for this is unknown, one theory suggests that it is a result of thick secretions obstructing the sphenoid ostium, causing inhibition of aeration and subsequently stunting the normal development of the sinus [2]. It has also been shown that CF patients that are homozygous for the delta-F508 mutation have a greater incidence of sphenoid hypoplasia than CF patients with other genotypes [9].

In addition, it should be noted that arachnoid granulations often occur in close proximity of the maxillary division of the trigeminal nerve in the pterygoid recesses of well-aerated sphenoid sinuses [2, 10]. This anatomic finding has been strongly associated with spontaneous cerebrospinal fluid leaks or meningoencephaloceles within the lateral recesses of well-aerated sphenoid sinuses [10]. A recent evaluation of radiographic findings of 77 sphenoid lateral recess encephaloceles in 59 patients, identified arachnoid pits in 93 %, anterior cranial fossa skull base attenuation in 80 %, and empty sella in 75 % of the cohort. Previously it was believed that sphenoid lateral recess encephaloceles arose congenitally in

"Sternberg's canal," a canal extending from the junction of the body of the sphenoid and lesser wing to the pharynx via a course medial to the superior orbital fissure. However, recent authors have refuted this claim as such a canal would lie medial to the foramen rotundum, but the vast majority of encephaloceles reported in the lateral sphenoid lie lateral to the foramen rotundum and therefore do not fulfill this critical criterion. The authors conclude that CSF leaks/encephaloceles at this location are likely the results of lateral pneumatization in the setting of an attenuated sphenoid sinus recess roof and development of arachnoid pits secondary to underlying intracranial hypertension [11].

Sphenoethmoidal cells, commonly referred to as Onodi cells, may also be present and should be identified preoperatively. These are posterior ethmoid cells that pneumatize posterior to the face of the sphenoid and may have direct communication with the optic nerve and/or carotid artery [10] (Fig. 27.4). Misidentification of sphenoethmoidal cells as being the sphenoid sinus could result in a significant complication to the vital surrounding neurovascular structures. Additionally, this variation emphasizes the importance of recognizing that the sphenoid does not simply lie posterior to the posterior ethmoid sinuses nor can it be safely identified by following the lamina papyracea [12, 13].

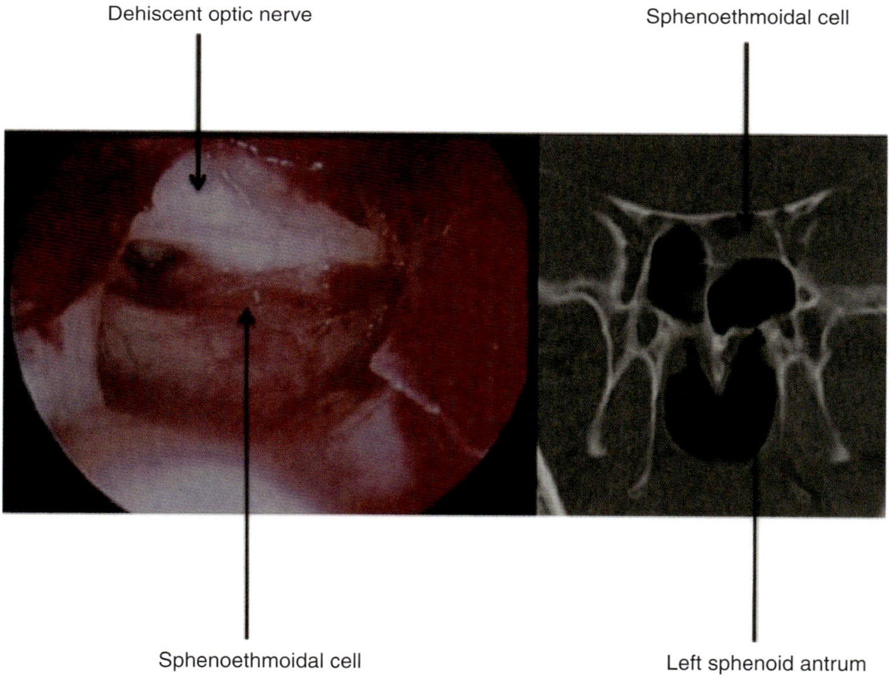

Fig. 27.4 Endoscopic view of a left sphenoethmoidal (Onodi) cell with dehiscent optic nerve localized to its lateral surface. A concurrent CT image reveals the classic radiographic findings of such a cell and pneumatization of the anterior clinoid, a feature common with dehiscence of the optic nerve

Indications

Sphenoid sinus surgery may be conducted for pathology directly related to the sphenoid sinus or pathology beyond the sphenoid sinus necessitating access for the purpose of exposure. The most common reason for sphenoid sinus surgery is sinusitis, either primary or revision surgery. Access to the surrounding neurovascular structures, including the pituitary gland, in addition to sellar, clival, or optic nerve lesions or tumors is also an indication for sphenoid sinus surgery. Furthermore, a common cause of isolated sphenoid sinus disease is occult or overt cerebrospinal fluid leaks. These may also be associated with an underlying meningoencephalocele.

Surgical Technique

A multitude of techniques exist to access the sphenoid sinus. These include open techniques (transseptal), transethmoid ("inside out"), transnasal ("outside in"), and transmaxillary transpterygoid for access to the lateral recess of the sphenoid sinus.

Traditional open techniques have been used mainly for access to the sella for pituitary lesions. The various techniques include the transantral ethmoidal approach via a Caldwell-Luc approach with concurrent ethmoidectomy, transethmoidal approach through an external ethmoidectomy, transnasal approach through an osteoplastic approach near the glabella, transpalatal approach, and transeptal approach through an extended submucous resection of the nasal septum [14]. The transseptal technique may be approached via either a sublabial or Killian incision. Once the incision is made, a submucoperichondrial dissection is conducted posteriorly to the face of the sphenoid sinus. The posterior vomer, perpendicular plate of the ethmoid bone, and sphenoid rostrum are then removed, giving access to one or both of the sphenoid sinuses. This may be combined with an open or endoscopic ethmoidectomy for increased exposure.

The transethmoid or "inside-out" technique is the most frequently utilized approach during endoscopic sinus surgery for inflammatory disease by the authors. Once the anterior and posterior ethmoid cavities have been dissected, the medial aspect of the posterior ethmoid cavity is addressed. After traversing the basal lamella of the middle turbinate, the superior turbinate is visualized medially within the ethmoid cavity. The inferior portion of the superior turbinate is then partially resected, providing visualization of the natural sphenoid ostium, located medial to the superior turbinate (Fig. 27.5). A stapes curette is then used to enter the natural ostium, directed in an inferomedial direction to widen the natural ostium. Next, a J-curette is used to further widen the ostium, again in an inferomedial vector to avoid vital neurovascular structures including the carotid artery and optic nerve, which lie laterally and superiorly, respectively. Once the ostium has been adequately widened, it may then be entered with a Kerrison rongeur, and the anterior face of the sphenoid is removed. Care should be taken to enter through the natural ostium, as entrance through another location may cause the mucosa to be inappropriately

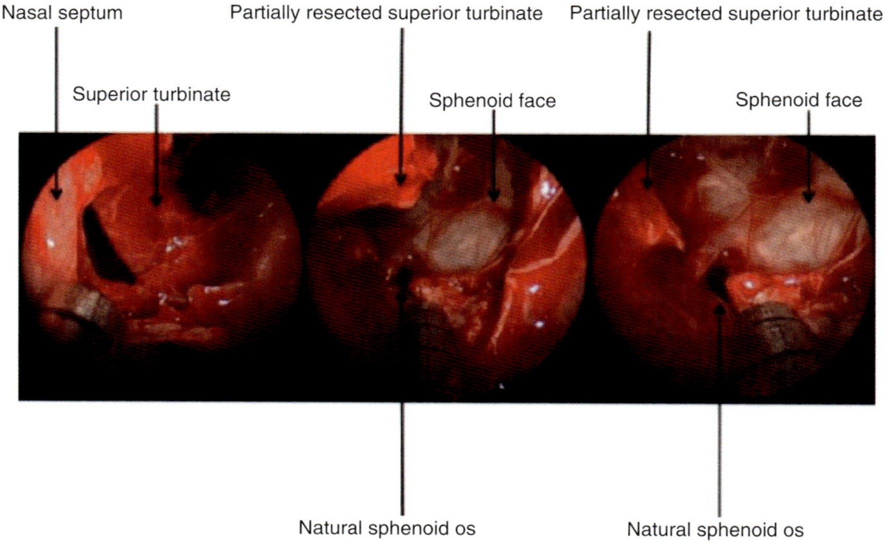

Fig. 27.5 Progressive identification of the left sphenoid ostium. The superior turbinate is visualized and isolated. Progressive sharp resection of the inferior aspect of the turbinate allows visualization of the sphenoid ostium, which is medial to the medial surface of the superior turbinate

separated from the underlying bone of the sphenoid sinus leading to marked oozing of blood. Once the ostium is widened, pathology within the sphenoid sinus can be addressed. This also allows identification of the skull base, to be followed anteriorly for completion of the ethmoidectomy portion of the endoscopic sinus surgery.

An additional technique that has been described to identify the sphenoid sinus during the ethmoid surgery is the concept of "Bolger's box." This is a parallelogram-shaped structure located at the posterior aspect of the posterior ethmoid cavity, delineated medially by the superior turbinate, superiorly by the posterior skull base, laterally by the medial orbital wall, and inferiorly by the basal lamella [15]. Identification of these key landmarks allows the surgeon excellent orientation for then locating the natural sphenoid ostium at the medial inferior corner of the box.

The transnasal (or "outside-in") approach is frequently utilized by the authors in the setting of isolated sphenoid disease or during endoscopic transsphenoidal approaches to the pituitary gland. This technique is conducted by first gently lateralizing the middle turbinate. The superior turbinate is then identified, which is also gently lateralized. A portion of the inferior aspect of the superior turbinate may be resected to improve visualization, if required. The natural sphenoid ostium is then identified and widened as aforementioned. In the setting of surgery of the sella, this may be combined with a posterior septectomy, allowing connection to the contralateral sphenoid ostium along with the removal of the sphenoid face/rostrum. This wide exposure allows excellent endoscopic visualization of the sella and related areas.

When access to the lateral recess of a well-pneumatized sphenoid sinus is necessary, a transmaxillary, transpterygoid approach may be required. This technique may be utilized for tumors, encephaloceles, or cerebrospinal fluid leaks, as the lateral recess is a common area for these to occur. The approach first requires a wide maxillary antrostomy, total ethmoidectomy, and wide sphenoidotomy. The posterior wall of the maxillary sinus is identified, as well as the inferior and medial walls of the orbit. These are critical landmarks used during the dissection. The sphenopalatine artery is identified and cauterized or ligated at the posteromedial aspect of the maxillary sinus. A high-speed drill is then used to remove the pterygoid wedge, and dissection continues to the area of the previously performed sphenoidotomy. Once these areas are connected, the vidian nerve is identified and is either preserved or transected, depending on the extent of the disease. Sacrifice of the vidian nerve is frequently necessary to gain access and visualization to the lateral and inferior aspects of the sphenoid sinus. Care should be taken to not violate the infratemporal fossa or the second division of the trigeminal nerve, if possible, during this approach. With more lateral lesions, however, this may be impossible.

In the setting of chronic or recurrent sphenoid disease that is refractory to medical management or traditional sphenoid surgery techniques, it is occasionally necessary to perform a "sphenoid nasalization" procedure. Typically, this is necessary in the setting of refractory infectious processes present in deep crypts of the sphenoid floor. The typical patient has had multiple previous sphenoid procedures with recalcitrant disease, often isolated in the sphenoid sinus. This procedure involves drilling out and removing the posterior septum, anterior sphenoid wall, clivus, intersinus septum, and sphenoid floor. This is then connected to the underlying nasopharynx. Wide drilling and exposure are often necessary to allow dependent drainage of the sphenoid into the nasopharynx. Depending on the extent of drilling, a nasoseptal flap from one or both sides of the septum may be necessary for mucosal coverage of the exposed bone.

Complications

As previously detailed, the anatomic variations of the sphenoid sinus place the adjacent neurovascular structures at varying degrees of risk. The optic nerve is of particular concern as direct injury is often irreversible. In a multitude of radiographic studies, intrasphenoidal prominence or dehiscence of the optic nerve was noted in 8–70.7 % of subjects [16–18]. In the largest of these studies, evaluation of 150 computed tomography scans revealed bulging of the optic nerve into the sphenoid sinus in 8 % of subjects. In all of these cases, an extremely thin osseous covering was noted with concurrent ipsilateral anterior clinoid process pneumatization [18]. Careful attention must be paid to preoperative imaging to identify such anatomic variations and lateral pneumatization that may place the optic nerve at increased risk. In the event of direct or suspected optic nerve injury, the optic nerve should be decompressed and ophthalmology consulted for concurrent management and serial examinations.

Local bleeding can occur during any endoscopic sinus procedure given the immense vascularity of the sinonasal tract. In addition to the aforementioned, catastrophic bleeding can occur in surgery of the sphenoid sinus given the position of the cavernous segment of the internal carotid artery and dehiscence of this segment in up to 23 % of cases [7]. During the surgical approach to the sphenoid sinus, the posterior ethmoid artery and posterior septal artery are of particular note. The posterior ethmoid artery is located a mean distance of 8.1 mm from the anterior wall of the sphenoid usually encased in the bone of the skull base. However, in some cases, it may hang below the skull base placing it at risk with excessive superior dissection of the sphenoid face. Moreover, with its origin off of the ophthalmic artery, there is increased propensity for intraorbital retraction and subsequent retrobulbar hematoma. In contrast, the posterior septal artery courses below the natural ostium of the sphenoid sinus, and dissection inferior to the horizontal plane of the superior turbinate places this vascular structure at risk [19, 20]. Injury to the internal carotid artery during sphenoid sinus surgery can be fatal and requires prompt identification and management. It is critical to ascertain the position of the internal carotid artery on preoperative imaging and discern the potential for dehiscence. Despite these measures, injury can occur with lateral dissection and particularly expanded approaches to the sellar and parasellar regions. In the event of injury, prompt action with inclusion of a multidisciplinary team is paramount. Attempts should be made to control the active bleed to allow for further diagnostic and therapeutic interventions as dictated by a particular center's resources. Such therapeutic interventions include open and/or endovascular control [20].

CSF leak is a known complication of any endoscopic sinus surgery. Classically, the lateral lamella of the cribriform plate is the most common site of skull base injury and resultant leakage [2]. During sphenoid sinus surgery, identification and often manipulation of the skull base are required resulting in the theoretic risk of CSF leak. If encountered, identification and repair are critical. A multitude of techniques have been described for skull base repair, and detailed description is beyond the scope of this chapter. Importantly, large systematic reviews have revealed primary repair success rates greater than 90 % [21].

While the previously noted complications require prompt identification and management to ensure the welfare of the patient, recurrent sphenoid disease is often a delayed complication of surgery in this locale resulting from surgical and patient factors. Recurrent disease requires an array of management techniques including antibiotic therapy, in-office treatments, and revision surgery ranging from revision sphenoidotomies to sphenoid nasalization in the most recalcitrant cases [20].

Conclusion

The sphenoid sinus displays a wide anatomic variance secondary to variable degree of pneumatization that can be directly affected by sinonasal pathology. This array of pneumatization significantly affects the osseous covering of the adjacent neurovascular structures, namely, the optic nerves and cavernous segments of the internal carotid arteries, which must be identified for safe surgical manipulation in this region. Understanding these key anatomic features allows surgical management of an array of extracranial and intracranial pathology in the region. Careful preoperative clinical and radiographic examinations significantly aid the surgical approach and allow the surgeon to be proactive rather than reactive when addressing the region.

References

1. Vidic B. The postnatal development of the sphenoidal sinus and its spread into the dorsum sellae and posterior clinoid processes. Am J Roentgenol Radium Ther Nucl Med. 1968;104(1):177–83.
2. Kennedy DW, Hwang PH. Rhinology: diseases of the nose, sinuses, and skull base. 1st ed. New York: Thieme Medical Publishers, Inc.; 2012.
3. Shah RK, Dhingra JK, Carter BL, Rebeiz EE. Paranasal sinus development: a radiographic study. Laryngoscope. 2003;113(2):205–9.
4. Hamberger CA, Hammer G, Norlen G, Sjogren B. Transantrosphenoidal hypophysectomy. Arch Otolaryngol. 1961;74:2–8.
5. Hamid O, El Fiky L, Hassan O, El Fiky S. Anatomic variations of the sphenoid sinus and their impact on trans-sphenoid pituitary surgery. Skull Base. 2008;18(1):9–15.
6. Rhoton Jr AL. The sellar region. Neurosurgery. 2002;51(1):335–74.
7. Kennedy DW, Zinreich SJ, Hassab MJ. The internal carotid artery as it relates to endonasal sphenoethmoidectomy. Am J Rhinol. 1990;4(1):7–12.
8. Batra PS, Citardi MJ, Gallivan RP, Roh HJ, Lanza DC. Software-enabled computed tomography analysis of the carotid artery and sphenoid sinus pneumatization patterns. Am J Rhinol. 2004;18(4):203–8.
9. Woodworth BA, Ahn C, Flume PA, Schlosser RJ. The delta F508 mutation in cystic fibrosis and impact on sinus development. Am J Rhinol. 2007;21(1):122–7.
10. Shetty PG, Shroff MM, Fatterpekar G, Sahani DV, Kirtane MV. A retrospective analysis of spontaneous sphenoid sinus fistula: MR and CT findings. AJNR Am J Neuroradiol. 2000;21(2):337–42.
11. Illing E, Schlosser RJ, Palmer JN, Cure J, Fox N, Woodworth BA. Spontaneous sphenoid lateral recess cerebrospinal fluid leaks arise from intracranial hypertension, not Sternberg's canal. Int Forum Allergy Rhinol. 2014;4:246–50.
12. Stammberger HR, Kennedy DW. Paranasal sinuses: anatomic terminology and nomenclature. The Anatomic Terminology Group. Ann Otol Rhinol Laryngol Suppl. 1995;167:7–16.
13. Onodi A. The optic nerve and the accessory sinuses of the nose. New York: William Wood & Co; 1910.
14. Lore JM, Medina JE. An atlas of head & neck surgery. 4th ed. Philadelphia: Elsevier Saunders; 2005.
15. Bolger WE, Keyes AS, Lanza DC. Use of the superior meatus and superior turbinate in the endoscopic approach to the sphenoid sinus. Otolaryngol Head Neck Surg. 1999;120(3): 308–13.
16. Teatini G, Simonetti G, Masala W, Decola GL. Computed tomography of the ethmoid labyrinth and adjacent structures. Ann Otol Rhinol Laryngol. 1987;96(3 pt 1):239–50.
17. Bansberg SF, Harmer SG, Forbes G. Relationship of the optic nerve to the paranasal sinuses as shown by computed tomography. Otolaryngol Head Neck Surg. 1987;96(4):331–5.
18. Dessi P, Moulin G, Castro F, et al. Protrusion of the optic nerve into the ethmoid and sphenoid sinus: prospective study of 150 CT studies. Neuroradiology. 1994;36:515–6.
19. Han JK, Becker SS, Bomeli SR, et al. Endoscopic localization of the anterior and posterior ethmoid arteries. Ann Otol Rhinol Laryngol. 2008;117:931–5.
20. Moeller CW, Welch KC. Prevention and management of complications of sphenoidotomy. Otolaryngol Clin North Am. 2010;43(4):839–54.
21. Soudry E, Turner JH, Nayak JV, Hwang PH. Endoscopic reconstruction of surgically created skull base defects: a systematic review. Otolaryngol Head Neck Surg. 2014;150(5):730–8.

Surgery for Nasal Polyposis

28

Joseph Brunworth and Peter John Wormald

Key Take-Home Points

- Although nasal polyposis in the setting of chronic rhinosinusitis (CRS) is a challenging disease process due to its higher rate of disease recurrence, research suggests that a few key surgical decisions and a more aggressive approach may help decrease the return of symptoms and rate of polyp recurrence [1–3].
- Even though a functional approach may be appropriate for straightforward osteomeatal complex obstruction and can be addressed with limited surgery (uncinectomy, maxillary antrostomy, restoration of adequate ventilation) [4, 5], a subset of patients including asthmatics and patients with eosinophilia, chronic rhinosinusitis with nasal polyposis, fungal sinusitis, a narrow frontal recess, and Samter's triad will require more extensive surgery [1].
- The mixture of polyps and mucin within the sinuses harbors large numbers of activated eosinophils and contributes to disease load. If these are not removed and persist within the sinuses, the capacity for rapid disease recurrence remains, and another exposure of the activating antigen can result in reactivation of the inflammatory cascade and result in significant disease recurrence.

J. Brunworth, MD
Department of Otolaryngology, St. Louis University Hospital,
6th Floor, Desloge Towers, 3635 Vista Avenue, St. Louis, MO 63110, USA
e-mail: brunworth@slu.edu

P.J. Wormald, FRACS, FCS(SA), FRCS(Ed), MD (✉)
Department of Otolaryngology – Head and Neck Surgery, University of Adelaide,
The Queen Elizabeth Hospital, 28 Woodville Road, Woodville, SA 5011, Australia
e-mail: peterj.wormald@adelaide.edu.au

P.S. Batra, J.K. Han (eds.), *Practical Medical and Surgical Management of Chronic Rhinosinusitis*, DOI 10.1007/978-3-319-16724-4_28

- The rate of polyp recurrence has been shown to be additive with the number of predisposing factors for recurrence [1] (e.g., a patient with a narrow anterior-posterior (AP) frontal diameter, a history of asthma, eosinophilic allergic fungal sinusitis, *plus* aspirin sensitivity). It is in these patients with multiple risk factors that the modified endoscopic Lothrop/Draf III procedure is an option to decrease the chance for polyp recurrence and the need for further surgery [1, 6].
- At this point in time, it is not currently recommended to perform primary frontal drill-outs on patients who have not had prior standard functional endoscopic sinus surgery (ESS). The current recommendation is to counsel patients with multiple predisposing factors about their increased chance of requiring future surgery, including the potential need for a frontal drill-out procedure.

Introduction

Nasal polyposis is a common disease that has a prevalence of 1–4 % of the population [7–9]. The pathogenesis of nasal polyps is poorly understood [10–13]. This distinctive disease process is now known to affect more than just primates, affecting other animals such as cats and even koalas [14, 15]. The nasal mucosa can exhibit a spectrum of disease ranging from edematous to polypoid to frank polyps, thus contributing to the difficulty in the research of this disease process [16, 17].

Surgery for nasal polyposis is perhaps one of the most challenging yet rewarding procedures performed by the otolaryngologist. Surgical difficulty is amplified by the increased rate of bleeding encountered during surgery, the thinning of the lamina papyracea due to expansion from the polyps, the obstructed view of the frontal recess during its dissection, and the propensity for polyps to distort anatomy near vital neurological and vascular structures [18]. However, the immediate relief of nasal obstruction with a high level of appreciation and increased quality of life found in most patients postoperatively accounts for the rewarding aspect of this surgery [19, 20].

The severity of nasal polyposis varies vastly from patient to patient. Although several attempts have been made to categorize polyps, their variability makes classification and grading a challenge [21]. The mucosa can exhibit a spectrum of disease ranging from edematous to true polyps even within the same nasal cavity. In addition, postoperative changes often mimic polyps in the initial healing phase after sinus surgery. In our research, we found it is important to differentiate between those who exhibited recurrent polyps that resolved on medical treatment and medically resistant recurrent polyps, because the latter group had a higher risk of ultimately requiring further surgical intervention [2].

Once a patient has been diagnosed with nasal polyps and other disease processes have been ruled out, a systematic investigation into the pathogenesis of the patient's disease is undertaken. A standard workup should include a complete history with a focus on past medical history (seasonal allergies, sinusitis, asthma, aspirin or non-steroidal anti-inflammatory [NSAID] sensitivity), sinus symptoms, family history (primary ciliary dyskinesia, cystic fibrosis, etc.), social history (smoking, environmental exposures), and prior therapies. Blood tests can help elucidate patients with high concentrations of eosinophils. Patient-specific allergens can be detected via immunoassay tests. Patients found to have specific allergens may benefit from additional skin allergy testing for higher sensitivity and specificity.

After a complete workup, a patient should be given options for his or her choice of treatment. In general, a trial of medical therapy is attempted prior to the decision to proceed with surgery. A portion of patients with minimal polyp disease will respond to medical therapy alone, while others may respond to surgery alone or surgery with continued medical therapy. Due to the fact that the pathogenesis of polyp disease is still incompletely known, it is important to counsel patients in regard to the long-term therapy for nasal polyposis and to dispel the preconceived notion that a single surgery will be curative.

Surgical Anatomy

In most patients with nasal polyposis, the nasal cavity is either partially or completely filled with polyps (Fig. 28.1). After decongestion and infiltration of the lateral nasal wall, the polyps are removed to reveal the underlying anatomy. A microdebrider is used to remove all the polypoid tissue from the middle turbinate with preservation of the turbinate itself. In previously unoperated patients, polyps from the middle meatus are debrided to expose the underlying uncinate and bulla

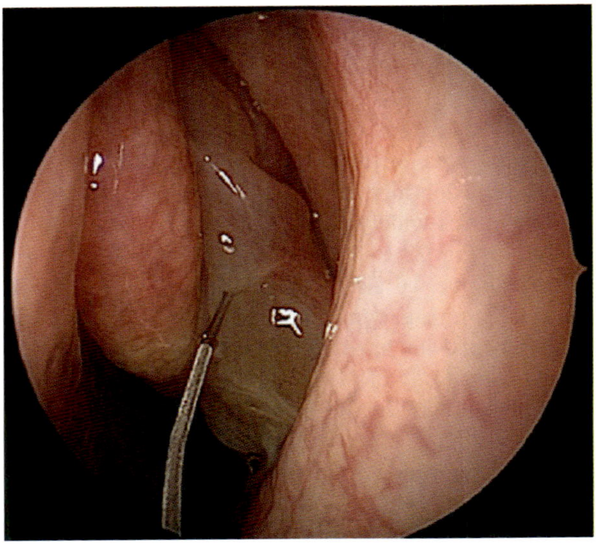

Fig. 28.1 Left nasal cavity showing polyp filling the middle meatus. In this revision case, residual uncinate is seen lateral to the polyp and must be addressed

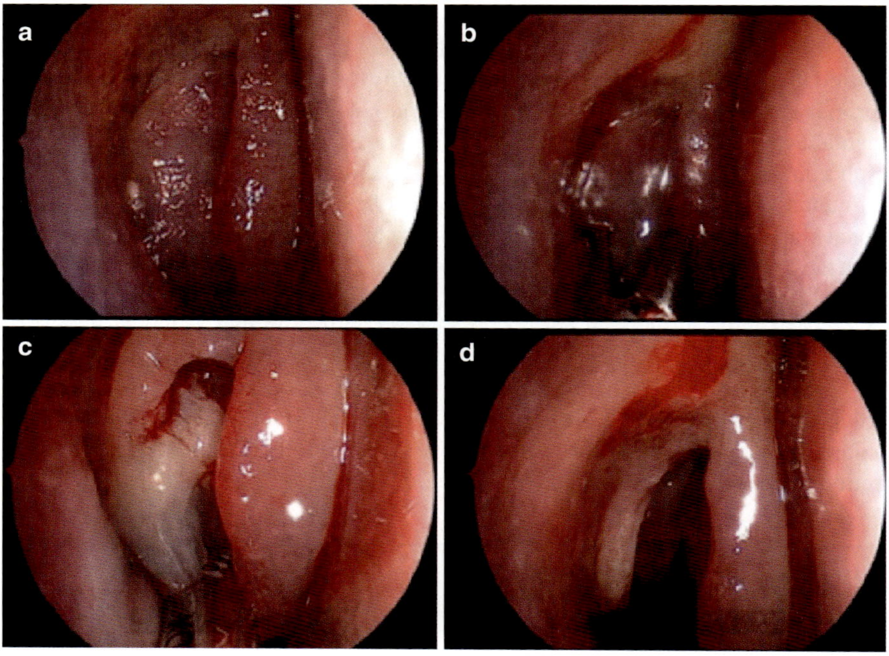

Fig. 28.2 Progression of surgery for polyps. (**a**) Polyps in the middle meatus. (**b**) Representative piece taken for histology. (**c**) Microdebrider usage. (**d**) Exposed uncinate and bulla ethmoidalis. The remainder of the surgery is carried out in the same manner as non-polyp patients

ethmoidalis (Fig. 28.2). The surgery is now conducted as if the patient did not have polyps and the anatomy is dealt with in the same way as patients without polyps. In patients who have had previous surgery, normal anatomical landmarks are often absent or obscured and surgery is conducted by first finding the most consistent landmarks. In these cases, the safest method is to start posteriorly and proceed along the skull base into the frontal sinus. First, the polyps are debrided and the middle turbinate or its remnant is identified. Next the posterior choanae are identified and the debrider is moved up the anterior face of the sphenoid until the sphenoid ostium is widely opened. This is continued superiorly until the skull base is identified (Fig. 28.3). Next, the skull base is followed anteriorly to the region of the anterior ethmoidal artery and the frontal ostium is identified and the entire skull base and lamina papyracea are cleared (Fig. 28.4).

In patients who have not previously undergone surgery, the easiest way to understand the anatomy of the frontal drainage pathway is to perform a careful analysis of the CT scans, identify each individual cell, and place them in their anatomical location so that a 3D conceptualization of the anatomy is achieved [18]. In general, cells that lie anterior to the drainage pathway are considered frontal ethmoidal cells, starting with the most anterior ethmoid air cell, the agger nasi. Cells posterior to the drainage pathway are typically suprabullar cells, and if they extend into the frontal sinus, they are denoted as frontal bullar cells.

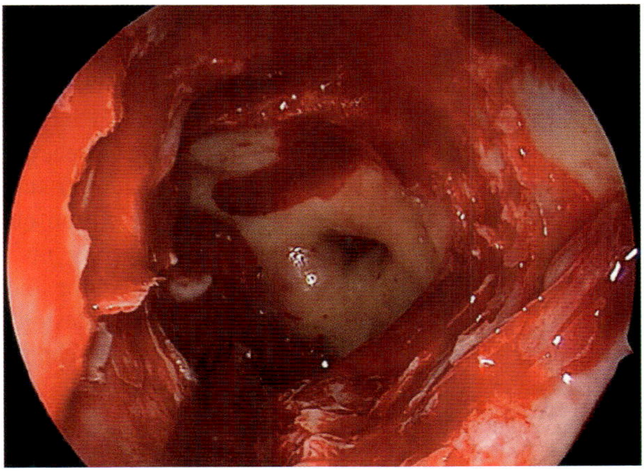

Fig. 28.3 Wide left sphenoidotomy showing the optico-carotid recess posterolaterally, skull base superiorly, and orbit laterally

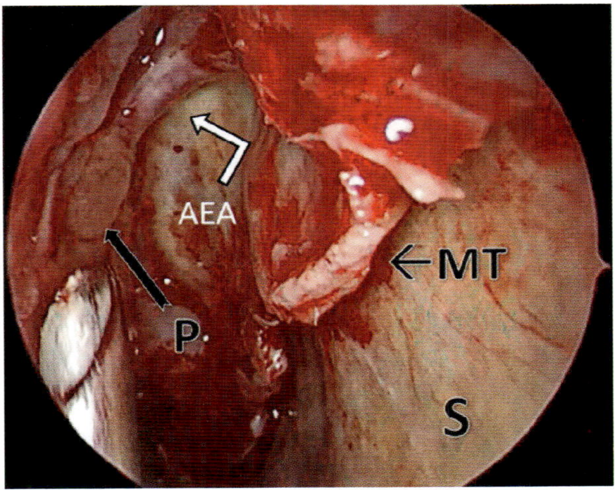

Fig. 28.4 Revision ESS for polyps requiring an aggressive approach. Picture shows the suction curette approaching the polypoid tissue (*P*) near the anterior ethmoidal artery (*AEA*) that lies on a mesentery along the skull base. This case required a frontal drill-out as well as trimming of the middle turbinate (*MT*). The septum (*S*) is marked for reference

Upon passing the axilla of the middle turbinate, the most commonly encountered drainage pathway is located posterior and medial to the agger nasi/frontal ethmoid cells. However, certain predisposing factors may cause the drainage pathway to run anterior or lateral such as an intersinus septal cell. In the case of polyps, the bony divisions on the preoperative CT scan can be difficult to discern and must be looked at with caution.

Indications

Indications to proceed with surgery for nasal polyposis are largely dependent on patient symptoms, the two most common symptoms being nasal airway obstruction and loss of the sense of smell. Other symptoms may include allergic symptoms (sneezing, ocular/nasal pruritus, rhinorrhea, etc.), recurrent bouts of sinusitis (colored nasal discharge, fevers, facial pain, etc.), or even a change in voice due to decreased resonance in the nasal airway. It is important to discuss the chronic nature of the disease with the patient. Although many of the symptoms that affect the patient may be improved by surgery, patients need to know the limitations of surgery. For example, nasal allergic symptoms and reactions to environmental triggers usually require ongoing medical management after surgery.

Although symptoms of polyp disease are often quite specific, there are some important exceptions to consider when working up a patient with polyps. Any patient with unilateral polyp disease should be biopsied to rule out papilloma, other benign tumors, or malignancy. Any suspicious lesion on endoscopy, a lesion that has a tendency to bleed, a polyp that does not respond to steroids, any expansile lesion seen clinically or radiographically, and especially any nasal mass that appears erosive or invasive also warrant a biopsy. If the clinical picture suggests a highly vascular tumor or an encephalocele, in-office biopsies are avoided and further workup is performed.

Once a patient is diagnosed with nasal polyps, a trial of maximal medical therapy is typically warranted prior to considering surgery. However, it has been increasingly recognized that patients with massive nasal polyps will have only short-term temporary relief [22], and the risks and benefits of offering a course of systemic steroids versus going straight to surgery need to be discussed with the patient. Initial treatment of polyps is often successful in reducing patient symptoms, but the frustration lies in the tendency for polyps to recur. Although systemic steroids are effective in reducing the size of polyps and improving symptoms, these medications have significant side effects, especially with long-term use. Recent research has looked at the risk-benefit of repeated steroid usage and found that the risks of steroid use start to outweigh the benefits once the steroids are used more than twice a year [23]. The most essential consideration in all patients is the importance of discussing the risks, benefits, and alternatives to the surgery so that expectations are fully anticipated and aligned with realistic goals.

Preoperative CT scans where surgery for nasal polyposis is to be performed are essential. However, the universal use of image guidance during polyp surgery is not an absolute and generally varies according to surgeon preference and image-guidance availability. Patients whose biopsy results show anything other than typical inflammatory polyposis will generally require an MRI and further workup prior to surgery, and their treatment will vary depending on the diagnosis.

Surgical Technique

For many centuries, nasal polyps have been written about, and records reflect the various attempts that have been made to eradicate them [24]. In the 1970s Messerklinger introduced the concept of nasal endoscopy [25, 26] followed by Stammberger's adaptation in the 1980s, popularizing a more functional approach to the sinuses [27–29]. Stammberger's technique is based on limited tissue resection with the aim of reestablishing the natural drainage pathways of the sinuses. It has

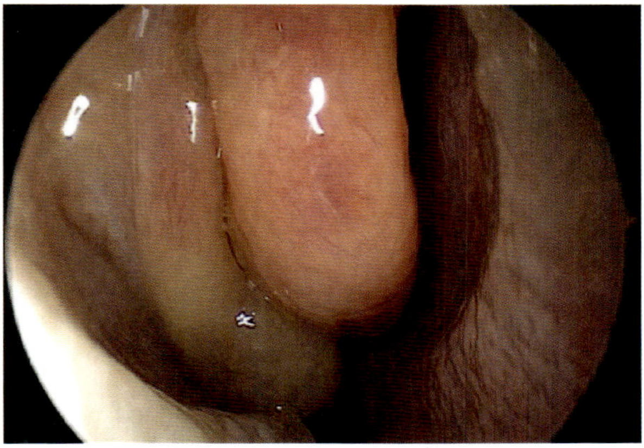

Fig. 28.5 Caution must be taken in polyp cases as the anatomy may initially be distorted. In this right nasal cavity, the uncinate process is retroflexed as well as polypoid

been shown to be effective in CRS patients but appears to be less effective in patients with a high disease load. In this patient group, usually defined as a Lund and MacKay score of more than 12 out of 24, a more radical approach has been shown to be more effective in reducing polyp recurrence. Inflammatory disease load is comprised of polyps and surrounding mucus. It is often thick, tenacious, and difficult to clear from the sinuses. The polyps have activated eosinophils that, if remain after surgery, quickly reactivate the inflammatory cascade and result in disease recurrence. The mucus, in turn, has bacteria often in the form of biofilms and may have superantigen producing *Staphylococcus aureus*. In subgroups of polyp patients, fungal elements promote inflammatory stimulation of the mucosa. These patients exhibit a high incidence of disease recurrence should the fungal mucus not be removed at the time of surgery.

Upon commencing surgery, the initial step is to take a representative polyp from each side and send this for histology. The microdebrider is then used to remove the intranasal polyps and delineate the middle turbinate and the uncinate process. Due to tendency of nasal polyps to compress nearby structures, the uncinate process is carefully assessed as it may be paper-thin and plastered against the orbit or it may be retroflexed upon itself (Fig. 28.5). A sickle knife is used to cut the upper region of the uncinate while a backbiter frees the inferior portion and a "swing-door" technique is used to finish the uncinectomy (a ball probe is used to fracture the uncinate forward; then a 45° through-biting forceps is used to remove the mobilized uncinate flush with its insertion on the frontal process of the maxilla).

Once an uncinectomy has been preformed, a 30° scope with a curved suction and right-angled ball probe is used to identify the natural ostium of the maxillary sinus. The ostium is enlarged into the posterior fontanelle and a 70° scope is used to assess the sinus for disease. In the author's hands, a fully diseased maxillary sinus with polyps throughout the sinus is best approached with a canine fossa trephination rather than a mega antrostomy in order to reach the anterior medial and lateral walls of the sinus. This allows for an efficient and thorough clearance of the maxillary sinus with effective, long-standing postoperative results [30]. The incidence of lip and teeth numbness if the correct landmarks are used for this procedure is around 3 % after 6 months. The landmark for canine fossa trephine is the mid-pupillary line and the floor of the nose.

The approach to the frontal sinus varies from surgeon to surgeon. In a previously unoperated patient, utilizing the axillary flap through the front face of the agger nasi cell allows a direct approach with good visualization while still predominately using the zero degree endoscope. Once the agger nasi and frontal ethmoidal cells have been removed, the pathway to the frontal sinus is cleared using a combination of angled instruments (giraffes, frontal punches, angled microdebriders, etc.) and angled scopes. All polyps are removed, the mucosa is trimmed but not stripped, and all partitions of the frontal recess are removed to ensure the maximal aperture of the frontal sinus.

Next the bulla ethmoidalis is opened and polyps are removed. The orbital wall is delineated with all partitions and polypoid mucosa trimmed down until flush with the lamina papyracea. Again, frequent palpation of the globe and careful attention is paid to the fact that the already thin lamina may be dehiscent in the case of polyps. The middle turbinate basal lamella is then opened medially at the junction of the horizontal and vertical portions of the lamella. An additional landmark is the level of the maxillary roof. The posterior ethmoids are visualized along with the superior turbinate, which will be in a medial and superior position. The inferior third of the superior turbinate is removed, thus exposing the sphenoid sinus natural ostium. Often polyps will need to be removed from the posterior nasal cavity inferior to the superior turbinate and even medial to the middle turbinate. Caution is taken to avoid the cribriform plate any time while working medially and superior in the nose. Next the sphenoid sinus is opened widely from the skull base to the level of the posterior septal artery. If the artery is transected, then suction cautery is used to achieve hemostasis. Polyps are removed from within the sphenoid sinus; powered instrumentation use is avoided within the sphenoid sinus near the optic nerve or internal carotid artery.

Traversing along the skull base from the sphenoid sinus toward the frontal sinus, the final partitions of the ethmoidal complex are removed, leaving mucosa on the roof while ensuring that all cells are open and the polyps are trimmed down to within approximately 1–2 mm of the bone. Caution is taken to identify and avoid the anterior ethmoidal artery should it be on a mesentery (Fig. 28.4) and therefore at risk for transection. The frontal recess and frontal ostium are again checked and cleared of any remaining polypoid tissue with maximization of the frontal ostium.

In patients in whom polyps recur, this is usually first seen in the frontal ostium/recess before the polyps and then spreads to the ethmoids. Why the recurrences start in this region and whether the narrow frontal ostial region predisposes to polyp formation are still unclear. In patients who have had a complete ESS with clearance of all polyps and ostia and who develop a recurrence, a modified Lothrop/Draf III or frontal drill-out may be required. This starts with complete clearance of all the other sinuses and a trimming of the lower half of the middle turbinate. This creates a much improved ventilation and topical therapy access to the posterior ethmoids and sphenoid region. Next the frontal drill-out is done. This creates a large common frontal ostium and allows effective topical application of steroids in the postoperative period. It improves the ventilation to the frontal region and, in a survey of outcomes from our department [2], has proved to be highly effective in reducing the incidence of polyp recurrence postoperatively. The frontal drill-out starts with a septal window with the posterior margin of the window formed by the anterior ends of the middle turbinates. The lower border of the window should allow an instrument to be passed from one side of the nose across the septum and under the axilla of the middle turbinate on the opposite side. The anterior margin is taken anteriorly until the frontal process of the maxilla anterior to the uncinate can be seen with an endoscope passed through the septal window via the opposite nostril. The upper rim of the window is taken onto the roof of the nose. Next, the frontal sinus mini-trephines are placed and fluorescein-stained saline is injected into the frontal sinuses so that the fluorescein can be seen draining through the natural frontal sinus ostium. This gives the surgeon the posterior landmark for the surgery. The drill is always kept anterior to the fluorescein. Drilling starts on the frontal process of the maxilla and progresses laterally until the skin is exposed giving the surgeon the lateral landmark. Drilling proceeds superiorly (not medially) until the floor of the frontal sinus is opened. This is done bilaterally; then the first olfactory neuron is identified determining the anterior projection of the skull base. This is confirmed with image guidance. The intersinus septum is taken down and the frontal "T" drilled back onto the skull base. An angled bur is used to take the superior edge of the neo-ostium away until the anterior wall of the frontal sinus runs smoothly out into the nose (Fig. 28.6).

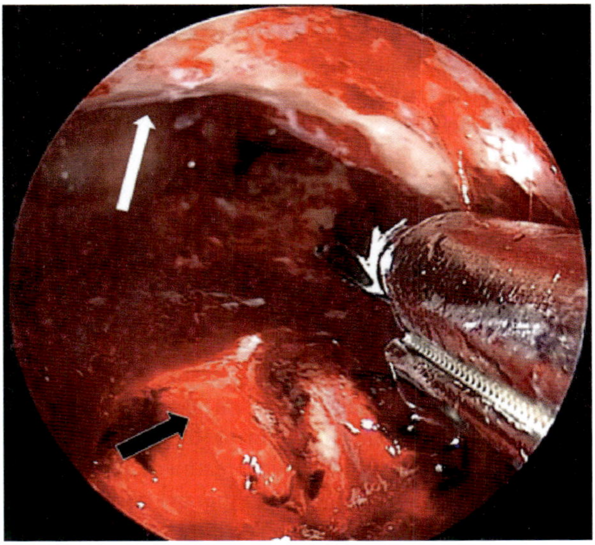

Fig. 28.6 Frontal drill-out being performed utilizing a high-speed 3 mm angled bur to ensure the frontal sinus drains smoothly into the nose (*white arrow*). The maximum anterior-posterior (AP) diameter is achieved by drilling the frontal "T" (*black arrow*) down to the anterior projection of the cribriform plate

In a study looking specifically at the recurrence rate of polyps after frontal sinus drill-out (Draf III) procedure compared to standard ESS with a Draf IIa frontal sinusotomy, the Draf III patients required significantly less revision surgeries [2]. This was even more evident in asthma and aspirin-intolerant patients. The overall revision rate was 18 % (follow-up duration >12 months, median = 29 months), with a 37 % revision rate in the ESS group versus 7 % in the Draf III group ($P < .001$). Survival analysis showed that the Draf III significantly reduced the risk of revision (hazard ratio = 0.258, $P = .0026$). We postulate that the more aggressive surgical approach to nasal polyps tends to maximize ostia size, clear the sinuses of the inflammatory load, and allow postoperative topical medications to reach all aspects of the sinuses and therefore reduce the incidence of polyp recurrence.

Complications

Before discussing iatrogenic complications of surgery for polyp disease, a brief overview of the possible complications that can arise from the polyps themselves is warranted and should also be discussed with patients. Left untreated, polyps have a wide range of natural growth patterns. In rare cases, polyps may resolve spontaneously. In other cases, polyps might grow to a certain size and remain stable; symptoms such as nasal blockage, rhinorrhea, postnasal drip, and hyposmia/anosmia may persist. However, in cases of more aggressive polyposis, more serious complications may arise. Firstly, polyps may grow large enough to block sinus outflow pathways and promote bacterial and fungal growth, thus leading to infectious sinusitis. Obstruction of sinus ostia may lead to mucocele formation with subsequent erosion of the orbit and/or skull base. Secondly, polyps may enlarge enough to cause complete bilateral nasal airway obstruction and even protrude from the nostrils. Lastly, benign nasal polyposis may also exhibit an aggressive growth pattern causing orbital violation or penetration into the skull base.

Alternatives to surgery should be discussed with patients as well. The most efficacious oral medications for treating nasal polyps, corticosteroids [31, 32], are fraught with side effects and occasionally cause permanent sequelae [33, 34]. Probably the most worrisome complication with enduring ramifications from corticosteroid usage is avascular necrosis of the hip joint. Although this has a known risk of 9–40 % when long-term therapy is needed, avascular necrosis is limited to case reports when used in 0.5 mg/kg doses for short-term treatment (less than 3 weeks) and is primarily found after intravenous usage [35–37]. In fact, in a survey by Madanagopal et al. of over 600 orthopedic physicians prescribing oral steroids, no cases of avascular necrosis were reported over a 2-year period [38]. Regardless, a brief discussion of the risks of steroids, antibiotics, or other medications used for treating nasal polyp patients should be included during the office visit. Considering the tendency for polyps to recur, a multimodality treatment approach is often necessary, and reviewing the risks and benefits of each therapy becomes essential (Table 28.1).

Despite a large percentage of patients having a temporary response to medical therapy, many will require surgery due to persistence of nasal polyposis.

Table 28.1 Risks of surgery, corticosteroids, or no intervention for nasal polyps

Surgery	Corticosteroids	No intervention
Visual impairment Blindness Vascular injury Death CSF leak Meningitis Anosmia Epiphora Need for further surgery Synechiae Return of polyps	Psychosis Insomnia Mood swings Nightmares Reflux/gastric ulcers Weight gain Moon facies/buffalo hump Avascular hip necrosis Increased blood sugars Immunosuppression Cataract development Temporary relief only	Continued nasal obstruction Worsening of nasal obstruction Anosmia Orbital extension Intracranial extension Sinus obstruction/infection Protrusion of polyps from nose

Table 28.2 Important predisposing risk factors for more common complications seen during surgery for nasal polyps [39, 55]

Complication	Predisposing factors
Violation of lamina papyracea (2 %)	Maxillary sinus hypoplasia (4 %) Ethmoid sinus hypoplasia (10 %) Laterally positioned natural ostium of maxillary sinus Dehiscence of lamina (0.5 %)
Bleeding (5 %)	History of bleeding disorder or tendency to bleed easily Pharmacological effects (i.e., platelet inhibitors, vitamin K antagonists, nonsteroidal anti-inflammatories, herbal medications) Polyp disease
Skull base violation (0.2–0.8 %)	Low riding ethmoid roof Asymmetry of ethmoid roof Deep cribriform plate Thin skull base bone density

Because of the tendency for polyps to distort nasal anatomy, utmost precaution must be taken during surgery for nasal polyposis. Although major complications are rare, their consequences can be permanent, devastating, and even lethal.

The types of complications encountered during surgery for nasal polyposis are analogous to those seen during other endoscopic sinus surgeries and have been written about extensively [39–45]. Bleeding may be as simple as a minor ooze during the surgery, can substantiate a blood transfusion, or can be as devastating as a carotid injury [46–48]. Orbital complications range from exposure of orbital fat exposure to blindness or permanent diplopia [49–52]. Intracranial penetration may entail an intraoperative repair of a CSF leak or can lead to extensive postoperative intracranial complications [53, 54].

In their review from 2013, Hosemann and Draf [39] quoted an overall minor complication rate of 5 % and major complication rate of 0.5–1 % during all routine endoscopic interventions. Certain predisposing factors may result in increased risk of particular complications (Table 28.2).

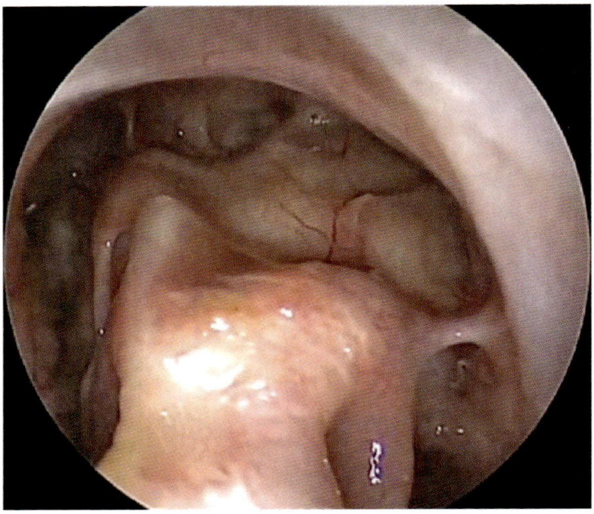

Fig. 28.7 Postoperative view of the frontal sinus 9 months after an endoscopic frontal drill-out for recurrent nasal polyps has been performed

Clinical Efficacy Data

The short- and long-term clinical efficacy of sinus surgery for adult chronic rhinosinusitis with and without nasal polyposis has been demonstrated in multiple reviews of the literature. Poetker et al. showed that significant improvements in patient-reported symptoms, quality-of-life surveys, endoscopy scores, medication use, and financial impact were found consistently throughout the literature across multiple institutions [56]. The data for nasal polyp surgery also shows significant improvements across multiple subjective and objective measures [19, 20, 57]. However, it is also well established that the recurrence rate for polyps is significantly higher than other forms of sinusitis, especially in the patients mentioned above with Samter's triad or similar predisposing conditions [58, 59]. In our review of 338 consecutive polyp patients [2], the incidence of a polyp recurring in the total cohort of all patients who were followed up for >12 months was 44.3 %. The incidence of polyp recurrence that persisted despite medical treatment for at least 3 months or more was significantly less, with 19.8 % in those followed up 6 months or longer and 22.7 % for those followed up 12 months or longer. When comparing the rate of polyp recurrence after standard ESS plus a Draf IIa (49 %) versus a Draf III procedure (36 %), the rate was found to be significantly less in those patients who underwent the Draf III (49 % vs 36 %). It is apparent that, although surgery for nasal polyposis is considered "non-curative" [60], the reduction of disease load in these patients appears to significantly affect the rate of recurrence and revision surgery (Fig. 28.7).

Conclusion

Surgery for nasal polyposis has proven to be an effective tool for improving patient symptoms as well as various other objective measures of success.

However, it does not always offer a cure for this chronic condition and many patients require multiple operations as well as continuation of additional treatment modalities. Patients that have a higher risk for recurrence include those with asthma, aspirin sensitivity, allergic fungal sinusitis, eosinophilia, narrowed frontal ostia (provided the polyp disease affects this region), or any combination of these factors. In these patients with a high likelihood of failure, a more aggressive surgery with complete clearance of all partitions from the sphenoid to the frontal outflow path, wide antrostomies, removal of all polyps, and trimming of the polypoid tissue to reduce inflammatory load has shown to improve results.

Sinus surgery, as an adjunct to medical therapy and allergy control or desensitization, has the potential to significantly improve the quality of life in patients with nasal polyposis. This is counterbalanced by the risks incurred during any of the aforementioned treatment options, and a thorough discussion is required with each patient in order to ensure patient understanding.

Considering the tendency for polyps to promote the harboring of bacteria, mucin, fungus, and eosinophils, we conclude that the wide clearance of sinus wall partitions and concurrent clearance of the polypoid tissue are of utmost importance. A total sphenoethmoidectomy, wide maxillary antrostomy (with canine fossa trephination when necessary), and wide access frontal clearance (Draf IIa) are performed as an initial procedure for polyp patients with subsequent Draf III reserved for revision cases with persistent polyp disease and symptoms. In this manner we can most efficiently provide access for delivery of postoperative topical medications and reduce the risk of polyp recurrence.

References

1. Naidoo Y, Bassiouni A, Keen M, Wormald PJ. Risk factors and outcomes for primary, revision, and modified Lothrop (Draf III) frontal sinus surgery. Int Forum Allergy Rhinol. 2013;3(5): 412–7.
2. Bassiouni A, Wormald PJ. Role of frontal sinus surgery in nasal polyp recurrence. Laryngoscope. 2013;123(1):36–41.
3. Bassiouni A, Naidoo Y, Wormald PJ. When FESS fails: the inflammatory load hypothesis in refractory chronic rhinosinusitis. Laryngoscope. 2012;122(2):460–6.
4. Stammberger H. Nasal and paranasal sinus endoscopy. A diagnostic and surgical approach to recurrent sinusitis. Endoscopy. 1986;18(6):213–8.
5. Stammberger H. Surgical treatment of nasal polyps: past, present, and future. Allergy. 1999;54 Suppl 53:7–11.
6. Gross WE, Gross CW, Becker D, Moore D, Phillips D. Modified transnasal endoscopic Lothrop procedure as an alternative to frontal sinus obliteration. Otolaryngol Head Neck Surg. 1995;113:427–34.
7. Settipane RA, Peters AT, Chiu AG. Chapter 6: Nasal polyps. Am J Rhinol Allergy. 2013;27 Suppl 1:S20–5.
8. Chaaban MR, Walsh EM, Woodworth BA. Epidemiology and differential diagnosis of nasal polyps. Am J Rhinol Allergy. 2013;27(6):473–8.
9. Rajguru R. Nasal polyposis: current trends. Indian J Otolaryngol Head Neck Surg. 2014;66 Suppl 1:16–21.
10. Bernstein JM, Gorfien J, Noble B. Role of allergy in nasal polyposis: a review. Otolaryngol Head Neck Surg. 1995;113(6):724–32.

11. Tos M, Sasaki Y, Ohnishi M, Larsen P, Drake-Lee AB. Fireside conference 2. Pathogenesis of nasal polyps. Rhinol Suppl. 1992;14:181–5.
12. Casale M, Pappacena M, Potena M, Vesperini E, Ciglia G, Mladina R, Dianzani C, Degener AM, Salvinelli F. Nasal polyposis: from pathogenesis to treatment, an update. Inflamm Allergy Drug Targets. 2011;10(3):158–63.
13. Van Cauwenberge P, Gevaert P, Van Hoecke H, Van Zele T, Bachert C. New insights into the pathology of nasal polyposis: the role of superantigens and IgE. Verh K Acad Geneeskd Belg. 2005;67(1):5–28; discussion 29–32.
14. Galler A, Shibly S, Bilek A, Hirt R. Chronic diseases of the nose and nasal sinuses in cats: a retrospective study. Schweiz Arch Tierheilkd. 2012;154(5):209–16.
15. Bercier M, Wynne J, Klause S, Stadler CK, Gorow A, Pye GW. Nasal mass removal in the koala (Phascolarctos cinereus). J Zoo Wildl Med. 2012;43(4):898–908.
16. Rizk HG, Ferguson BJ. Categorizing nasal polyps by severity and controller therapy. Arch Otolaryngol Head Neck Surg. 2012;138(9):846–53.
17. Czerny MS, Namin A, Gratton MA, Antisdel JL. Histopathological and clinical analysis of chronic rhinosinusitis by subtype. Int Forum Allergy Rhinol. 2014;4:463–9.
18. Wormald PJ. Endoscopic sinus surgery – anatomy, three-dimensional reconstruction, and surgical technique. 3rd ed. New York: Thieme; 2012.
19. Khademi B, Gandomi B, Tarzi M, Yeganeh F. Quality of life, pulmonary spirometry, and dosage of steroid in asthmatic patients with polyposis after endoscopic sinus surgery. Iran J Otorhinolaryngol. 2013;25(71):103–6.
20. Dufour X, Bedier A, Ferrie JC, Gohler C, Klossek JM. Diffuse nasal polyposis and endonasal endoscopic surgery: long-term results, a 65-case study. Laryngoscope. 2004;114(11):1982–7.
21. Durr ML, Pletcher SD, Goldberg AN, Murr AH. A novel sinonasal endoscopy scoring system: the discharge, inflammation, and polyps/edema (DIP) score. Int Forum Allergy Rhinol. 2013;3(1):66–72.
22. Van Zele T, Gevaert P, Holtappels G, Beule A, Wormald PJ, Mayr S, Hens G, Hellings P, Ebbens FA, Fokkens W, Van Cauwenberge P, Bachert C. Oral steroids and doxycycline: two different approaches to treat nasal polyps. J Allergy Clin Immunol. 2010;125(5):1069–1076.e4.
23. Leung RM, Dinnie K, Smith TL. When do the risks of repeated courses of corticosteroids exceed the risks of surgery? Int Forum Allergy Rhinol. 2014;4:871–6.
24. Wright J. History of laryngology and rhinology. St Louis: Lea and Febiger; 1893. p. 57–9.
25. Messerklinger W. Endoscopy of the nose. Monatsschr Ohrenheilkd Laryngorhinol. 1970;104(10):451–6.
26. Messerklinger W. Techniques and possibilities of nasal endoscopy. HNO. 1972;20(5):133–5.
27. Stammberger H. Endoscopic endonasal surgery–concepts in treatment of recurring rhinosinusitis. Part I. Anatomic and pathophysiologic considerations. Otolaryngol Head Neck Surg. 1986;94(2):143–7.
28. Stammberger H. Personal endoscopic operative technic for the lateral nasal wall–an endoscopic surgery concept in the treatment of inflammatory diseases of the paranasal sinuses. Laryngol Rhinol Otol (Stuttg). 1985;64(11):559–66.
29. Tos M, Drake-Lee AB, Lund VJ, Stammberger H. Treatment of nasal polyps–medication or surgery and which technique. Rhinol Suppl. 1989;8:45–9.
30. Seiberling KA, Church CA, Tewfik M, Foreman A, Chang D, Ghostine M, Wormald PJ. Canine fossa trephine is a beneficial procedure in patients with Samter's triad. Rhinology. 2012;50(1):104–8.
31. Poetker DM, Jakubowski LA, Lal D, Hwang PH, Wright ED, Smith TL. Oral corticosteroids in the management of adult chronic rhinosinusitis with and without nasal polyps: an evidence-based review with recommendations. Int Forum Allergy Rhinol. 2013;3(2):104–20.
32. Howard BE, Lal D. Oral steroid therapy in chronic rhinosinusitis with and without nasal polyposis. Curr Allergy Asthma Rep. 2013;13(2):236–43.

33. Poetker DM, Smith TL. What rhinologists and allergists should know about the medico-legal implications of corticosteroid use: a review of the literature. Int Forum Allergy Rhinol. 2012;2(2):95–103.
34. Richards RN. Side effects of short-term oral corticosteroids. J Cutan Med Surg. 2008;12(2): 77–81.
35. Weinstein RS. Glucocorticoid-induced osteonecrosis. Endocrine. 2012;41(2):183–90.
36. van Schaardenburg D, van den Brink HR, Wieringa HJ. Short-term steroid therapy, sometimes with long-term sequelae. Ned Tijdschr Geneeskd. 2001;145(37):1769–73.
37. Taylor LJ. Multifocal avascular necrosis after short-term high-dose steroid therapy. A report of three cases. J Bone Joint Surg Br. 1984;66(3):431–3.
38. Madanagopal SG, Kovaleski JE, Pearsall 4th AW. Survey of short-term oral corticosteroid administration by orthopaedic physicians in college and high school athletes. J Sports Sci Med. 2009;8(1):37–44.
39. Hosemann W, Draf C. Danger points, complications and medico-legal aspects in endoscopic sinus surgery. GMS Curr Top Otorhinolaryngol Head Neck Surg. 2013;12:Doc06.
40. Fokkens W, Lund V, Mullol J, European Position Paper on Rhinosinusitis and Nasal Polyps group. European position paper on rhinosinusitis and nasal polyps 2007. Rhinol Suppl. 2007;20:1–136.
41. Dalziel K, Stein K, Round A, Garside R, Royle P. Endoscopic sinus surgery for the excision of nasal polyps: a systematic review of safety and effectiveness. Am J Rhinol. 2006;20(5): 506–19.
42. Stankiewicz JA, Lal D, Connor M, Welch K. Complications in endoscopic sinus surgery for chronic rhinosinusitis: a 25-year experience. Laryngoscope. 2011;121(12):2684–701.
43. Siedek V, Pilzweger E, Betz C, Berghaus A, Leunig A. Complications in endonasal sinus surgery: a 5-year retrospective study of 2,596 patients. Eur Arch Otorhinolaryngol. 2013;270(1):141–8.
44. Rombout J, de Vries N. Complications in sinus surgery and new classification proposal. Am J Rhinol. 2001;15(6):363–70.
45. May M, Levine HL, Mester SJ, Schaitkin B. Complications of endoscopic sinus surgery: analysis of 2108 patients–incidence and prevention. Laryngoscope. 1994;104(9):1080–3.
46. Valentine R, Wormald PJ. Controlling the surgical field during a large endoscopic vascular injury. Laryngoscope. 2011;121(3):562–6.
47. Valentine R, Wormald PJ. Carotid artery injury after endonasal surgery. Otolaryngol Clin North Am. 2011;44(5):1059–79.
48. Valentine R, Wormald PJ. A vascular catastrophe during endonasal surgery: an endoscopic sheep model. Skull Base. 2011;21(2):109–14.
49. Maharshak I, Hoang JK, Bhatti MT. Complications of vision loss and ophthalmoplegia during endoscopic sinus surgery. Clin Ophthalmol. 2013;7:573–80.
50. Ilieva K, Evens PA, Tassignon MJ, Salu P. Ophthalmic complications after functional endoscopic sinus surgery (FESS). Bull Soc Belge Ophtalmol. 2008;308:9–13.
51. Bhatti MT, Stankiewicz JA. Ophthalmic complications of endoscopic sinus surgery. Surv Ophthalmol. 2003;48(4):389–402.
52. Rene C, Rose GE, Lenthall R, Moseley I. Major orbital complications of endoscopic sinus surgery. Br J Ophthalmol. 2001;85(5):598–603.
53. Davis DH, Laws Jr ER, McDonald TJ, Salassa JR, Phillips 2nd LH. Intraventricular tension pneumocephalus as a complication of paranasal sinus surgery: case report. Neurosurgery. 1981;8(5):574–6.
54. Clevens RA, Bradford CR, Wolf GT. Tension pneumocephalus after endoscopic sinus surgery. Ann Otol Rhinol Laryngol. 1994;103(3):235–7.
55. Wright ED, Agrawal S. Impact of perioperative systemic steroids on surgical outcomes in patients with chronic rhinosinusitis with polyposis: evaluation with the novel Perioperative Sinus Endoscopy (POSE) scoring system. Laryngoscope. 2007;117(11 Pt 2 Suppl 115):1–28.

56. Poetker DM, Smith TL. Adult chronic rhinosinusitis: surgical outcomes and the role of endoscopic sinus surgery. Curr Opin Otolaryngol Head Neck Surg. 2007;15(1):6–9.
57. Klossek JM, Peloquin L, Friedman WH, Ferrier JC, Fontanel JP. Diffuse nasal polyposis: postoperative long-term results after endoscopic sinus surgery and frontal irrigation. Otolaryngol Head Neck Surg. 1997;117(4):355–61.
58. Jankowski R, Pigret D, Decroocq F, Blum A, Gillet P. Comparison of radi- cal (nasalisation) and functional ethmoidectomy in patients with severe sinonasal polyposis. A retrospective study. Rev Laryngol Otol Rhinol (Bord). 2006;127:131–40.
59. Wynn R, Har-El G. Recurrence rates after endoscopic sinus surgery for massive sinus polyposis. Laryngoscope. 2004;114:811–3.
60. Hopkins C, Browne JP, Slack R, Lund V, Topham J, Reeves B, Copley L, Brown P, van der Meulen J. The national comparative audit of surgery for nasal polyposis and chronic rhinosinusitis. Clin Otolaryngol. 2006;31(5):390–8.

Surgery for Allergic Fungal Rhinosinusitis

29

Jessica W. Grayson and Bradford A. Woodworth

Key Take-Home Points

- AFRS is a subtype of CRS with characteristic features: type 1 hypersensitivity to fungus; hyperdense opacification on CT scan often accompanied by bone erosion, nasal polyps, eosinophilic mucin without fungal invasion; and a positive fungal stain.
- Surgical management includes endoscopic sinus surgery with wide antrostomies to eliminate fungal debris and provide exposure for topical steroid treatment.
- Desensitization to fungal antigens should be considered postoperatively to decrease recurrence.

J.W. Grayson, MD
Department of Surgery/Division of Otolaryngology –
Head and Neck Surgery, University of Alabama at Birmingham,
BDB 563; 1720 2nd Avenue South,
Birmingham, AL 35294, USA
e-mail: jgrayson@uabmc.edu

B.A. Woodworth, MD, FACS (✉)
Department of Surgery/Division of Otolaryngology – Head and Neck Surgery,
Gregory Fleming James Cystic Fibrosis Research Center,
University of Alabama at Birmingham,
BDB 563; 1720 2nd Avenue South, Birmingham, AL 35294, USA
e-mail: bwoodwo@hotmail.com

P.S. Batra, J.K. Han (eds.), *Practical Medical and Surgical Management of Chronic Rhinosinusitis*, DOI 10.1007/978-3-319-16724-4_29

Background

Chronic rhinosinusitis (CRS) is a common chronic condition, particularly in the United States. CRS occurs in 1 out of 8 American adults [1]. There are two different subtypes of CRS – CRS with nasal polyps and CRS without nasal polyps [2]. Allergic fungal rhinosinusitis (AFRS) is in the CRS with nasal polyps category under the subtype of eosinophilic chronic rhinosinusitis (along with aspirin-exacerbated respiratory disease) instead of the neutrophilic CRS that is present in cystic fibrosis patients [3]. Of these different subtypes of CRS with nasal polyposis, AFRS accounts for approximately 6–9 % of cases that will require an operation. Of note, aspirin-exacerbated respiratory disease is still considered to be the most refractive to medical therapy [4].

The original requirements for diagnosis of CRS were presented in 1997 by the Rhinosinusitis Task Force and required the following: two major or one major and two minor criteria for a period greater than 12 weeks. The major criteria included facial pressure, nasal obstruction or blockage, hyposmia or anosmia, and purulent nasal drainage. The minor criteria included headache, fever, halitosis, cough, dental pain, fatigue, and ear pain or pressure [4, 5]. The subset of AFRS was defined by Bent and Kuhn, and despite further discussion into histopathologic, endoscopic, and/or treatment criteria, these have remained the standard diagnostic criteria with slight modifications over the last 20 years. A diagnosis of AFRS requires the presence of the following: history of atopy, nasal polyps, characteristic CT scan findings, eosinophilic mucin without fungal invasion, and a positive fungal stain [6, 7]. Characteristic CT scan findings include unilateral (up to 50 %) or bilateral opacification of the sinuses with areas of hyperattenuation representing allergic mucin often with concomitant erosion of surrounding bone (Fig. 29.1a, b). T2-weighted signal intensity "dropout" on MRI scan is typically pathognomonic for fungus (Fig. 29.1c, d). These patients will often also present with elevated levels of IgE and eosinophilic mucin that have been described as "peanut butter" in consistency with cascading eosinophils and Charcot-Leyden crystals on the periphery (Fig. 29.2) [4].

Epidemiology

AFRS is usually identified in patients who are young adults with a long history of nasal congestion, immunocompetence, unilateral or asymmetric involvement of the paranasal sinuses, nasal casts, hyposmia or anosmia, and facial pressure without significant pain. These findings cannot be used for diagnosis of AFRS, but they are usually present in people who have AFRS [6, 7]. Studies have estimated that anywhere from 5 to 10 % of patients who have been diagnosed with CRS are actually suffering from AFRS. AFRS is much more common in the southeastern and southwestern portion of the United States, including the Mississippi River basin. This geographical predominance is linked to the areas with a temperate climate and

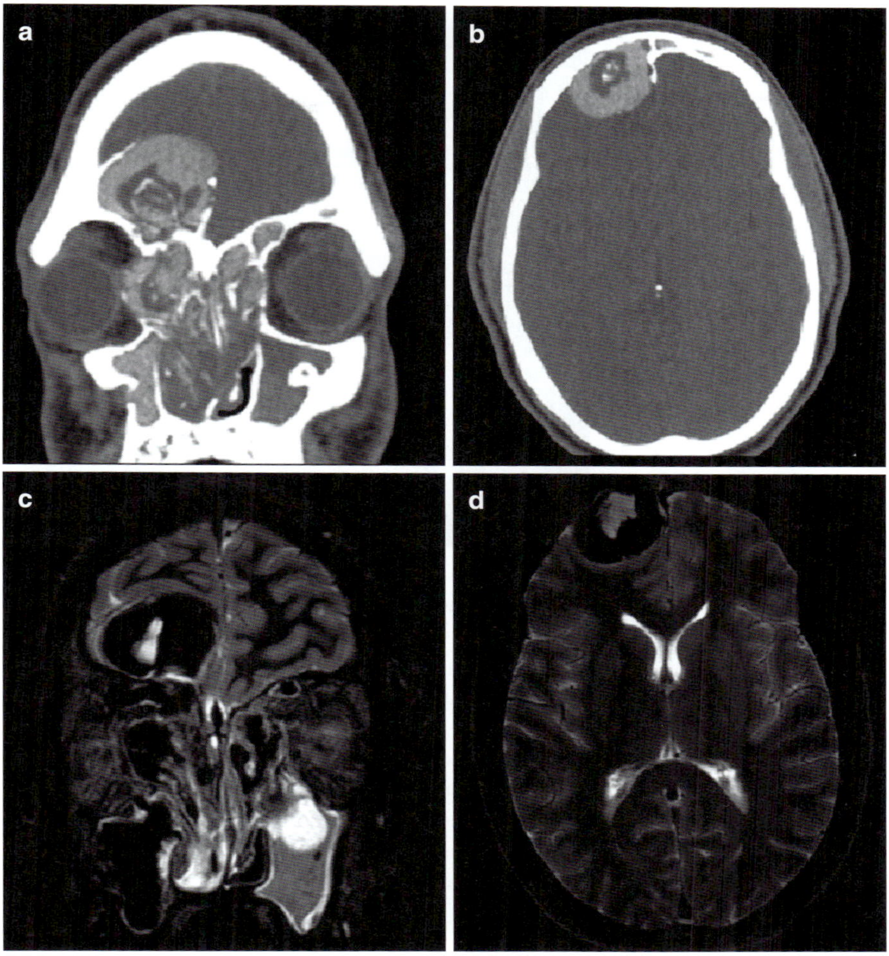

Fig. 29.1 A patient with massive right frontal sinus posterior table erosion on coronal (**a**) and axial (**b**) CT scans with heterogeneous densities suggesting AFRS. The corresponding coronal (**c**) and axial (**d**) T2-weighted MRI scans show complete dropout of the signal in these areas

increased humidity, which is more conducive for the fungus to flourish [8]. In the southeastern portion of the country, up to one third of the people undergoing functional endoscopic sinus surgery are found to have fungal sinusitis [6]. AFRS is associated with a type 1 hypersensitivity reaction and has been likened to allergic bronchopulmonary aspergillosis (ABPA) in that they are both chronic inflammatory conditions utilizing the same facets of the immune response. Both of these disease processes are set in motion by an allergic response to small numbers of fungus present in the respiratory tract [4].

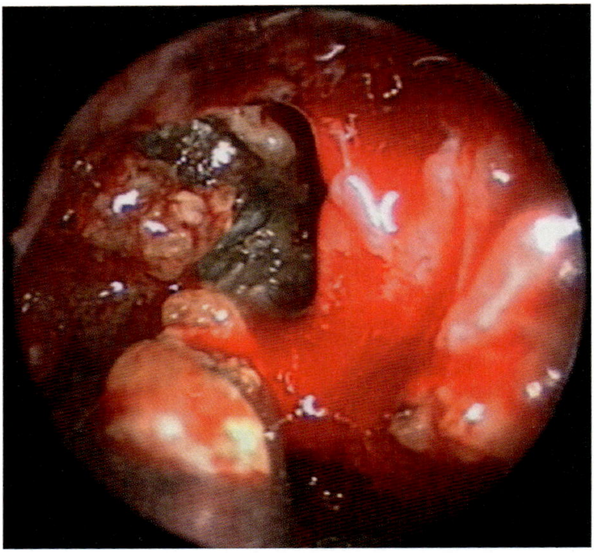

Fig. 29.2 Transnasal endoscopic view of allergic fungal mucin being removed from the frontal sinus. Note the peanut butter viscosity typical of AFRS

Pathophysiology

Increasing evidence over the years indicates that allergens and fungus play a large role in the pathogenesis of CRS. However, many questions regarding the cause of nasal polyposis remain unanswered. The development of CRS with nasal polyps may be associated with allergens – a claim bolstered by immunological evidence that Th2 (helper T cells) and eosinophils are the predominant cell types present. In contrast, acute rhinosinusitis due to bacterial causes or mucociliary dysfunction (e.g., cystic fibrosis) is associated with a neutrophilic response [9–13]. In some cases, it is thought that fungus incites an inflammatory response that is a separate trigger for CRS in the absence of a type 1 IgE hypersensitivity reaction [14]. Although the exact mechanism of a noninvasive allergic response in AFRS is still uncertain, the most well-accepted theory on the development of the disease is as follows: (1) a previously atopic patient is exposed to a fungus, (2) the fungus incites an antigenic inflammatory response via type 1 and type 3 hypersensitivity reactions in the nasal airway leading to eosinophilic accumulation and mucosal hypertrophy, (3) the fungus is able to propagate in a closed system when coupled with previously present mechanical or anatomical obstructions (occluded ostia or polyposis), (4) the propagation of the fungus leads to the eosinophilic mucin that continues to obstruct the drainage of the paranasal sinuses, and (5) further proliferation of the fungus stimulates a vicious inflammatory cycle [8, 15]. In contrast to that theory, Ponikau [16] suggested that fungus was present in nearly all nasal mucosa of CRS patients. Further studies of these patients noted that they did not have a fungal-specific antigenic or inflammatory response and that the response did not depend on IgE-mediated reactions but instead was secondary to T-lymphocyte-mediated inflammatory cascades that ultimately incite eosinophilic chemotaxis and activation. Regardless of controversies over fungal etiology, individuals with classical AFRS have type I hypersensitivity to molds that are usually very robust and will be the focus of the current chapter.

Medical Treatment

The recurrence rate of AFRS is considered high in patients with incomplete treatment. Therapy consists of both surgical (where fungal load should be removed) and postoperative medical interventions [8]. Medical therapy alone may not be enough for treatment of AFRS.

Oral Steroids

Like ABPA, oral steroid therapy is a mainstay of treatment for AFRS preoperatively due to the similarities in the pathophysiology of the two conditions. Corticosteroids limit the inflammatory reaction and cell recruitment to the mucosa by biochemically limiting IL-5, which is necessary for eosinophil chemotaxis and decrease vessel permeability [17]. In studies performed on AFRS patients, all patients eventually suffered a recurrence of AFRS if they were not treated with corticosteroids, and the time to surgical revision was extended for those that continued steroids for an extended period of time (1 year) [17, 18]. While systemic corticosteroids have been shown to be beneficial, risks are high with long-term and high-dosage therapy. These complications can include the following: growth retardation, diabetes mellitus, hypertension, psychotropic effects, gastrointestinal side effects, cataracts, glaucoma, osteoporosis, and aseptic necrosis of the femoral head [17]. Separating administration of systemic steroids to 3-month intervals can reduce the risks of the deleterious side effects but should be performed with informed decision from the patient. However, in a study by Schubert and Goetz [17], there were no complications reported with systemic corticosteroid treatment in the short term. Recommendations for preoperative and postoperative treatment with systemic steroids have been proposed. One of the accepted regimens for preoperative treatment is 0.5–1.0 mg/kg prednisone per day for 1 week before surgery to minimize inflammation and polyp volume [19]. It is also routinely accepted that steroids provided for greater than 2 weeks should be tapered over a period of time to prevent an Addisonian crisis.

Topical Steroids

Similar to systemic corticosteroids, topical corticosteroids limit the recruitment of inflammatory cells to the mucosa and reduce the edema and swelling that occurs in response to fungal antigen presentation. However, they have fewer complications than systemic steroids since the topical steroids have minimal systemic absorption. Unfortunately, topical steroid use is limited in the preoperative period because of poor penetration into the sinuses secondary to obstructive polyps and mucin.

Postoperative administration is considered a critical therapy for AFRS because of the smaller side effect profile and limited systemic absorption when compared to oral steroids. Overall, the safety profile of the newer generation nasal corticosteroids is excellent, but there is still a risk of nasal bleeding and septal perforation. The risk of hypothalamic pituitary axis dysfunction can be seen with topical steroid when inhalational steroids are used in asthmatic patients [8]. When possible, patients should be provided nasal steroids with the smallest amount of systemic absorption (e.g., mometasone) for long-term administration. Because the allergy to molds will remain unless durable desensitization is performed, many individuals with AFRS may require prolonged treatment. Another option for acute exacerbations is the local application of steroid to the sinuses in an absorbable vehicle such as triamcinolone in carboxymethylcellulose foam [20].

Nasal Saline Irrigation

Nasal saline irrigation is a cheap and well-tolerated adjunct to other medical therapies for CRS with and without polyps, including AFRS. Randomized, controlled trials have found that sinus symptoms were reduced, and quality of life measures were improved with the use of saline irrigation. Compounded mometasone or budesonide mixed in saline rinse has become an attractive option for treatment because delivery to the sinus mucosa is greatly improved, while overall exposure to the drug may be less than a nasal steroid spray. This has become standard therapy in many institutions due to the belief that better treatment outcomes occur with more widespread sinus treatment [21].

Systemic and Topical Antifungal Therapy

Antifungal therapy was initially used for treatment because of the repeated findings that people without any conjugate treatment following surgery were very likely to relapse. Amphotericin B, with its high side effect profile, was exchanged for the drugs itraconazole and ketaconazole. Historical studies suggested antifungals used in the treatment of ABPA resulted in decreasing IgE levels and reduced need for corticosteroids [22]. This data was used as evidence to support this treatment option for individuals with AFRS [23]. However, the risk of drug-related morbidity and the cost of the drugs limit how useful they may be in clinical practice [22]. The effectiveness of antifungal therapy has also been questioned due to the lack of histological evidence of any tissue invasion [24]. Topical antifungal therapy with amphotericin B has also been suggested for treatment of AFRS due to a low toxicity profile. Theoretically, antifungal therapy could help prevent recurrence of AFRS by decreasing the fungal burden, which would reduce antigen exposure in an atopic individual [25]. A recent meta-analysis regarding antifungal therapies for CRS concluded that there was no support for treatment with this modality [26]. However, studies generally did not separate AFRS patients from other forms of CRS.

Immunotherapy

Initial concerns that immunotherapy would be harmful in the treatment of AFRS were unfounded. Studies conducted by Mabry [27, 28] found that there was no decline in patient outcomes or increase in patient symptoms within the first year of treatment with immunotherapy. Some patients were able to forego systemic corticosteroid therapy and eventually discontinue topical corticosteroid therapy. Furthermore, subjects who maintained the regimen had a smaller likelihood of recurrence up to 2 and 3 years of clinical follow-up [28]. Recurrence rates were also significantly lowered in patients who received surgical treatment and immunotherapy when compared to a surgical cohort alone [29].

Hypersensitivities to fungal and non-fungal antigens are usually treated in AFRS. Antigens are delivered separately, with fungal antigens in one vial and non-fungal antigens in a separate vial with separate spots of injection. This allows for monitoring of any allergic or delayed hypersensitivity reactions and the ability to discern which injection is causing the local reaction. Once maintenance level dosages have been reached, the two vials can be combined to decrease the number of injections and improve efficiency of the process [8]. Dosage adjustment follows the guidelines for other allergy shots, and the duration of treatment is typically 3–5 years [30].

Originally, it was suggested that immunotherapy be directed against the fungal antigens that were cultured out of the paranasal sinuses, but this overlooked a crucial aspect of fungal culturing. There is a noted inconsistency and unreliability to culture technique and fungal spore numbers on culture (e.g., high detection with PCR). This could lead to incomplete treatment [8, 28].

Risks of immunotherapy include increasing the patient inflammatory response if they continue to be exposed to a large antigen load while receiving immunotherapy injections [8]. Previous small-scale studies looking at the comparison of treatment with immunotherapy before and after surgery found that patients who received injections prior to surgery began to get worse with treatment or failed to improve, while those postsurgery had better outcomes [8]. If AFRS and ABPA concurrently exist in the same patient, immunotherapy can be risky because there is no good surgical intervention to remove ABPA (aside from bronchoscopy) [31].

Surgical Intervention

Because clinical and radiographic findings of AFRS may include "invasive" features such as orbital/skull base erosion or cranial neuropathies, destructive surgical procedures were often employed (Fig. 29.3). Osteoplastic flaps, cranializations, lateral rhinotomies, and facial degloving procedures were intended to eliminate the disease and the mucosa because of "invasion" into surrounding structures. Even with less aggressive intranasal procedures (e.g., sphenoethmoidectomy), the intent was to completely remove the mucosa [32]. These approaches carried high morbidity, symptoms would return, and patients required further surgery [33, 34]. For

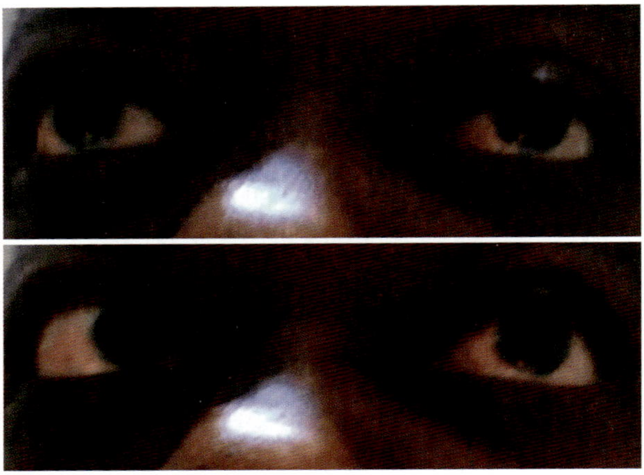

Fig. 29.3 A patient presents with a left abducens palsy on leftward gaze secondary to compression from skull base erosion at the petrous apex

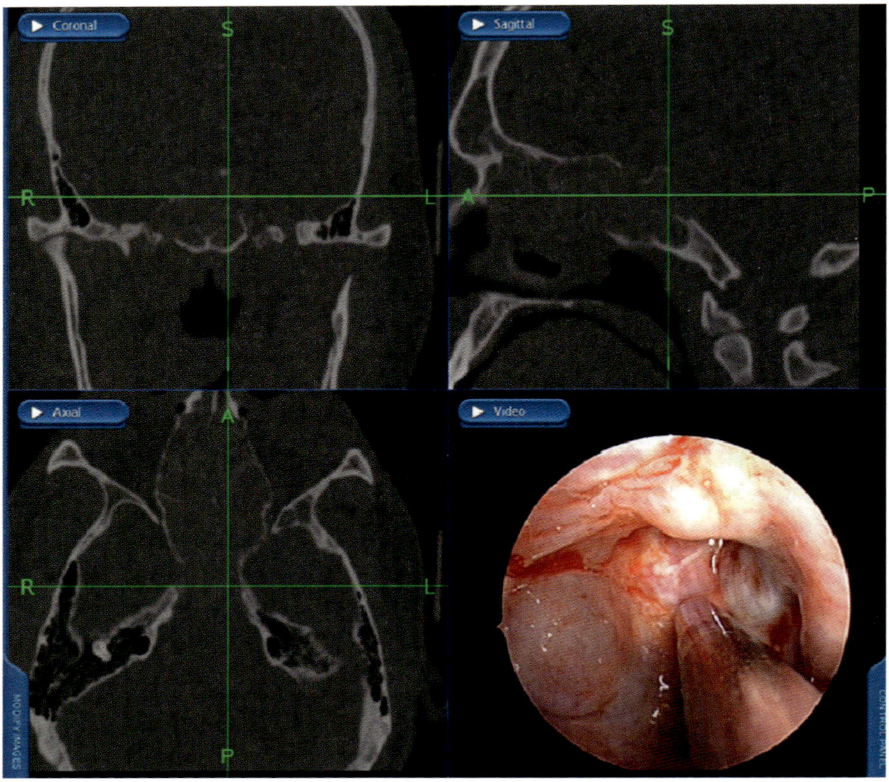

Fig. 29.4 Triplanar CT image guidance and endoscopic view of the sphenoid sinus after removal of extensive allergic fungal mucin. Note the large dehiscence in the posterior sphenoid over the brain stem

example, Sarti et al. describe a subject diagnosed with "paranasal aspergillosis" that was "invading the sella turcica and the anterior cranial fossa." Despite no histological demonstration of invasion into the mucosa, a craniofacial resection was performed, and the patient subsequently died due to a thromboembolism [35].

The gradual accumulation of allergic mucin in the sinus cavity causes the bony remodeling and decalcification that can resemble "invasion" on radiographic images. The areas of the bone that demineralize and the expansive areas of disease are directed by the inflammatory process in the area and the pressure of the accumulating mucin (Fig. 29.4) [35]. This expansile disease process can lead to exophthalmos, intracranial extension, and facial dysmorphia. Craniofacial changes occur gradually over time and are often not noticed by the patient or their family [36]. However, the expansive disease may expand ostia and provide large passageways to eliminate fungal mucin when performing functional endoscopic sinus surgery (FESS). Because of the lack of invasion and orbital and skull base remodeling that occurs over time following appropriate treatment of the disease, FESS is the gold standard treatment [37]. As the treatment of this disease requires access for topical steroid treatment, "full house" FESS is the technique of choice (Fig. 29.5) [38]. This includes a complete sphenoethmoidectomy with large maxillary antrostomies and frontal sinusotomies. There is no role for balloon sinuplasty alone in AFRS because

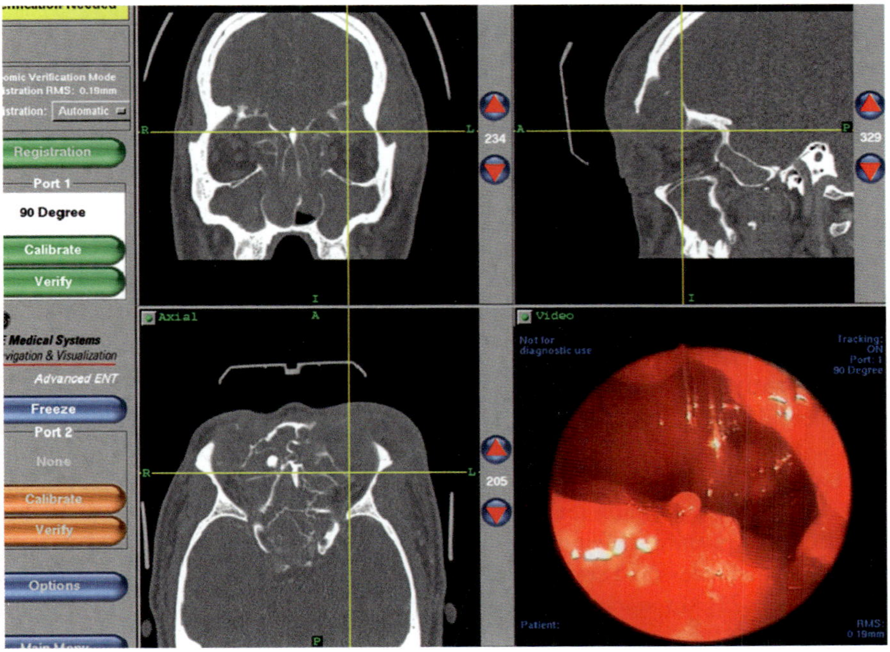

Fig. 29.5 "Full-house" endoscopic sinus surgery is the surgical intervention of choice for AFRS. CT image guidance and 70° endoscopic view of the left frontal sinus after evacuation of fungal mucin provide large openings for medical treatment and postoperative surveillance while leaving the mucosal lining intact

all fungal mucin must be evacuated, although some find it useful as a tool to find the frontal ostia.

Operative intervention can be difficult when there is a loss of surgical landmarks and bony dehiscences increase the risk for iatrogenic injury. Increased bleeding from nasal polyps can also cause disorientation [37]. Thus, the use of intraoperative image guidance is recommended for all cases of AFRS.

In order to prevent or decrease recurrence of AFRS, complete fungal eosinophilic mucin removal and reduction of the underlying inflammatory response via previously mentioned medical therapies are critical. There are three goals of surgical intervention as described by Marple [8]. First, completely remove all allergic mucin and fungal hyphae to rid the sinuses of the antigenic material within an atopic individual. This should be performed endoscopically, and external approaches are rarely needed. The second goal of surgical intervention should be permanent ventilation and drainage of the sinuses to prevent the buildup of fungal hyphae and the cycle of obstruction and proliferation of allergic mucin. Mucosa should be left intact in the lining of the sinuses, because fungal hyphae do not histologically invade the mucosa, and removal leads to neo-osteogenesis and recalcitrant disease. The use of newer instrumentation and microdissectors allows for the clearance of polyps and mucin and marsupialization of the diseased areas without injury to the mucosa [39]. Care should be taken around the orbit and cranial fossa because of the bone dissolution in response to the disease [37]. The final goal of surgery is to maintain access to the previously diseased areas for medical treatment and office-based surveillance of recurrence.

The largest risks of these surgical procedures lie in the risk for iatrogenic injury due to the decreased visibility and obscured anatomic boundaries. Recent literature states that there is minimal risk of fungal invasion in an immunocompetent host without iatrogenic injury. There have been several cases reporting invasive aspergillosis brain abscesses following endoscopic surgical intervention [34]. However, it is not clear if this was secondary to the invasive nature of the fungus or unnoticed compromise of the dura during FESS. Exposure of the dura without injury only rarely results in the development of an encephalocele [40].

Postoperative Treatment

Oral steroid tapers are recommended to diminish postoperative inflammation in AFRS. Topical steroid irrigations have become a mainstay of postoperative treatment, with 0.6 mg of mometasone or 0.5 mg of budesonide mixed in 100–240 ml of saline as the most common remedies [41]. Delivery of topical steroid drops in the inverted head position (Mygind's position) allows delivery of the topical steroid into the frontal recess and sinus, which has been noted to have a high rate of recurrent polyps [21]. Immunotherapy is also recommended after several weeks of recovery.

Postoperative surveillance includes endoscopic evaluation and subjective complaints indicating disease recurrence. Every patient should undergo nasal endoscopy at each clinic visit because polyps and mucosal edema can be visualized prior to an increase or change in symptomatology. Individuals with previous surgical intervention can undergo clinic-based debridement of mucin and polypoid edema. If using long-term corticosteroids, patients should be evaluated at regular intervals to assess for any side effects to steroid therapy. Postoperative surveillance is also useful for monitoring improvements in cosmetic effect (i.e., proptosis and facial dysmorphia).

Outcomes

Some of the signs and symptoms of AFRS include proptosis with diplopia and visual loss due to the slowly expanding allergic mucin proliferating and compressing against the orbit and lamina papyracea. Stonebracker and Schlosser [42] conducted a retrospective study of proptotic surgical patients compared to CRS patients without orbital involvement and found that clinical proptosis resolved after FESS without orbital reconstruction. As the sinus disease improves after medical and surgical treatment, the orbital volumes slowly diminish over the course of 6–12 months.

Immunotherapy outcomes were included in a study by Mabry [27, 28, 30, 43–45], who evaluated at a 4-year retrospective trial of people using immunotherapy as suppressive therapy postoperatively. During the first year of treatment with immunotherapy, these patients had a decrease in polyp size and formation, allergic mucin, and nasal crusting, and none experienced problems with immune complex deposition. During the course of the study, only two of the patients required use of corticosteroids and repeat operations. When compared to the control group, they required less corticosteroid therapy and had better physical exams. In this study, even after the termination of immunotherapy, patients went without recurrence of significant disease for 17 months. At this time, there is still a need for double-blind, placebo-controlled studies evaluating fungal desensitization in AFRS patients.

Conflict of Interest/Financial Disclosures Bradford A. Woodworth, MD is a consultant for ArthroCare ENT, Olympus, and Cook Medical.

References

1. Hamilos D. Chronic rhinosinusitis: epidemiology and medical management. J Allergy Clin Immunol. 2011;128(4):693–707.
2. Chaaban MR, Walsh EM, Woodworth BA. Epidemiology and differential diagnosis of nasal polyps. Am J Rhinol Allergy. 2013;27(6):473–8.
3. Kern R, Conley D, Walsh W. Perspectives on the etiology of chronic rhinosinusitis: an immune barrier hypothesis. Am J Rhinol. 2008;22(6):549–59.
4. Schubert M. Allergic fungal sinusitis: pathophysiology, diagnosis, and management. Allergy Asthma Clin. 2009;47(Supplement I):S324–30.
5. Lanza D, Kennedy D. Adult rhinosinusitis defined. Otolaryngol Head Neck Surg. 1997;117(3): S1–7.
6. Laury A. Allergic fungal rhinosinusitis. Am J Rhinol. 2013;27(3):S26–7.
7. Glass D, Amedee R. Allergic fungal rhinosinusitis: a review. Oschner J. 2011;11:271–5.

8. Marple B. Allergic fungal rhinosinusitis: current theories and management strategies. Laryngoscope. 2001;111:1006–19.
9. Benninger M. Adult chronic rhinosinusitis: definitions, diagnosis, epidemiology, and pathophysiology. Otololaryngol Head Neck Surg. 2003;129(3):S1–3.
10. Zele TV. Differentiation of chronic sinus disease by measurement of inflammatory mediators. Allergy. 2006;61(11):1280–9.
11. Jiang X. The characterization of IL-17A expression in patients with chronic rhinosinusitis with nasal polyps. Am J Rhinol. 2011;25(5):e171–5.
12. Chaaban MR, Kejner A, Rowe SM, Woodworth BA. Cystic fibrosis chronic rhinosinusitis: a comprehensive review. Am J Rhinol Allergy. 2013;27(5):387–95.
13. Virgin F, Rowe SM, Wade MB, Gaggar A, Leon KJ, Young KR, et al. Extensive surgical and comprehensive postoperative medical management for severe, recalcitrant cystic fibrosis chronic rhinosinusitis. Am J Rhinol Allergy. 2012;26(1):70–5.
14. Bachert C. Presence of IL-5 protein and IgE antibodies to staphylococcal enterotoxins in nasal polyps is associated with comorbid asthma. J Allergy Clin Immunol. 2010;126(5):962–8, 8, e1–6.
15. Manning S. Allergic aspergillosis: a newly recognized form of sinusitis in the pediatric population. Laryngoscope. 1989;99:681–5.
16. Ponikau J. The diagnosis and incidence of allergic fungal sinusitis. Mayo Clin Proc. 1999;74: 877–84.
17. Schubert M, Goetz D. Evaluation and treatment of allergic fungal sinusitis. II. Treatment and follow-up. J Allergy Clin Immunol. 1998;102(3):395–402.
18. Bent J. Allergic fungal sinusitis/polyposis. Allergy Asthma Proc. 1996;17:259–68.
19. Marple B, Mabry R. Comprehensive management of allergic fungal sinusitis. Am J Rhinol. 1998;12:263–8.
20. Chaudhry A, Chaaban MR, Ranganath NK, Woodworth BA. Topical triamcinolone acetonide/carboxymethylcellulose foam for acute exacerbations of chronic rhinosinusitis/nasal polyposis. Am J Rhinol Allergy. 2014;28:341–4.
21. Bhalla R, Payton K, Wright E. Safety of budesonide in saline sinonasal irrigations in the management of chronic rhinosinusitis with polyposis: lack of significant adrenal suppression. J Otolaryngol Head Neck Surg. 2008;37:821–5.
22. Ferguson B. What role do systemic corticosteroids, immunotherapy, and antifungal drugs play in the therapy of allergic fungal rhinosinusitis? Arch Otolaryngol Head Neck Surg. 1998;124: 1174–7.
23. Denning D, Wye J, Lewiston N. Adjunctive treatment of allergic bronchopulmonary aspergillosis with itraconazole. Chest. 1991;100:813–9.
24. Schubert M. Medical treatment of allergic fungal sinusitis. Ann Allergy Asthma Immunol. 2000;85:90–8.
25. Andes D, Proctor R, Bush R, Pasic T. Report of successful prolonged antifungal therapy for refractory allergic fungal sinusitis. Clin Infect Dis. 2000;31(1):202–4.
26. Sacks PL, Harvey RJ, Rimmer J, Gallagher RM, Sacks R. Antifungal therapy in the treatment of chronic rhinosinusitis: a meta-analysis. Am J Rhinol Allergy. 2012;26(2):141–7.
27. Mabry R, Mabry C. Immunotherapy for allergic fungal sinusitis: the second year. Otolaryngol Head Neck Surg. 1997;117:367–71.
28. Mabry R, Marple B, Folker R, Mabry C. Immunotherapy for allergic fungal sinusitis: three years' experience. Otolaryngol Head Neck Surg. 1998;119:648–51.
29. Folker R, Marple B, Mabry R, Mabry C. Treatment of allergic fungal sinusitis: a comparison trial of postoperative immunotherapy with specific fungal antigens. Laryngoscope. 1998;108: 1623–7.
30. Mabry R, Marple B, Mabry C. Outcomes after discontinuing immunotherapy for allergic fungal sinusitis. Otolaryngol Head Neck Surg. 2000;122:104–6.

31. Greenberger P, Atkinson NF Jr., Yunginger JW, Busse WW. Allergic bronchopulmonary aspergillosis. In: Middleton E, Reed C, Ellis E, et al, eds. Allergy principles and practice. St. Louis: Mosby; 1993:1395–414.
32. McGuirt W, Harrill J. Paranasal sinus aspergillosis. Laryngoscope. 1979;89:1563–8.
33. Kupferberg S, Bent J, Kuhn F. The prognosis of allergic fungal sinusitis. Otolaryngol Head Neck Surg. 1997;117:35–51.
34. Tsimakas S, Hollingsworth H, Nash G. Aspergillus brain abscess complication allergic aspergillus sinusitis. J Allergy Clin Immunol. 1994;94:264–7.
35. Sarti E, Blaugrun S, Lin P, Camins M. Paranasal sinus disease with intracranial extension: aspergillosis versus malignancy. Laryngoscope. 1988;98:632–5.
36. Klapper S, Lee A, Patrinely J, Stewart M, Alford E. Orbital involvement in allergic fungal sinusitis. Ophthalmology. 1997;104:2094–100.
37. Marple B. Allergic fungal sinusitis: surgical therapy. Otolaryngol Clin N Am. 2000;33:409–19.
38. Conger Jr BT, Illing E, Bush B, Woodworth BA. Management of lateral frontal sinus pathology in the endoscopic era. Otolaryngol Head Neck Surg. 2014;151:159–63.
39. Mirante J, Krouse J, Munier M. The role of powered instrumentation in the surgical treatment of allergic fungal sinusitis. Ear Nose Throat J. 1998;77:678–82.
40. Jackson C, Pappas D, Manolidis S. Brain herniation into the middle ear and mastoid: concepts in the diagnosis and surgical management. Am J Otol. 1997;18:198–206.
41. Welch KC, Thaler ER, Doghramji LL, Palmer JN, Chiu AG. The effects of serum and urinary cortisol levels of topical intranasal irrigations with budesonide added to saline in patients with recurrent polyposis after endoscopic sinus surgery. Am J Rhinol Allergy. 2010;24(1):26–8.
42. Stonebracker A, Schlosser R. Orbital volumetric analysis of allergic fungal sinusitis patients with proptosis before and after endoscopic sinus surgery. Am J Rhinol. 2005;19(3):302–6.
43. Mabry R, Manning S, Mabry C. Immunotherapy in the treatment of allergic fungal sinusitis. Otolaryngol Head Neck Surg. 1997;116:31–5.
44. Doellman M, Dion G, Weitzel E, Reyes E. Immunotherapy in allergic fungal sinusitis: the controversy continues. A recent review of the literature. Allergy Rhinol. 2013;4(1):e32–5.
45. Bent J, Kuhn F. Diagnosis of allergic fungal sinusitis. Otolaryngol Head Neck Surg. 1994;111:580–8.

Surgery for Pediatric Rhinosinusitis

30

Hassan H. Ramadan

Key Take-Home Points

- Surgery for complicated acute sinusitis can be emergent.
- Surgery is reserved for children with chronic sinusitis who fail maximal medical therapy.
- Several procedures are available to be considered in a stepwise approach.
- Adenoidectomy is an integral part of our surgical therapy.
- Balloon dilatation +/– sinus wash can be considered prior to sinus surgery.
- Endoscopic sinus surgery in children is safe, with low complication rate, and has an excellent outcome.

Introduction

Rhinosinusitis is classified into four categories:

1. Acute rhinosinusitis: symptoms lasting up to 2 weeks but not more than 4 weeks.
2. Subacute rhinosinusitis: symptoms last 2–4 weeks but not more than 3 months. This represents a transition between acute and chronic stages and needs to be dealt with accordingly.
3. Chronic rhinosinusitis: symptoms last more than 3 months.
4. Recurrent acute rhinosinusitis: four or more episodes per year of acute rhinosinusitis.

H.H. Ramadan, MD, MSc, FACS
Department of Otolaryngology – Head and Neck Surgery, RCBHSCS,
West Virginia University, PO Box 9200, Morgantown, WV 26506, USA
e-mail: hramadan@hsc.wvu.edu

P.S. Batra, J.K. Han (eds.), *Practical Medical and Surgical Management of Chronic Rhinosinusitis*, DOI 10.1007/978-3-319-16724-4_30

Chronic sinusitis in children is defined as signs and symptoms lasting more than 3 months. Those symptoms include nasal stuffiness, nasal discharge, cough, and facial pain. Other symptoms can include hyposmia, postnasal drip, sore throat, and halitosis. Examination of nasal cavity in children can be difficult. Anterior rhinoscopy most often is unable to demonstrate sinonasal pathology. Performing nasal endoscopy on a child can be challenging, but finding of colored discharge can be very helpful in determining the diagnosis. Nasal endoscopy can help examine the adenoids for infection or hypertrophy. The presence of nasal polyps on examination is extremely important; if polyps were noted, then cystic fibrosis is an important consideration in the workup of the child [1].

Chronic adenoiditis can give signs and symptoms that are exactly the same as chronic sinusitis. Differentiating between the two conditions can prove very helpful in deciding which surgical approach to recommend for the child. To do that clinically is almost impossible; however, a CT scan of the sinuses can provide that information [2].

Children who are refractory to medical therapy, which includes oral antibiotics, topical steroid nasal sprays, and topical nasal saline sprays, should have an allergy workup, an immune workup, and a ciliary biopsy as well as sweat chloride test especially if nasal polyps were seen on nasal exam or endoscopy [3].

Imaging studies should be reserved to those with complicated sinusitis or those who have failed medical therapy and are considered for surgery. Plain X-rays have very low specificity and sensitivity and are not recommended. CT scan is the imaging modality of choice, since it can provide a road map for surgery as well as excellent anatomy of the sinuses. MRI may be used in complicated cases of sinusitis or when evaluating a mass or an invasive fungal infection in the sinuses [4].

In young children the ethmoid and maxillary sinuses are usually the ones involved, since the frontal and sphenoid sinuses will not be developed until later in life. Pathogenesis is secondary to bacterial adenoiditis or blockage of the sinus ostia whether anatomical or secondary to allergies or viral upper respiratory infections [1]. Knowledge of the development and surgical anatomy of the sinuses is extremely important before performing sinus surgery on children.

Surgical Anatomy

The nasal cavity can be narrower in children since it is still in development. The ethmoid and maxillary sinuses are the only sinuses present at birth, but the sizes are different than that of adults. Also the pneumatization of the ethmoid sinuses is more simple in early childhood years. The frontal and sphenoid sinuses will develop later in childhood.

The septum divides the nose into left and right nasal cavities that are a mirror image in details. The posterior inferior walls of the nasal cavity lead to the posterior choanae and adenoids which are an integral part of sinusitis in children.

The lateral nasal walls house the sinus cavities and their openings. The lateral nasal walls have fixtures that are the turbinates – the inferior, middle, superior, and in some instances supreme turbinates. Below each turbinate is a meatus, the inferior meatus has the opening of the nasolacrimal duct, and the middle meatus is what is important for sinus surgeons because it has the openings of the ethmoid and maxillary sinuses as well as frontal sinuses. The superior meatus allows drainage of the posterior ethmoid and the sphenoethmoid recess has the opening of the sphenoid sinus ostium.

The ostiomeatal complex (OMC) is the main culprit in children with chronic sinusitis. Since the OMC is the area of drainage of the ethmoid and maxillary sinuses, which are often involved in children, surgery is directed mainly to this area.

The OMC contains the uncinate process, a crescent-shaped bone that projects from the inferior turbinate and palatine bone and runs along the lateral nasal bone. Just posterior to it is the hiatus semilunaris, which is the space between the uncinate process and the ethmoid bulla. The opening into the hiatus is the infundibulum. The hiatus semilunaris is where the maxillary sinus ostium opens posteriorly and the frontal sinus ostium opens superiorly. In children, identification of the ostium of the maxillary sinus is of utmost importance and has ramifications on surgical outcome as we will discuss later. The size of the uncinate process is proportionately larger in children than in adults. Also the nasolacrimal duct, to which the uncinate process is anteriorly attached to, can be very prominent and often mistaken for the uncinate process. It is also important to be familiar with fontanelle, which is the medial wall of the maxillary sinus that separates the sinus from the nasal cavity.

The ethmoid sinus then fills the space between the lateral wall of the middle turbinate and the bony lamina of the orbit. Ethmoid sinuses are divided into anterior and posterior ethmoid air cells. The major anterior ethmoid is made of multiple air cells that are arranged in a honeycomb fashion, while the posterior ethmoid can be a single large cell in young children. The anterior and posterior ethmoids are separated by the basal lamella, which is the posterior attachment of the middle turbinate. This makes the basal lamella an important landmark when performing sinus surgery.

Other cells that are relevant for sinus disease in children are the Haller cells, agger nasi cells, and concha bullosa involving the middle turbinate. The Haller cells, or now better known as infraorbital cells, are ethmoid air cells that are present inside the maxillary sinus just inferior to the orbital wall. Their significance is that they can narrow or block the ostium of the maxillary sinus into the hiatus semilunaris. Similarly the agger nasi cells, which are ethmoid cells that are anterior to the ethmoid bulla, can possibly encroach the frontal sinus ostium. A pneumatized middle turbinate known as a concha bullosa can block the ostiomeatal complex if it is large and highly pneumatized [5, 6].

Surgical Indications

There are no available guidelines or consensus regarding the surgical treatment of pediatric sinusitis. Most agree that once medical treatment has failed, surgery should be considered. Several surgical options are available for our use. Adenoidectomy is the mainstay of treatment and is performed alone or in conjunction with other surgical options. Those include sinus lavage, balloon sinus dilatation, or endoscopic sinus surgery [7–9].

Surgical indications can be divided into two categories: the absolute vs. relative indications.

Absolute Indications

Most otolaryngologists agree that the following are absolute indications for surgery [10].

1. Orbital complications, most commonly subperiosteal abscess
2. Central nervous system complications
3. Severe nasal polyposis
4. Suspected benign lesions, tumor, or fungal infection

Surgical procedure in these situations consists of sinus surgery, whether endoscopic vs. open technique depends on the involved sinus as well as the expertise of the surgeon.

Relative Indications

This group includes children who have signs and symptoms of chronic sinusitis and have failed maximal medical therapy. Several surgical procedures are available; however, there are no guidelines or consensus on how to proceed and which surgical option is appropriate [11]. The following are the surgical indications:

1. Chronic rhinosinusitis with anatomical abnormalities
2. Children with symptoms of asthma secondary to refractory CRS who are not responding to systemic steroids
3. Children with immotile cilia or immune deficiency who are not responding to medical treatment of culture and irrigation

Contraindications

1. Children with chronic rhinitis without evidence of rhinosinusitis
2. Children with normal CT scan of the sinuses

Surgical Technique

There is agreement that surgery should be a last resort, and most physicians tend to start with adenoidectomy as a first line [7, 8]. The problem though is that adenoidectomy alone has an overall success rate of around 50 % and even less in children with asthma (<30 %). Adenoids play a major role in the signs and symptoms of chronic sinusitis. It is mainly the chronic adenoiditis rather than the adenoid size [12]. The issue is that these children invariably will have an adenoiditis, but some will have sinusitis as well. Those with chronic adenoiditis but no sinusitis, based on CT scan score, will have a great success with adenoidectomy alone (65 %). However, those children with adenoiditis as well as sinusitis will have a poor success rate

(43 %) and in particular if these kids have asthma. Then adenoidectomy will be successful in only 28 % of these children [13]. The following surgical procedures have been used for treatment of chronic sinusitis in children:

1. Adenoidectomy
2. Balloon dilatation +/– sinus wash
3. Endoscopic sinus surgery
4. Combination of the above

Adenoidectomy

The procedure is done under general anesthesia with the patient in supine position. Most use a transoral approach, with mouth opened using a McIvor retractor with red rubbers inserted in nasal cavities to retract the palate. Using suction cautery ablation of the adenoids is usually done. Other approaches are to use a shaver or curettes to remove the adenoids and then use cautery for hemostasis. There have been reports of removing the adenoids endoscopically; the surgeon will use a rigid zero-degree scope, and using a shaver the adenoids will be removed transnasally. Hemostasis was controlled with suction cautery [14, 15].

Balloon Sinus Dilatation

Balloon catheter dilatation has been shown to be an effective treatment of CRS in adults [16, 17]. Results from adult studies demonstrate an excellent safety profile with a major complication rate of 0.0035 % per sinus or 0.01 % per patient. More recently it has been also shown that balloon dilatation can be performed safely and effectively in children [9]. Balloon sinus dilatation can be offered as a treatment alternative at time of adenoidectomy or prior to endoscopic sinus surgery after an adenoidectomy has failed [18]. A CT scan of sinuses is a requirement prior to performing balloon dilatation.

Two balloon companies have different versions for dilatation of sinuses. Irrespective of which balloon catheter you are using, procedure is performed under general anesthesia. The nasal cavities are initially packed with oxymetazoline pledgets. Afterward using preferably the 4 mm rigid scope, the pledgets are removed, and the nasal septum, middle turbinate, and uncinate process are injected with 1 % lidocaine with 1:100,000 epinephrine.

Procedure

Both devices at this point come in one package. The Acclarent system has a guide catheter for the respective sinuses (maxillary, frontal, and sphenoid), whereas the Entellus system has a probe that can be fashioned according to which sinus is targeted.

- Appropriate guide catheter/probe are introduced under direct endoscopic visualization.

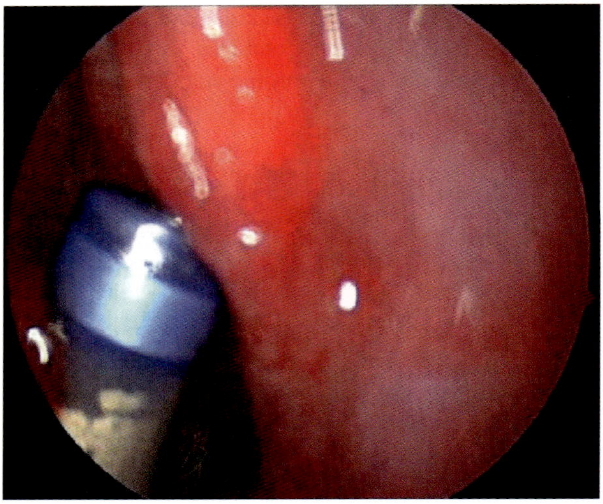

Fig. 30.1 The sinus balloon is passed over the guidewire

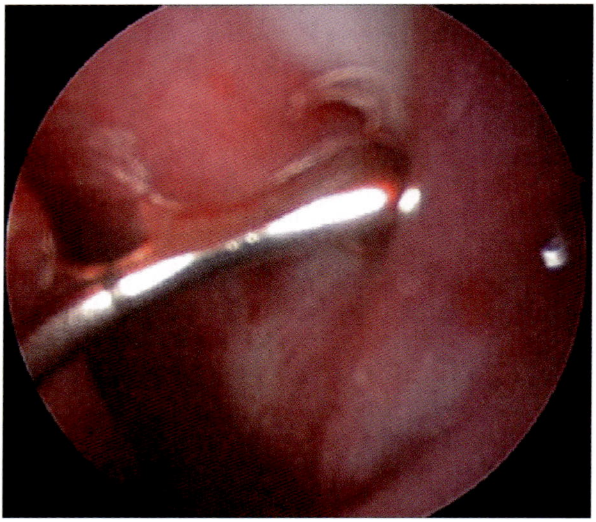

Fig. 30.2 Markers are used on the sinus balloon to ensure proper placement

- Guidewire is passed through the catheter/probe into the intended sinus.
- Confirmation that the guidewire is in the sinus with transillumination (except sphenoid sinus).
- The sinus balloon is passed over the guidewire (Fig. 30.1).
- Use markers on balloon to ensure proper placement (Fig. 30.2).
- Inflate the balloon to 12 atmospheric pressure with special inflation device for the Acclarent balloon, or just use the special inflation device in the Entellus package.
- Irrigation/wash of sinus as needed.
- Remove balloon and wire and then remove guide.

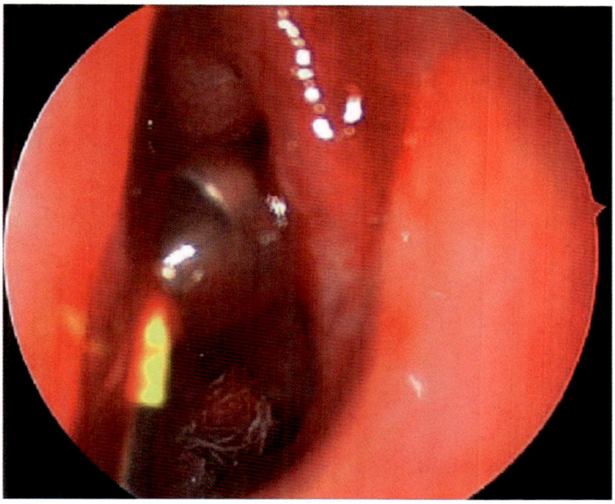

Fig. 30.3 Hold tension on the sinus balloon while inflated to prevent the inflated balloon from slipping inside/outside the sinus

- Confirm dilatation of ostium with direct visualization.
- MeroGel packing (Medtronic, Jacksonville, Florida) is typically sufficient.

Pitfalls and Tips

- Create an accessory ostium.
- Strip the mucosa posteriorly, thus collapsing the whole lining anteriorly.
- Significant injury to ostium and uncinate process to the extent that an antrostomy may be needed.
- Guide catheter/probe is introduced tip up (personal preference for children).
- Hold tension on balloon while inflated to prevent inflated balloon from slipping inside/outside the sinus (Fig. 30.3).

Postoperative Care

- Child is discharged after a period of observation.
- Oral antibiotics are given for 7 days postoperatively.
- Avoid nose blowing.
- Follow up in 2 weeks.

Contraindications to Balloon Catheter Dilatation in Children

- Previous sinonasal surgery in target ostia
- Cystic fibrosis
- Extensive sinonasal osteoneogenesis
- Sinonasal tumors or obstructive lesions
- History of facial trauma that distorts sinus anatomy and precludes access to the sinus ostium
- Ciliary dysfunction
- Hypoplastic sinus as these have been shown to be more difficult to cannulate [9] (Fig. 30.4)

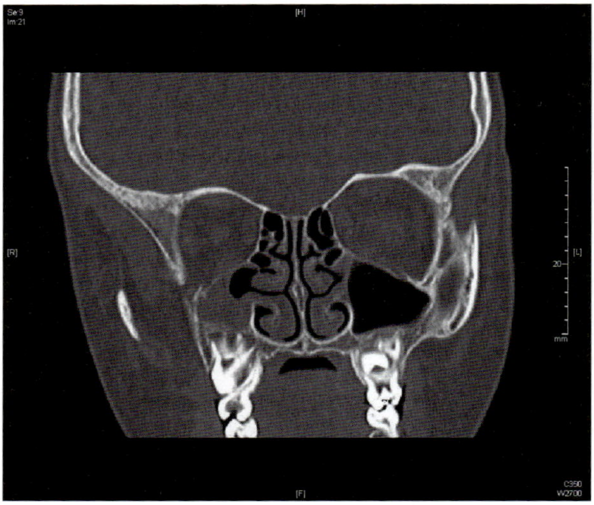

Fig. 30.4 A contraindication to balloon catheter dilation is hypoplastic sinus as these have been shown to be more difficult to cannulate [9]

It is also helpful to have experience with balloons in adults prior to working on children.

Endoscopic Sinus Surgery

The procedure is indicated for complicated rhinosinusitis, nasal polyposis, fungal sinusitis, and children with CRS after failure of medical treatment. A CT scan prior to surgery is mandatory. The CT scan will allow for evaluation of anatomy and extent of disease. CT scan should be available in the operating room at all times during the procedure. Image-guided surgery can be performed for cases with polyps, complicated sinusitis, or revision cases. A special consideration should also be given for cystic fibrosis patients. The following are required instrumentation for the procedure:

1. 0°, 30°, and 70° rigid scopes preferably 4 mm in size
2. Straight and upturned Blakesley forceps of different sizes
3. Straight and upturned through-cutting forceps
4. Double-blind ostium seeker
5. Short and long curved antrum cannula
6. Right-side and left-side backward punch cutting forceps
7. 3, 5, and 7 French Frazier suction tubes
8. Cottle elevator
9. If needed, powered microdebrider with aggressive 2.9 and 4 mm blades
10. Additional instruments as deemed appropriate by the surgeon for frontal sinus and sphenoid surgery

Prior to start of the procedure, the following preparations are necessary:

1. ESS in children is done under general anesthesia.
2. Oxymetazoline 0.5 % solution-impregnated pledgets are used for topical vasoconstriction.
3. Injection of the middle turbinates, the uncinate processes, bulla ethmoidalis, and septum adjacent to the middle turbinates with 1 % lidocaine solution with 1:100,000 epinephrine.
4. Child is placed supine with the head of the table slightly elevated.
5. The surgeon should be facing the patient with the monitor facing the surgeon.

We routinely give the patient Decadron 0.15 mg/kg IV bolus.

Procedure

1. The 0° 4 mm scope is introduced into the nasal cavity after the pledgets have been removed.
2. If more injection is needed, it can be performed at this stage.
3. Using the Cottle elevator the middle turbinate is mediatized until the uncinate process and bulla are visualized.
4. Using the seeker the area of the maxillary sinus ostium is found and the ostium palpated. This can be performed in a retrograde or anterograde manner. I prefer the anterograde technique because it prevents the posterior maxillary mucosa from stripping.
5. The ostium can then be widened posteriorly by removing the inferior edge of the uncinate process with a straight cutting forceps. For retrograde technique the right-sided backbiter can be used to remove the uncinate process anteriorly. Care should be taken not to injure the nasolacrimal duct with this technique.
6. A curved angled cannula is then introduced into the maxillary sinus for suction. Polyps, cysts, or other debris can be suctioned and removed. All attempts should be made not to strip the mucous membrane of the sinus.
7. The remainder of the uncinate process is then removed using up- and backbiting forceps.
8. The ethmoid bulla should be now fully visualized. A straight biter is used to enter the bulla inferiorly and medially. These cells are then removed using straight and up-biting forceps.
9. The lamina papyracea and skull base should be visualized during this procedure to avoid any injuries.
10. If a posterior ethmoidectomy is needed, the ground lamella of the middle turbinate should be identified. Penetration through the lamella with a 5 mm Frazier suction can be performed. Any pathologic contents inside can be suctioned or removed. The anterior table of the posterior ethmoid can be widened. Removal of the mucous membrane of the sinus is not encouraged.

11. A posterior to anterior dissection is then performed along the skull base which is easily identified in the posterior ethmoid air cells. This can be facilitated by using a 30° 4 mm endoscope. Exenteration of these cells along skull base can be performed using the J-curette.
12. Using an up-biting forceps, these cells can be removed under visualization.
13. If a posterior ethmoidectomy is not needed, then identification of the skull base can be done anterior to the basal lamella and a similar posterior to anterior dissection is then done.
14. At this point if the frontal sinus is diseased, then opening of the frontal recess and ostium is needed.
15. In most instances, once the uncinectomy is performed, a small residual piece superiorly can be identified. The seeker is used to palpate just posterior to that piece (if not present, palpation in that area is done) to enter into the frontal sinus opening.
16. A curved suction cannula is then introduced into the sinus for inspection.
17. In most instances, the surgeon will alternate between right and left nasal cavities using pledgets impregnated with 0.5 % oxymetazoline solution for control of hemostasis while performing part of the procedure on the other side.
18. Once the procedure is complete, the cavities are packed with hyaluronic pledgets rolled up in thirds and placed in the ethmoid cavity next to the middle turbinate.
19. A nasal drip pad is placed on the nose.
20. The eyes are then inspected for any swelling, edema, increased pressure, or ecchymosis.

Complications

The complications of balloon dilatation have been very rare. No major complications have been reported thus far after balloon dilatation in children. Complications after ESS in children have also been rare. A recent meta-analysis has shown incidence of major complications to be 1.4 % [8]. These complications can occur either intraoperatively or postoperatively. The intraoperative complications can be dealt with immediately during the procedure. Some of the major complications include:

- CSF leak
  This needs to be recognized immediately during the procedure and repaired.
- Orbital entry with fat herniation
  In most instances the procedure can be completed, and no intervention is necessary if no increased intraorbital pressure is detected.
- Orbital hemorrhage with increased pressure
  An immediate lateral canthotomy with removal of all the packing in the ethmoid sinus on that side. An ophthalmology consult should be obtained.
- Stripping of the maxillary sinus mucosa

This needs to be recognized; otherwise, even though the bony ostium is open, the mucosa inside the sinus will be collapsed with no ventilation of the inside of the sinus.

- Inadvertent injury to the middle turbinate
  All attempts should be made to preserve it in place.
- Bleeding
  If it is impairing visualization considerably, the procedure should be aborted. There is no need to put the patient at risk for blood transfusion and potentially cause an intraoperative complication due to poor visualization. Once the bleeding is excessive with respect to the blood volume of the child, then the procedure should also be aborted.

Majority of postoperative complications are minor and include:

- Bleeding
  In most instances it is self-contained. Rarely packing or exam in the operating room is needed.
- Adhesions
  Those can be very common depending on the age of the child. If they are not causing any symptoms, then they can be left alone. If symptomatic and severe, a relook to deal with them would be appropriate.
- Orbital swelling and ecchymosis
  If eye pressure is high, then proceed as in intraoperative increased pressure. If pressure is normal and child is cooperative enough, remove the packing and observe.

Clinical Efficacy Data

ESS has been performed in children for over two decades. Initially there was some concern about major complications such as CSF leak, eye injury, and blindness that prevented early adoption of the procedure. However, as more surgeries were performed and lack of significant potential complications, ESS gained wide acceptance for treatment of CRS in children [11]. Several publications are available regarding the success of ESS in children. Makary and Ramadan [8] in a Cochrane review in 2014 found that ESS was successful between 82 and 100 % of cases with complication rate of 1.4 %. Bothwell et al. [19] found that there was no impact on facial growth development in those children who had ESS after 10 years of follow-up. ESS is a safe and successful procedure when performed on appropriate patients.

Balloon dilatation of the sinuses was first described in children in 2008 after several studies have shown the success the procedure had in adults [9]. The procedure was found to be safe and feasible in children. Later it was reported that balloon dilatation had an 87 % success rate in children who had CRS and failed medical therapy. It was also noted that balloon dilation was successful after failure of adenoidectomy as an alternative to ESS [18]. There have been no reported cases of major complications with balloon dilation to date. The procedure is indicated either at the time of adenoidectomy or prior to ESS after an adenoidectomy has failed.

Conclusion

Surgery for pediatric CRS should be reserved to those children who have failed maximal medical therapy. Several surgical options are available which include adenoidectomy, balloon dilation of sinuses with irrigation, and ESS or a combination of all of them. Adenoidectomy should be considered as an initial approach specifically for younger children (less than 5 years of age), those with chronic adenoiditis (Lund-MacKay CT score less than five), and children with no asthma. Balloon dilation should be considered in specific indications due to lack of enough evidence to support its use in children. ESS has been shown to be an effective procedure for the treatment of children with CRS. It is also a safe procedure with low incidence of major complications.

References

1. Fokkens WJ, Lund VJ, Mullol J, et al. European position paper on rhinosinusitis and nasal polyps 2012. Rhinol Suppl. 2012;23:3.
2. Bhattacharyya N, Jones DT, Hill M, Shapiro NL. The diagnostic accuracy of computed tomography in pediatric chronic rhinosinusitis. Arch Otolaryngol Head Neck Surg. 2004;130(9):1029–32.
3. Sedaghat AR, Phipatanakul W, Cunningham MJ. Prevalence of and associations with allergic rhinitis in children with chronic rhinosinusitis. Int J Pediatr Otorhinolaryngol. 2014; 78(2):343–7.
4. Setzen G, Ferguson BJ, Han JK, Rhee JS, Cornelius RS, Froum SJ, Gillman GS, Houser SM, Krakovitz PR, Monfared A, Palmer JN, Rosbe KW, Setzen M, Patel MM. Clinical consensus statement: appropriate use of computed tomography for paranasal sinus disease. Otolaryngol Head Neck Surg. 2012;147(5):808–16.
5. Scuderi AJ, Harnsberger HR, Boyer RS. Pneumatization of the paranasal sinuses: normal features of importance to the accurate interpretation of CT scans and MR images. AJR Am J Roentgenol. 1993;160(5):1101–4.
6. Laine FJ, Smoker WR. The ostiomeatal unit and endoscopic surgery: anatomy, variations, and imaging findings in inflammatory diseases. AJR Am J Roentgenol. 1992;159(4):849–57.
7. Brietzke SE, Brigger MT. Adenoidectomy outcomes in pediatric rhinosinusitis: a meta-analysis. Int J Pediatr Otorhinolaryngol. 2008;72(10):1541–5.
8. Makary CA, Ramadan HH. The role of sinus surgery in children. Laryngoscope. 2013;123(6): 1348–52.
9. Ramadan H, McLaughlin K, Josephson G, et al. Balloon catheter sinuplasty in children. Am J Rhinol Allergy. 2010;24(1):e54–6.
10. Conrad S, Buwalda J. Surgical or medical management of subperiosteal orbital abscess in children: a critical appraisal of the literature. Rhinology. 2009;47:18–23.
11. Ramadan HH. Surgical management of chronic sinusitis in children. Laryngoscope. 2004;114(12):2103–9.
12. Lee D, Rosenfeld RM. Adenoid bacteriology and sinonasal symptoms in children. Otolaryngol Head Neck Surg. 1997;116(3):301–7.

13. Ramadan HH, Makary CA. Can CT score predict outcome of adenoidectomy for chronic rhinosinusitis in children. Am J Rhinol Allergy. 2014;28(1):80–2.
14. Wynn R, Rosenfeld RM. Outcomes in suction coagulator adenoidectomy. Arch Otolaryngol Head Neck Surg. 2003;129(2):182–5.
15. Somani SS, Naik CS, Bangad SV. Endoscopic adenoidectomy with microdebrider. Indian J Otolaryngol Head Neck Surg. 2010;62(4):427–31.
16. Levine HL, Sertich 2nd AP, Hoisington DR, Weiss RL, Pritikin J. Multicenter registry of balloon catheter sinusotomy outcomes for 1,036 patients. Ann Otol Rhinol Laryngol. 2008;117(4):263–70.
17. Weiss RL, Church CA, Kuhn FA, Levine HL, Sillers MJ, Vaughan WC. Long-term outcome analysis of balloon catheter sinusotomy: two-year follow-up. Otolaryngol Head Neck Surg. 2008;139(3 Suppl 3):S38–46.
18. Ramadan HH, Tiu J. Failures of adenoidectomy for chronic rhinosinusitis in children: for whom and when do they fail? Laryngoscope. 2007;117(6):1080–3.
19. Bothwell MR, Piccirillo JF, Lusk RP, Ridenour BD. Long-term outcome of facial growth after functional endoscopic sinus surgery. Otolaryngol Head Neck Surg. 2002;126(6):628–34.

Surgery of the Nasal Septum and Turbinates

31

Phillip S. LoSavio and Thomas R. O'Toole

Key Take-Home Points

- Preoperative assessment of the patient's nasal pathology is critical to surgical success.
- Unrecognized internal nasal valve incompetence remains one of the most common reasons for failure after septal and turbinate surgery.
- Determine whether the patient can be treated with a standard endonasal approach or requires an open septorhinoplasty technique.
- Conditions that may necessitate an open approach include severe dorsal septal twisting or deviations contributing to airway obstruction, nasal tip ptosis, severe caudal septal deflections, and deficient nasal valve architecture requiring open cartilage grafting.
- Meticulous attention to subperichondrial and subperiosteal septal injections will greatly facilitate subsequent flap elevation.
- Modify the initial incision and septoplasty technique as needed to address the location of the septal pathology.
- Pay attention to maintain adequate caudal and dorsal septal support. This may require removal of severely deviated tissue with replacement of cartilage grafts.
- Current medical evidence supports using quilting sutures alone without nasal packing or nasal splints.

P.S. LoSavio, MD, MS (✉)
Section Head – Sleep Surgery, Department of Otorhinolaryngology – Head and Neck Surgery, Rush University Medical Center, 1611 W. Harrison Street, Suite 550, Chicago, IL 60612, USA
e-mail: phillip_losavio@rush.edu

T.R. O'Toole, MD
Department of Otorhinolaryngology – Head and Neck Surgery, Rush University Medical Center, 1611 W. Harrison Street, Suite 550, Chicago, IL 60612, USA
e-mail: totoole@rush.edu

P.S. Batra, J.K. Han (eds.), *Practical Medical and Surgical Management of Chronic Rhinosinusitis*, DOI 10.1007/978-3-319-16724-4_31

Introduction

The dawn of modern-day nasal septal surgery dates back to the final years of the late nineteenth century. Prior to this time, the most common surgery in the United States to correct nasal septal deformities was the Bosworth operation. This technique involved removing septal spurs and deformities along with the overlying mucosa on one side using an intranasal saw. In 1896, both Dr. E. B. Gleason and Dr. Arthur W. Watson presented reports of a new nasal septal operation. In their work, one can see the early origins of key concepts including perichondrial flap elevation, local anesthesia using cocaine, cartilage repositioning, and avoidance of iatrogenic septal perforation [1]. Advances in this field progressed over the next half century, with major contributions from pioneers including Freer, Killian, Metzenbaum, Cottle, Goldman, and Converse [2].

Overall, nasal operations are quite common today in the United States. Bhattacharyya [3] published a review of the 2006 National Survey of Ambulatory Surgery. In that year, it is estimated that there were about 340,405 (±3.6 % S.E.) septoplasty and/or turbinate surgeries in the United States. Overall, these two procedures account for the majority (56 %) of all sinonasal procedures (nasal/turbinate surgery, sinus surgery, cosmetic nasal surgery, treatment of nasal fractures, nasal biopsy, and operative control of epistaxis). The mean age of patients undergoing these types of procedures is 40.4 years with the largest age distribution in the 15–44-year-old age group. There is an estimated slight male predominance of 53.7 % [3].

Septal surgery has evolved over time from the traditional submucous resection to more contemporary septoplasty techniques. At the same time, turbinate surgery continues to move in the same direction with an emphasis on mucosal and structural preservation. For the purposes of this discussion, we will focus on intranasal septoplasty techniques and its outcomes. Open rhinoplasty techniques and surgical intervention for acute nasal trauma are also important adjunct procedures and have their role for treating patients with nasal obstruction.

Surgical Anatomy

Functional Anatomy

The nasal septum divides the nasal cavity into two separate anatomic compartments starting at the nasal vestibule and ending at the choanae and sphenoid rostrum. Deviation of the nasal septum from the midline appears to be a common finding among the general population. Published estimates of the prevalence of nasal septal deviation in the population of otolaryngology patients may reach almost 90 % [4]. The etiology of septal deviation is not entirely clear although traumatic nasal injury seems to contribute in some instances to septal deviations. Skull base remodeling, birth trauma, and iatrogenic insult have also been implicated [4, 5]. A tendency for inferior turbinate hypertrophy to occur contralateral to a unilateral septal deviation

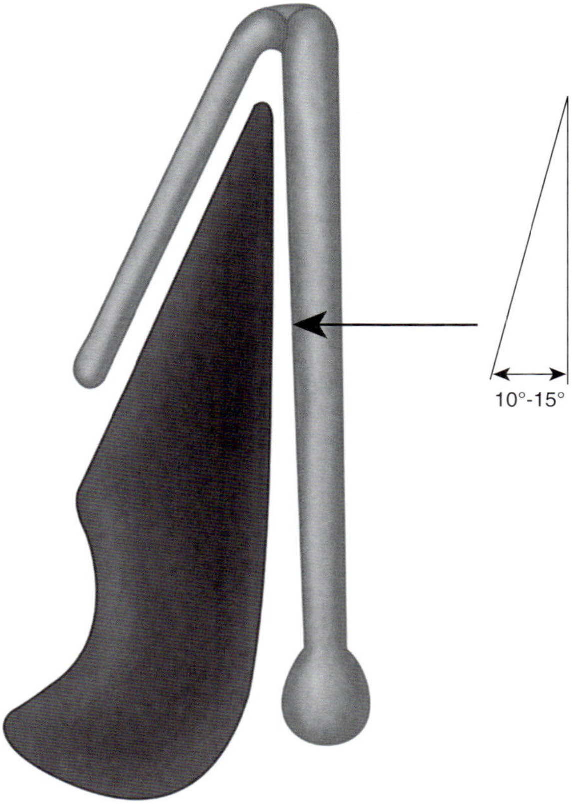

Fig. 31.1 The anatomy of the internal nasal valve showing the relationship of the most anterior portion of the inferior turbinate, the caudal aspect of the upper lateral cartilage, and the nasal septum (Reprinted from Schlosser and Park [8], February 1999, with permission from Elsevier). The image required enhancement and adaptation for final publication

is well recognized. Systems to classify nasal septal deviations have been described, and observations concerning specific subtypes of nasal septal deviations have provided evidence that at least some anterior septal deviations may be hereditary [6].

The internal nasal valve is described as the region between the caudal edge of the upper lateral cartilage, the head of the inferior turbinate, and the nasal septum. It represents an area of maximal nasal airway resistance [7]. Anatomic obstruction of the internal nasal valve can occur not only with nasal valve incompetence but can be exacerbated due to high septal pathology. This area should be noted during any standard nasal exam (Fig. 31.1) [8].

Structural Anatomy

The majority of the nasal septum is composed of bone and cartilage covered on both sides by mucosal epithelium. The most caudal portion of the nasal septum, the membranous septum, is covered by skin with associated hair follicles, vibrissae, and it is continuous inferiorly with the columella. By pushing the membranous septum laterally in either direction, the most caudal portion of the nasal septal, or quadrangular, cartilage may be identified. A transition of the epithelium from hair-bearing skin to mucosa occurs near the junction of the membranous septum and the nasal septal cartilage. The nasal septal cartilage provides structural support to the nasal dorsum. Lack of support in this area will lead to a saddle nose deformity or supratip depression. The anterior nasal spine of the maxilla and the maxillary crest provide an inferior attachment for the nasal septal cartilage at or near the midline. Unilateral deficiency of the nasal spine and maxillary crest on one side, as can be found in unilateral cleft palate, may be associated with deviation of the cartilaginous septum away from the deficient side [9].

The perpendicular plate of the ethmoid bone lies posterior and superior to the nasal septal cartilage. It continues further superiorly to join the skull base at the thin cribriform plate of the ethmoid bone. The vomer sits posterior and inferior to the septal cartilage. Inferiorly, the vomer is attached to the hard palate by the maxillary crest and the crest of the palatine bone. The posterior superior aspect of the vomer is attached to the anterior face of the sphenoid bone in the midline. Aeration of the sphenoid bone extending into the posterior septum can occur. Spurs and bony septal deflections are prone to occur near the junction of the vomer and the perpendicular plate of the ethmoid bone. The actual amount of contact between these two bones is dependent upon the amount of intervening nasal septal cartilage. The frontal bones also make small contributions to the bony portion of the nasal septum.

Blood Supply

The nasal septum has a robust submucosal blood supply which receives contributions from the internal carotid artery by way of the anterior and posterior ethmoidal arteries as well as from branches of the external carotid artery. These include the sphenopalatine artery via the posterior septal artery, a contribution from the greater palatine artery traveling through the incisive foramen, and the facial artery from the septal branch of the superior labial artery. Kiesselbach's plexus (Fig. 31.2) [10], a

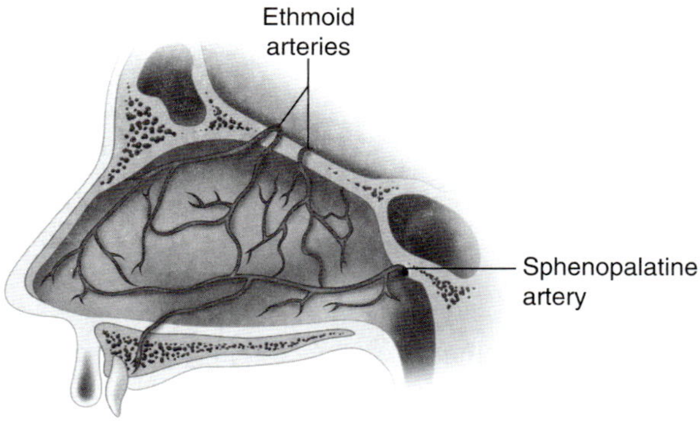

Fig. 31.2 The arterial blood supply and the confluence of blood vessels in Kiesselbach's area of the nasal septum (Image reprinted with permission from Watson [10]. University of California, San Diego, School of Medicine). The image required enhancement and adaptation for final publication

confluence of superficial terminal arterial branches along the caudal nasal septum, is a common location for anterior epistaxis [11].

A bloodless dissection along the nasal septal cartilage can be accomplished by entering the subperichondrial plane. This is possible because the nutrient supply to the chondrocytes within the cartilage occurs via diffusion down the concentration gradients from the vascular perichondrium through the avascular extracellular matrix of the cartilage [12].

Anatomy of the Inferior Turbinates

The inferior turbinates consist of a solitary bone, the inferior nasal concha, which is covered with a thick mucous membrane. This membrane contains cavernous tissue which is active in the nasal cycle, a periodic swelling of the nasal mucous membranes. In addition to its physiologic role in regulating humidification and nasal airflow, the nasal cycle may contribute to the perception of nasal airway obstruction, and often individuals with significant nasal septal deviation will have a heightened awareness of their own nasal cycle.

Innervation

The nasal cavities including the septum and the inferior turbinates have a complex pattern of innervation related to the multiple functions of the mucosal lining of the nose. The superior portion of the nasal cavity including a portion of the superior nasal septum is covered with olfactory epithelium which transmits neurons through the olfactory bulbs along CN I. General sensory innervation from the remaining nasal cavity is transmitted by way of branches of CN V1 and V2. The anterior and superior portions of the nasal septum are innervated by branches of V1 via the anterior ethmoidal nerve which arises as a branch of the nasociliary nerve within the bony orbit, while the inferior and posterior portions of the nasal septum and the inferior turbinates are supplied by branches of V2 arising from the sphenopalatine and greater palatine nerves [12]. Autonomic innervation of the nasal cavity occurs along branches of V2 which distribute both postganglionic parasympathetic and postganglionic sympathetic fibers.

Indications

The evaluation of a patient for septal and/or turbinate surgery starts with a thorough history and physical exam evaluation. Some patients will present with a diagnosis already established or suggested by a referring physician that needs confirmation. However, most will be seen with a chief complaint of nasal obstruction that then requires a full otolaryngologic evaluation. In addition to a standard medical history, the physician should specifically ask questions regarding time onset, laterality of

Table 31.1 Differential diagnosis of nasal obstruction

Structural/anatomic
Nasal septal deviation
Internal nasal valve collapse
External nasal valve insufficiency
Nasal tip ptosis
Nasal turbinate hypertrophy
Septal perforation
Empty nose syndrome
Neoplastic
Malignant
Benign
Inflammatory
Nasal polyposis
Rhinosinusitis
Allergic rhinitis
Nonallergic rhinitis
Hormonal (e.g., rhinitis of pregnancy, hypothyroidism)
Primary vasomotor rhinitis
Rhinitis medicamentosa
Granulomatous and autoimmune disease
Granulomatosis with polyangiitis (Wegener's granulomatosis)
Sarcoid
Churg-Strauss syndrome
Foreign body
Medications
Intranasal illicit drug use
Congenital
Choanal atresia (unilateral or bilateral)
Nasolacrimal duct cyst
Encephalocele

symptoms, time variation (intermittent vs. constant), epistaxis, facial pain or hypesthesia, improvement with prior use of nasal medications or antihistamines, as well as symptoms suggestive of atopy (e.g., seasonal variation, environmental triggers, sneezing, rhinorrhea, ocular symptoms, eczema). The past medical and social history should include an inquiry regarding the history of preceding or ongoing illness, recurrent sinusitis, confirmed diagnosis of environmental allergies, facial trauma, abuse of topical decongestants, or intranasal illicit drug use. The differential diagnosis for a patient with nasal obstruction is outlined in Table 31.1.

The physical exam is a key aspect of the initial evaluation. The exam should start with close attention to the external anatomy looking for potential areas of structural deficits contributing to the patient's symptoms of nasal obstruction. While patients may present with a chief complaint of functional limitations, they may also have further expectations regarding cosmetic outcomes from nasal surgery. It is best to establish up front the purpose of a septoplasty in order to avoid any misunderstandings about the ultimate goals of therapy.

Major external structures to examine include the nasal tip, nasal dorsum, and nasal valve regions. Nasal tip ptosis is more common with advanced age and requires open rhinoplasty techniques to correct. Severe dorsal septal deflections as well may require open techniques. One of the initial key elements in deciding on a septoplasty approach is to first determine if the patient would be better served by an open septorhinoplasty. Most importantly, the nasal valve region should be examined carefully since this is a major reason for failed outcomes after surgery. The most traditional maneuver used to evaluate nasal valve collapse is the Cottle maneuver. The examiner places his or her hand along the nasolabial groove to provide tension and pull the nasal wall lateral while the patient takes an inspiratory breath through the nose. A subjective improvement in nasal airflow can indicate potential internal nasal valve collapse [13]. Becker et al. [2] performed a large review of 577 patients who underwent septoplasty looking at outcome failures and identifying risk factors in patients who required revision surgery. Multivariate analysis confirmed that patients who had nasal valve surgery in conjunction with their primary septoplasty were significantly less likely to undergo revision surgery. For those that did require revision septoplasty surgery, 40 % had nasal valve surgery done at the time of the second procedure [2]. Overall, there is a lack of strong primary evidence in the literature regarding outcomes in nasal valve surgery with many uncontrolled observational studies. This is an area for future research as cited by the most recent clinical consensus statement by the American Academy of Otolaryngology – Head and Neck Surgery (AAO-HNS) [14].

The examination proceeds to anterior rhinoscopy after completing the external nasal examination. Direct anterior rhinoscopy with a nasal speculum provides a working perspective of the anterior nasal anatomy. Attention is first brought to the caudal septum and the degree of deformity that may exist. This portion of the examination requires direct visualization with the speculum removed and while inserted gently in the nose. Palpation is also useful to determine the structural pathology present in this region. The anterior half of the septum and particularly the nasal valve region can be visualized well along with the inferior turbinates. This should be done before instilling any decongestant solution so as to appreciate a true understanding of the degree of visible nasal obstruction. While posterior septal deflections can be partially viewed using adequate illumination along with appropriate nasal decongestion, a complete examination for complaints of nasal obstruction typically necessitates a formal nasal endoscopy. Both rigid and flexible techniques are acceptable with flexible endoscopy allowing for further evaluation of the lower pharynx and larynx at the same time if clinically indicated. Flexible instrumentation may also be necessary for patients with severe septal deflections in order to fully visualize the middle meatus and posterior anatomic structures. Most importantly, a nasal endoscopy examination will provide a complete evaluation of the entire nasal cavity to identify any synchronous pathology such as nasal polyps, rhinosinusitis, or nasal tumors.

Clinical indicators developed by the AAO-HNS for septoplasty surgery include nasal airway obstruction, frequent epistaxis, atypical facial pain of nasal origin (rhinogenic or contact point headaches), and deformity that prevents surgical access for other nasal procedures including functional endoscopic sinus surgery and skull base operations [15]. Clinical indicators outlined by the AAO-HNS for inferior turbinate surgery include a history of chronic nasal obstruction, failure of directed medical management, failure of treatment of rhinitis medicamentosa, or symptoms of OSA [16]. Septal deviation has been identified as a risk factor in patients with epistaxis. O'Reilly et al. [17] studied a group of 54 patients with recurrent epistaxis compared to controls. They demonstrated a significant association with nasal septal deviation ($p <.001$) [17]. Another study determined that 16/75 patients with intractable epistaxis had a septal deviation near the site of bleeding [18]. Patients with post-traumatic epistaxis are also more likely to demonstrate an external nasal deformity [19]. Contact point or rhinogenic headaches have been a topic of interest for some time with many studies published on the topic. Harrison and Jones [20] completed a systematic review of the topic in 2013. They identified 65 potential studies with 22 included in the final analysis. They concluded that nasal contact points can be identified in many asymptomatic subjects. Also, the literature that supports the removal of contact points is mostly retrospective and uncontrolled in design and does not consistently use the International Headache Society criteria [20]. For now, it is a continuing topic of clinical interest and further research. Septoplasty can be necessary as an adjunct procedure for surgical access during endoscopic sinus procedures. Rudmik et al. [21] reviewed 221 patients undergoing endoscopic sinus surgery. All patients had chronic rhinosinusitis (CRS) without nasal polyposis. Approximately half (108/221) required a septoplasty. Compared to those patients who did not have septal surgery, concurrent septoplasty did not appear to affect surgical outcomes (CRS-related HRQoL) [21]. Van Lindert et al. [22] reviewed 185 patients undergoing endoscopic transsphenoidal pituitary surgery. About 50 % of patients had a deformity of the nasal septum or anterior septal spine. Overall, 16 patients (8.6 %) required some form of surgical correction to allow for anatomic access to the sphenoid sinus [22]. Nasal surgery is playing a growing role in the treatment of patients with obstructive sleep apnea (OSA). Overall, studies to date have demonstrated limited efficacy of nasal surgery in improving objective polysomnographic measures of OSA disease. However, studies have shown improvement in subjective measures including snoring, quality of life, and sleepiness [23–28]. It should be noted, though, that the literature is limited to uncontrolled case series and there is continued interest in regard to the use of nasal surgery in multilevel sleep apnea surgery. The efficacy of nasal surgery in improving CPAP compliance use has also been investigated in the literature with promising results [29–31].

For septoplasty surgery, the AAO-HNS clinical indicators [15] state that nasal endoscopy and CT scan are optional tests in the preoperative period. We would encourage the use of nasal endoscopy in the preoperative workup as emphasized above in our discussion. Radiologic testing is not typically done routinely for every patient presenting for nasal obstruction especially given the increasing concerns regarding the risk of iatrogenic radiation exposure. Karatas et al. [32] did a study of patients who underwent septoplasty with preoperative screening CT scan. The most common findings were concha bullosa, inferior turbinate hypertrophy, and chronic sinusitis [32]. Given the cost and inherent risks of CT, it is most appropriate to reserve this testing for patients with specific clinical indications. For nasal turbinate surgery, the AAO-HNS [16] lists an allergy evaluation, rhinomanometry, and acoustic rhinometry as optional tests in the preoperative setting. Allergy testing is appropriate when clinically suspected and the patient does not respond to conventional medical therapy. The use of rhinomanometry and acoustic rhinometry in the conventional ambulatory clinical setting is limited and typically reserved for research purposes.

Surgical Technique

Preoperative Decision Making

While precision technique and experience are critical to a successful surgical outcome, strategic preoperative planning is the most important step in the care of these patients. The nasal surgeon should not prescribe to any one septoplasty "style." The vast array of different septal pathology demands an armamentarium of surgical approaches and techniques to manage the individual patient. While a classic submucous resection is certainly no longer necessary for every patient, at the same time, an overly conservative septoplasty can leave inadequate results. The first step after performing your evaluation is to decide if the patient can be approached using an endonasal vs. open septorhinoplasty technique. Conditions that may necessitate an open approach include severe dorsal septal twisting or deviations contributing to airway obstruction, nasal tip ptosis, severe caudal septal deflections, and deficient nasal valve architecture requiring open cartilage grafting. Standard incisions involve either a hemitransfixion or Killian's incision and should be adapted to the individual patient (Fig. 31.3) [10].

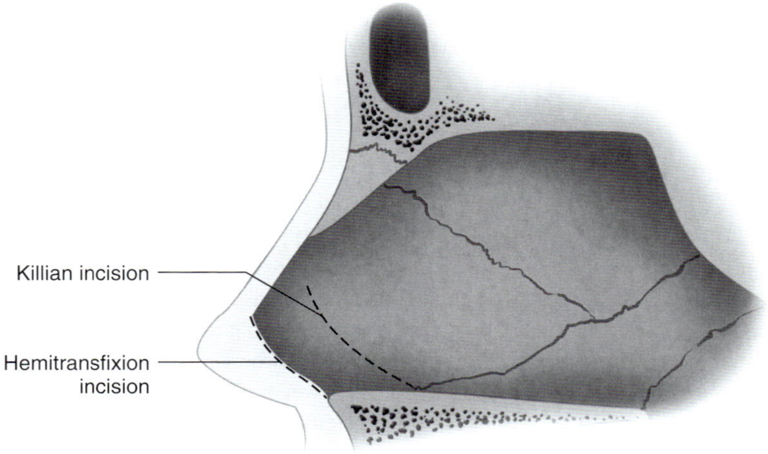

Fig. 31.3 Common septoplasty incisions [10] (Image reprinted with permission from Watson [10]. University of California, San Diego, School of Medicine). The image required enhancement and adaptation for final publication

Surgical Preparation

Surgery can be performed using either general anesthesia or local techniques with/without sedation. After anesthesia induction, a throat pack is typically placed to prevent the collection of blood in the hypopharynx and stomach. However, there is no evidence that this reduces postoperative nausea and vomiting. Recent work suggests it may be more efficacious to remove blood using an orogastric tube at the end of surgery [33]. The septum is prepped in the same fashion regardless of whether the patient receives general anesthesia. The two main purposes of a septal injection are hydrodissection and vasoconstriction. This is critical and the first technique taught to anyone learning the art of septal surgery. A topical solution of oxymetazoline (0.05 %) is placed in the nasal cavity bilaterally using nasal pledgets or cotton balls. Next, 1 % lidocaine with 1:100,000 solution is injected using a 25-gauge needle or smaller along the septum in a subperiosteal and subperichondrial plane. A stepwise injection technique is used where the edge of the dissection bleb from the prior injection is used as a starting point to develop the next area of hydrodissection. The oxymetazoline pledgets are then replaced while scrubbing and prepping the patient to allow time for adequate effect. Higgins et al. [34] completed a systematic review of topical vasoconstrictors used in nasal surgery. They emphasized safe and judicious use of these medications and recommended avoiding topical phenylephrine if possible along with cautious use of topical cocaine [34]. Beta-blockers should be avoided to treat hypertension during cases using alpha adrenergic agonists to avoid unintended development of pulmonary edema [35, 36].

The efficacy of hydrostatic injections is controversial. Studies do demonstrate that the perichondrial layer provides the largest amount of tensile strength and thus a subperichondrial dissection is logical and favored [37]. However, the technique of hydrodissection has been questioned. A cadaveric study by Dubach et al. [38] demonstrated only 25 % (5/20) of experimental cases with injections performed in the correct dissection plane. Most injections were either in the perichondrium itself or supra-perichondrial [38]. This may be an area for further investigation and research.

Submucous Resection

The traditional submucous resection of the septum dates back over half a century with the instrumentation and surgical technique mostly unaltered over time. After appropriate surgical preparation, the procedure begins with one of the traditional incisions (Fig. 31.3). Typically, for a classical submucous resection, a Killian's incision is made on the left side of the septum. This approach is generally taken due to the predominance of right-handed surgeons. However, a right-sided incision can be made as well if deemed necessary for the particular clinical circumstance. A no. 15 blade knife is used to incise through the mucosa and perichondrium. This is a key part of the procedure, and much time will be saved later in the procedure if some additional patience and attention are paid to this step. If the dissection starts in the incorrect surgical plane, the operation will inevitably be more difficult with an increased likelihood of mucosal tears and loss of subsequent flap integrity. The proper plane of dissection is determined by visualization and tactile feedback with the instrumentation. With modern-day halogen headlights used in the operating room, the septal cartilage will reflect back almost a slight bluish hue that is bright white in color. With proper vasoconstriction, the subperichondrial plane should be avascular with minimal bleeding. Excessive bleeding from inside the flap indicates that the dissection may be progressing at the incorrect depth. It is even acceptable to begin dissecting just slightly into the superficial layer of the cartilage itself to ensure that one is deep enough within the plane of dissection and then back off into the proper layer. In an atraumatic patient with no prior nasal surgery, the subperichondrial plane will dissect quite easily also providing an indicator of a correct surgical dissection level. After incising with the scalpel, a sharp elevator is used such as a Cottle elevator or Tebbetts™ septal elevator. Carefully, the flap is elevated using this instrumentation until an adequate length of flap is raised to allow for the introduction of a nasal speculum in a vertical orientation. At this point, one can use a less aggressive instrument such as a Freer elevator if preferred or continue with a sharp elevator if needed to continue flap dissection. The dissection is carried posterior to the bony-cartilaginous junction. There is usually a small area of flap adhesion at this line that requires some careful elevation. Once dissection proceeds to the bone, the surgeon needs to reconfirm if he or she is working in the correct plane. At any point in the dissection, when transitioning between different bones or from cartilage to bone, there is usually a small amount of flap adhesion at these suture lines. As the surgery proceeds along the perpendicular plate of the ethmoid bone, care is taken to avoid dissection near the cribriform plate but high enough so that all areas of structural deviation are addressed. The flap is elevated down to the floor of the nose. The septal flaps may fold over and sit deeply in the groove between the quadrangular cartilage and maxillary crest. Therefore, this area of flap elevation should typically be done last. A Pierce elevator may be useful in this circumstance especially with more inferiorly located spurs. Next, a transcartilaginous incision is created along the caudal septal cartilage. Care is taken to leave at least a 1-cm caudal strut. This can be performed using a scalpel knife or sharp elevator. Typically, an elevator is adequate and less likely to create a contralateral perforation in the mucosa. A contralateral flap is raised on the opposite side similar in fashion to the initial dissection. A long nasal speculum is then inserted fully back to the face of the sphenoid rostrum once the flaps have been fully developed. At this point, a swivel knife can be used to remove a large section of deviated cartilage and set aside for later replacement if necessary. Deviated portions of the perpendicular ethmoid plate and vomer are removed using Jansen-Middleton cutting forceps. Care is taken not to use any torsional force when removing these superior portions of the bone to avoid a CSF leak. Once the superior attachments are free, the lower sections of the bone and spurs can be removed more aggressively using a grasping instrument such as Takahashi forceps. Large 90° oriented spurs that prevented adequate flap elevation earlier in the procedure can now be fractured off the floor of the nose using an elevator and gently teased away from the attached mucosa. Anterior, there is typically a strip of cartilage still in place along the maxillary crest that can be removed using a

Freer elevator. Small deviations in the maxillary crest are typically not responsible for symptomatic nasal airway obstruction as opposed to high septal deviations along the nasal valve region. Aggressive removal of the maxillary crest can lead to subsequent postoperative dental anesthesia. Therefore, discretion must be used in judging whether to remove portions of this bone. If necessary, a 4-mm chisel and mallet can be utilized to remove any deviated sections. Care should be taken throughout the procedure to preserve a 1-cm caudal and dorsal strut for structural support and prevention of postoperative nasal tip ptosis and/or dorsal saddle nose deformities. Upon completion of the resection, the amputated cartilage graft can be reformed and flattened using a press and replaced between the flaps. This is generally more important in scenarios where a bilateral opposing septal mucosal tear exists after flap elevation. Care must be taken upon closure to not allow the cartilage graft to "slip" inferior and sit alongside the remaining maxillary crest creating a new postoperative septal deformity. The incision can be closed using absorbable suture such as 4–0 chromic gut. Especially if a cartilage graft was replaced, quilting sutures are recommended using absorbable suture such as 4–0 plain gut with a straight needle to avoid mucosal trauma. Running quilting sutures should be used with caution which can cause strangulation of the septal mucosa if done in a circumferential fashion. Sutures placed in an interrupted fashion can avoid this potential problem. If a mucosal tear does not already exist from the prior dissection, a drainage incision needs to be created posterior-inferior to prevent postoperative hematoma formation. Use a scalpel blade to create a puncture site in conjunction with angled scissors.

Septoplasty

Evolution from the days of Gleason and Watson to the contemporary septoplasty has been slow and stepwise. The modern-day septoplasty emphasizes structural support and tissue conservation. A hemitransfixion incision is typically utilized to open the caudal septum, but some variation starting more posterior is also appropriate depending on the location of the pathology. Again, emphasizing that every septum is unique, thus the surgery should be tailored and adapted to the individual patient. A subperichondrial flap is raised again on the left side typically as with the submucous resection. However, instead of removing the quadrangular cartilage, the bony-cartilaginous junction is identified and divided using the Freer elevator with contralateral flap elevation. At this point, deviated sections of bone are removed using cutting forceps. Since the cartilage is still in place, this dissection takes place in a smaller space. Care must be taken not to perforate the posterior superior flap and injure the middle turbinate. Surgical treatment of the anterior cartilage is an expansive topic with volumes of text written on individual subunits such as the caudal septum. Techniques emphasize different variations of conservative cartilage removal with repositioning of the remaining structural elements. Commonly, an inferior thin strip of cartilage is removed allowing the cartilage to realign into proper position classically known as the "swinging door" technique. Remaining memory might require further scoring using a sharp instrument such as a Freer knife. Curvature can still remain in a severely deviated septum, and many times, it is also prudent to raise a contralateral flap anterior through the hemitransfixion incision fully isolating the anterior cartilage and removing any attachments of the opposing mucosa. Despite cartilage scoring techniques, the contralateral mucosa can remain a barrier to allowing the cartilage to relax into a neutral position. Further suturing may be required to hold the septum in position along the maxillary crest. A caudal septal deviation can be a challenging and vexing problem. If treated through an endonasal septoplasty approach rather than an open rhinoplasty, full bilateral flap elevation is typically necessary. The question at this point is whether to remove the cartilage and replace it with a reformed cartilage graft or try to realign the cartilage in situ. If cartilage segments are removed from the caudal septum, it can be difficult to replace these grafts in an endonasal fashion. Some authors have advocated the use of polydioxanone (PDS) foil (Ethicon Inc, Johnson & Johnson) as an adjunct to septal reconstruction [39–42]. Sections of resected cartilage are laid out on a piece of PDS foil and sutured in place. A second piece of foil can be placed on the opposite side for further support. The graft is then sutured in place between the septal flaps. The incisions are closed in a standard fashion as with a traditional submucous resection.

Endoscopic Septoplasty/Blended Techniques

Endoscopic septoplasty is a newer technique that has come about with the advent of endoscopic sinus surgery. The ideal candidate for a minimally invasive pure endoscopic septoplasty is the patient with an isolated posterior bony spur or anatomic deformity. The area is injected directly with local anesthetic solution to hydrodissect the mucosa off the bone. This is done under direct endoscopic guidance using either a long 25-gauge spinal needle or tonsil needle. A small limited mucosal flap is raised off the spur exposing the bone. The spur can be directly removed using a small diamond burr. Otherwise the section of deformed bone can be fully cut out and isolated with dissection off the contralateral flap. The small mucosal flap is just laid down without any suturing. If done in conjunction with sinus surgery, the middle turbinate can many times be sutured in place against this area for support. A "blended" or "back-and-forth" technique is now becoming more common [43]. A variation of endoscopic septoplasty, the septal incisions are made through a traditional approach, but the endoscope is used between the flaps intermittently throughout the procedure to provide magnified visualization of the posterior structures and assistance in raising flaps in challenging areas.

Traditional Submucous Turbinate Resection

Aggressive partial or complete inferior turbinate resection including the overlying mucosa can lead to long-term complications of atrophic rhinitis or "empty nose syndrome." This procedure is not advocated by the authors and will not be detailed for that reason. A traditional submucous resection involves first injecting the turbinate in a submucosal fashion along its length on each side using a standard local anesthetic solution used in septal surgery. An incision is made along the anterior two-thirds of the turbinate and a mucosal flap raised along the bone. Cutting instruments such as a Jansen-Middleton forceps or long scissors are used to remove a section of the bone. The flaps are then laid back in position and not typically sutured in place. The turbinates can be outfractured to provide additional expansion of the airway.

Microdebrider-Assisted Turbinate Reduction

Microdebrider-assisted turbinate reduction is widely used today to address inferior turbinate pathology. The technology is readily available during endoscopic sinus surgery cases further lending to its convenience and surgeon comfort with the device. The anterior turbinate head and body are again injected with local anesthetic solution, allowing time to have its effect. Under direct endoscopic visualization, the tip of the blade can be used to make a puncture incision along the anterior head of the turbinate and subsequently raise a small submucosal pocket as far posterior as necessary to address the degree of turbinate hypertrophy. Alternatively, a no. 15 blade knife can be used to make a small anterior incision with a standard Freer elevator then utilized to raise the flap. As the flap is raised, care must be taken not to tear a lengthwise flap or create posterior perforation sites. Various microdebrider blades exist from different manufacturers with some designed specifically for inferior turbinate use. In general, the blade is passed into the pocket with the cutting edge of the blade facing lateral. Debridement is performed posterior to anterior but can move back and forth if necessary. Attention should be paid anterior-superior to the area of the internal nasal valve. The blade needs to be angled superior to reach this area when moving anterior, which can be a critical area of obstruction. The turbinates are then outfractured if deemed necessary.

Radio-frequency Turbinate Ablation

Radio-frequency ablation can be done alone as an office-based procedure or in the same setting as other concurrent nasal surgery. Again, settings for the equipment vary based on the manufacturer. The general principle involves making multiple passes using a needle electrode tip device in a submucosal plane along the length of the turbinate. Energy is delivered through the tip to the surrounding tissue. Care must be taken not to burn the edge of the nasal vestibule when using these devices.

Perioperative Care

Perioperative care in nasal surgery has been an active source of debate over the years regarding the use of corticosteroids, antibiotics, nasal packing, and airway splints. There is limited evidence looking at the role of corticosteroids in the perioperative care of nasal surgery patients. One recent randomized double-blind trial demonstrated decreased pain and improved postoperative nausea and vomiting when a single 8-mg dose of dexamethasone was given at induction of anesthesia [44]. Multiple studies have looked at the role of perioperative antibiotic usage in nasal surgery [45–48]. Georgioiu et al. [49] concluded in a literature review that the rate of postoperative infection is very low and recommended antibiotic usage in cases of complicated revision surgery, prolonged nasal packing placement, and patients at risk for infection. More recently, Ricci and D'Ascanio [50] conducted a prospective randomized clinical trial of 630 patients undergoing septoplasty. There was no significant difference in outcomes or complication rates regardless of antibiotic administration [50]. Other studies have also shown that systemic antibiotics do not protect against *S. aureus* colonization in the postoperative period [51]. However, another study by Bandhauer et al. [52] demonstrated that packing soaked in antibiotic ointment may impede the growth of *S. aureus*. Gioacchini et al. [53] performed the most recent contemporary review and meta-analysis of the topic in 2014. They were able to identify two studies for statistical review (including the above RCT). The meta-analysis showed no association between postoperative infection and use of antibiotics. They conclude there is limited evidence to support the use of routine antibiotic prophylaxis; however, they do note that there are only three studies to date that include a nontreatment group (no antibiotics) [53].

Traditionally, nasal packing was tightly placed in each nasal cavity after septal surgery using petroleum jelly-soaked gauze. The role of nasal packing after septal surgery has been investigated over the past three decades [54–62]. Recent contemporary reviews have attempted to clarify its efficacy [52, 62–64]. A systematic review and meta-analysis was completed in 2012 comparing transseptal suturing methods to traditional packing. They concluded that postoperative pain and headache were significantly lower in non-packing patients and that packing conferred no advantage over transseptal suturing alone in regard to postoperative complications [63]. A meta-analysis in 2013 looking at the efficacy of nasal packing demonstrated no postoperative benefit [64]. A systematic review from 2013 compared various methods of postoperative care (quilting sutures, nasal packing, nasal splints, fibrin glue). They concluded that the studies demonstrated no benefit of different packing methods over quilting sutures alone. However, the authors did note a lack of high-quality studies and significant bias in many articles [65]. Finally, the aforementioned review by Gioacchini et al. [53] also looked at the role of nasal packing. They also concluded no advantage to the use of packing and point to the possible increased risk of complications.

As with nasal packing, the role of septal splints has also been debated over the decades [66–71]. A review done in 2012 identified six randomized trials looking at the use of intranasal splints. They concluded there is no benefit to the routine use of splints [72]. A study investigating the timing of splint removal demonstrated equal outcomes when splints were removed at 24 h or 5 days [73]. This further suggests there may be no benefit to their use in nasal surgery.

Complications

There is a paucity of good prospective data regarding complication rates during septoplasty and turbinate surgery. Most studies are either retrospective or relate to some type of intervention (e.g., nasal packing). Potential complications after septal and turbinate surgery are listed in Table 31.2.

Reported rates of septal perforation range between less than 1 and 5 % [74, 75]. Many asymptomatic perforations are probably underreported overall. Cosmetic deformities are uncommon after septoplasty surgery [76]. However, minor subclinical cosmetic changes in the postoperative period may be more common than previously reported. Daudia et al. [77] found a high rate of minor cosmetic deformities when measured using standardized objective measures. However, these findings had no correlation with subjective patient perceptions [77]. Infections overall are rare after septal and turbinate surgery. There are case reports of toxic shock syndrome (TSS) after use of nasal packing [78] and intranasal splints [79]. Cerebrospinal fluid (CSF) rhinorrhea after septoplasty is a rare but serious complication [80, 81]. Prevention is most important with care taken when resecting high deviations. Encephaloceles have been rarely reported to form as a result of septoplasty [82]. Anosmia overall is a rare complication, but temporary hyposmia has been seen in patients undergoing both septoplasty and inferior turbinate surgery [83–85]. Limited studies have been done to investigate the rate of dental anesthesia of the upper incisors after septoplasty surgery, but it is a potential complication. Ocular complications are very rare, but reports do exist [86, 87].

For patients with OSA undergoing multilevel surgery, Pang et al. [88] reviewed 487 cases and found a complication rate of 7.1 % overall. Only 1 patient had postoperative upper airway obstruction [88]. A more recent study also affirmed these findings [89]. In addition, patients with OSA undergoing nasal surgery alone may have a temporary worsening of OSA parameters if nasal packing is placed in the postoperative period [90].

Table 31.2 Complications after septal and turbinate surgery

Septal surgery
Hemorrhage/septal hematoma
Infection/septal abscess/toxic shock syndrome
Septal perforation
Cerebrospinal fluid leak
Anosmia
Tooth anesthesia
Structural deformity (saddle nose, nasal tip ptosis)
Ocular complications
Cardiac/medical complications
Turbinate surgery
Hemorrhage
Infection
Atrophic rhinitis

Atrophic rhinitis has been attributed to overly aggressive turbinate resection with chronic symptoms of nasal crusting, mucosal atrophy, and nasal congestion. Primary and secondary forms exist with the later being associated with trauma or prior nasal surgery [91]. Empty nose syndrome is a similar entity more specifically referring to the symptoms of paradoxical nasal congestion [92].

More serious medical complications can occur as well after septoplasty. A recent review in 2014 demonstrated no convincing evidence of increased cardiac complications with nasal packing after septoplasty [93]. Turhan et al. [94] studied 43 patients who underwent septoplasty with a normal preoperative apnea-hypopnea index (AHI). Patients who underwent nasal packing had an increased AHI post-op as well as more severe oxygen desaturations [94]. Patients undergoing nasal packing have been seen to be at least three times more likely to have respiratory distress in the postoperative period [95]. Reports of death exist in the literature due to skull base injury as well [96]. Fortunately, this is quite rare.

Clinical Efficacy Data

Nasal airway obstruction is a common presenting complaint in rhinologic practice, and nasal septal reconstruction, either alone or combined with a procedure to reduce the size of the inferior turbinates, remains one of the most commonly performed surgical procedures in the practice of otolaryngology. Historically, septoplasty was performed for patients with persistent complaints of nasal airway obstruction and evidence of nasal septal deviation on physical examination. Although most practitioners would likely agree that the majority of patients who underwent septoplasty with or without turbinate reduction for this indication received benefit, difficulty exists in comparing surgical outcomes between studies. Outcomes are measured using an array of metrics, the surgical procedures both between and within studies are variable, and the criteria used when making the decision to proceed with surgery are inconsistent. Due to pressure on the surgical community from multiple sources, a method to standardize the reporting of surgical outcomes as well as identification of the patients most likely to benefit from nasal septal reconstruction and/or inferior turbinate reduction is desirable.

Quality of Life (QoL) Outcomes

It is believed that nasal septal deviation is widely prevalent in the general population, but surgical intervention is reserved for patients who in one manner or another are symptomatic. This idea provides the basis for the use of quality of life (QoL) instruments to assess the benefit of nasal septal surgery. The SNOT-22, a 22-question sinonasal outcome test, was used in a prospective study by Buckland et al. [97] with 75 % of individuals undergoing septoplasty or SMR with or without turbinate reduction reporting an improvement on the questions related to nasal obstruction. Similarly, Arunachalam et al. [98] conducted a prospective study of septoplasty with or without turbinate reduction for nasal obstruction. They utilized the Fairley nasal symptom score, a validated measure of nasal symptoms, finding significant improvement in nasal obstruction symptoms in 74 % of their patients at 6 weeks postoperatively [98]. A study by Konstantinids et al. [99] also demonstrated improvement in Fairley nasal symptom scores especially for those patients that rated their nasal obstruction as being more severe preoperatively. Neither of these studies demonstrated significant change in general health questionnaire scores between the preoperative and postoperative assessments.

Neither the SNOT-22 nor the Fairley nasal symptom score is a specific measure of nasal obstruction. In 2004, Stewart et al. [100] published the NOSE (Nasal Obstruction Symptom Evaluation) questionnaire as a validated, disease-specific instrument for measuring the severity of nasal obstruction symptoms. Since its publication [100], multiple prospective studies have been conducted that demonstrate significant improvement in NOSE scores following septoplasty [101–103]. In a follow-up prospective study written by Stewart et al. [101], 59 patients undergoing septoplasty alone or septoplasty and turbinate reduction were found to have significant overall improvement in NOSE scores 3 months after surgery. The magnitude of this improvement was maintained and did not change significantly at an assessment 6 months postoperatively indicating that the results were durable. No statistically significant difference in NOSE scores was seen between patients receiving septoplasty alone versus those that also underwent turbinate reduction. However, only 16 of the 59 patients underwent septoplasty as an isolated procedure [101].

Retrospective studies have also been performed utilizing the NOSE instrument. In one study by Toyserkani and Frisch [104] that had an 11-year follow-up, 68 % of patients who had undergone septoplasty reported symptomatic improvement on the NOSE scale, while those who reported the worst preoperative nasal obstruction were noted to have the largest improvement in their scores [104]. Other retrospective studies have also reported significant benefit in patient-reported symptoms of nasal obstruction [105, 106].

Patient Factors

As QoL measures are composed of a subjective self-reporting of a patient's own symptoms and patient-reported satisfaction with a surgical procedure relies on an individual's own judgment of the value of the procedure, it seems intuitive that any number of patient factors may influence the results of these measures. In the study by Toyserkani and Frisch [104], the authors noted that patients who continued to smoke at follow-up were noted to be less satisfied with their nasal surgery. However, other prospective studies have found no correlation between smoking and NOSE score reduction following septoplasty [107].

Mondina et al. [107] in a prospective study of septoplasty without inferior turbinate surgery observed that while age, gender, and BMI were not predictive factors in postoperative NOSE and RhinoQoL score improvement, the presence of allergic rhinitis (AR) did have a statistically significant impact. Another prospective study by Karatzanis et al. [108] also reported decrease in NOSE score improvement in patients with allergic rhinitis that underwent septoplasty alone. They also documented a decreased improvement in acoustic rhinometry measurements on the side of the septal deviation in patients with allergic rhinitis when compared to those without AR [108]. At least two other prospective trials examining the outcome of septoplasty with or without inferior turbinate surgery failed to show statistically significant differences in measured outcomes between subjects with AR and those without [101, 109]. This provides some evidence to support the importance of lateral nasal wall surgery in patients with AR.

One prospective study that evaluated personality traits of patients undergoing endoscopic sinus surgery with septoplasty and inferior turbinate reduction noted that the subgroup of patients with attachment anxiety did not have a statistically significant patient-reported QoL improvement following surgery while the overall group did. This supports the idea that subjective self-reporting on QoL measures may be influenced by psychological factors in addition to disease- and surgery-specific factors [110].

Objective Measures of Nasal Patency

Other objective measures of nasal patency such as acoustic rhinometry and active rhinomanometry are attractive for their ease of comparison, but they have shown inconsistent correlation with QoL measures and reports of symptom severity. In a follow-up on their 11-year retrospective study, Toyserkani et al. [111] did find that patients who reported that they were either satisfied or very satisfied with their surgery had a greater improvement in some measures on postoperative acoustic rhinometry but there was no correlation with NOSE scores. One prospective study also demonstrated improvement in postoperative rhinomanometry following septoplasty alone. Again, a significant correlation between NOSE score reduction and individual nasal airflow was not identified [108].

Comparison of Turbinate Surgeries and Outcomes of Septoplasty ± Turbinate Surgery

A single randomized controlled trial examined surgical outcomes of patients with nasal obstruction due to septal deviation with compensatory inferior turbinate hypertrophy. Earlier postoperative improvement in symptomatic nasal obstruction and improved acoustic rhinometry findings on the side of turbinate hypertrophy at both 3 and 6 months postoperatively were found in patients who underwent septoplasty with submucous resection of the inferior turbinate as opposed to septoplasty alone [112]. This study used a technique of submucous resection with powered instrumentation for turbinate reduction, but many different techniques to manage turbinate hypertrophy exist. Several studies have aimed to compare these various techniques.

A prospective three-way comparison of submucosal monopolar cauterization, Coblation, and ultrasound-assisted turbinate reduction demonstrated effectiveness of all procedures in improving acoustic rhinometry, active rhinomanometry, and nasal obstruction symptom self-reporting. Evidence that the ultrasound technique performed superior to the traditional monopolar cautery technique for all three measures was also provided [113]. Other authors have reported superiority of submucosal microdebrider-assisted turbinate reduction over conventional cautery and radio-frequency ablation over partial turbinectomy [114, 115].

Conclusions

Many prospective studies have documented improvement in nasal obstruction symptoms following septoplasty. Validated disease-specific quality of life measures for nasal obstruction exist and have been adopted for quality of life outcome reporting. There is evidence to suggest that turbinate reduction with septoplasty may be especially beneficial in patients with allergic rhinitis or compensatory turbinate hypertrophy. Multilevel upper airway surgery may improve treatment utilization in patients who are intolerant of nasal CPAP due to nasal obstruction. Objective measures of nasal patency have inconsistently shown correlation with quality of life measures or symptom reporting but can be consistently affected by surgical intervention on the internal nasal valve area. Multiple methods of managing inferior turbinate hypertrophy have been described, and the effectiveness of these methods has been documented.

The techniques involved in nasal septal and turbinate surgery have undergone much evolution and refinement over time while still adhering to time-honored principles. Contemporary nasal surgery is precise with an emphasis and focus on tissue preservation. While the indications are expanding into the frontiers of endoscopic sinus surgery, sleep surgery, and skull base operations, it still remains a cornerstone of surgical treatment for nasal airway obstruction. It is now over a century since the days of the Bosworth operation and the early work of Gleason and Watson. Despite this, nasal septal and turbinate surgery continues to be an active source of academic discussion, personal opinion, and ongoing efforts to improve patient outcomes.

References

1. Bailey BJ. Nasal septal surgery 1896–1899: transition and controversy. Laryngoscope. 1997; 107(1):10–6.
2. Becker SS, Dobratz EJ, Stowell N, Barker D, Park SS. Revision septoplasty: review of sources of persistent nasal obstruction. Am J Rhinol. 2008;22(4):440–4.
3. Bhattacharyya N. Ambulatory sinus and nasal surgery in the United States: demographics and perioperative outcomes. Laryngoscope. 2010;120(3):635–8.
4. Mladina R, Cujic E, Subaric M, Vukovic K. Nasal septal deformities in ear, nose, and throat patients: an international study. Am J Otolaryngol. 2008;29(2):75–82.

5. Gray LP. Deviated nasal septum. Incidence and etiology. Ann Otol Rhinol Laryngol Suppl. 1978;87(3 Pt 3 Suppl 50):3–20.
6. Mladina R, Subaric M. Are some septal deformities inherited? Type 6 revisited. Int J Pediatr Otorhinolaryngol. 2003;67(12):1291–4.
7. Moche JA, Palmer O. Surgical management of nasal obstruction. Oral Maxillofac Surg Clin North Am. 2012;24(2):229–37, viii.
8. Schlosser RJ, Park SS. Functional nasal surgery. Otoloaryngol Clin North Am. 1999;32(1): 37–51. Figure 1A. The upper lateral cartilage (ULC), nasal septum, head of the inferior turbinate, and floor of the nose; p. 38.
9. Sandham A, Murray JA. Nasal septal deformity in unilateral cleft lip and palate. Cleft Palate Craniofac J. 1993;30(2):222–6.
10. Watson D. Septoplasty. Published by Medscape Reference (http://www.emedicine.medscape.com/). 2014. Available at: http://www.emedicine.medscape.com/article/877677-overview.
11. Oneal RM, Beil Jr RJ, Schlesinger J. Surgical anatomy of the nose. Otolaryngol Clin North Am. 1999;32(1):145–81.
12. Gray H, Standring S, Ellis H, Berkovitz BKB. Gray's anatomy: the anatomical basis of clinical practice. 39th ed. Edinburgh/New York: Elsevier Churchill Livingstone; 2005.
13. Bloching MB. Disorders of the nasal valve area. GMS Curr Top Otorhinolaryngol Head Neck Surg. 2007;6:Doc07.
14. Rhee JS, Weaver EM, Park SS, Baker SR, Hilger PA, Kriet JD, et al. Clinical consensus statement: diagnosis and management of nasal valve compromise. Otolaryngol Head Neck Surg. 2010;143(1):48–59.
15. Clinical Indicators: Septoplasty. In: Clinical Indicators Compendium of the American Academy of Otolaryngology – Head and Neck Surgery. Available at: http://www.entnet.org/Practice/Septoplasty.cfm (2014). Accessed 14 May 2014.
16. Clinical Indicators: Inferior Turbinate Surgery. In: Clinical Indicators Compendium of the American Academy of Otolaryngology – Head and Neck Surgery. Available at: http://www.entnet.org/Practice/Inferior-Turbinate-Surgery.cfm (2014). Accessed 14 May 2014.
17. O'Reilly BJ, Simpson DC, Dharmeratnam R. Recurrent epistaxis and nasal septal deviation in young adults. Clin Otolaryngol Allied Sci. 1996;21(1):12–4.
18. Jackson KR, Jackson RT. Factors associated with active, refractory epistaxis. Arch Otolaryngol Head Neck Surg. 1988;114(8):862–5.
19. Daniel M, Raghavan U. Relation between epistaxis, external nasal deformity, and septal deviation following nasal trauma. Emerg Med J. 2005;22(11):778–9.
20. Harrison L, Jones NS. Intranasal contact points as a cause of facial pain or headache: a systematic review. Clin Otolaryngol. 2013;38(1):8–22.
21. Rudmik L, Mace J, Ferguson BJ, Smith TL. Concurrent septoplasty during endoscopic sinus surgery for chronic rhinosinusitis: does it confound outcomes assessment? Laryngoscope. 2011;121(12):2679–83.
22. Van Lindert EJ, Ingels K, Mylanus E, Grotenhuis JA. Variations of endonasal anatomy: relevance for the endoscopic endonasal transsphenoidal approach. Acta Neurochir (Wien). 2010;152(6):1015–20.
23. Meen EK, Chandra RK. The role of the nose in sleep-disordered breathing. Am J Rhinol Allergy. 2013;27(3):213–20.
24. Victores AJ, Takashima M. Effects of nasal surgery on the upper airway: a drug-induced sleep endoscopy study. Laryngoscope. 2012;122(11):2606–10.
25. Takahashi R, Ohbuchi T, Hohchi N, Takeuchi S, Ohkubo J, Ikezaki S, et al. Effect of septoplasty and turbinectomy on obstructive sleep apnea syndrome. Nihon Jibiinkoka Gakkai Kaiho. 2013;116(7):789–92.
26. Verse T, Maurer JT, Pirsig W. Effect of nasal surgery on sleep-related breathing disorders. Laryngoscope. 2002;112(1):64–8.
27. Li HY, Lee LA, Wang PC, Fang TJ, Chen NH. Can nasal surgery improve obstructive sleep apnea: subjective or objective? Am J Rhinol Allergy. 2009;23(6):e51–5.

28. Koutsourelakis I, Georgoulopoulos G, Perraki E, Vagiakis E, Roussos C, Zakynthinos SG. Randomised trial of nasal surgery for fixed nasal obstruction in obstructive sleep apnoea. Eur Respir J. 2008;31(1):110–7.
29. Friedman M, Tanyeri H, Lim JW, Landsberg R, Vaidyanathan K, Caldarelli D. Effect of improved nasal breathing on obstructive sleep apnea. Otolaryngol Head Neck Surg. 2000;122(1):71–4.
30. Poirier J, George C, Rotenberg B. The effect of nasal surgery on nasal continuous positive airway pressure compliance. Laryngoscope. 2014;124(1):317–9.
31. Powell NB, Zonato AI, Weaver EM, Li K, Troell R, Riley RW, et al. Radiofrequency treatment of turbinate hypertrophy in subjects using continuous positive airway pressure: a randomized, double-blind, placebo-controlled clinical pilot trial. Laryngoscope. 2001;111(10): 1783–90.
32. Karatas D, Yuksel F, Senturk M, Dogan M. The contribution of computed tomography to nasal septoplasty. J Craniofac Surg. 2013;24(5):1549–51.
33. Korkut AY, Erkalp K, Erden V, Teker AM, Demirel A, Gedikli O, et al. Effect of pharyngeal packing during nasal surgery on postoperative nausea and vomiting. Otolaryngol Head Neck Surg. 2010;143(6):831–6.
34. Higgins TS, Hwang PH, Kingdom TT, Orlandi RR, Stammberger H, Han JK. Systematic review of topical vasoconstrictors in endoscopic sinus surgery. Laryngoscope. 2011;121(2): 422–32.
35. Groudine SB, Hollinger I, Jones J, DeBouno BA. New York State guidelines on the topical use of phenylephrine in the operating room. The Phenylephrine Advisory Committee. Anesthesiology. 2000;92(3):859–64.
36. Schwalm JD, Hamstra J, Mulji A, Velianou JL. Cardiogenic shock following nasal septoplasty: a case report and review of the literature. Can J Anaesth. 2008;55(6):376–9.
37. Kim DW, Egan KK, O'Grady K, Toriumi DM. Biomechanical strength of human nasal septal lining: comparison of the constituent layers. Laryngoscope. 2005;115(8):1451–3.
38. Dubach P, Mantokoudis G, Banz Y, Herrmann G, Caversaccio M. Hydrodissection for subperichondrial septoplasty – an experimental anatomical study. Rhinology. 2010;48(2): 195–200.
39. Tweedie DJ, Lo S, Rowe-Jones JM. Reconstruction of the nasal septum using perforated and unperforated polydioxanone foil. Arch Facial Plast Surg. 2010;12(2):106–13.
40. Rimmer J, Ferguson LM, Saleh HA. Versatile applications of the polydioxanone plate in rhinoplasty and septal surgery. Arch Facial Plast Surg. 2012;14(5):323–30.
41. Boenisch M, Nolst Trenite GJ. Reconstruction of the nasal septum using polydioxanone plate. Arch Facial Plast Surg. 2010;12(1):4–10.
42. Gerlinger I, Karasz T, Somogyvari K, Szanyi I, Rath G, Moricz P, et al. Extracorporeal septal reconstruction with polydioxanone foil. Clin Otolaryngol. 2007;32(6):465–70.
43. Trimarchi M, Bellini C, Toma S, Bussi M. Back-and-forth endoscopic septoplasty: analysis of the technique and outcomes. Int Forum Allergy Rhinol. 2012;2(1):40–4.
44. Eftekharian A, Roozbahany NA. Use of intravenous steroids at induction of anesthesia for septoplasty to reduce post-operative nausea and vomiting and pain: a double-blind randomized controlled trial. Indian J Otolaryngol Head Neck Surg. 2013;65 Suppl 2:216–9.
45. Caniello M, Passerotti GH, Goto EY, Voegels RL, Butugan O. Antibiotics in septoplasty: is it necessary? Braz J Otorhinolaryngol. 2005;71(6):734–8.
46. Rechtweg JS, Paolini RV, Belmont MJ, Wax MK. Postoperative antibiotic use of septoplasty: a survey of practice habits of the membership of the American Rhinologic Society. Am J Rhinol. 2001;15(5):315–20.
47. Yoder MG, Weimert TA. Antibiotics and topical surgical preparation solution in septal surgery. Otolaryngol Head Neck Surg. 1992;106(3):243–4.
48. Weimert TA, Yoder MG. Antibiotics and nasal surgery. Laryngoscope. 1980;90(4):667–72.
49. Georgiou I, Farber N, Mendes D, Winkler E. The role of antibiotics in rhinoplasty and septoplasty: a literature review. Rhinology. 2008;46(4):267–70.

50. Ricci G, D'Ascanio L. Antibiotics in septoplasty: evidence or habit? Am J Rhinol Allergy. 2012;26(3):194–6.
51. Karaman E, Alimoglu Y, Aygun G, Kilic E, Yagiz C. Effect of septoplasty and per-operative antibiotic prophylaxis on nasal flora. B-ENT. 2012;8(1):13–9.
52. Bandhauer F, Buhl D, Grossenbacher R. Antibiotic prophylaxis in rhinosurgery. Am J Rhinol. 2002;16(3):135–9.
53. Gioacchini FM, Alicandri-Ciufelli M, Kaleci S, Magliulo G, Re M. The role of antibiotic therapy and nasal packing in septoplasty. Eur Arch Otorhinolaryngol. 2014;271(5):879–86.
54. Mane RS, Patil B, Mohite A. Comparison of septoplasty with and without nasal packing and review of literature. Indian J Otolaryngol Head Neck Surg. 2013;65 Suppl 2:406–8.
55. Bernardo MT, Alves S, Lima NB, Helena D, Conde A. Septoplasty with or without postoperative nasal packing? Prospective study. Braz J Otorhinolaryngol. 2013;79(4):471–4.
56. Yilmaz MS, Guven M, Elicora SS, Kaymaz R. An evaluation of biodegradable synthetic polyurethane foam in patients following septoplasty: a prospective randomized trial. Otolaryngol Head Neck Surg. 2013;148(1):140–4.
57. Kim YS, Kim YH, Kim NH, Kim SH, Kim KR, Kim KS. A prospective, randomized, single-blinded controlled trial on biodegradable synthetic polyurethane foam as a packing material after septoplasty. Am J Rhinol Allergy. 2011;25(2):e77–9.
58. Walikar BN, Rashinkar SM, Watwe MV, Fathima A, Kakkeri A. A comparative study of septoplasty with or without nasal packing. Indian J Otolaryngol Head Neck Surg. 2011;63(3):247–8.
59. Awan MS, Iqbal M. Nasal packing after septoplasty: a randomized comparison of packing versus no packing in 88 patients. Ear Nose Throat J. 2008;87(11):624–7.
60. Von Schoenberg M, Robinson P, Ryan R. Nasal packing after routine nasal surgery–is it justified? J Laryngol Otol. 1993;107(10):902–5.
61. Illum P, Grymer L, Hilberg O. Nasal packing after septoplasty. Clin Otolaryngol Allied Sci. 1992;17(2):158–62.
62. Guyuron B. Is packing after septorhinoplasty necessary? A randomized study. Plast Reconstr Surg. 1989;84(1):41–4; discussion 45–6.
63. Certal V, Silva H, Santos T, Correia A, Carvalho C. Trans-septal suturing technique in septoplasty: a systematic review and meta-analysis. Rhinology. 2012;50(3):236–45.
64. Banglawala SM, Gill M, Sommer DD, Psaltis A, Schlosser R, Gupta M. Is nasal packing necessary after septoplasty? A meta-analysis. Int Forum Allergy Rhinol. 2013;3(5):418–24.
65. Quinn JG, Bonaparte JP, Kilty SJ. Postoperative management in the prevention of complications after septoplasty: a systematic review. Laryngoscope. 2013;123(6):1328–33.
66. Jung YG, Hong JW, Eun YG, Kim MG. Objective usefulness of thin silastic septal splints after septal surgery. Am J Rhinol Allergy. 2011;25(3):182–5.
67. Malki D, Quine SM, Pfleiderer AG. Nasal splints, revisited. J Laryngol Otol. 1999;113(8): 725–7.
68. Cook JA, Murrant NJ, Evans KL, Lavelle RJ. Intranasal splints and their effects on intranasal adhesions and septal stability. Clin Otolaryngol Allied Sci. 1992;17(1):24–7.
69. Von Schoenberg M, Robinson P, Ryan R. The morbidity from nasal splints in 105 patients. Clin Otolaryngol Allied Sci. 1992;17(6):528–30.
70. Campbell JB, Watson MG, Shenoi PM. The role of intranasal splints in the prevention of post-operative nasal adhesions. J Laryngol Otol. 1987;101(11):1140–3.
71. Doyle DE, House LF, Hall WP. Description of a new device: an intranasal airway/splint. Laryngoscope. 1977;87(4 Pt 1):608–12.
72. Tang S, Kacker A. Should intranasal splints be used after nasal septal surgery? Laryngoscope. 2012;122(8):1647–8.
73. Aksoy E, Serin GM, Polat S, Kaytaz A. Removing intranasal splints after septal surgery. J Craniofac Surg. 2011;22(3):1008–9.
74. Bateman ND, Woolford TJ. Informed consent for septal surgery: the evidence-base. J Laryngol Otol. 2003;117(3):186–9.

75. Topal O, Celik SB, Erbek S, Erbek SS. Risk of nasal septal perforation following septoplasty in patients with allergic rhinitis. Eur Arch Otorhinolaryngol. 2011;268(2):231–3.
76. Yeo NK, Jang YJ. Rhinoplasty to correct nasal deformities in postseptoplasty patients. Am J Rhinol Allergy. 2009;23(5):540–5.
77. Daudia A, Alkhaddour U, Sithole J, Mortimore S. A prospective objective study of the cosmetic sequelae of nasal septal surgery. Acta Otolaryngol. 2006;126(11):1201–5.
78. Jacobson JA, Kasworm EM. Toxic shock syndrome after nasal surgery. Case reports and analysis of risk factors. Arch Otolaryngol Head Neck Surg. 1986;112(3):329–32.
79. Wagner R, Toback JM. Toxic shock syndrome following septoplasty using plastic septal splints. Laryngoscope. 1986;96(6):609–10.
80. Onerci TM, Ayhan K, Ogretmenoglu O. Two consecutive cases of cerebrospinal fluid rhinorrhea after septoplasty operation. Am J Otolaryngol. 2004;25(5):354–6.
81. Leong AC, Patel T, Rehman F, Oyarzabal M, Gluckman P. Cerebrospinal fluid rhinorrhea complicating septoplasty: a novel mechanism of injury. Ear Nose Throat J. 2010;89(1):27–9.
82. Gulsen S, Yilmaz C, Aydin E, Kocbiyik A, Altinors N. Meningoencephalocele formation after nasal septoplasty and management of this complication. Turk Neurosurg. 2008;18(3):281–5.
83. Pfaar O, Huttenbrink KB, Hummel T. Assessment of olfactory function after septoplasty: a longitudinal study. Rhinology. 2004;42(4):195–9.
84. Briner HR, Simmen D, Jones N. Impaired sense of smell in patients with nasal surgery. Clin Otolaryngol Allied Sci. 2003;28(5):417–9.
85. Damm M, Eckel HE, Jungehulsing M, Hummel T. Olfactory changes at threshold and suprathreshold levels following septoplasty with partial inferior turbinectomy. Ann Otol Rhinol Laryngol. 2003;112(1):91–7.
86. Atighechi S, Alimohammadi SH, Baradaranfar MH, Mirvakili SA. Temporary adduction deficit after nasal septoplasty and radiofrequency ablation of the inferior turbinate. J Neuroophthalmol. 2009;29(1):29–32.
87. Rao GN, Rout K, Pal A. Central retinal artery occlusion and third cranial nerve palsy following nasal septoplasty. Case Rep Ophthalmol. 2012;3(3):321–6.
88. Pang KP, Siow JK, Tseng P. Safety of multilevel surgery in obstructive sleep apnea: a review of 487 cases. Arch Otolaryngol Head Neck Surg. 2012;138(4):353–7.
89. Banuchi V, Cohen JC, Kacker A. Safety of Concurrent Nasal and Oropharyngeal Surgery for Obstructive Sleep Apnea. Ann Otol Rhinol Laryngol. 2014;123:619–22.
90. Friedman M, Maley A, Kelley K, Leesman C, Patel A, Pulver T, et al. Impact of nasal obstruction on obstructive sleep apnea. Otolaryngol Head Neck Surg. 2011;144(6):1000–4.
91. Moore EJ, Kern EB. Atrophic rhinitis: a review of 242 cases. Am J Rhinol. 2001;15(6):355–61.
92. Coste A, Dessi P, Serrano E. Empty nose syndrome. Eur Ann Otorhinolaryngol Head Neck Dis. 2012;129(2):93–7.
93. Banglawala SM, Gill MS, Dhillion N, Khan JS, Gupta MK, Psaltis A, et al. Nasal packing after septoplasty: cardiopulmonary impact. JAMA Otolaryngol Head Neck Surg. 2014;140(3):253–8.
94. Turhan M, Bostanci A, Akdag M, Dinc O. A comparison of the effects of packing or transseptal suture on polysomnographic parameters in septoplasty. Eur Arch Otorhinolaryngol. 2013;270(4):1339–44.
95. Cayonu M, Acar A, Horasanli E, Altundag A, Salihoglu M. Comparison of totally occlusive nasal pack, internal nasal splint, and transseptal suture technique after septoplasty in terms of immediate respiratory distress related to anesthesia and surgical complications. Acta Otolaryngol. 2014;134(4):390–4.
96. Peyvandi A, Roozbahany NA. Skull base injury leading to death after conventional septoplasty. Am J Forensic Med Pathol. 2013;34(1):5–6.
97. Buckland JR, Thomas S, Harries PG. Can the Sino-nasal Outcome Test (SNOT-22) be used as a reliable outcome measure for successful septal surgery? Clin Otolaryngol Allied Sci. 2003;28(1):43–7.

98. Arunachalam PS, Kitcher E, Gray J, Wilson JA. Nasal septal surgery: evaluation of symptomatic and general health outcomes. Clin Otolaryngol Allied Sci. 2001;26(5):367–70.
99. Konstantinidis I, Triaridis S, Triaridis A, Karagiannidis K, Kontzoglou G. Long term results following nasal septal surgery. Focus on patients' satisfaction. Auris Nasus Larynx. 2005;32(4):369–74.
100. Stewart MG, Witsell DL, Smith TL, Weaver EM, Yueh B, Hannley MT. Development and validation of the Nasal Obstruction Symptom Evaluation (NOSE) scale. Otolaryngol Head Neck Surg. 2004;130(2):157–63.
101. Stewart MG, Smith TL, Weaver EM, Witsell DL, Yueh B, Hannley MT, et al. Outcomes after nasal septoplasty: results from the Nasal Obstruction Septoplasty Effectiveness (NOSE) study. Otolaryngol Head Neck Surg. 2004;130(3):283–90.
102. Bezerra TF, Stewart MG, Fornazieri MA, Pilan RR, Pinna Fde R, Padua FG, et al. Quality of life assessment septoplasty in patients with nasal obstruction. Braz J Otorhinolaryngol. 2012;78(3):57–62.
103. Gandomi B, Bayat A, Kazemei T. Outcomes of septoplasty in young adults: the Nasal Obstruction Septoplasty Effectiveness study. Am J Otolaryngol. 2010;31(3):189–92.
104. Toyserkani NM, Frisch T. Are too many septal deviations operated on? A retrospective patient's satisfaction questionnaire with 11 years follow-up. Rhinology. 2012;50(2):185–90.
105. Schwentner I, Dejakum K, Schmutzhard J, Deibl M, Sprinzl GM. Does nasal septal surgery improve quality of life? Acta Otolaryngol. 2006;126(7):752–7.
106. Durr DG. Endoscopic septoplasty: technique and outcomes. J Otolaryngol. 2003;32(1): 6–11.
107. Mondina M, Marro M, Maurice S, Stoll D, de Gabory L. Assessment of nasal septoplasty using NOSE and RhinoQoL questionnaires. Eur Arch Otorhinolaryngol. 2012;269(10): 2189–95.
108. Karatzanis AD, Fragiadakis G, Moshandrea J, Zenk J, Iro H, Velegrakis GA. Septoplasty outcome in patients with and without allergic rhinitis. Rhinology. 2009;47(4):444–9.
109. Velasco LC, Arima LM, Tiago RS. Assessment of symptom improvement following nasal septoplasty with or without turbinectomy. Braz J Otorhinolaryngol. 2011;77(5):577–83.
110. Saragusty C, Berant E, Yaniv E. Association of attachment anxiety and satisfaction with nasal surgery. Rhinology. 2011;49(1):117–20.
111. Toyserkani NM, Frisch T, Von Buchwald C. Postoperative improvement in acoustic rhinometry measurements after septoplasty correlates with long-term satisfaction. Rhinology. 2013;51(2):171–5.
112. Devseren NO, Ecevit MC, Erdag TK, Ceryan K. A randomized clinical study: outcome of submucous resection of compensatory inferior turbinate during septoplasty. Rhinology. 2011;49(1):53–7.
113. Gindros G, Kantas I, Balatsouras DG, Kaidoglou A, Kandiloros D. Comparison of ultrasound turbinate reduction, radiofrequency tissue ablation and submucosal cauterization in inferior turbinate hypertrophy. Eur Arch Otorhinolaryngol. 2010;267(11):1727–33.
114. Joniau S, Wong I, Rajapaksa S, Carney SA, Wormald PJ. Long-term comparison between submucosal cauterization and powered reduction of the inferior turbinates. Laryngoscope. 2006;116(9):1612–6.
115. Garzaro M, Landolfo V, Pezzoli M, Defilippi S, Campisi P, Giordano C, et al. Radiofrequency volume turbinate reduction versus partial turbinectomy: clinical and histological features. Am J Rhinol Allergy. 2012;26(4):321–5.

Index

P.S. Batra, J.K. Han (eds.), *Practical Medical and Surgical Management of Chronic Rhinosinusitis*, DOI 10.1007/978-3-319-16724-4

Printing: Ten Brink, Meppel, The Netherlands
Binding: PHOENIX PRINT, Würzburg, Germany